Surgical Management OF Obesity

Surgical Management OF Obesity

Henry Buchwald, M.D., Ph.D.

Professor of Surgery and Biomedical Engineering
Owen H. and Sarah Davidson Wangensteen Chair in Experimental Surgery, Emeritus
Department of Surgery
University of Minnesota Medical School
Minneapolis, Minnesota

George S.M. Cowan, Jr., M.D.

Professor Emeritus
University of Tennessee Health Science Center, College of Medicine
Medical Director
Obesity Wellness Center
Memphis, Tennessee

Walter J. Pories, M.D.

Professor of Surgery and Biochemistry
Department of Surgery
East Carolina University School of Medicine
Greenville, North Carolina

SAUNDERS

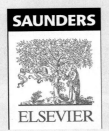

ELSEVIER

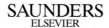

SAUNDERS
ELSEVIER

1600 John F. Kennedy Blvd.
Suite 1800
Philadelphia, PA 19103-2899

SURGICAL MANAGEMENT OF OBESITY   ISBN-13:978-1-4160-0089-1
Copyright © 2007 by Saunders, an imprint of Elsevier Inc.   ISBN-10:1-4160-0089-5

Library of Congress Cataloging-in-Publication Data
Surgical management of obesity / [edited by] Henry Buchwald, George S.M. Cowan Jr.,
Walter Pories. —1st ed.
    p. ; cm.
Includes index.
ISBN 1-4160-0089-5
1. Morbid obesity–Surgery. 2. Jejunoileal bypass. I. Buchwald, Henry. II. Cowan,
George S.M., III. Pories, Walter J.
[DNLM: 1. Obesity, Morbid–surgery. 2. Bariatric Surgery–methods. 3. Treatment
Outcome. WD 210 S9659 2007]
RD540.S87 2007
17.4'3–dc26   2006041808

Acquisitions Editor: Judith Fletcher
Developmental Editor: Martha Limbach
Publishing Services Manager: Tina Rebane
Project Manager: Mary Anne Folcher
Design Direction: Karen O'Keefe Owens

Printed in the United States of America

Last digit is the print number: 9 8 7 6 5 4 3 2 1

To my life companion, my wife, Emilie D. Buchwald. Herself a writer and publisher, she has tried to teach me to be graceful, as well as informative, in my writing. Not only would my career not have been possible without her support, but also the pleasure in my career, as well as in my children and in my grandchildren.

HB

Anne Cowan, my wife and dearest friend, personifies unconditional love which, once learned, is an immense joy to share, as she has inspired me to do with my patients, and many others, over the 40+ years of our lives together. This book is dedicated as a token of my boundless gratitude to her for this and so very much more.

GSMC

To Mary Ann Rose (Pories), professor, nurse, karate teacher, professional horticulturist, musician, baker, mother, wife, and constant friend without whom my whole career would not have been possible.

WJP

Contributors

Subhi Abu-Abeid, M.D.
Deputy Chair of General Surgery and Consultant, Tel Aviv University Sourasky Medical Center; Consultant, Tel Aviv, Israel

Chapter 44, *Resolution of Bariatric Comorbidities: Sleep Apnea*

Peter Ako, M.D.
Center for Surgical Treatment of Obesity, Tri-City Regional Medical Center, Hawaiian Gardens, California

Chapter 27, *Banded Gastric Bypass*

John C. Alverdy, M.D.
Professor of Surgery, University of Chicago: The Pritzker School of Medicine, Chicago, Illinois

Chapter 12, *Patient Selection for Bariatric Surgery*

Mitiku Belachew, M.D.
Head, Surgical Department and University Service, Centre Hospitalier Hutois, Huy, Belgium

Chapter 19, *Laparoscopic Adjustable Gastric Banding*

Kumar G. Belani, M.B.B.S., M.S.
Professor of Anesthesiology, Medicine and Pediatrics; Professor, Division of Environmental Sciences, Schollos of Medicine and Public Health, University of Minnesota, Minneapolis; Consultant Anesthesiologist, Fairview University Medical Center, University Children's Hospital, Fairview, Minnesota

Chapter 14, *Anesthesia Consideration in the Obese*

Peter N. Benotti, M.D., F.A.C.S.
Director of General Surgery, Department of Surgery, Geisinger Health System, Danville, Pennsylvania

Chapter 13, *Preoperative Preparation of the Bariatric Surgery Patient*

Jeanne D. Blankenship, M.S., R.D.
Department of Surgery, University of California, Davis Medical Center, Sacramento, California

Chapter 9, *Dietary Management of Obesity*

Claude Bouchard, Ph.D.
Executive Director, Pennington Biomedical Research Center, Baton Rouge, Louisiana

Chapter 3, *Etiology of Obesity*

George A. Bray, M.D.
Chronic Disease Prevention, Pennington Biomedical Research Center, Baton Rouge, Louisiana

Chapter 10, *Drug Management of Obesity*

Stacy A. Brethauer, M.D.
Fellow, Advanced Laparoscopic and Bariatric Surgery, Cleveland Clinical Foundation, Cleveland, Ohio

Chapter 23, *Current Status of Laparoscopic Gastric Bypass*

Robert E. Brolin, M.D.
Adjunct Professor of Surgery, University of Pittsburgh Medical Center, Pittsburgh, Pennsylvania; Director of Bariatric Surgery, University Medical Center at Princeton, Princeton; Director, Bariatric Surgery Program, Saint Peter's University Hospital, New Brunswick, New Jersey

Chapter28, *Long-Limb Roux Gastric Bypass*

Henry Buchwald, M.D., Ph.D.
Professor of Surgery and Biomedical Engineering, Owen H. and Sarah Davidson Wangensteen Chair in Experimental Surgery, Emeritus, Department of Surgery, University of Minnesota Medical School, Minneapolis, Minnesota

Chapter 5, *Obesity Comorbidities;*

Chapter 18, *Evolution of Bariatric Procedures and Selection Algorithm*

Marie-Claire Buckley, M.D.
Assistant Professor, Division of Plastic and Reconstructive Surgery, University of Minnesota Medical School, Minneapolis, Minnesota

Chapter 38, *Body Contouring After Massive Weight Loss*

Giovanni Camerini, M.D.
Assistant Professor of Surgery, Università di Genova, Ospedale San Martino, Genoa, Italy

Chapter 29, *Biliopancreatic Diversion*

J.K. Champion, M.D., F.A.C.S.

Clinical Professor of Surgery, Mercer University School of Medicine, Macon, Georgia; Director of Bariatric Surgery, Emory-Dunwoody Medical Center, Atlanta, Georgia

> *Chapter 21, Laparoscopic Vertical Banded Gastroplasty*

Paul T. Cirangle, M.D., F.A.C.S.

Laparoscopic Associates of San Francisco, San Francisco, California

> *Chapter 31, Laparoscopic Duodenal Switch and Sleeve Gastrectomy Procedures*

G. Wesley Clark, M.D.

Alvarado Center for Surgical Weight Loss, San Diego, California

> *Chapter 25, Laparoscopic Gastric Bypass Using the Circular Stapler*

Matthew M. Clark, Ph.D.

Professor of Psychology, Mayo Clinic College of Medicine; Health Psychologist, Department of Psychiatry and Psychology, Mayo Clinic, Rochester, Minnesota

> *Chapter 51, Multidisciplinary Team in a Bariatric Surgery Program*

Maria L. Collazo-Clavell, M.D.

Assistant Professor, Department of Internal Medicine, Mayo Clinic College of Medicine; Consultant, Division of Endocrinology, Diabetes, Metabolism and Nutrition, Mayo Clinic, Rochester, Minnesota

> *Chapter 51, Multidisciplinary Team in a Bariatric Surgery Program*

George S.M. Cowan, Jr., M.D.

Professor Emeritus, Department of Surgery, University of Tennessee Health Sciences Center, College of Medicine, Memphis, Tennessee

> *Chapter 11, Nonsurgical Methods of Weight Loss;*
>
> *Chapter 34, Principles of Revisional Bariatric Surgery*

Paul R.G. Cunningham, M.D.

Professor of Surgery, State University of New York Upstate Medical University; Chair, Department of Surgery, University Hospital, Syracuse, New York

> *Chapter 16, Postoperative Care of the Bariatric Surgery Patient*

Mervyn Deitel, M.D., F.I.C.S., C.R.C.S.C., F.A.C.N., D.A.B.S.

Editor in Chief, *Obesity Surgery*
Formerly, Professor of Surgery and Nutritional Sciences, University of Toronto, Toronto, Ontario, Canada

> *Chapter 56, The Requirements for Medical Writing: Reporting Bariatric Surgical Outcomes*

Joseph D. DiRocco, M.D.

Resident, General Surgery, State University of New York Upstate Medical University, Syracuse, New York

> *Chapter 16, Postoperative Care of the Bariatric Surgery Patient*

John B. Dixon, M.B.B.S., Ph.D., F.R.A.C.G.P.

Head, Clinical Research, Center of Obesity Research and Education, Monash University, Alfred Hospital, Melbourne, Victoria, Australia

> *Chapter 41, Nutritional Outcomes of Bariatric Surgery;*
>
> *Chapter 45, Orthopedic Conditions and Obesity: Changes with Weight Loss*

Basil Felahy, M.D.

Center for Surgical Treatment of Obesity, Tri-City Regional Medical Center, Hawaiian Gardens, California

> *Chapter 27, Banded Gastric Bypass*

John J. Feng, M.D., F.A.C.S.

Laparoscopic Associates of San Francisco, San Francisco, California

> *Chapter 31, Laparoscopic Duodenal Switch and Sleeve Gastrectomy Procedures*

Latham Flanagan, Jr., M.D., F.A.C.S.

The Oregon Center for Bariatric Surgery, Eugene, Oregon

> *Chapter 48, Practical Training of the Bariatric Surgeon*

Louis Flancbaum, M.D., F.A.C.S., F.C.C.M., F.C.C.P.

Chair, Department of Surgery; Director, Bariatric Services, North Shore University Hospital at Glen Cove, Glen Cove, New York

> *Chapter 46, Metabolic Outcomes of Bariatric Surgery*

M.A.L. Fobi, M.D.

Medical Director, Surgeon, Center for Surgical Treatment of Obesity, Tri-City Regional Medical Center, Hawaiian Gardens, California

> *Chapter 27, Banded Gastric Bypass*

Nicole N. Fobi, M.D.
Center for Surgical Treatment of Obesity, Tri-City
Regional Medical Center, Hawaiian Gardens, California

Chapter 27, Banded Gastric Bypass

Katherine Mary Fox, R.N., M.P.H.
CEO, Surgical Weight Loss Clinic, Tacoma,
Washington; CEO, Surgical Weight Loss Clinic of
Eastern Washington, Richland, Washington; Director
of Education, Fill Centers USA, Snowflake, Arizona

*Chapter 49, Nursing Care of the Bariatric
Surgery Patient*

S. Ross Fox, M.D.
St. Francis Community Hospital, Federal Way,
Washington

*Chapter 36, Leaks and Gastric Disruption in
Bariatric Surgery*

Victor F. Garcia, M.D.
Professor of Surgery, Pediatrics, University of Cincinnati
School of Medicine; Pediatric Surgeon, Cincinnati
Children's Hospital Medical Center, Cincinnati, Ohio

Chapter 37, Adolescent Bariatric Surgery

John J. Gleysteen, M.D.
Professor of Surgery, University of Alabama in
Birmingham; Chief, Surgical Service, Birmingham VA
Medical Center, Birmingham, Alabama

*Chapter 53, Requisite Facilities for Bariatric
Surgical Practice*

Jeanne E. Grant, R.D.
Clinical Dietician, Mayo Clinic, Rochester, Minnesota

*Chapter 51, Multidisciplinary Team in a Bariatric
Surgery Program*

Robert J. Greenstein, M.D., F.A.C.S., F.R.C.S.
Department of Surgery, Veterans Affairs
Medical Center, Bronx, New York

Chapter 17, Surgery in the Morbidly Obese Patient

Ward O. Griffen, Jr., M.D., Ph.D.
Professor of Surgery (Retired), University of Kentucky
College of Medicine, Lexington, Kentucky

Chapter 22, Open Roux-en-Y Gastric Bypass

John D. Halverson, M.D.
Professor of Surgery, State University of New York
Upstate Medical University, Syracuse, New York;
Director, Surgical Bariatric Center, Syracuse,
New York

*Chapter 16, Postoperative Care of the Bariatric
Surgery Patient*

Emanuel Hell, M.D.
Professor of Surgery, Krankenhaus Hallein,
Hallein, Austria

Chapter 7, Social Implications of Obesity

Douglas S. Hess, M.D.
Clinical Assistant Professor, Department of Surgery,
Medical College of Ohio, Toledo; Wood County
Hospital, Bowling Green, Ohio

*Chapter 30, Biliopancreatic Diversion with
Duodenal Switch*

Kelvin D. Higa, M.D.
Valley Surgical Specialists, Fresno, California

*Chapter 26, Laparoscopic Roux-en-Y Gastric Bypass:
Hand-Sewn Gastrojejunostomy Technique*

Neil E. Hutcher, M.D., F.A.C.S.
Clinical Associate Professor of Surgery, Medical College
of Virginia; Medical Director, Bariatric Program,
BonSecours St. Mary's Hospital, Richmond, Virginia

Chapter 2, Incidence, Prevalence, and Demography of Obesity

Sayeed Ikramuddin, M.D.
Associate Professor of Surgery, Co-Director of
Minimally Invasive Surgery, University of Minnesota
Medical School, Minneapolis, Minnesota

*Chapter 4, Energy Metabolism and Biochemistry
of Obesity;*

*Chapter 24, Laparoscopic Roux-en-Y Gastric Bypass:
The Linear Technique*

Andrew C. Jamieson, M.D.
Honorary Senior Lecturer, Department of Surgery,
Monash University Medical School, Melbourne; Head
of Surgical Unit, Box Hill Hospital, Victoria, Australia

Chapter 20, Vertical Banded Gastroplasty

Gregg H. Jossart, M.D., F.A.C.S.
Laparoscopic Associates, San Francisco, California

*Chapter 31, Laparoscopic Duodenal Switch and
Sleeve Gastrectomy Procedures*

Daniel Kaufman, M.D.
Department of Surgery, State University of New York
Downstate Medical Center, Brooklyn, New York

Chapter 47, Academic Training of Bariatric Surgeons

Michael L. Kendrick, M.D.
Assistant Professor of Surgery, Mayo Clinic College
of Medicine; Senior Associate Consultant, Division of
Gastroenterologic and General Surgery, Mayo Clinic,
Rochester, Minnesota

*Chapter 51, Multidisciplinary Team in a Bariatric
Surgery Program*

Joseph Klausner, M.D.
Professor and Head of Surgery, Tel Aviv Sourasky
Medical Center, Tel Aviv, Israel

> *Chapter 44, Resolution of Bariatric Comorbidities:
> Sleep Apnea*

John G, Kral, M.D., Ph.D.
Professor of Surgery and Medicine, State University
of New York Downstate Medical Center, Brooklyn,
New York

> *Chapter 47, Academic Training of Bariatric Surgeons*

Hanna-Maaria Lakka, M.D., Ph.D.
Assistant Professor of Public Health, Kuopio University,
Kuopio, Finland; Pennington Biomedical Research
Center, Baton Rouge, Louisiana

> *Chapter 3, Etiology of Obesity*

Crystine M. Lee, M.D.
Laparoscopic Associates of San Francisco,
San Francisco, California

> *Chapter 31, Laparoscopic Duodenal Switch and Sleeve
> Gastrectomy Procedures*

Hoil Lee, M.D.
Center for Surgical Treatment of Obesity,
Tri-City Regional Medical Center,
Hawaiian Gardens, California

> *Chapter 27, Banded Gastric Bypass*

Kenneth G. MacDonald, Jr., M.D.
Professor of Surgery; Chief, Gastrointestinal Surgery and
Surgical Endoscopy; Director, Surgical Obesity Program;
Brody School of Medicine at East Carolina University,
Greenville, North Carolina

> *Chapter 43, Resolution of Bariatric Comorbidities:
> Hypertension*

Jane L. Mai, R.N.
Physician Extender, Mayo Medical Center,
Rochester, Minnesota

> *Chapter 51, Multidisciplinary Team in a Bariatric
> Surgery Program*

Giuseppe M. Marinari, M.D.
Assistant Professor of Surgery, Università di Genova,
Ospedale San Martino, Genoa, Italy

> *Chapter 29, Biliopancreatic Diversion*

Louis F. Martin, M.D., F.A.C.S., F.C.C.M.
Professor of Surgery, Department of Surgery,
Louisiana State University Health Sciences Center,
New Orleans, Louisiana

> *Chapter 8, Economic Implications of Obesity*
> *Chapter 15, Perioperative Management of the Bariatric
> Surgery Patient*

Tracy Martinez, R.N., B.S.N.
Program Director, Wittgrove Bariatric Center, Scripps
Memorial Hospital, La Jolla, California

> *Chapter 50, Patient Support Groups in Bariatric Surgery*

Edward E. Mason, M.D., Ph.D., F.A.C.S.
Emeritus Professor, University of Iowa College of
Medicine, Iowa City, Iowa

> *Chapter 1, Historical Perspectives*

Samer G. Mattar M.D., F.A.C.S.
Associate Professor, Indiana University School of
Medicine, Indianapolis; Medical Director, Clarian
Bariatric Center, Clarian North Medical Center,
Carmel, Indiana

> *Chapter 23, Current Status of Laparoscopic
> Gastric Bypass*

W. Scott Melvin, M.D.
Professor of Surgery; Chief, Division of General Surgery;
Director, Center for Minimally Invasive Surgery;
Ohio State University College of Medicine and Public
Health, Columbus, Ohio

> *Chapter 54, Laparoscopic Suites and Robotics in
> Bariatric Surgery*

Karl A. Miller, M.D.
Professor of Surgery, Krankenhaus Hallein,
Hallein, Austria

> *Chapter 7, Social Implications of Obesity*

Ido Nachmany, M.D.
Resident, Tel Aviv University Sourasky
Medical Center, Tel Aviv, Israel

> *Chapter 44, Resolution of Bariatric Comorbidities:
> Sleep Apnea*

Erik Näslund, M.D., Ph.D.
Professor, Department of Clinical Sciences, Karolinska
Institutet, Danderyd Hospital, Stockholm, Sweden

> *Chapter 6, Longevity and Obesity*

Michelle A. Neseth
Secretary to Obesity Program Director, Department of
Surgery, Mayo Medical Center, Rochester, Minnesota

> *Chapter 51, Multidisciplinary Team in a Bariatric
> Surgery Program*

Matthew E. Newlin, M.D.
Clinical Instructor, Center for Minimally Invasive
Surgery, Ohio State University Medical School,
Columbus, Ohio

> *Chapter 54, Laparoscopic Suites and Robotics in
> Bariatric Surgery*

Ninh T. Nguyen, M.D.

Associate Professor of Surgery, University of California Irvine School of Medicine, Irvine; Chief, Division of Gastrointestinal Surgery, University of California Irvine Medical Center, Orange, California

Chapter 33, *Open Versus Laparoscopic Bariatric Surgery*

Paul E. O'Brien, M.D., F.R.A.C.S.

Director, Center for Obesity Research and Education, Monash University Medical School, Alfred Hospital, Melbourne, Victoria, Australia

Chapter 41, *Nutritional Outcomes of Bariatric Surgery;*

Chapter 45, *Orthopedic Conditions and Obesity: Changes with Weight Loss*

J. Patrick O'Leary, M.D.

Professor of Surgery; Chair, Department of Surgery, Louisiana State University School of Medicine, New Orleans, Louisiana

Chapter 15, *Perioperative Management of the Bariatric Surgery Patient*

Horacio E. Oria, M.D., F.A.C.S.

Private Practice, Department of Surgery, Spring Branch Medical Center, Houston, Texas

Chapter 40, *Long-Term Follow-Up and Evaluation of Results in Bariatric Surgery*

John T. Paige, M.D.

Assistant Professor of Clinical Surgery, Louisiana State University School of Medicine, New Orleans, Louisiana

Chapter 15, *Perioperative Management of the Bariatric Surgery Patient*

Francesco Papadia, M.D.

Assistant Professor of Surgery, Università di Genova, Ospedale San Marino, Genoa, Italy

Chapter 29, *Biliopancreatic Diversion*

John R. Pender, IV, M.D.

Clinical Assistant Professor of Surgery, Brody School of Medicine at East Carolina University; Attending Surgeon, Pitt County Memorial Hospital, Greenville, North Carolina

Chapter 43, *Resolution of Bariatric Comorbidities: Hypertension*

Athanassios Petrotos, M.D.

Attending Surgeon, Greenwich Hospital, Greenwich, Connecticut

Chapter 46, *Metabolic Outcomes of Bariatric Surgery*

Jessica Planer, R.D., C.D.N.

Dietician, Surgical Bariatric Center, State University of New York Upstate Medical University Hospital, Syracuse, New York

Chapter 16, *Postoperative Care of the Bariatric Surgery Patient*

Walter J. Pories, M.D., F.A.C.S.

Professor of Surgery and Biochemistry, Department of Surgery, East Carolina University School of Medicine, Greenville, North Carolina

Chapter 42, *Resolution of Bariatric Comorbidities: Diabetes*

Vivek N. Prachand, M.D.

Assistant Professor of Surgery, University of Chicago Hospitals and Health System, Chicago, Illinois

Chapter 12, *Patient Selection for Bariatric Surgery*

Lipi Ramchandani, M.B.B.S.

Visiting Research Scholar, Department of Anesthesiology, Medical School of the University of Minnesota, Minneapolis, Minnesota

Chapter 14, *Anesthesia Considerations in the Obese*

Stewart E. Rendon, M.D.

Formerly, Department of Surgery, East Carolina University School of Medicine, Greenville, North Carolina

Chapter 42, *Resolution of Bariatric Comorbidities: Diabetes*

Hector Rodriguez, M.D.

Department of Anesthesia, Valley Hospital, Ridgewood, New Jersey

Chapter 13, *Preoperative Preparation of the Bariatric Surgery Patient*

Tomasz Rogula, M.D., Ph.D.

Clinical Instructor of Surgery, Department of Surgery, Minimally Invasive Surgery Center, University of Pittsburgh Medical Center, Pittsburgh, Pennsylvania

Chapter 23, *Current Status of Laparoscopic Gastric Bypass*

Martin Sanguinette, M.D.

Center for Surgical Treatment of Obesity, Tri-City Regional Medical Center, Hawaiian Gardens, California

Chapter 27, *Banded Gastric Bypass*

Heena Santry, M.D.

Resident, General Surgery, University of Chicago: The Pritzker School of Medicine, Chicago, Illinois

Chapter 12, *Patient Selection for Bariatric Surgery*

Michael G. Sarr, M.D.

Professor of Surgery, Mayo College of Medicine; Consultant and Surgeon, Director, Obesity Surgery Program, Mayo Medical Center, Rochester, Minnesota

Chapter 51, Multidisciplinary Team in a Bariatric Surgery Program

Philip R. Schauer, M.D.

Professor of Surgery, Director, Advanced Laparoscopic and Bariatric Surgery, The Cleveland Clinic Foundation, Cleveland, Ohio

Chapter 23, Current Status of Laparoscopic Gastric Bypass

Bruce David Schirmer, M.D.

Stephen H. Watts Professor of Surgery, Vice-Chair, Program Director, Department of Surgery, University of Virginia Health System, Charlottesville, Virginia

Chapter 35, Strictures and Marginal Ulcers in Bariatric Surgery

Nicola Scopinaro, M.D.

Professor of Surgery, Università di Genova, Ospedale San Martino, Genoa, Italy

Chapter 29, Biliopancreatic Diversion

Scott A. Shikora, M.D.

Professor of Surgery, Tufts University School of Medicine, Tufts-New England Medical Center, Boston, Massachusetts

Chapter 32, Implantable Gastric Stimulation for the Treatment of Morbid Obesity

Myur S. Srikanth, M.D.

St. Francis Community Hospital, Federal Way, Washington

Chapter 36, Leaks and Gastric Disruption in Bariatric Surgery

Thomas A. Stellato, M.D., M.B.A.

Professor of Surgery, Charles A. Hubay Professor of Surgery, Case University School of Medicine; Director, Division of General Surgery, University Hospitals of Cleveland, Cleveland, Ohio

Chapter 39, Ancillary Procedures in Bariatric Surgery

Amir Szold, M.D.

Senior Staff, Department of Surgery, Tel Aviv Sourasky Medical Center; Sacular School of Medicine, Tel Aviv University, Tel Aviv, Israel

Chapter 44, Resolution of Bariatric Comorbidities: Sleep Apnea

Janos Taller, M.D.

Laparoscopic Associates of San Francisco, San Francisco, California

Chapter 31, Laparoscopic Duodenal Switch and Sleeve Gastrectomy Procedures

Paul A. Thodiyil, M.D., F.R.C.S.

Assistant Professor of Surgery, University of Pittsburgh School of Medicine; Attending Staff, Assistant Professor, University of Pittsburgh Medical Center, Magee Women's Hospital, Pittsburgh, Pennsylvania

Chapter 23, Current Status of Laparoscopic Gastric Bypass

Jarl S. Torgerson, M.D., Ph.D.

Associate Professor, Goteborg University, Göteborg, Sweden; Head, Department of Medicine, Northern Alvsborg Hospital, Trollhattan Sweden

Chapter 6, Longevity and Obesity

Mary Lou Walen

Bariatric Program Director, Lenox Hill Hospital, New York, New York

Chapter 52, Allied Science Team in Bariatric Surgery

Marguerite Walser, F.N.P.

Clinical Coordinator, State University of New York Upstate Medical University, Surgical Bariatric Center, Syracuse, New York

Chapter 16, Postoperative Care of the Bariatric Surgery Patient

Otto L. Willbanks, M.D., F.A.C.S.

Clinical Professor, University of Texas Health Science Center at Dallas: Baylor University Medical Center, Dallas, Texas

Chapter 55, Liability Issues in Bariatric Surgery

Michael Williams, M.D.

Staff Surgeon, Emory-Dunwoody Medical Center, Atlanta, Georgia

Chapter 21, Laparoscopic Vertical Banded Gastroplasty

Bruce M. Wolfe, M.D.

Professor of Surgery; Chief, Division of Gastrointestinal and Laparoscopic Surgery, University of California, Davis, Medical Center, Sacramento, California

Chapter 9, Dietary Management of Obesity;

Chapter 33, Open Versus Laparoscopic Bariatric Surgery

Preface

In this first decade of the 21st century there are three unassailable facts concerning obesity: (1) There is a global epidemic of obesity and, in particular, of morbid obesity. (2) The disciplines of behavior modification, diet management, exercise, and drug therapy have not, alone or in combination, come close to dealing with this epidemic for the long-term. Surgery – bariatric surgery – is the only current treatment with proven long-term efficacy. And, (3) bariatric surgery, since its origin about 50 years ago, is in a constant state of flux.

Since there are multiple physiologic, and possibly biochemical, hormonal, and neurogenic, approaches in the surgical armamentarium, and since the techniques for performing a given operative approach are multiple, there is no 'gold standard' operation. And, therefore, this book – *Surgical Management of Obesity* – is in part a history in order to give the reader an insight into the present; in part an overview of the current field of bariatric surgery and its relationship to society; in part a guide to how the common operative procedures are performed; and, throughout, is concerned with how to approach patient care to achieve safe and excellent outcomes, with humanity and evolving knowledge.

This resource text is a comprehensive coverage of bariatric surgery, featuring the work of more than 90 international experts. The contents of their chapters reflect their thoughts and not necessarily the concepts or practices of others in the field. For example, the criteria for patient selection (Chapter 12) work well for the authors and are helpful guidelines; other groups may follow different guidelines that are also effective. The 56 chapters of this book are divided into the following sections: Background; Consequences; Nonoperative Management; Preoperative, Perioperative, and Postoperative Patient Care; Operative Procedures; Reoperations and Complications; Special Considerations; Outcomes; and Education, Practice, and Reporting.

Surgical Management of Obesity begins with a thorough examination of the history, incidence, demography, etiology, biology, comorbidities, longevity, and social and economic implications of obesity. It then discusses pre-, peri-, and postoperative issues of importance before detailing how to perform the complete range of bariatric procedures. The discussion of the evolution of bariatric procedures is followed by individual chapters that examine laparoscopic adjustable gastric banding, vertical banded gastroplasty, gastric bypass, biliopancreatic diversion and duodenal switch, and other surgical approaches. This includes a full section devoted to the topic of reoperation in bariatric surgery and possible complications.

The outcomes of bariatric surgery with respect to nutrition, diabetes, hypertension, sleep apnea, orthopedic conditions, and metabolism are enumerated in considerable detail. The growing incidence of childhood obesity is highlighted with a chapter focusing on adolescent bariatric surgery patients. Since bariatric surgery has become a multidisciplinary specialty, we offer guidance on practical and academic training of the bariatric surgeon, patient support groups, importance of the team approach, managed care, allied health staff assistance, laparoscopic suites and robotics, liability issues, and more. This book equips the reader with the essential knowledge to understand the field of bariatrics and to provide patients with the best possible results.

Why is this book timely? Bariatric surgery, though a proven entity today, is resisted, restrained, and relatively sparsely utilized. The 200,000 bariatric procedures performed annually in the United States may sound like a large number. When one considers, however, that there are about twenty million eligible patients who qualify under the current standard for operative selection of a body mass index (BMI) over 40 kg/m^2 or over 35 kg/m^2 in the presence of significant co-morbidities, then 200,000 represents only two percent of the *treatable* population. In many other nations, even two percent is a high value and, in some nations, the percent of qualified individuals who qualify for operative care and are allowed bariatric surgery within their nation's health system is zero. Would the health care system in the United States, or any other progressive nation, tolerate treating only two percent or fewer of its patients with diabetes, its patients with cancer, or those with clinically significant coronary heart disease? The United States is often criticized for not having a policy for management of AIDS around the globe. But its policy on bariatric surgery is criticized by only a handful of individuals for lacking a national policy of universal bariatric surgery coverage for all who qualify and request therapy.

Although operative and perioperative (30-day) mortality for bariatric surgery is extremely low, actually lower than the 30-day mortality for other major abdominal procedures, a bariatric surgery death, or severe complication, frequently attracts massive media attention, and an unfairly balanced condemnation of the field as dangerous, rather than life-saving and life-affirming.

It is common for a patient with morbid obesity to exhibit the co-morbid conditions of type 2 diabetes, hyperlipidemia, hypertension, and obstructive sleep apnea. Today's nonoperative therapy for this patient would be diets for the obesity (as a rule, ineffectual), oral hypoglycemics or insulin for the diabetes (palliative), statins for the hyperlipidemia (palliative), drugs for the hypertension (palliative), and continuous positive airway pressure (CPAP) machines for the obstructive sleep apnea (palliative). Over time, the expense for these multiple therapies becomes exorbitant and possibly prohibitive, and the diseases of morbid obesity, diabetes, hyperlipidemia, hypertension, and obstructive sleep apnea persist or progress until premature death. Bariatric surgery offers this same individual resolution and possibly a "cure" for all five of these diseases through one procedure, with no need for a lifetime of palliative therapy.

Not only is bariatric surgery still struggling for affirmative recognition, but the very disease of obesity, and in particular morbid obesity, is struggling for legitimate recognition as a disease. We designate drug addiction, alcoholism, compulsive gambling, and smoking as diseases. Yet, only recently have national health agencies designated obesity a disease, against considerable opposition. While addiction to substances or disease-inducing life-styles are considered diseases, treated as diseases, and freed from the stigma of being considered a character fault subject to condemnation, a person with a genetic predisposition to obesity by the overconsumption of food, the matter of life-sustenance

for all humans, is still met with derision, ostracism, and shunning. Truly, ridicule of the obese is the last public and legally permitted, at times even encouraged, prejudice in Western society. As yet, we do not live in communities where obesity is accepted as a disease.

The only permanent freedom from ignorance and bias lies in knowledge. We hope that, in some modest manner, this comprehensive text will provide knowledge to a struggling field emerging from its infancy with great potential to do good and to provide for progress. If *Surgical Management of Obesity* can advance the acceptance of obesity as a disease, and of bariatric surgery as a solution to this disease, we will have done our job, and we will have been of service to the medical community.

Henry Buchwald, M.D., Ph.D.
George S.M. Cowan, Jr., M.D.
Walter J. Pories, M.D.

Acknowledgments

First and foremost, the editors wish to thank the chapter contributors, who represent the pioneers and leaders of bariatric surgery worldwide. Their contributions provide up-to-date knowledge regarding their respective subjects; historical perspectives; detailed techniques; discussions of the patient; and social, economic, and scholarly aspects of the topics in *Surgical Management of Obesity*. We have avoided uniformity of style and idiom in this text, and we have allowed the chapter authors to speak in their own voices, in order to give the reader a flavor of the unique personalities of these individuals and the formulation of their thought processes.

Editing is crucial, however, for a readable book, and we are most grateful to Jane N. Buchwald of MEDWRITE Communications, Inc., for her painstakingly precise reading and substantive editing of each chapter. We could not have done this book without her.

We thank Stewart E. Rendon, M.D., and John R. Pender, M.D., who were of considerable help in the substantive editing.

We needed, and thoroughly appreciated, the guidance and organizational abilities of Ms. Danette Oien, secretary to Dr. Buchwald, a constant source of efficiency and communication skills.

The staff of Elsevier have been a pleasure to work with. We wish to thank, in particular, Joe Rusko for acquiring this book for Elsevier; Janine Kusza for nearly keeping us on schedule; Mary Anne Folcher for making all parts into a whole; and, above all, Judy Fletcher for her professionalism, support, sound advice, and accommodating manner.

Contents

BACKGROUND

1

Historical Perspectives

Edward E. Mason, M.D., Ph.D., F.A.C.S.

The surgical treatment of obesity began with the simple concept that by restricting intake, producing malabsorption, or both, one could reduce body weight and maintain that reduction. The first operation was intestinal bypass, which made use of the "short gut syndrome," a result of extensive bowel resection for cancer or loss of intestinal blood supply. Because the intestine was bypassed instead of removed, the operation was reversible, which established an important guideline for all subsequent operations used to control body weight.

In 1954, when the use of intestinal bypass was first mentioned at a meeting of the American Surgical Association, obesity was not recognized as a disease.[1] The concept that obesity was a disease that could be successfully treated by an operation was accepted first by the severely obese; they welcomed relief from their morbidity, their repeated failures in dieting, and the disrespect shown them by society. The medical profession gradually accepted obesity surgery when they found that it provided a solution for complications and morbidity that needed treatment, which until then they had been unable to provide.

In December 1994, we sent questionnaires to all academic surgery departmental chairs in America. Their answers indicated acceptance of obesity surgery by 74% of those who responded (also 74%).[2] This was far less than the mandatory status of surgical treatment for cancer or many other morbid and lethal diseases. However, in many hospitals, more operations on the stomach are now performed for obesity than for any other disease, and the percentage reported in 1996[2] has probably increased markedly.

The prevalence of body mass index (BMI) of 30.0 kg per m² or higher was about 15% of the population in the United States between 1960 and 1980, according to the National Health and Nutrition Examination Survey (NHANES). The prevalence began to increase after 1980, and by 1999-2000 the prevalence had reached 30.5% of the population.[3] Flegal and Troiano observed that the increase in weight was at the heavy end of the distribution.[4] This suggested a combination of profound environmental determinants and a highly susceptible population. Also, the patients operated upon are heavier each year.[5]

The first operations used in treating obesity were not entirely new. They were founded on experience, following the tradition of Claude Bernard's *Introduction to Experimental Medicine* of 1865. We knew about many of the complications that needed to be prevented, diagnosed, or treated. The bypass component was new, and it led to new problems, primarily bacterial overgrowth in the bypassed bowel, which contributed to liver failure, cirrhosis, renal disease, autoimmune disease, and other complications peculiar to intestinal bypass. This issue led to almost complete replacement of intestinal bypass by operations on the stomach.

The creation of impaired ingestion, digestion, and absorption of essential nutrients with bypass of intestine (1954) or of the upper digestive tract (1966) introduced potential for complications such as protein malnutrition, fluid and electrolyte imbalance, metabolic bone disease, and neurologic damage (Wernicke-Korsakoff syndrome). Surgeons were therefore required to become experts in the prevention, recognition, and management of malnutrition as well as of obesity. Patients needed information about the risks and benefits of the operations that were recommended. The accumulation of outcome data from each surgeon's experience increased in importance. An annual meeting of surgeons committed to the care of the severely obese culminated, in 1983, in the incorporation of the American Society for Bariatric Surgery. In 1986, the National Bariatric Surgery Registry was established to assist surgeons in the collection, analysis, and comparison of results (with a later change in name to the International Bariatric Surgery Registry). There are now many national obesity surgery societies, an International Federation for Surgery of Obesity, and two obesity surgery journals (*Obesity Surgery and Surgery of Obesity and Related Diseases*).

▶ INTESTINAL BYPASS

In 1954 Kremen and colleagues presented the results of a study in dogs that compared bypass of jejunum with bypass of ileum, with and without the ileocecal valve.[1] Kremen mentioned that a patient had been treated with intestinal bypass for obesity. Kremen was concerned about the effects of extensive loss of small bowel function, but the ultimate result of the study was the surgical treatment of obesity. Kremen's mentor at the University of Minnesota, where this study was performed, was Richard L. Varco. Owen H. Wangensteen had asked for Varco's assistance with the treatment of malnutrition that followed the extensive removal of intestine required in the treatment of cancer and other diseases. Kremen's experimental design made it possible to make comparisons within animals instead of between animals because the bypassed jejunum (or ileum) was maintained as a Thiry-Vella fistula, which could then be exchanged for the other half. John Linner, whose patient was operated on for obesity, assisted Kremen in the laboratory work and later became one of the early leaders in surgical treatment of obesity. According to Buchwald, a patient of Varco was actually the first to have an intestinal bypass.[6]

Payne and colleagues popularized intestinal bypass as a treatment for obesity. They first bypassed most of the small bowel and part of the colon by anastomosis of jejunum to transverse colon.[7] The initial plan was to restore bowel continuity after the patient reached a normal weight. Rapid regain in weight soon caused a change to the use of a permanent jejunoileal bypass. Payne mentioned V. Henrickson of Gothenberg, who resected "an appropriate amount of small intestine" because of obesity and induced weight loss but realized a situation of difficult nutritional balance. Payne and many other surgeons studied varying lengths of functioning jejunum and ileum. Eventually, 14 inches of jejunum and 4 inches of ileum became the most common measurements.

The literature gradually changed from studies of optimum design and early results to the reporting of complications. There was no combination of lengths that would provide the desired weight reduction without an excess of complications. Fat digestion and absorption were impaired to the extent that calcium soaps formed; this allowed oxalate (which is normally precipitated by calcium and excreted in the feces) to be absorbed and excreted by the kidneys, where it combined with calcium in the kidney tissues and as stones in the urinary collection system. Autoimmune disease (caused by absorption of bacterial and protein breakdown products in the bowel) also damaged the kidneys, and some patients required dialysis and renal transplantation. Protein malnutrition developed and contributed to liver damage due to the accumulation of fat. There was damage resulting from the bacterial overgrowth products that arrived in portal blood to cause cirrhosis and the occasional need for liver transplantation. Anastomosis of the gallbladder to the upper end of the bypassed bowel decreased diarrhea and decreased bacterial overgrowth.[8,9] Cleator closed the upper end of the bypassed bowel but anastomosed the lower end to the stomach to decrease the backwash of bacteria.[10] Oxalate stones remained a complication with Cleator's jejunoileal bypass and ileogastrostomy.

▶ GASTRIC BYPASS

Billroth II gastrectomy (BII) was the antecedent to gastric bypass and provided more than 50 years of literature regarding its use in the treatment of cancer and peptic ulcer.

One of the complications that caused surgeons to quit using BII for treating ulcers was excessive weight loss, which was explained as an intake deficiency. The dumping syndrome resulting from loss of pyloric control of passage of food into the small bowel was a part of the explanation for decreased intake. Another was the loss of gastric capacity for a meal. Blowout of the duodenal stump was an early postoperative complication of BII gastrectomy for ulcer disease. Bypass of the duodenum in BII gastrectomy led to late complications of iron-deficiency anemia and metabolic bone disease. Loop gastroenterostomy caused gastritis due to bile and alkaline pancreatic juice entering the pouch. However, the dictum was to use a "short loop," retrocolic gastroenterostomy to provide buffering of the acid at the site of entry of acid into the jejunum.

The first gastric bypass for treatment of obesity was a copy of the operation used by Wangensteen for treatment of peptic ulcer, except that the stomach was bypassed instead of removed.[11] Ten years after the first gastric bypass, Hornberger wrote about the "technically difficult and tedious procedure done in the attic of the peritoneal cavity." He concluded that "with careful attention to pre-, intra-, and postoperative detail, it is reasonably safe, effective, and relatively free from unmanageable complications."[12] During the early years the stomach was divided and inverted above and below the division with two rows of interrupted sutures. The introduction of linear staplers was a great advance. Alden further simplified the operation by performing a high gastroenterostomy as the first step in the operation, followed by stapling the stomach in continuity immediately below the anastomosis.[13] Stapling in continuity reduced the operative risk because if there was breakdown of the staple line, the result was a fistula between pouch and stomach instead of peritonitis. However, a more secure partition was important. Harris and colleagues found that four rows of staples with a 2-mm space between rows provided the most secure partition.[14] This was made possible by the commercial production of a stapler with a cartridge containing four rows of staples, specifically designed for use in obesity surgery.

Terry began measuring the pouch.[15] During the entire history of gastrectomy there had never been an effort to measure pouch volume. For treatment of obesity, this was essential. With unmeasured pouches, patients would lose weight for months or a year and then they would begin to gain. When a revision was performed, the pouch would measure a surprising 800 ml or more. The pouch was then reduced to a measured 60 ml at a pressure of 70 cm of water, and weight again decreased. We learned that pouches not only had to be measured but they needed to be small. It required a number of years of these observations, extending over experience with gastric bypass and gastroplasty, before we arrived at a pouch of 30 ml or less for gastric bypass and 20 ml or less for gastroplasty. Mechanical application of the law of LaPlace (i.e., wall tension [T] is proportional to the product of intraventricular pressure [P] and ventricular radius [r]: $T \sim P \times r$) was again discovered to be important. Wangensteen taught us that the reason the cecum was the site of perforation in colon obstruction was that the tension on the wall that caused the tear was related to the radius. For obesity surgery, the larger the pouch the more it stretched, because the tension was related to the radius.

The only safe way to keep a pouch small was to make it small in the beginning. Cummings has called our attention to the location of the powerful orexigenic (hunger) hormone, ghrelin, upon the construction of the pouch.[16] In theory, the fundus should be excluded from the pouch in order to reduce ghrelin secretion to as low a level as possible. Ghrelin is highest in concentration in the fundus. Either a very small pouch or a longer vertical pouch along the lesser curvature of the stomach should exclude the fundus.

Stomal Ulcers Resulting From Exclusion

Before gastric bypass could be used for treatment of obesity it was necessary to determine its effect upon the secretion of acid and stomal ulceration. Eiselberg, a trainee and colleague of Billroth, began in 1895 to divide the stomach above the antrum in patients with inoperable cancers. He closed the antrum and anastomosed the upper stomach to a loop of jejunum. He also used this operation for treatment of peptic ulcer in two patients. Wangensteen reviewed the history of stomal ulcer production by exclusion operations, including studies at the University of Minnesota that showed that vagotomy did not prevent such ulcers.[17]

Stomal ulcer was common when gastroenterostomy was used for treatment of duodenal ulcer. After gastric bypass, if a communication between the stomach pouch and the distal stomach developed, the incidence of stomal ulcer was so high that closure of the fistula was recommended even before an ulcer developed.[18] This is an argument for division of the stomach and interposition of the alimentary limb between the pouch and the distal stomach when a Roux-en-Y gastric bypass (RYGB) is performed.[19]

Suppressing Gastrin

The first experiment in the laboratory at the University of Iowa was designed to study acid secretion stimulated by a standard meal before and after gastric bypass. Pavlov pouches were created and acid secretion determined following a meal. A series of operations made it possible to make comparisons within rather than between animals. The Pavlov pouches secreted very little acid after a two-thirds distal gastric bypass, which included considerable parietal cell (acid-secreting) mucosa in the excluded segment. The parietal-cell-bearing tissue was then removed, leaving only antrum, which resulted in an intestinal-phase type of acid secretion following a meal. The antrum was then removed, which created a BII gastric resection and abolished acid-secretory response to a meal. Final proof that gastric bypass preserved enough acid secretion in the distal stomach to suppress gastrin secretion came later, after the gastrin assay was available. We found that plasma gastrin increased following a meal before gastric bypass and was significantly less stimulated by a meal after gastric bypass.[20]

▶ REFINEMENT OF GASTRIC BYPASS

The first gastric bypass operations were based upon what I had learned as a surgical intern about gastrectomy for ulcer as practiced by Wangensteen in 1945, except that the distal stomach was left in place and weight loss was made a virtue instead of a complication. Reconstruction was performed using a short afferent loop, retrocolic end-to-side gastrojejunostomy, performed between the greater curvature end of the divided stomach pouch and an area of the jejunum overlapping the spot where the ligament of Treitz had been divided. The stomach was divided and the distal end closed with a double row of interrupted sutures. The mesocolon was sutured to the gastric pouch above the gastroenterostomy. All sites for potential internal hernias were closed. The first report of any experience with gastric bypass outside of Iowa City was made in 1976 by Hornberger, based on his private-practice experience in Waterville, Maine.[12] A number of papers from other surgeons began appearing in 1977, and one of these was a comparison by Griffen and colleagues between RYGB and intestinal bypass.[21] Griffen preferred the Roux-en-Y reconstruction to the loop gastrojejunostomy because it prevented bile and pancreatic juice from entering the stomach pouch. If a leak occurred from the pouch, it was easier to manage without bile and pancreatic juice draining from the area. Buckwalter published another comparison between intestinal and gastric bypass.[22] Both of these studies led to an early preference for gastric bypass and jejunoileal bypass. The patients with gastric bypass felt stronger and were able to eat an adequate diet sooner. Diarrhea was infrequent after gastric bypass but frequent after intestinal bypass.

Laparoscopic Roux-en-Y Gastric Bypass

Wittgrove introduced laparoscopic RYGB in 1994.[23] There had been an earlier increase in the use of RYGB because of a desire for more weight loss than could be obtained using purely restrictive operations. There is no reason to believe that the long-term effects of the operation will be any different for having been performed laparoscopically except for (1) the avoidance of large incisional hernias and (2) the decreased formation of adhesions. Exposure is usually excellent and does not exhaust the surgeons.

Bypass Complications

The complications resulting from BII gastrectomy, the antecedent operation to gastric bypass, were the reason for developing gastroplasty, beginning in 1971. The duodenum is normally the chief site of iron absorption, so bypass usually results in a decrease in total body iron and hemoglobin. Oral iron is commonly required in treatment and, occasionally, parenteral iron and blood transfusions are necessary. A few patients require restoration of duodenal passage of food. Because there is the possibility of duodenal ulcer as a cause of iron deficiency anemia, access to the duodenum for endoscopy and radiologic study is a concern. A long pediatric endoscope can be passed retrograde into the area. Some surgeons have placed a radiopaque marker at the site of a temporary distal gastrostomy for use in percutaneous injection of contrast or even for passage of a gastroscope.[24] Severe bleeding may require an emergency operation with a tentative diagnosis of duodenal ulcer.

Calcium is also normally absorbed most efficiently in the duodenum. As a result, gastric bypass increases the risk of metabolic bone disease.[25] Unlike anemia, bone depletion can occur without symptoms until pathologic fractures appear in ribs, spine, or hips. Secondary hyperparathyroidism is appearing in case reports and should be looked for during follow-up so that it can be treated before severe bone changes occur.[26] The informed patient is often the only one who can ensure that lifelong monitoring takes place. During early weight loss, the bones provide calcium because of the decrease in bone mass. Later, after weight is stable, inadequate intake and absorption of calcium and vitamin D may result in continued bone loss. Osteoporosis and osteomalacia must be diagnosed and treated before irreversible changes occur and before patients begin to have bone pain and pathologic fractures of ribs, spine, or hips. The more effective the operation is in reducing weight, the more risk there is of developing metabolic bone disease.

There are complications peculiar to bypass operations, such as bleeding ulcers in the stoma and duodenum, that are uncommon but can rapidly become lethal unless diagnosed and operated on emergently. Distal gastric dilatation, after gastric bypass, took the place of the duodenal stump rupture that complicated BII gastrectomy during the early postoperative days. Distal gastric dilatation occurs in about one in a thousand patients during the first month following operation, but it remains a risk as long as the operation remains in place. Obstruction of the biliopancreatic limb creates a closed segment and rapid distention by gastric juice, bile, and pancreatic juice. Pressure necrosis of the walls of these structures can lead to perforation and death within a day if it is not recognized and the walls decompressed. The correct diagnosis is more likely if those seeing the patient are aware of its possibility and are making deliberate efforts to rule out distal gastric dilatation. Patient awareness of the anatomic basis of a closed obstruction of the bypassed segment and the need for early detection and prompt operative treatment could mean the difference between life and death.[27] The patient would need to be made aware of these signs and symptoms; however, that is a lot to expect a patient to remember for a lifetime.

Biliopancreatic Diversion

Biliopancreatic diversion (BPD) was introduced by Scopinaro in Genoa in 1976.[27] It is a combination of BII gastrectomy and intestinal bypass and provides the greatest weight reduction and best maintenance of the lower weight, but it requires the greatest lifelong care by both patients and physicians. Scopinaro visited Iowa City during his early use of BPD. He and I discussed the similarity of his operation to one used by Mann and Williamson in 1923 for the experimental production of chronic ulcers in the animal laboratory. The difference was that Scopinaro removed much of the distal stomach and emptied the remaining small gastric pouch into the distal small bowel, whereas the Mann-Williamson procedure emptied the entire stomach into the distal small bowel. The similarity was the wide separation of the areas where acid and alkaline digestive juices enter and can mix in the small bowel.

Normally, the pylorus allows small amounts of gastric contents to enter the duodenum, where it mixes with bile and pancreatic juice. The acid is neutralized and rendered harmless. In the treatment of peptic ulcer, Wangensteen emphasized the short-loop retrocolic gastroenterostomy so that the duodenal juices would be close and available for buffering acid at the stoma. BPD placed most of the small bowel between the sites of acid and alkaline juice entrance. Scopinaro observed stomal ulcers after BPD and found that they responded to medical management, seldom required an operation, and decreased in frequency over time.

BPD requires close adherence to the recommended pouch size and limb lengths as developed by Scopinaro. The gastric pouch is between 200 and 500 ml, depending upon a number of patient characteristics. The pouch is larger than that in other operations because the patient is required to eat as much as 150 g of protein a day to prevent protein malnutrition. Prevention of bone disease requires that the patient take large amounts of calcium and vitamin D. Scopinaro provides a large retinue of physicians to assist with the care of these patients and has emphasized the hazards of changing the operation. There is more information about the long-term effects of BPD than there is about any other operation for obesity. The conversion of an operation with a small pouch and a long common limb into an operation with a small pouch and a short common limb increases the risk for protein malnutrition. Fobi and colleagues reported a 23% incidence of albumen less than 3 g after such conversions were performed to increase weight loss.[28] This effect can be prevented or treated either by increasing the size of the gastric pouch or by lengthening the common limb. The variability in patient response to such changes in pouch size and limb length means that further surgery may be required.

Biliopancreatic Diversion With Duodenal Switch

This modification of BPD maintains the normal sequence of lesser curvature of stomach, a full width of antrum, the pyloric muscle, and the duodenum just above the entrance of the bile and pancreatic ducts. At this point, the duodenum is divided and an anastomosis is made end-to-end between the short segment of duodenum and the last 250 cm of ileum. The duodenum just above the ampulla of Vater is closed, and the long, bypassed biliopancreatic limb is anastomosed end-to-side to the ileum about 100 cm from the cecum. This would be close to the Mann-Williamson operation for experimental production of chronic peptic ulcer were it not for the removal of most of the acid-secreting stomach. To decrease the risk of peptic ulcer, a sleeve resection is performed, removing the greater-curvature side of the stomach from the esophagus to the antrum. A long lesser-curvature tube is created, similar to that of Tretbar in his gastroplasty for obesity, but the volume is 250 ml and there must be no restriction of passage of food by the long pouch. Like Scopinaro's BPD, the partial gastric resection is not reversible. However, control of gastric emptying by the pyloric muscle is preserved. Whether the small segment of duodenum left in the food stream improves the absorption of iron and calcium over that of BPD or RYGB is not yet known. Hess[29] introduced BPD with duodenal switch, and

Marceau and colleagues have provided considerable experience with it.[30]

There are inherent risks in BPD with duodenal switch and gastric sleeve resection. Dissection near the bile duct, pancreatic ducts, and duodenum risks injury to these structures. The total length of divided and stapled stomach and bowel increases the risk for leak, peritonitis, abscess, and fistula.

▶ GASTROPLASTY

The initiation of gastroplasty in early 1971 at the University of Iowa was intended to minimize the complications of gastric bypass.[31] By the end of the year, it was evident that patients were not losing enough weight, and we returned to performing gastric bypass. Gomez resurrected horizontal gastroplasty.[32] The pouch was measured and smaller than in 1971, and a mesh collar was placed around the outlet and sutured to the end of the staple line. Obstruction occurred, and Gomez concluded that the mesh was stimulating excessive scar tissue, which caused obstruction. He then substituted a running, nonabsorbable, seromuscular suture for the mesh. A 32F tube was placed in the lumen to provide calibration while the stoma was fashioned. The suture occasionally resulted in an outlet that was too tight but, in time, the suture would migrate into the lumen and the outlet would then become too large.

Unpublished experience by John Kroyer of Long Beach, California, led me to use polypropylene mesh for the gastroplasty collar, although without any sutured attachment to the stomach. Later, I learned that Grace had been using the same technique as Kroyer with horizontal gastroplasty.[33] Ultimately, all horizontal gastroplasties were abandoned. It was difficult to visualize and to dilate the outlet endoscopically. A pouch was needed that did not require two right-angle turns of the gastroscope. At the University of Iowa, the reason for discontinuing the use of horizontal gastroplasty in 1971, after 1 year, and again in 1980, after 3 years of use, was a reoperation rate of 15% per year.

Vertical Gastroplasty

In 1979, Tretbar tried to reduce the capacity of the stomach by wrapping the greater curvature around the lesser curvature like a long, slipped Nissen fundoplication. The stomach unwrapped, but the idea of a long vertical pouch had been implanted in Tretbar's thinking, and he began using an 18-cm staple line extending from the angle of His and parallel to the lesser curvature.[34] There was no stabilizing collar. In retrospect, this operation should probably be considered an 18-cm outlet without a pouch.

Laws introduced a gastroplasty with a 50-ml pouch and an outlet on the lesser curvature. This resulted in the linear staple line that was almost vertical, although he did not use the word *vertical* and did not mention the angle of His. A 2.2-mm outside diameter Silastic tube 42 mm long was used to stabilize the outlet. The tubing was threaded twice with a polypropylene suture that was passed through the lower end of the staple line.[35] This was tied down over a 32F bougie.

Laws mentioned nothing about the tension on the suture as it was tied. Laws reported his early results at our June 1982 meeting in Iowa City. He was following 117 patients at the time, and in 101 of these patients, the Silastic ring gastroplasty was the initial operation for obesity. The patients were in the hospital for an average of 6.7 days, which allowed some time for teaching as they began to take fluids and pureed foods. Of those, 20 patients required intravenous therapy for excessive vomiting. There was erosion of the ring into the lumen in 5 patients and staple-line breakdown in 3. In some patients it was unclear whether erosion or staple-line breakdown had occurred first. The weight loss was comparable to that obtained with RYGB for the 15 months during which these patients were observed. In retrospect, the outlet was probably too small in many of these patients. It was possible to obtain weight loss equal to that obtained with RYGB but at the risk of obstruction.

Laws gave Woodward credit for the idea that the ultimate size of the outlet was dependent upon the tightness of the tie of the encircling suture that held the tubing in place.[36] Laws also gave Daniel Fabito credit for the change from horizontal to vertical in gastroplasty. Fabito had been working with Gomez. He noticed the lesser curvature was thicker and better suited for a meal-limiting pouch. Fabito used a 2-0 polypropylene suture for stabilization of the outlet and no tubing to cover the suture. Laws visited Gomez and Fabito in February 1980 and was impressed with the simplicity of the technique. He proceeded to develop his own vertical gastroplasty with Silastic tubing added to keep the suture from migrating through the stomach wall into the lumen.

▶ LONG GASTROPLASTY

Michael Long, in Victoria, Australia, moved the outlet from the greater to the lesser curve in 1977 and gradually changed the staple line from horizontal to vertical, reaching the angle of His in 1980, and using two bare sutures through the staple line, encircling the outlet at the lower end.[37] Jamieson, who was a surgical resident working with Long, took the operation into his own practice and added a third suture, which extended the outlet to 22 mm. The longer outlet improved weight loss. During the next 20 years Jamieson continued to perform the operation and followed more than 3000 of these patients; they had what he considered to be highly satisfactory results.[38] The operation has not been adapted to laparoscopic surgery, which will be necessary if it is to gain acceptance by patients and surgeons. Jamieson's technique must be followed closely, especially with regard to the calibration of the outlet. Placing a 36F to 38F bougie in the outlet when the three sutures are tied prevents obstruction of the outlet.

Vertical Banded Gastroplasty

Long presented his results at a meeting in Genoa hosted by Scopinaro in the fall of 1980. I began performing vertical banded gastroplasty (VBG) after that meeting. I decided to use a circular window stapled into the stomach near the lesser curvature for placement of the linear stapler and a polypropylene mesh collar that would not be sutured to the stomach wall.[39] The first collars were 5 cm in circumference. A few patients were readmitted because of vomiting. The collar was then increased to 5.5 cm, and a greater effort was made to teach the patients how to begin eating with smaller bites by using a medicine glass to measure the food. Patients were in the hospital for 6 days after the operation so they had time to think about their new eating pattern and protect the small pouch by chewing all food until it was liquid before swallowing. A return was made to the 5-cm collar in 1981, and it was well tolerated. It was then decided to use a 4.5-cm collar for the super obese (225% of ideal weight or greater). The super obese with the 4.5-cm collar complained about inability to eat fibrous foods and felt they were forced to eat what they considered junk food. The smaller collar increased the need for reoperation due to disrupted staple lines. All patients, regardless of weight, were then provided with 5-cm collars.

MacLean began his study of obesity surgery with the goal of reducing all patients to within 50% of ideal weight, or a BMI of less than 35 kg per m^2. In the effort to achieve that goal with VBG, he used two layers of mesh measured at less than 5 cm in length. The result was a reoperation rate that far exceeded that of any other report.[40] This final paper in the series describes a randomized trial comparing VBG with RYGB and explains that, in their experience, VBG has been unsatisfactory mainly as the result of the breakdown of the vertical staple line. No other surgeon has performed VBG with two layers of mesh in the collar, so MacLean's results cannot be generalized. By setting the weight loss goal at a higher level than was realistic and defining failure as the failure to reach that goal, the outcome of the randomized trial was preordained.

The weight-loss goal is only one variable in determining a satisfactory operation. We must obtain much more information about the long-term complications of bypass and purely restrictive operations before establishing a weight-loss goal. Vertical gastroplasty appears to be as effective as laparoscopic gastric banding and uses far less foreign material. Today, laparoscopic methods for VBG are available. Patients need to have a simple restrictive operation as an option if they wish to avoid the complications of bypass operations. For surgeons who wish to avoid the window and mesh of VBG, the Long operation as performed by Jamieson is attractive, but adaptation to the laparoscopic approach is necessary. The history and the future of gastroplasty have been reviewed in greater detail.[41]

GASTRIC BANDING

Shortly after vertical gastroplasty was begun, Knolle, Bo, and Stadias at Ulleval Hospital in Oslo began gastric banding.[42] A tube was passed through the mouth; it had an attached balloon so that the pouch could be calibrated at 50 ml in volume with an outlet of 9 mm in diameter. A lockable nylon band enclosed in a Dacron vascular prosthesis was wrapped around the upper stomach and secured. The operation required no cutting or stapling of the stomach. Kuzmak developed an adjustable band and a tensometer that was inserted through the mouth into the stomach for controlling the tension and therefore the diameter of the outlet when the band was tightened and locked into place.[43] The outlet was 12.5 mm in diameter. The adjustable band was constructed with an inflatable bladder on the inner surface that was connected by tubing to an injection port under the skin on the upper anterior abdominal wall. The Lap-Band (BioEnterics, Carpinteria, CA) and the Swedish Adjustable Band (Ethicon Endo-Surgery, a Johnson & Johnson Company, Cincinnati, OH) are the two bands that have been used extensively in Europe. The Lap-Band was limited to use under strict protocol in the United States until June of 2001. At that time the Food and Drug Administration approved the Lap-Band for use in the United States following a multi-institutional study.

Because there is no adherence of the adjustable band to the stomach wall, there has been a problem of slippage of stomach wall into the pouch and of the tilting of the band, producing obstruction of the outlet. This has been largely overcome by placement of the band above the peritoneal reflection behind the stomach and by the use of imbricating sutures placed to cover the band with stomach wall anteriorly. Migration of the band into the lumen also has been reported. One of the main attractions of the procedure to patients is placement by laparoscopic approach; ease of removal for reversal by the laparoscopic approach is also attractive.

RECAPITULATION AND EXPLORATION

In 1977, during a gastric bypass workshop in Iowa City, George Blackburn raised a recurring question: "Is it out of place to ask Dr. Drenick for input as to what our obligation is to treatment for these massively obese people? He has probably done as much as anyone in the field." E. J. Drenick, an internist devoted to the study of obesity, was a regular attendee at these yearly meetings. There followed a friendly exchange that is too long to include here, but toward the end Blackburn asked, "Would you randomize now?" Drenick responded, "I think that we have to separate very, very clearly what our desires are and what the patient's desires are. They are totally different perspectives. Your desire is to furnish objective scientific information and criteria. The patient is not interested in that. He knows that he cannot get a job, that he has been unemployed for the last 10 years, and that he wants to finally live."

In the United States in 2003, surgeons, the medical profession, third-party payers, and our society are confronted with at least 8 million potential candidates for surgical treatment. Not infrequently, the question is raised about treatment choices, randomization, and all that is involved in improving outcomes. We certainly need centers for intensive study and continued development of improved techniques and patient care. We must also continue to save lives and improve living by use of the simple restrictive and bypass operations that have been in use now for 30 years.

In 1977, we had data from our first year of a National Bypass Registry with central data entry. There were 8 surgical practices and sets of data from 108 patients. There had been 3 early deaths. Now in the International Bariatric Surgery Registry, with distributed data entry, we have

111 surgeons at 76 surgical sites and data from 30,000 patients collected over 17 years. The 30-day operative mortality is 0.4%. Operative weight continues to increase. Simple restrictive operations have given way to bypass operations, which produce weight loss more rapidly. The bypass operations carry lifelong risks, which require more follow-up and treatment.

The surgeon's first duty is to serve the patient, as Drenick stated. The patient is responsible for making the choice of treatment. In order to advise patients, the surgeon must know the lifelong effects of recommended operations, as Blackburn stated. This requires lifelong follow-up, data management and analysis, and education of patients regarding the results of surgery at the time that they make an informed decision. Surgical treatment is incomplete unless it includes the necessary monitoring, prevention, and treatment for life. Accomplishing this may require additional changes in our medical care system that may constitute an important contribution to the history of obesity surgery.

Surgery made obesity a disease. Obesity surgery can change the medical care system so that lifelong disease is treated for life.

▶ REFERENCES

1. Kremen AJ, Linner JH, Nelson CH: An experimental evaluation of the nutritional importance of proximal and distal small intestine. Ann Surg 1954;140:439-444.
2. Mason EE: Acceptance of surgery for obesity by academic surgeons in North America. Obes Surg 1996;6:218-223.
3. Flegal KM, Carroll MD, Ogden CL, et al: Prevalence and trends in obesity among US adults, 1999-2000. JAMA 2002;288:1723-1727.
4. Flegal K, Troiano RP: Changes in the distribution of body mass index of adults and children in the US population. Int J Obes 2000;24:807-818.
5. Mason EE, Tang S, Renquist KE, et al: A decade of change in obesity surgery. Obes Surg 1997;7:189-197.
6. Buchwald H: Overview of bariatric surgery. J Am Coll Surg 2002;194:367-375.
7. Payne JH, DeWind LT, Commons RR: Metabolic observations in patients with jejunocolic shunts. Am J Surg 1963;106:273-289.
8. Hallberg DA, Holmgren U: Bilio-intestinal shunt for treatment of obesity. Acta Chir Scand 1979;145:405-408.
9. Eriksson F: Biliointestinal bypass. Int J Obes 1981;5:437-447.
10. Cleator IGM, Gourlay RH: Ileogastrostomy for morbid obesity. Can J Surg 1988;31:114-116.
11. Mason EE, Ito C: Gastric bypass in obesity. Surg Clin North Am 1967;47:1345-1351.
12. Hornberger HR: Gastric bypass. Am J Surg 1976;131:415-418.
13. Alden JF: Gastric and jejunoileal bypass. A comparison in the treatment of morbid obesity. Arch Surg 1977;112:799-806.
14. Harris P, Freedman BE, Bland KI, et al: Collagen content, histology, and tensile strength: determinants of wound repair in various stapling devices in a canine gastric partition model. J Surg Res 1987;42:411-417.
15. Alder RL, Terry BE: Measurement and standardization of the gastric pouch in gastric bypass. Surg Gynecol Obstet 1977;144:762-763.
16. Cummings DE, Shannon MH: Roles for ghrelin in the regulation of appetite and body weight. Arch Surg 2003;138:389-396.
17. Wangensteen OH, Wangensteen SD: The Rise of Surgery from Empiric Craft to Scientific Discipline, pp. 157-159. Minneapolis, MN, University of Minnesota Press, 1978.
18. Jordan JH, Hocking MP, Rout WR, et al: Marginal ulcer following gastric bypass for morbid obesity. Am Surg 1991;57:286-288.
19. MacLean LD, Rhode BM, Nohr C, et al: Stomal ulcer after gastric bypass. J Am Coll Surg 1997;185:1-7.
20. Mason EE, Munns JR, Kealey GP, et al: Effect of gastric bypass on gastric secretion. Am J Surg 1976;131:162-168.
21. Griffen WO, Young VL, Stevenson CC: A prospective comparison of gastric and jejunoileal bypass procedures for morbid obesity. Ann Surg 1977;186:500-509.
22. Buckwalter JA: A prospective comparison of the jejunoileal and gastric bypass operations for morbid obesity. World J Surg 1977;1:757-768.
23. Wittgrove AC, Clark GW, Tremblay LJ: Laparascopic gastric bypass, Roux en-Y: preliminary report of five cases. Obes Surg 1994;4:353-357.
24. Fobi MAL, Chicola K, Lee H: Access to the bypassed stomach after gastric bypass. Obes Surg 1998; 8: 289-295.
25. Shaker JL, Norton AJ, Woods MF, et al: Secondary hyperparathyroidism and osteopenia in women following gastric exclusion surgery for obesity. Osteoporos Int 1991;1:177-181.
26. Goldner WS, O'Dorisio T, Mason EE: Case report: severe metabolic bone disease as a long-term complication of obesity surgery. Obes Surg 2002;12:685-692.
27. Scopinaro N, Gianetta E, Civalleri D, et al: Bilio-pancreatic by-pass for obesity: II. Initial experience in man. Br J Surg 1979;66:619-620.
28. Fobi MA, Lee H, Igwe D Jr, et al: Revision of failed gastric bypass to distal Roux-en-Y gastric bypass: a review of 65 cases. Obes Surg 2001;11:190-195.
29. Hess DS: Biliopancreatic diversion with a duodenal switch procedure. Obes Surg 1994;4:106 (abstract).
30. Marceau P, Biron S, Bourque RA, et al: Biliopancreatic diversion with a new type of gastrectomy. Obes Surg 1993;3:29-35.
31. Printen KJ, Mason EE: Gastric surgery for the relief of morbid obesity. Arch Surg 1973;106:428-431.
32. Gomez CA: Gastroplasty in the surgical treatment of morbid obesity. Am J Clin Nutr 1980;33(2 suppl):406-415.
33. Grace DM: The demise of horizontal gastroplasty. In Mason EE, Nyhus LM (eds): Surgical Treatment of Morbid Obesity, vol 9, pp. 260–265. Philadelphia, JB Lippincott, 1992.
34. Tretbar LL, Sifers EC: Vertical stapling: a new type of gastroplasty. Int J Obes 1981;5:538 (abstract).
35. Laws HL: Standardized gastroplasty orifice. Am J Surg 1981;141:393-394.
36. Laws HL: The origin of the vertical Silastic ring gastroplasty. In Mason EE (guested), Nyhus LM (eds): Surgical Treatment of Morbid Obesity, vol 9, pp. 276-279. Philadelphia, JB Lippincott, 1992.
37. Long M, Collins JP: The technique and early results of high gastric reduction for obesity. Aust N Z J Surg 1980;50:146-149.
38. Jamieson AC: Determinants of weight loss after gastroplasty. In Mason EE (guested), Nyhus LM (eds): Surgical Treatment of Morbid Obesity, vol 9, pp. 290-297. Philadelphia, JB Lippincott, 1992.
39. Mason EE: Vertical banded gastroplasty for obesity. Arch Surg 1982; 117: 701-706.
40. MacLean LD, Rhode BM, Forse RA, et al: C: Surgery for obesity: an update of a randomized trial. Obes Surg 1995;5:145-151.
41. Mason EE: Development and future of gastroplasties for morbid obesity. Arch Surg 2003;138:361-366.
42. Check W: Yet another variation on surgery for obesity. JAMA 1982;248:1939.
43. Kuzmak LI: Stoma adjustable silicone gastric banding. In Mason EE, Nyhus LM (eds): Surgical Treatment of Morbid Obesity, vol 9, pp. 298-317. Philadelphia, JB Lippincott, 1992.

2

Incidence, Prevalence, and Demography of Obesity

Neil E. Hutcher, M.D., F.A.C.S.

On December 13, 2001, United States Surgeon General David Satcher, M.D., issued an alarm in his Call to Action. Health problems related to obesity could reverse many of the health gains achieved in the United States in recent decades.[1] Overweight and obesity are escalating as the worldwide threat of atherosclerotic disease, for example, has diminished because of improved treatment, prevention, and the modification of risk factors, including hypertension and hyperlipidemia. The downward-trend shift in atherosclerotic disease was instigated by widespread education and outreach efforts,[2] but ignorance of the risk factors for obesity has led to a marked rise in its incidence and prevalence around the world. The obesity epidemic now surpasses the threat of atherosclerotic disease in many parts of the world, and it is spreading rapidly.[3]

Dr. Satcher identified 15 activities as national priorities for immediate action. He clearly stated that obesity is a crisis concerning health, not appearance. The crisis is figured both in health costs and in economic losses.[1] The overall cost in lives is estimated to have reached more than 300,000 deaths, with economic costs exceeding $117 billion per year.[1] Others have estimated the cost at $700 per individual for the entire population of the United States.[4] Quesenberry and colleagues found that in a closely managed health maintenance organization, an individual with a body mass index (BMI; kg/m^2) of 30.0 to 34.9 had a 25% greater cost per year than one with a BMI of 20.0 to 24.9. When the BMI was 35, the cost increased to 44% per year more than that of individuals of normal weight.[5]

The costs to health and years of life expectancy are alarming. Table 2-1 lists the disease entities that have a relationship with obesity.[6] Fontaine and colleagues reported that life expectancy for 20-year-olds with BMIs of 45 is 13 years lower for Caucasian men and 20 years lower for African-American men compared with that of people of normal weight. These effects were somewhat lower for obese Caucasian women (8 years) and African-American women (5 years).[7]

Although the percentage of overweight is highest in the United States, at 61%, this crisis is an issue not only in the United States but also in the world as a whole. The World Health Organization began sounding the alarm in the 1990s.[8] The term *globesity* was coined to warn that between 1995 and 2000, the number of obese adults had increased from 200 million to 300 million worldwide.[3] It was estimated that at least 115 million adults suffer from obesity-related problems, especially type 2 diabetes, heart disease, and obesity-related cancers.

▶ DEFINITION OF OBESITY

The current standard for reporting weight-related statistics is the BMI, which was initially described as Quetelet's Index,[9] after Adolphe Quetelet, a Belgian mathematician,

Table 2-1	POTENTIAL HEALTH CONSEQUENCES OF BMIs OF 25 OR HIGHER

- High blood pressure, hypertension
- High blood cholesterol, dyslipidemia
- Type 2 (non-insulin-dependent) diabetes
- Insulin resistance, glucose intolerance
- Hyperinsulinemia
- Coronary heart disease
- Angina pectoris
- Congestive heart failure
- Stroke
- Gallstones
- Cholecystitis and cholelithiasis
- Gout
- Osteoarthritis
- Obstructive sleep apnea, respiratory problems, and asthma
- Some types of cancer (such as endometrial, breast, prostate, and colon)
- Complications of pregnancy
- Poor female reproductive health (such as menstrual irregularities, infertility, irregular ovulation)
- Bladder control problems (such as stress incontinence)
- Uric acid nephrolithiasis
- Psychological disorders (such as depression, eating disorders, distorted body image, and low self-esteem).

Table 2-2	BMIs AND ASSOCIATED RISK LEVELS	
	BMI	RISK FOR COMORBIDITIES
Normal	18.5-24.9	Average
Overweight:		
Preobese	25.0-29.9	Increased
Obesity class I	30.0-34.9	Moderate
Obesity class II	35.0-39.9	Severe
Obesity class III	40	Very severe

combined the disciplines of mathematics and sociology to study population-based issues in the 1830s. The BMI is a ratio of weight, adjusted for height, expressed as weight in kilograms divided by height in meters squared. There are several inherent problems associated with use of the BMI because it allows no adjustment for body-fat composition or age.

Table 2-2 lists the 1998 National Institutes of Health Clinical Guidelines on the Identification, Evaluation, and Treatment of Overweight and Obesity in Adults into Class I (BMI 30.0 kg/m² to 34.9 kg/m²); Class II (BMI 35.0 kg/m² to 39.9 kg/m²); and Class III (BMI = 40 kg/m²) values for normal weight, overweight, obesity, and severe obesity.[10] It is important to use these terms appropriately because each has its own implications. In children in particular, it is important to note differences in gender and in age. BMI for age is plotted on gender-specific charts and reported as a percentile. Figure 2-1 is an example of such a chart.[10]

It is also important to have knowledge of the composition of body fat. A well-conditioned athlete may appear to have an elevated BMI but be in excellent condition because of increased muscle mass. It is valuable to distinguish the difference between overweight and the degrees of obesity, terms that are often used interchangeably but have dramatically different implications. Overweight (BMI 25.0 to 29.9) is commonly a step in the progression to obesity, but it has few health implications of its own. The impact of obesity (BMI 30.0 to 34.9) and severe or morbid obesity (BMI = 35.0) has been expressed in many forms. No matter the method of expression, the implication is clear: obesity has a dramatic adverse effect on health and on economic costs.

The Centers for Disease Control and Prevention estimate that 47 million Americans suffer from the "metabolic syndrome," which is characterized by obesity, insulin resistance, increased abdominal fat mass (central obesity), high blood sugar, high serum lipids, and hypertension.[11] This constellation of obesity and comorbidities accelerates a decrease in life expectancy. It is, therefore, clear that the current obesity epidemic and its continued rapid increase has catastrophic implications for global health.

Obesity in the United States

Much of the information used by researchers and health care planners comes from a series of surveys from the National Health and Nutrition Examination Survey (NHANES)[10] as well as from data reported by Flegal and Mokdad and their colleagues.[12,13] Between 1960 and 1994,

in the United States, the prevalence of obesity increased geometrically, from 12.8% in 1962 to 22.5% in 1994 in the 20- to 74-year-old age-adjusted population,[10] increasing to 27% in the most recent (2002) NHANES IV report for 1999.[14] The number of obese individuals in the United States has nearly doubled in the past 20 years.[14]

Childhood obesity begins when a child exceeds the 85th percentile for age but is below the 95th percentile. A child is obese when the 95th percentile is exceeded. Table 2-3 shows that between l963 and 2000, there has been an increase of almost 400% (from 4% to 15%) in overweight children 6 to 11 years old. In adolescents 12 to 19 years of age, this increase has been 300% (from 5% to 15%).[15]

Changes in diet and activity levels are the primary contributors to this increase in childhood obesity. Anderson and colleagues have shown a correlation between television viewing and increased weight.[15] This is but one of many contributing factors, which include, but are not limited to, the use of computers and video games, the decrease in school-based physical education, and the popularity of fast foods, especially in school cafeterias.[16] The adverse implications of childhood obesity are many. These children have been shown to be at increased risk for insulin resistance, hypertension, respiratory difficulties, arthritic conditions, and dyslipidemia. Two or more of these risk factors are found in 58% of obese children. These children have become physiologically old beyond their years, prematurely acquiring the health problems of middle-aged and older adults. Further, obese children have greater difficulty in interpersonal relationships and educational attainment. These as well as other psychological problems commonly persist into adulthood.[17,18]

Table 2-4 shows statistics from the Behavioral Risk Factor Surveillance System (BRFSS) (1991-2001).[19] This survey indicates the magnitude of the problem among adults, showing that in a single decade, there was a staggering 61% increase in the prevalence of obesity. This increase was similar in men and women and spanned every age group. Obesity was by far a greater problem for African-American, non-Hispanic people than for any other racial group. Even though the total percent of obesity in Asians was significantly lower than in other races, it still doubled during the decade and was mirrored by increased comorbidity, especially type 2 diabetes. Those with partial or completed college educations showed a lower overall rate of obesity; however, their rate also doubled in one decade.[19]

Mokdad and colleagues, in a series of publications, have shown the fattening of the United States by state and region.[20,21] As depicted in Figure 2-2, in 1990, no state had a rate of obesity greater than or equal to 20%. The Southeast, Southwest, and Midwest had the greatest incidence, with obesity rates between l5% and l9%. By 2000, as shown in Figure 2-3, 20 states had obesity rates of 20%. Colorado was the only state with an incidence of less than 15%. South Carolina led the way with a 101.8% increase. New Mexico was next, with an increase of 89.3%. Maryland, Florida, and Virginia were close behind, with increases greater than 70%. Regionally, the southern Atlantic (67.2%) and the Pacific (66.8%) areas led the nation in the rate of increase. These trends are alarming, particularly because

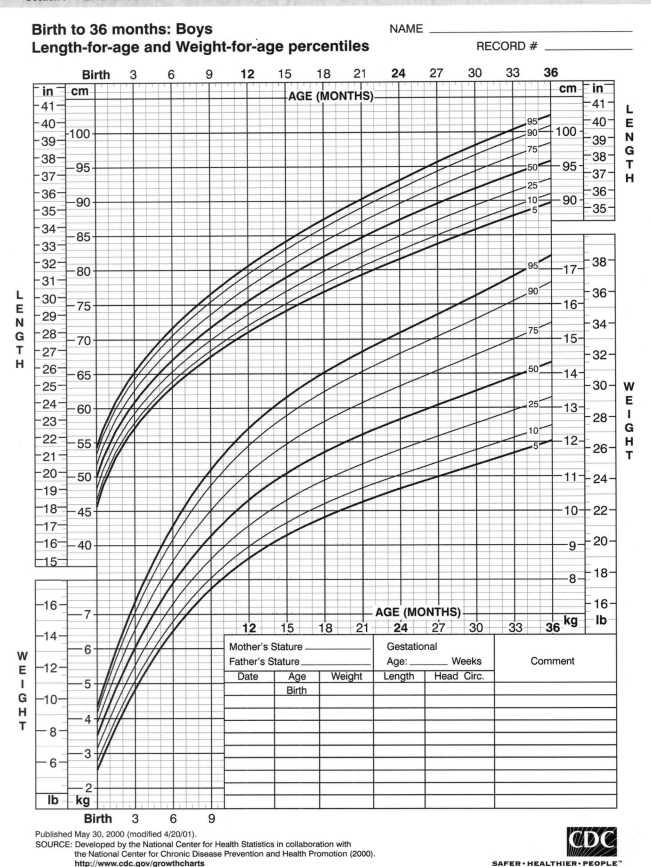

Figure 2-1. Gender-specific body mass index growth chart. (From National Health and Nutrition Examination Survey: Centers for Disease Control and Prevention Growth Charts for the United States, 2000. cdc.gov/growthcharts. By permission.)

Table 2-3	OVERWEIGHT IN CHILDREN

AGE (years)	1963-1965 1966-1970	1971-1974	1976-1980	1988-1994	1999-2000
6-11	4	4	7	11	15
12-19	5	6	5	11	15

Data from [15] Hammer

Table 2-4	PERCENTAGES OF OBESITY

CHARACTERISTICS	PERCENT OBESE					
	1991	**1995**	**1998**	**1999**	**2000**	**2001**
Total	12.0	15.3	17.9	18.9	19.8	20.9
Gender						
Men	11.7	15.6	17.7	19.1	20.2	21.0
Women	12.2	15.0	18.1	18.6	19.4	20.8
Age groups						
18-29	7.1	10.1	12.1	12.1	13.5	14.0
30-39	11.3	14.4	16.9	18.6	20.2	20.5
40-49	15.8	17.9	21.2	22.4	22.9	24.7
50-59	16.1	21.6	23.8	24.2	25.6	26.1
60-69	14.7	19.4	21.3	22.3	22.9	25.3
>70	11.4	12.1	14.6	16.1	15.5	17.1
Race, ethnicity						
White, non-Hispanic	11.3	14.5	16.6	17.7	18.5	19.6
Black, non-Hispanic	19.3	22.6	26.9	27.3	29.3	31.1
Hispanic	11.6	16.8	20.8	21.5	23.4	23.7
Other	7.3	9.6	11.9	12.4	12.0	15.7
Education level						
Less than high school	16.5	20.1	24.1	25.3	26.1	27.4
High school degree	13.3	16.7	19.4	20.6	21.7	23.2
Some college	10.7	15.1	17.8	18.1	19.5	21.0
College or above	8.0	11.0	13.1	14.3	15.2	15.7
Smoking status						
Never smoked	12.0	15.2	17.9	19.0	19.9	20.9
Ex-smoker	14.0	17.9	20.9	21.5	22.7	23.9
Current smoker	9.9	12.3	14.8	15.7	16.3	17.8

Data from Behavioral Risk Factor Surveillance System (1991-2001). cdc.gov/needphp/dnpa/obesity/trend/prev-char.htm

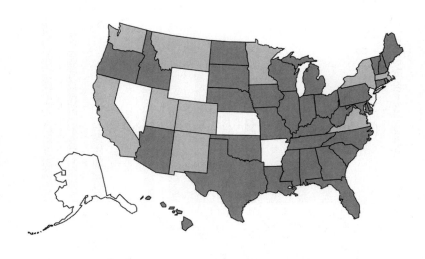

Figure 2-2. Obesity trends among U.S. adults: Behavioral Risk Factor Surveillance System (BRFSS), 1990, self-reported data. BMIs are 30 or higher, or approximately 30 lb overweight for a woman 5'4". (From Mokdad AH, Bowman BA, Ford ES, et al: The continuing epidemics of obesity and diabetes in the United States. JAMA 2001;286:1195-1200. By permission.)

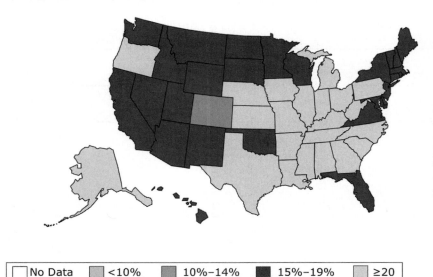

Figure 2-3. Obesity trends among U.S. adults: Behavioral Risk Factor Surveillance System (BRFSS), 2000, self-reported data. BMIs are 30 or higher, or approximately 30 lb overweight for a woman 5'4". (From Mokdad AH, Bowman BA, Ford ES, et al: The continuing epidemics of obesity and diabetes in the United States. JAMA 2001;286:1195-1200. By permission.)

| □ No Data | ▨ <10% | ▨ 10%–14% | ■ 15%–19% | ▨ ≥20 |

there is no indication of a slowing in the rates of incidence or prevalence of obesity.

The overall percent of minorities in the general population has grown. Obesity has increased most rapidly in minorities, especially in minority women. The rate and severity of obesity-related diabetes, heart disease, and hypertension have become a national health emergency.

Between 1960 and 1999, the prevalence of those having BMIs of 30.0 has doubled.[22] This dramatically illustrates the sudden surge in the incidence of obesity recorded over the past 30 years. Between 1962 and 1980, the incidence of obesity increased only from 12.8% to 14.5%. The 20-year period from 1980 to 1999 showed an increase of 14.5% to 27%. This means that in the segment of the population between 20 and 74 years of age, the incidence of obesity doubled; one in four individuals is currently obese. Monteforte and Torkelson, using data from the 2000 United States Census, estimated that 50 million U.S. adults are obese.[22] Of these, more than 15 million have BMIs of 35 kg per m^2, and 5 to 6 million have BMIs of 40 kg per m^2.

▶ WORLDWIDE TRENDS IN OBESITY

Obesity in other developed, as well as underdeveloped, countries is also on the rise. Only in areas such as sub-Saharan Africa and Asia is there a low and steady rate

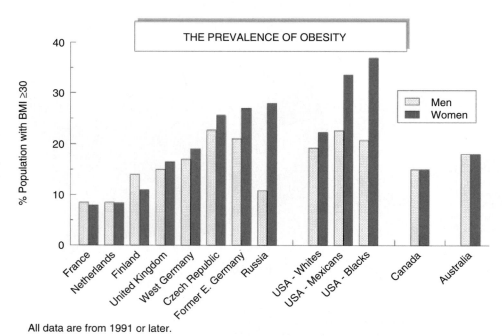

Figure 2-4. Prevalence of obesity in U.S. and European populations with BMIs of 30, post-1991. (From Grummer-Strawn L, Hughes M, Kahn LK, et al: Obesity in women from developing countries. Eur J Clin Nutr 2000; 54: 247-252. By permission.)

All data are from 1991 or later.

Table 2-5	PERCENTAGE OF OBESITY IN SELECTED COUNTRIES				
	UNITED STATES	CHINA	RUSSIA	SOUTH AFRICA	BRAZIL
	1988-91	1993	1994-95	1994	1989
Girls	24.2	12.2	17.8	20.3	10.5
Boys	21.3	14.1	25.6	25.0	12.8

of obesity.[23] Throughout most of Latin America, Europe, North Africa and the Middle East, the rate of obesity is high. Figure 2-4 shows the percentage of the population with BMIs greater than 30 kg per m^2 by country and gender and, for the United States, by race.[23]

Table 2-5 shows relative rates of overweight and obesity in children in the United States and selected countries. Data for children are less complete and harder to come by than data for adults. Figure 2-5 shows the trends in overweight in children in the United States by age and gender. Table 2-6 further breaks down the trends by age, gender, and ethnicity.[10] These trends will probably be reflected throughout the world. Figure 2-6 illustrates a survey indicating why Americans feel they are not successful in maintaining their desired weight. This survey is appropriate because it addresses the two main issues of physical activity and caloric intake.[24]

Figure 2-5. Trends in overweight in U.S. children with BMIs in the 95th percentile. (From Centers for Disease Control and Prevention, National Center for Health Statistics NHANES IV Report. www.cdc.gov/nchs/product/pubs/pubd/hestats/obes/obese99.htm2002. By permission.)

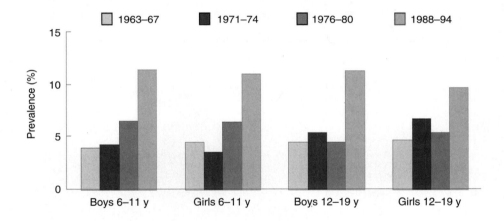

Table 2-6	PERCENTAGE OF OVERWEIGHT CHILDREN AND ADOLESCENTS BY SEX AND RACE-ETHNIC GROUP, UNITED STATES, 1988-94	
SEX AND RACE ETHNIC GROUP	6-11 YEARS	12-19 YEARS
Boys		
Total	11.8	11.3
Non-Hispanic white	10.9	11.6
Non-Hispanic black	12.3	10.7
Mexican American	17.7	14.1
Girls		
Total	11.0	9.7
Non-Hispanic white	9.8	8.9
Non-Hispanic black	17.1	16.3
Mexican American	15.3	13.5

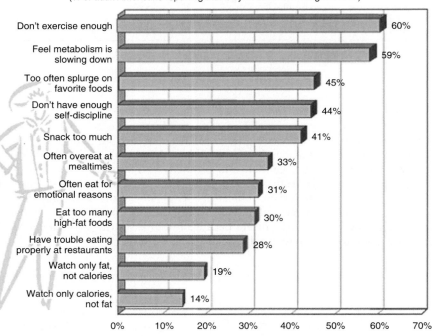

Why Do We Fail?

Reasons Americans are not successful at
losing desired weight

(% of adult Americans reporting that they need to lose weight who…)

Source: Calorie Control Council National Consumer Survey, 2004.

Figure 2-6. Ideal-weight-maintenance failure reported in the United States, 2000. (From Calorie Control Council National Survey, 2004. Reasons Why Americans Are Not Successful at Maintaining Their Desired Weight. www.caloriecontrol.org/reasonswhy.html)

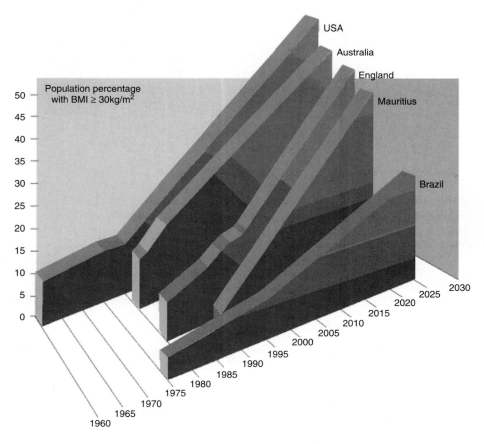

Figure 2-7. Projected obesity trends to the year 2025. (From The Global Challenge of Obesity and the International Obesity Task Force.www.iuns.org/features/obesity/tabfig.html)

Figure 2-7 projects obesity trends to the year 2030 in selected countries.[25] These trends give no reason for optimism as far as future control of the obesity epidemic. Statistical analyses of the incidence, prevalence, and demography of obesity clearly show that this problem has become global and undeniable.

▶ REFERENCES

1. US Department of Health and Human Services: The Surgeon General's Call to Action to Prevent and Decrease Overweight and Obesity. Rockville, MD, US Department of Health and Human Services, Public Health Service, Office of the Surgeon General, 2001.
2. Ford ES, Giles WH, Mokdad AH: The distribution of 10-year risk for coronary heart disease among US adults: findings from the National Health and Nutrition Examination Survey III. J Am Coll Cardiol 2004;43(10):1791-1796.
3. Worldwatch Institute: Chronic hunger and obesity epidemics eroding global progess. www.worldwatch.org. Accessed Sept 9, 2002.
4. Allison DB, Fontaine KR, Manson JE, et al: Annual deaths attributable to obesity in the United States. JAMA 1999;282: l530-1538.
5. Quesenberry CP Jr, Caan B, Jacobson A: Obesity, health services use, and health care costs among members of a health maintenance organization. Arch Intern Med 1998;158:466-472.
6. Stunkard AJ, Wadden TA (eds): Obesity. Theory and Therapy, ed 2. New York, Raven Press, 1993.
7. Fontaine KR, Redden DT, Wang C, et al: Years of life lost due to obesity. JAMA 2003;289:l87-l93.
8. World Health Organization: The global challenge of obesity, 2002. www.who.int/nut/obs.htm. Accessed July 7, 2003.
9. Stigler SM. Adolphe Quetelet. Encyclopedia of Statistical Sciences. New York, John Wylie, 1986.
10. National Health and Nutrition Examination Survey: Centers for Disease Control and Prevention Growth Charts for the United States, 2000: www.cdc.gov/growthcharts. Accessed May 6, 2003.
11. Ford ES, Giles WH, Dietz WH: Prevalence of the metabolic syndrome among US adults. JAMA 2002;287:356-359.
12. Flegal KM, Carol MD, Kuczmarski RJ, Johnson CL: Overweight and obesity in the United States: prevalence and trends, l960-1994. Int J Obes 1998;22:39-47.
13. Mokdad AH, Ford ES, Bowman BA, et al: Prevalence of obesity, diabetes and obesity-related health risk factors, 2001. JAMA 2003;289:76-79.
14. Centers for Disease Control and Prevention: The National Center for Health Statistics NHANES IV Report. www.cdc.gov/nchs/product/pubs/pubd/hestats/obes/obese99.htm2002. Accessed Sept 9, 2002.
15. Hammer LD, Kraemer HC, Wilson DM, et al: Standardized percentile curves of body mass index for children and adolescents. Am J Dis Child 1991;145:259-263.
16. Anderson RE, Crespo CJ, Bartlett SJ, et al: Relationship of physical activity and television watching with body weight and level of fatness among children. JAMA 1998;279:938-942.
17. Whitaker RC, Wright JA, Pepe MS, et al: Predicting obesity in young adulthood from childhood and parental obesity. N Engl J Med 1997;337:869-873.
18. Breaux CW. Obesity surgery in children. Obes Surg 1995;5: 279-284.
19. Behavioral Risk Factor Surveillance System (1991-2001): Self-reported data. www.cdc.gov/nccdphp/dnpa/obesity/trend/prev_char.htm. Accessed July 2, 2003.
20. Mokdad AH, Serdula MK, Dietz WH, et al: The spread of the obesity epidemic in the United States, 1991-1998. JAMA 1999;282: 1519-1922.
21. Mokdad AH, Bowman BA, Ford ES, et al: The continuing epidemics of obesity and diabetes in the United States. JAMA 2001;286: 1195-1200.
22. Monteforte MJ, Torkelson CM. Bariatric surgery for morbid obesity. Obes Surg 2000;10:391-401.
23. Grummer-Strawn L, Hughes M, Kahn LK, et al: Obesity in women from developing countries. Eur J Clin Nutr 2000;54:247-252.
24. Calorie Control Council National Survey, 2004: Reasons why Americans are not successful at maintaining their desired weight. www.caloriecontrol.org/reasonswhy.html. Accessed May 27, 2004.
25. International Union of Nutritional Sciences, The Global Challenge of Obesity and International Obesity Task Force: Projected prevalence of obesity in adults by 2025. www.iuns.org/features/obesity/tabfig.html. Accessed July 7, 2003.

3

Etiology of Obesity

Hanna-Maaria Lakka, M.D., Ph.D. and Claude Bouchard, Ph.D.

Obesity is a chronic disease that causes personal suffering for affected individuals and major costs to public health systems and societies. In the United States alone, more than 100 million people are overweight (that is, having a body mass index [BMI] ≥25 kg/m^2) or obese (BMI ≥30 kg/m^2), and the prevalence of obesity continues to increase. Based on a recent survey of American adults, the prevalence of obesity (BMI ≥30 kg/m^2) was 20.9% in 2001 as opposed to 19.8% in 2000, an increase of 5.6%.[1] By one estimate, obesity and related disorders are currently responsible for the death of 300,000 persons per year in the United States alone. Around the world, the costs of obesity range from 2% to 10% of total health care costs.[2,3]

Obesity results from a long-term imbalance between energy intake and energy expenditure, which favors positive energy balance. When energy intake chronically exceeds energy expenditure, the resulting imbalance causes expansion of adipose tissue lipid storage and favors adipogenesis, that is, an increase in the number of fat cells. The etiology of obesity is complex and multifactorial in nature, and numerous biological and behavioral factors can affect the energy balance equation.

The past decade has seen a remarkable increase in our understanding of the molecular mechanisms that regulate energy homeostasis, the molecular mediators of energy homeostasis in the brain and the periphery, and the genetics of obesity. However, given the epidemic level of obesity, a level reached within a short time, it is obvious that environmental and lifestyle factors are playing a strong role.

▶ ADIPOSITY AND RISK FOR DISEASE

Abdominal Obesity

Overweight and obesity are not homogeneous phenotypes because individuals differ in terms of the regional distribution of the excess weight or fat. A body of data supports the notion that fat located in the abdominal area is associated with a higher risk for adverse health consequences than fat in other depots. Abdominal fat consists of abdominal subcutaneous fat and intraabdominal fat. Intraabdominal adipose tissue is composed of intraperitoneal or visceral fat, which is composed primarily of omental and mesenteric fat and of retroperitoneal fat.

Abdominal obesity has been hypothesized to affect carbohydrate and lipid metabolism adversely through the increased lipolytic activity of omental adipocytes, a depot that drains directly into the portal-venous system. The release of free fatty acids into the portal vein is thought to result in alterations in hepatic functions, especially insulin clearance, and in hepatic glucose and very low density lipoprotein production. It has been suggested that these alterations result in insulin resistance in the liver and skeletal muscle. According to this "portal hypothesis," visceral fat, in distinction to peripheral fat, is more closely linked with insulin resistance and its associated metabolic derangements.[4]

Since the portal hypothesis was proposed, a body of observational evidence has accumulated in support of the concept that increased visceral adipose tissue mass is associated with increased risk for developing metabolic derangements, diabetes, and cardiovascular disease.[5] However, there is a lack of experimental evidence to support this hypothesis in humans. Moreover, several studies have shown that subcutaneous abdominal adipose tissue is also a strong contributor to these metabolic alterations.[6,7] Therefore, the pathophysiologic significance of these abdominal fat depot subdivisions remains to be fully clarified.

Ectopic Fat Deposition

Given the apparent problems with the portal hypothesis, alternative hypotheses have been suggested.[7] In addition to lipid storage in adipose tissue, lipid deposition in skeletal muscle, liver, and other organs has been shown to be a powerful determinant of insulin sensitivity.[8,9] As the ability of peripheral adipocytes to store fat is exceeded, the fat cells become insulin resistant, resulting in increased lipolysis, release of fatty acids into the blood stream, and decreased uptake of fatty acids. This is thought to favor storage of lipids in liver, skeletal muscle, pancreas, heart, and possibly other tissues. This spillover of lipids has been said to be at the origin of lipotoxic diseases.[10]

There is evidence to support the hypothesis that when adipose tissue is unable to proliferate and expand to accommodate excess calories, ectopic fat deposition with insulin resistance and ultimately type 2 diabetes are the consequences.[10,11] Several lines of evidence provide support for this scenario. The lack or severe depletion of adipose tissue in mice or humans (i.e., lipodystrophy) results in severe insulin resistance and diabetes, most probably because of the ectopic storage of lipid in liver, skeletal muscle, and the pancreatic insulin-secreting beta cells. In patients infected with the human immunodeficiency virus who have the lipodystrophy associated with antiretroviral therapy, the severity of the insulin resistance syndrome is related to the extent of fat accumulation in the liver rather than in the intraabdominal region. Fat accumulation in the liver may therefore play a causative role in the development of insulin resistance in these patients.[12] Several studies have demonstrated that intramyocellular lipid content and the degree of lipid infiltration into liver, measured by nuclear magnetic resonance spectroscopy, are strong determinants of insulin resistance in humans, independent of obesity.[8,9] Finally, increased fat-cell size is associated with insulin resistance and the development of diabetes.[13] Increased fat-cell size may represent the failure of the adipose tissue mass to expand to accommodate a growing demand for lipid storage.

Adipose Tissue Secretions

Another alternative is the endocrine hypothesis. Adipose tissue is not a passive organ of fat storage; it is now considered an endocrine organ that secretes a wide variety of hormones and metabolically active substances. A central feature of the endocrine hypothesis is that as the adipose organ increases in size, there is a change in the circulating concentrations of several endocrine signals. Numerous hormones, cytokines, and polypeptides secreted by adipose tissue have been identified and linked with components of the metabolic syndrome. These include leptin, resistin, adiponectin, tumor necrosis factor alpha, angiotensinogen, interleukin-6, and plasminogen activator inhibitor-1. Confirming the endocrine hypothesis, obese humans show increased serum leptin levels; furthermore, circulating leptin and insulin levels are correlated with each other.

▶ DETERMINANTS OF ENERGY BALANCE

Human energy balance over long periods is determined by energy intake, energy expenditure, partitioning of nutrients, and adipogenesis. Positive energy balance occurs when energy intake is greater than energy expenditure; it promotes an increase in body fat stores. Conversely, negative energy balance occurs when intake is less than expenditure, promoting a decrease in energy stores. Under normal circumstances, the energy balance oscillates from meal to meal, day to day, and week to week, without any major change in body stores or weight. Multiple physiologic mechanisms act to match overall energy intake with overall energy expenditure and to keep body weight stable in the long term. Thus, it is only when positive energy balance prevails for a considerable period that obesity is

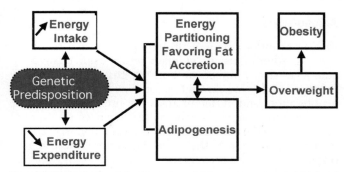

Figure 3-1. Diagram of the determinants of positive energy balance and fat deposition, with indication of the sites of action of a genetic predisposition. (From Bouchard C, Perusse L, Rice T, et al: Genetics of human obesity. In Bray GA, Bouchard C (eds): Handbook of Obesity, ed 2, New York, M. Dekker, in press. By permission.)

likely to develop. Figure 3-1 shows a model integrating various determinants of positive energy balance and the paths leading to obesity, with indication of the sites of action of a genetic predisposition.

Energy Intake

Total energy intake refers to all energy consumed as food and drink that can be metabolized inside the body. Fat provides the most energy per unit weight (9 kcal/g), and carbohydrate (4 kcal/g) and protein (4 kcal/g) provide the least. Fiber undergoes bacterial degradation in the large intestine to produce fatty acids that are then absorbed and used as energy (1.5 kcal/g). Alcohol intake can be a major contributor to energy balance in some individuals (7 kcal/g).

Energy Expenditure

Total energy expenditure can be defined in terms of the following three components: basal and resting metabolic rates; thermic effect of food (dietary thermogenesis); and physical activity (spontaneous physical activity and other physical activities of daily living). In sedentary adults, the basal and resting metabolic rates account for about 60% to 70% of total energy output, the thermic effect of food for around 10%, and physical activity for the remaining 20% to 30%. In those engaged in heavy manual work or demanding exercise training, total energy expenditure accounted for by physical activity may rise to as much as 50% of the total daily energy expenditure.

Nutrient Partitioning

An imbalance between energy intake and energy expenditure does not explain all of the variance in body-weight gain. Energy or nutrient partitioning is emerging as an important determinant of long-term energy balance. Under conditions of positive energy balance, individuals who are more likely to gain weight partition more energy for storage in adipose tissue, whereas the low gainers partition relatively more for oxidation by skeletal muscle and other tissues. These phenotypes are typically reflected by differences in respiratory quotient and skeletal muscle lipoprotein lipase activity.

Adipogenesis

Adipocyte differentiation, or adipogenesis, is a regulated process. Alterations in fat mass result from changes in adipocyte size, number, or both. A change in adipocyte number is achieved through a complex interplay between proliferation and differentiation of preadipocytes. The balance among signals to which preadipocytes are exposed appears to determine whether these cells undergo adipogenesis. In addition to the endocrine system, these signals originate from the preadipocytes themselves and operate as part of feedback loops involving mature adipocytes. In general, the factors that regulate adipogenesis may employ either process.[14,15]

▶ PHYSIOLOGIC REGULATION OF BODY WEIGHT

A major organ in the regulation of energy homeostasis is the brain, although multiple organ systems participate in the process.[16,17] Signaling molecules produced in the periphery circulate in the bloodstream and provide feedback to the brain. Key peripheral signals, such as leptin, insulin, and ghrelin, have been linked to hypothalamic neuropeptide neurons, and the anatomic and functional networks that integrate these neurons have begun to be elucidated (Fig. 3-2). Long-term body-weight regulation is best understood in terms of a regulatory loop with three distinct steps: (1) a sensor that provides information about adipose tissue mass and energy storage; (2) hypothalamic centers that receive and integrate the signals from the periphery, particularly adipose tissue; and (3) effector systems that influence energy intake and energy expenditure.[18]

Impaired control of food intake plays a major role in the causes of obesity. When assessing the control of food intake, it is commonly recognized that one needs to take into account three markers characterized by different time scales: (1) satiation, the suppression of hunger that induces the end of the meal; (2) satiety, the period of time characterized by absence of hunger between meals; and (3) the long-lasting control of food intake, which arises from hormonal signals such as leptin.[18] Certain of the key hormones and neuropeptides contributing to the regulation of energy homeostasis have been identified.

Peripheral Molecules

LEPTIN

Leptin is a hormone secreted by adipocytes; its circulating levels are proportional to adipose tissue mass. Leptin reduces food intake by upregulating anorexigenic (appetite-reducing) neuropeptides, such as α-melanocyte-stimulating hormone (α-MSH), and by downregulating orexigenic (appetite-stimulating) factors, primarily neuropeptide Y (NPY). Leptin provides a functional link between the adipose tissue and the brain, where it is involved in energy-balance-regulating processes, particularly in the defense against low-body-fat stores.[19]

INSULIN

Insulin is a hormone secreted by pancreatic β cells. It regulates glucose homeostasis through its ability to stimulate glucose uptake, glycogen synthesis, and other pathways of fuel storage in peripheral tissues. Insulin also serves as a peripheral indicator of energy status, and it binds to

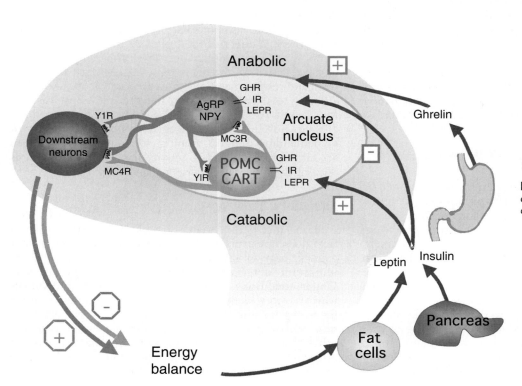

Figure 3-2. Central pathways contributing to the regulation of energy intake and energy expenditure.

receptors in the arcuate nucleus in the hypothalamus. Insulin inhibits eating through its action in the brain but increases it by decreasing the blood glucose level.[19]

CHOLECYSTOKININ

Cholecystokinin (CCK) is released into the bloodstream from intestinal endocrine cells in response to a meal. It binds to receptors on the afferent vagus nerve and helps to terminate feeding. CCK is also produced in the brain, where it functions as a neuropeptide participating in the regulation of behavior.[19]

GHRELIN

Ghrelin is a hormone secreted primarily from the stomach and proximal small intestine. Circulating ghrelin levels increase before meals, contributing to meal initiation, and decline postprandially, contributing to satiety.[20] Ghrelin receptors are expressed in the hypothalamus, where their activation stimulates food intake. In addition to being an orexigenic signal, ghrelin may also have long-term effects on the regulation of body adiposity. Plasma ghrelin levels increase after diet-induced weight loss,[21] supporting the hypothesis that ghrelin has a role in the long-term regulation of body weight. A recent study demonstrated that in morbidly obese subjects who lost weight after gastric bypass surgery, serum ghrelin levels were markedly suppressed and were lower than in normal-weight subjects and in obese subjects who had lost weight through conventional dieting.[21] This study suggested that the lowering of serum ghrelin levels may be involved in the mechanism that induces weight loss after gastric bypass surgery, possibly by affecting appetite and the initiation of meals.[21]

NEUROPEPTIDES

The growing number of putative appetite-regulating neuropeptides includes orexigenic and anorectic peptides. The major orexigenic neuropeptides are NPY; melanin-concentrating hormone (MCH); orexin A and B (also known as hypocretin-1 and -2); dynorphin; β-endorphin; galanin; and agouti-related peptide (AgRP). On the other hand, many anorectic peptides have been discovered, including α-MSH; corticotropin releasing hormone (CRH); CCK; cocaine and amphetamine regulated transcript (CART); neurotensin; glucagon-like peptide 1 (GLP-1); urocortin; neuromedin U; calcitonin; amylin; enterostatin; and bombesin.[22,23]

In brief, in the hypothalamic, the arcuate nucleus, the AgRP/NPY neurons, and the proopiomelanocortin (POMC) and CART neurons act as primary sites for receiving humoral signals that reflect body-fat stores. They then transduce those signals into behavioral and metabolic responses that promote the maintenance of body-fat stores at a constant level (see Fig. 3-2).

▶ DIETARY FACTORS AND PHYSICAL ACTIVITY PATTERNS

Dietary Factors

Dietary factors (that is, caloric intake and the macronutrient composition of the diet) and dietary patterns (such as daily eating pattern and eating disorders) can influence energy balance. The consumption of foods high in energy (excess calories) and low in essential nutrients has a potential to promote positive energy balance, overweight, and obesity. It is commonly accepted that the amount of the energy consumed in relation to physical activity and the quality of the food consumed are key determinants of nutrition-related chronic diseases such as obesity.[2,24] In the following paragraphs, the dietary factors and practices that have been proposed as playing a role in the cause of obesity are briefly defined.

ENERGY-DENSE, MICRONUTRIENT-POOR FOODS

Energy-dense foods tend to be high in fat (e.g., butter, oils, fried foods), sugars, or starch, whereas energy-diluted foods have a high water content (e.g., fruits and vegetables).[24] High intake of energy-dense foods promotes weight gain. In high-income countries (but increasingly in developing countries too), energy-dense foods are not only highly processed (low nonstarch polysaccharide and fiber content) but are also micronutrient-poor, further diminishing their nutritional value.

SUGAR-SWEETENED BEVERAGES

Diets that are low in fat are typically higher in carbohydrate (including variable amounts of sugars) and are often associated with protection against weight gain. However, a high intake of free sugars in beverages is thought to promote weight gain.[24] Increasing consumption of sugar-sweetened drinks by children is of serious concern because they play a role in the development of obesity in children.[25] The physiologic effects of energy intake on satiation and satiety appear to be quite different for solid foods as opposed to fluids. This may be caused by several factors, such as reduced gastric distension and the faster transit time for fluids.

PORTION SIZE

Large portion sizes are typically thought to contribute to weight gain.[26] The marketing of "supersize" portions, particularly in fast-food outlets, is now common practice in many countries. At the same time, the portion size for food consumed at home is also increasing—a shift that indicates marked changes in eating behavior in general.[26]

PALATABILITY

In the short-term regulation of energy intake, a positive drive to eat arises from the sight, smell, and palatability of food. The palatability of food, or pleasantness of taste, has an important influence on behavior and is positively associated with the energy intake of single foods.[27] The presence of fat in food is particularly enjoyable and is associated with a pleasurable mouth-feel. Sweetness is also one of the most powerfully pleasurable tastes. Sweetened foods with high fat content are likely to be conducive to excess consumption because palatability is enhanced by both sweetness and mouth-feel, and fat has only a small suppressive effect on appetite and food intake.[27]

FIBER

High intake of nonstarch polysaccharides (dietary fiber) may be related to the regulation of body weight through mechanisms involved in the control of hunger, satiation, satiety, and energy intake. Two recent reviews of randomized, controlled trials have concluded that the majority of studies show that a high intake of dietary fiber promotes weight loss and that fiber-rich diets containing nonstarchy vegetables, fruits, whole grains, legumes, and nuts may be effective in the prevention and treatment of obesity, although the effect is likely to be moderate.[28,29]

LOW AND HIGH GLYCEMIC INDEX

The glycemic index (GI) is defined as the incremental area under the glucose response curve after a standard amount of carbohydrate from a test food (either white bread or glucose) is consumed. The GI of the average diet in the Westernized world appears to have risen in recent years because of increases in carbohydrate consumption and changes in food-processing technology. It has been suggested that the decreased circulating concentrations of metabolic fuels in the mid-postprandial period after a high-GI meal would be expected to result in increased hunger and food intake as the body attempts to restore energy homeostasis.[30] Some studies, but not all, suggest that low-GI foods may protect against weight gain.[31] However, there are no long-term clinical trials that examine the effects of dietary GI on body weight regulation.[24,30,31]

BREASTFEEDING

Several reports have suggested that breast-feeding may prevent childhood obesity, even though negative findings have also been published.[32] There are probably multiple confounding factors, and the mechanism by which breast-feeding may protect against overweight and obesity remains uncertain.

DIETARY PATTERNS

In one study, the dietary pattern defined as *flexible restraint* was associated with lower risk for weight gain, whereas a *rigid restraint/periodic disinhibition* pattern was associated with a higher risk.[24] A recent study showed that a healthful dietary pattern (defined as consuming a diet high in fruit, vegetables, reduced-fat dairy, and whole grains, but low in red and processed meat, fast food, and soda) was associated with smaller gains in BMI and waist circumference, compared with four other eating patterns (white bread, alcohol, sweets, meat and potatoes).[33] Because foods are not consumed in isolation, dietary-pattern research based on observations in natural eating settings may be useful in understanding the dietary causes of obesity and in helping individuals to control their weight.[33]

Eating Disorders

Eating disorders are divided into three diagnostic categories: anorexia nervosa, bulimia nervosa, and atypical eating disorders, or eating disorders not otherwise specified.[34] Eating disorders that result in excess energy intake relative to requirements have been observed in obese people, but it is uncertain whether obesity is a result or an underlying cause of such disorders.

Binge-Eating Disorder

Binge-eating disorder (BED) is a newly proposed category of eating disorders in the fourth edition of the *Diagnostic and Statistical Manual of Mental Disorders*. People with the BED syndrome have binge-eating episodes, as do subjects with bulimia nervosa, but unlike the latter, they do not engage in compensatory behavior (e.g., self-induced vomiting or the misuse of laxatives and diuretics). BED seems to be highly prevalent among subjects seeking weight-loss treatment (a range of 1.3% to 30.1%).[35] Among patients undergoing bariatric surgery, the rates of BED were 27%, 38%, 43%, and 47% in four reports.[36]

Night Eating Syndrome

Night eating syndrome (NES) is a stress-related, eating, sleeping, and mood disorder that is associated with disordered neuroendocrine function.[36] It follows a characteristic circadian pattern and has responded to an agent that enhances serotonin function. NES is uncommon in the general population (1.5%). It is present in the nonobese but is more prevalent in the obese. The prevalence of NES was 8.9%, 15%, and 43% in three studies in obesity clinic patients, and 10%, 27%, and 42% in studies in obese patients who were evaluated for surgical treatment.[36]

Physical Activity

Physical activity is an important part of total daily energy expenditure. A decrease in energy expenditure through decreased physical activity is generally recognized as one of the major factors contributing to the global epidemic of overweight and obesity.

There is evidence that regular physical activity protects against weight gain, whereas sedentary lifestyles (sedentary occupations and inactive leisure-time activities, such as watching television, working at a computer, or playing video games) promote weight gain. Most studies that include data on physical activity collected at follow-up have found an inverse association between physical activity and long-term weight gain.[37] Results from prospective studies in which physical activity is measured at baseline and from randomized weight-reduction interventions are less consistent, probably because of low adherence over long periods.[37] Therefore, it is the current physical activity level, rather than previous physical activity or enrollment in an exercise program, that appears to offer some protection against unhealthful weight gain.

Physical activity influences body composition—the amount of fat, muscle, and bone tissue. A recent review assessed whether exercise-induced weight loss was associated with corresponding reductions in total adiposity and abdominal and visceral fat in a dose-response manner.[38] In well-controlled, short-term trials of increasing physical activity, expressed as energy expended per week, reductions in total adiposity occurred in a dose-response manner. However, although physical activity was associated with a reduction in abdominal and visceral fat, there was insufficient evidence to assess whether there is a dose-response relationship.[38]

How much physical activity is enough to prevent unhealthful weight gain? The current physical activity guideline for adults of 30 minutes of moderately intense activity daily, preferably all days of the week, focuses on limiting health risks for a number of chronic diseases, including coronary heart disease and diabetes.[39] However, for preventing weight gain or regain, that is likely to be insufficient for many individuals in the current environment, as stipulated by an expert panel brought together recently by the International Association for the Study of Obesity.[40] There is evidence that prevention of weight regain in formerly obese individuals may require as much as 60 to 90 minutes of moderate-intensity activity per day. Although definitive data are lacking, it seems likely that moderate-intensity activity of approximately 45 to 60 minutes per day, or a 1.7 physical activity level (PAL) value, is required to prevent the transition to overweight or obesity. For children, even more activity time is recommended.[40]

▶ CULTURAL AND SOCIETAL FACTORS

Cultural Influences

Culture is a learned system of categories, rules, and plans that people use to guide their behavior. A person's culture permeates every aspect of life, including thinking about fatness and thinness, eating behaviors, and physical activity patterns. Cultural values and norms about body weight vary considerably. Few cross-cultural analyses have examined perceptions about body weight. However, those that have suggest that most cultures in the world value moderate fatness and not extreme thinness. The male body ideal is most often related to "bigness" (large structure and muscularity) but not necessarily to fatness. In women, increased body weight and girths have been viewed as signs of health, reproductive health, and prosperity. This is still the case in many cultures. In contrast, in many industrialized countries, thinness in women has come to symbolize competence, success, control, and sexual attractiveness, whereas obesity represents laziness, self-indulgence, and lack of willpower.

People who live in economically developed societies are more likely to be obese than their counterparts in developing societies. However, people are now becoming fatter in developing countries as well. In general, there are more obese people in high socioeconomic classes in poor countries and more obese people in low socioeconomic classes in rich countries. Migration from one part of the world to another is also an important factor; it typically transplants people into new food systems and new social and economic environments. The major migration stream is from less-developed to more-developed economies. Migration and acculturation are associated with increases in body weight for height.

Societal Factors

In its effort to develop a model defining a big picture of the causes of obesity, the International Obesity Task Force has produced a causal-web diagram integrating the many social factors contributing to obesity (Fig. 3-3).[41] The many arrows define the factors bearing on individual behavior and the numerous interactions among them. When read from left to right, the model identifies the multisectoral factors that, whether or not acknowledged, are latent influences on an individual's energy input and output. The shaded rectangle after the first column stands for the cultural filter, which represents influences ranging from traditional customs and practices to media and advertising influences.

Many intervention strategies can potentially influence the physical, economic, policy or sociocultural environments, but the evidence base for these interventions is small.[41-43] Multisector, broad-based, and adequately resourced public health approaches will be required to stop and eventually reverse the current trends of increasing obesity prevalence. Political support, intersector collaboration, and community participation will be essential for success. The key settings for interventions are schools, homes, workplaces, neighborhoods, communities, and primary health care services. The key sectors for interventions include transport and urban infrastructure, media, food, and health care services.

Between the completion of the second and third National Health and Nutrition Examination Surveys (NHANES II and NHANES III) in 1980 and 1994, the number of children and adolescents considered overweight increased by 100% in the United States. Despite the obvious importance of the roles of parents and home environments on children's eating habits and physical activity, there is very little hard evidence available to support this view.[24,44] It appears that access and exposure to a range of fruits and vegetables in the home is important for the development of preferences for these foods. Parental knowledge of and attitudes and behaviors related to healthy diet and physical activity are also likely to play significant roles, even though the evidence is currently incomplete. More data are available about the impact of the school environment on nutrition knowledge, eating patterns and physical activity at school, and sedentary behaviors at home.[44] Some studies have shown an effect of school-based interventions on obesity prevention.[44]

Improving the general socioeconomic conditions for disadvantaged, marginalized, or poor populations is also a central strategy for obesity prevention. Classically, the pattern of the progression of obesity through a population starts with middle-aged women in high-income groups, but as the epidemic progresses, obesity becomes more common in people (especially women) in lower socioeconomic groups. The relationship may even be bidirectional, setting up a vicious circle (i.e., lower socioeconomic status promotes obesity, and obese people are more likely to end up in groups with low socioeconomic status). The mechanisms by which socioeconomic status influences food and activity patterns are probably multiple, and elucidation is necessary. However, people living in circumstances of low socioeconomic status may be more at the mercy of the obesogenic environment because their eating and activity behaviors are more likely to be the default choices. The evidence for an effect of low socioeconomic status on the prevalence of obesity is consistent (in higher income countries) across a number of cross-sectional and longitudinal studies.[24]

Individual and Biological Predisposition

BIOLOGICAL PREDISPOSITION

Sex

A number of physiologic processes contribute to an increased storage of fat in females. Such fat deposits are believed to be essential in ensuring female

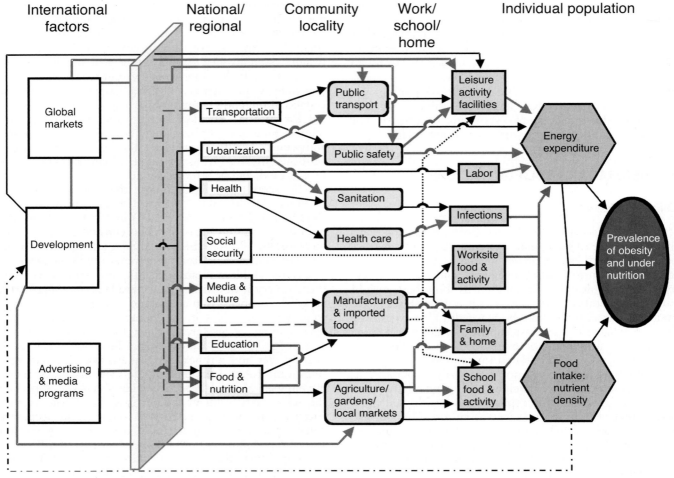

Figure 3-3. Societal policies and processes with direct and indirect influences on the prevalence of obesity and undernutrition.

reproductive capacity. Sex differences in the prevalence of obesity vary within populations and among ethnic groups.

Ethnicity

Minority ethnic groups in many industrialized countries appear to be especially susceptible to the development of obesity.[2] This may be due to a genetic predisposition to obesity that becomes apparent only when such groups are exposed to a more affluent lifestyle, or it may be because of their lower socioeconomic circumstances, as outlined earlier. Examples of this trend include Pima Indians of Arizona, Australian Aboriginals, and South Asians (Bangladeshi, Indians, and Pakistani) living overseas, as well as African-Americans and Mexican-Americans in the United States.[2]

Critical Periods for Weight Gain

Even though the evidence is at times contradictory, some studies suggest that poor intrauterine growth can increase the risk of obesity in later life.[45] Furthermore, adiposity rebound around the ages of 5 to 7 years may be associated with an increased risk for overweight later in life. In adolescence, increased autonomy may bring about

lifestyle changes that, combined with physiologic changes, promote increased fat deposition, particularly in females. Early adulthood is usually a period of marked reduction in physical activity, and that may cause weight gain. In the lifespan of women, pregnancies and menopause are critical periods for weight gain. The average weight gain after a pregnancy is almost 1 kg, although the range is wide. In many developing countries, consecutive pregnancies at short intervals often result in weight loss rather than weight gain. Menopausal women are prone to rapid weight gain.

Other Individual Factors Promoting Weight Gain

SMOKING CESSATION

The health consequences of cigarette smoking are well established. One of the many factors that may encourage smoking, despite its health risks, is the influence of smoking on body weight. Adult smokers weigh less than nonsmokers (on average, 3 kg) after many years of smoking. However, among adolescents and young adults, weight differences are small or nonexistent, and smoking initiation is not associated with weight loss. Nonetheless, smoking for weight control is frequently reported, particularly in young women. On average, quitting smoking increases one's weight to the level expected for a nonsmoker.

EXCESS ALCOHOL INTAKE

In many developed countries, the average alcohol intake of those who drink is about 10 to 30 g per day, or 3% to 9% of the total daily energy intake. Moderate alcohol consumers usually add alcohol to their daily energy intake rather than substituting it for food. However, the relationship between alcohol consumption and weight gain or the risk of obesity is inconclusive. There are undoubtedly many confounding factors that influence the association. In a recent prospective study in middle-aged men, heavy alcohol intake (30 g/d) was associated with increased weight gain.[46] The findings support the concept that greater alcohol consumption contributes directly to weight gain and obesity.[46]

DRUG TREATMENT

Weight gain is a common but often overlooked side effect of many widely used drugs, such as corticosteroids and certain antidepressant, antipsychotic, anticonvulsant, and antidiabetic agents.[47] Weight gain can have a serious impact on medication compliance with an otherwise beneficial treatment.

DISEASE STATES

Certain endocrinologic conditions such as hypothyroidism, Cushing's disease, and hypothalamic tumors can cause weight gain. However, these are rare causes of obesity, accounting for only a very small proportion of the obesity in the population.

MAJOR REDUCTION IN ACTIVITY

In some individuals, a major and often sudden reduction in activity without a compensatory decrease in habitual energy intake may be the major cause of increased adiposity. Examples of this phenomenon include sports or other injuries, retirement from active competition by an elite athlete, and development of physically limiting conditions such as arthritis.

CHANGES IN PERSONAL, SOCIAL, AND ENVIRONMENTAL CIRCUMSTANCES

Marriage, the birth of a child, the taking of a new job, or the loss of a job can lead to undesirable changes in eating patterns and to weight gain.

Genetic Predisposition

GENETIC EPIDEMIOLOGY, HERITABILITY LEVELS

The interest in the genetics of obesity has increased considerably in recent times. There is a significant familial aggregation of many obesity phenotypes, including excess body mass or percent body fat, excess abdominal total, subcutaneous and visceral fat, and excess gluteofemoral fat. Genetic epidemiology has been helpful in defining the magnitude of the genetic contribution to obesity from a population perspective. The level of heritability, which has been considered in a large number of twin, adoption, and family studies, is the fraction of variation in a population of a trait (e.g., BMI) that can be explained by genetic transmission. The estimates of heritability level depend on how the studies are designed and on the types of relatives on whom they are based. For instance, studies conducted with monozygotic and dizygotic twins, or monozygotic twins reared apart, have yielded the highest heritability levels, with values clustering around 70%. In contrast, adoption studies have generated the lowest heritability estimates, about 10% to 30%. Family studies have generally found levels of heritability intermediate between twin and adoption study reports.

Recent surveys undertaken with the collaboration of severely obese and morbidly obese subjects, together with information obtained about their parents, siblings, and spouses, suggest that the genetic contribution to obesity may account for about 25% to 40% of the individual differences in BMI. Based on the recent dramatic increases in the prevalence of obesity, serious doubts have been raised concerning high heritability values for weight-for-height phenotypes such as BMI.

Familial Risk for Obesity

The risk for becoming obese when a first-degree relative is overweight or obese can be quantified using a statistics method called the lambda coefficient (λ), which is defined as the ratio between the risk for being obese when a biological relative is obese and the risk for obesity in the population at large, that is, the prevalence of obesity. Estimates of λ for obesity based on data about BMI have been reported. Age- and gender-standardized risk ratios obtained from 2349 first-degree relatives of 840 obese probands and 5851 participants in the National Health and Nutrition Examination Survey III revealed that the prevalence of obesity is twice as great in families of obese individuals as it is in the population at large.[48] Moreover, the risk increases with the severity of obesity in the proband. Thus, the risk for extreme obesity (BMI $\geq$45 kg/m^2) is about eight times higher in families of extremely obese subjects.[48] The results of a study in a Canadian population were concordant with regard to extremely or morbidly obese subjects, as estimated by BMI percentile cutoffs.[49] However, λ estimates were also significant when the analyses were performed with pairs of spouses and were actually higher in spouses than in first-degree relatives for subcutaneous fat. This suggests that caution is warranted when interpreting λ values based only on biological relatives, as the familial risk does not depend on genetic causes alone.[49]

Monogenic Forms of Obesity

MENDELIAN DISORDERS

As of October 2002, 37 Mendelian syndromes of relevance to human obesity have been mapped to a genomic region, and the causal genes or strong candidate genes have been identified for 23 of these syndromes.[50] Such syndromes include Prader-Willi syndrome, Bardet-Biedl syndromes, Berardinelli-Seip congenital lipodystrophy-1, and Albright hereditary osteodystrophy.

OTHER HUMAN SINGLE-GENE MUTATIONS

Several mutations in human genes that have homology to obesity-causing genes in mice, and in genes involved in the same metabolic pathways, have been identified. In such cases, obesity is the dominant feature and is largely independent of environmental factors. Although these cases are rare, they have led to a better understanding of the physiologic regulatory pathways of appetite and energy homeostasis. Finding that mutations in a gene cause similar phenotypes in rodents and humans underscores the fundamental and highly conserved nature of the pathway that regulates energy balance. The genes in which these mutations have been reported include leptin (LEP), leptin receptor (LEPR), proopiomelanocortin (POMC), carboxypeptidase E (Cpe), prohormone convertase-1 (PCSK1), and melanocortin-4 receptor (MC4R).[50]

Polygenic and Common Forms of Obesity

Individuals affected with Mendelian obesity syndromes or single-gene disorders represent only a small fraction of the obese population and cannot explain the magnitude of the obesity problem that industrialized societies are facing today. Human studies to identify the specific genes involved in common obesity are currently dominated by three strategies. One approach is the candidate-gene approach, which relies on the current understanding of the physiopathology of obesity. The candidate genes are selected on the basis of their perceived role or function in biochemical pathways related to the regulation of energy balance or to adipose tissue biology. A second approach is to perform genome-wide linkage scans with a view to identifying chromosomal regions of interest, the so-called quantitative trait loci (QTLs), and eventually genes within these QTLs. The third approach is based on tissue-specific gene expression profiling that compares lean and obese individuals and other informative samples.

ASSOCIATION STUDIES

The evidence for associations between candidate genes and obesity-related phenotypes is summarized in the most recent version of the Human Obesity Gene Map.[50] A total of 222 studies covering 71 candidate genes have reported significant associations. In general, however, the results of these studies have been somewhat disappointing, with small sample size, small effect size, and lack of replication studies or failure to replicate being the most common problems. For certain candidate genes, the positive findings have been replicated in independent studies; they include the uncoupling protein (UCP1, UCP2, UCP3), adrenoceptor (β2–AR, 3–AR, α2–AR), peroxisome proliferator-activated receptor γ (PPARγ), LEP, and LEPR receptor genes.

LINKAGE STUDIES

Another strategy used to identify genes and mutations responsible for the predisposition to obesity has been to perform genome-wide scans with a view to identifying chromosomal regions of interest. These studies have typically been performed with pairs of siblings, sometimes whole nuclear families or pedigrees, and have been based on about 300 or more microsatellite markers. On the Human Obesity Gene Map,[50] a total of 68 QTLs for obesity-related phenotypes have been identified in genomic scans of the human genome performed thus far. In addition, significant linkage peaks with candidate genes and other polymorphic markers have been identified in targeted linkage studies. Putative loci affecting obesity-related phenotypes can be found on all chromosomes except chromosome Y.

Genotype-Environment Interactions

GENETIC PREDISPOSITION AND INTERACTIONS WITH THE ENVIRONMENT

Genotype-environment interaction (G × E) arises when the response of a phenotype to environmental changes is determined by the genotype of the individual. Although it is well known that there are interindividual differences in the responses to various dietary interventions, few attempts have been made to test whether these differences are genotype dependent, particularly for obesity-related phenotypes. Results of experiments performed with monozygotic twins have revealed that the response to a positive or negative energy balance intervention is very heterogeneous among twin pairs but quite homogeneous in members of the same pair.[51,52]

Obesity is clearly a genetic disorder in some relatively rare cases. When obesity is caused by an invalidated gene that results in the lack of a competent protein to affect a pathway impacting on the regulation of energy balance, obesity is a disorder with a genetic origin. In such cases, the environment has only a permissive role in the severity of the phenotype. It is difficult to arrive at a firm conclusion about the number of cases of genetic obesity, as there remain a large number of genes to be evaluated in this regard. Based on the body of data accumulated to date, it would seem that genetic obesity could represent as much as 5% of obesity cases and a large percentage of the very severely obese.[53]

We have proposed dividing the more common forms of obesity into those with a strong genetic predisposition and those with a slight genetic susceptibility. In contrast with the first category (genetic obesity), those with a strong genetic predisposition are not characterized by a clearly defective biology that can be reduced to a gene and a mutation or some other abnormalities. The strong predisposition results from susceptibility alleles at a number of loci. In an environment that does not favor obesity, these individuals would probably be overweight. They become obese and potentially severely obese in an obesogenic environment. A third group is arbitrarily defined as having inherited a slight predisposition to obesity. In a restrictive environment, they may be of normal weight or slightly overweight. An obesogenic environment will cause a large fraction of them to become obese. Finally, a fourth group includes those who are genetically resistant to obesity. They remain of normal weight or almost normal weight in a wide range of obesogenic conditions. These four types are depicted with respect to differences in obesogenic conditions in Figure 3-4.

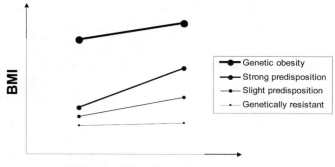

Figure 3-4. Four levels of genetic susceptibility to becoming obese in relation to differences in obesogenic conditions. (From Kumanyika S, Jeffery RW, Morabia A, et al, Public Health Approaches to the Prevention of Obesity [PHAPO] Working Group of the International Obesity Task Force [IOTF]: Obesity prevention: the case for action. Int J Obes Relat Metab Disord 2002; 26: 425-436.)

▶ CONCLUSIONS

Overweight and obesity represent a major and growing threat to the health of populations worldwide. Our understanding of the molecular mechanisms that regulate energy homeostasis and of the genetics of obesity has increased rapidly in recent times. Genes are important in determining a person's susceptibility to weight gain. However, given the epidemic level of obesity, a level reached within a short time, it is clear that environmental and lifestyle factors are playing an important role. The human body is designed to store energy efficiently for times of shortage, an adaptation that has become a liability in modern times. If the current obesogenic environment persists, obesity rates will continue to increase. Complex cultural and societal factors interact to create living conditions that favor a low level of physical activity and the consumption of more calories than are needed.

▶ REFERENCES

1. Mokdad AH, Ford ES, Bowman BA, et al: Prevalence of obesity, diabetes, and obesity-related health risk factors, 2001. JAMA 2003; 89:76-79.
2. World Health Organization: Obesity: preventing and managing the global epidemic. Report of a WHO consultation. WHO Technical Report Series, 894. Geneva, World Health Organization, 2000.
3. National Institutes of Health: Clinical guidelines on the identification, evaluation and treatment of overweight and obesity in adults. Evidence report. NIH Publication No. 98-4083. Bethesda, MD, National Institutes of Health, 1998.
4. Bjorntorp P. "Portal" adipose tissue as a generator of risk factors for cardiovascular disease and diabetes. Arteriosclerosis 1990;10:493-496.
5. Wajchenberg BL. Subcutaneous and visceral adipose tissue: their relation to the metabolic syndrome. Endocr Rev 2000;21:697-738.
6. Kelley DE, Thaete FL, Troost F, et al: Subdivisions of subcutaneous abdominal adipose tissue and insulin resistance. Am J Physiol 2000;278:E941.
7. Smith SR, Lovejoy JC, Greenway F, et al: Contributions of total body fat, abdominal subcutaneous adipose tissue compartments, and visceral adipose tissue to the metabolic complications of obesity. Metabolism 2001;50:425-435.
8. Krssak M, Falk Petersen K, Dresner A, et al: Intramyocellular lipid concentrations are correlated with insulin sensitivity in humans: a 1H NMR spectroscopy study. Diabetologia 1999;42:113-116.
9. Seppala-Lindroos A, Vehkavaara S, Hakkinen AM, et al: Fat accumulation in the liver is associated with defects in insulin suppression of glucose production and serum-free fatty acids independent of obesity in normal men. J Clin Endocrinol Metab 2002;87:3023-3028.
10. Ravussin E, Smith SR: Increased fat intake, impaired fat oxidation, and failure of fat cell proliferation result in ectopic fat storage, insulin resistance, and type 2 diabetes mellitus. Ann N Y Acad Sci 2002;967:363-378.
11. McGarry JD: Banting lecture 2001: dysregulation of fatty acid metabolism in the etiology of type 2 diabetes. Diabetes 2002;51:7-18.
12. Sutinen J, Hakkinen AM, Westerbacka J, et al: Increased fat accumulation in the liver in HIV-infected patients with antiretroviral therapy-associated lipodystrophy. AIDS 2002;16:2183-2193.
13. Weyer C, Foley JE, Bogardus C, et al: Enlarged subcutaneous abdominal adipocyte size, but not obesity itself, predicts type II diabetes independent of insulin resistance. Diabetologia 2000;43:1498-1506.
14. MacDougald OA, Mandrup S: Adipogenesis: forces that tip the scales. Trends Endocrinol Metab 2002;13:5-11.
15. Gregoire FM: Adipocyte differentiation: from fibroblast to endocrine cell. Exp Biol Med (Maywood) 2001;226:997-1002.
16. Schwartz MW, Woods SC, Porte D Jr, et al: Central nervous system control of food intake. Nature 2000;404:661-671.
17. Barsh GS, Schwartz MW: Genetic approaches to studying energy balance: perception and integration. Nat Rev Genet 2002;3:589-600.
18. Jequier E: Pathways to obesity. Int J Obes Relat Metab Disord 2002;26(suppl 2):12-17.
19. Havel PJ: Peripheral signals conveying metabolic information to the brain: short-term and long-term regulation of food intake and energy homeostasis. Exp Biol Med (Maywood) 2001;226:963-977.
20. Cummings DE, Purnell JQ, Frayo RS, et al: A preprandial rise in plasma ghrelin levels suggests a role in meal initiation in humans. Diabetes 2001;50:1714-1719.
21. Cummings DE, Weigle DS, Frayo RS, et al: Plasma ghrelin levels after diet-induced weight loss or gastric bypass surgery. N Engl J Med 2002;346:1623-1630.
22. Tritos NA, Maratos-Flier E: Two important systems in energy homeostasis: Melanocortins and melanin-concentrating hormone. Neuropeptides 1999;33:339-349.
23. Ravussin E, Bouchard C: Human genomics and obesity: finding appropriate drug targets. Eur J Pharmacol 2000;410:131-145.
24. World Health Organization: Diet, nutrition and the prevention of chronic diseases. Report of a joint WHO/FAO expert consultation. WHO Technical Report Series, 916. Geneva, World Health Organization, 2003.
25. Ludwig DS, Peterson KE, Gortmaker SL: Relation between consumption of sugar-sweetened drinks and childhood obesity: a prospective, observational analysis. Lancet 2001;357:505-508.
26. Nielsen SJ, Popkin BM: Patterns and trends in food portion sizes, 1977-1998. JAMA 2003;289:450-453.
27. Drewnovski A: Taste preferences and food intake. Annu Rev Nutr 1997;17:237-253.
28. Pereira MA, Ludwig DS: Dietary fiber and body-weight regulation: observations and mechanisms. Pediatr Clin North Am 2001;48:969-980.
29. Howarth NC, Saltzman E, Roberts SB: Dietary fiber and weight regulation. Nutr Rev 2001;59:129-139.
30. Ludwig DS: The glycemic index: physiological mechanisms relating to obesity, diabetes, and cardiovascular disease. JAMA 2002;287:2414-2423.
31. Brand-Miller JC, Holt SH, Pawlak DB, et al: Glycemic index and obesity. Am J Clin Nutr 2002;76:281S-285S.
32. Dietz WH: Breastfeeding may help prevent childhood overweight. JAMA 2001;285:2506-2507.
33. Newby PK, Muller D, Hallfrisch J, et al: Dietary patterns and changes in body mass index and waist circumference in adults. Am J Clin Nutr 2003;77:1417-1425.
34. Fairburn CG, Harrison PJ: Eating disorders. Lancet 2003;361:407-416.
35. Dingemans AE, Bruna MJ, van Furth EF: Binge eating disorder: a review. Int J Obes Relat Metab Disord 2002;26:299-307.
36. Stunkard AJ, Allison KC: Two forms of disordered eating in obesity: binge eating and night eating. Int J Obes Relat Metab Disord 2003;27:1-12.

37. Fogelholm M, Kukkonen-Harjula K: Does physical activity prevent weight gain: a systematic review. Obes Rev 2000;1:95-111.

38. Ross R, Janssen I: Physical activity, total and regional obesity: dose-response considerations. Med Sci Sports Exerc 2001;33:S521-S527; discussion S528-S529.

39. U. S. Department of Health and Human Services: Physical Activity and Health: A Report of the Surgeon General. Atlanta, GA, Department of Health and Human Services, Centers for Disease Control, National Center for Chronic Disease Prevention and Health Promotion, 1996.

40. Saris WH, Blair SN, van Baak MA, et al: How much physical activity is enough to prevent unhealthy weight gain? Outcome of the IASO 1st Stock Conference and consensus statement. Obes Rev 2003;4:101-114.

41. Kumanyika S, Jeffery RW, Morabia A, et al, Public Health Approaches to the Prevention of Obesity (PHAPO) Working Group of the International Obesity Task Force (IOTF): Obesity prevention: the case for action. Int J Obes Relat Metab Disord 2002;26:425-436.

42. Jackson Y, Dietz WH, Sanders C, et al: Summary of the 2000 Surgeon General's listening session: toward a national action plan on overweight and obesity. Obes Res 2002;10:1299-1305.

43. French SA, Story M, Jeffery RW: Environmental influences on eating and physical activity. Annu Rev Public Health 2001;22:309-335.

44. Dietz WH, Gortmaker SL: Preventing obesity in children and adolescents. Annu Rev Public Health 2001;22:337-353.

45. Oken E, Gillman MW: Fetal origins of obesity. Obes Res 2003;11: 496-506.

46. Wannamethee SG, Shaper AG: Alcohol, body weight, and weight gain in middle-aged men. Am J Clin Nutr 2003;77:1312-1317.

47. Breum L, Fernstrom MH: Drug-induced obesity. In Bjorntorp P (ed): International Textbook of Obesity. Chichester, UK, John Wiley, 2001.

48. Lee JH, Reed DR, Price RA: Familial risk ratios for extreme obesity: implications for mapping human obesity genes. Int J Obes Relat Metab Disord 1997;21:935-940.

49. Katzmarzyk PT, Perusse L, Rao DC, et al: Familial risk of obesity and central adipose tissue distribution in the general Canadian population. Am J Epidemiol 1999;149:933-942.

50. Chagnon YC, Rankinen T, Snyder EE, et al: The human obesity gene map: the 2002 update. Obes Res 2003;11:313-367.

51. Bouchard C, Tremblay A, Despres JP, et al: The response to long-term overfeeding in identical twins. N Engl J Med 1990;322: 1477-1482.

52. Bouchard C, Tremblay A, Despres JP, et al: The response to exercise with constant energy intake in identical twins. Obes Res 1994;2:400-410.

53. Bouchard C, Perusse L, Rice T, et al: Genetics of human obesity. In Bray GA, Bouchard C (eds): Handbook of Obesity, ed 2. New York, M. Dekker, in press.

4

Energy Metabolism and Biochemistry of Obesity

Sayeed Ikramuddin, M.D.

In 2001 the Centers for Disease Control and Prevention contacted the Center for Medicare and Medicaid Services (CMMS) to request that it modify the terminology in the National Coverage Document to reflect the threat of obesity.[1] On July 15, 2004, Secretary of Health Tommy Thompson stated that the CMMS would delete the wording "obesity is not an illness" in the CMMS manual.[2] This is perhaps the first governmental recognition in the history of our society that the epidemic of obesity is not just a cultural phenomenon but, rather, is an epidemic resulting from a survival mechanism gone astray.

Human survival has been dependent on the capacity to overcome starvation. Scarcity of food, or starvation, induces migration, creating the foundation for a hunter-gatherer lifestyle. In such an environment, individuals with the capacity to store food efficiently in the form of fat fare better than those who cannot. Efficient storage of calories in the form of fat makes individuals "fit," in the Darwinian sense, into an environment of scarcity. However, in the current Western dietary environment, many of these individuals suffer from morbid obesity. The individual who can "eat anything" and *not* gain weight fares the best in our modern setting, replete as it is with abundant calories, and in our modern lifestyle, one that is largely sedentary. Genetic predisposition, developmental factors, and environmental influences combined with molecular interactions impede the obese in their quest for weight loss.[3]

Intense scientific effort over the past 20 years has given us a glimpse into these mechanisms. Currently, we have a reasonable understanding of the causes of many diseases, and our knowledge of disease biology allows us to target multiple aspects of a disease's developmental process and tailor treatment accordingly; such is the case with colon cancer and melanoma. In contrast, our understanding of obesity is still in its infancy. One of the problems in dealing with obesity is the overall lack of attention paid to it. Even within the medical community, many circles do not recognize obesity as anything more than the result of a lack of self-control. Still today, reports emerge that downplay the significance of obesity.

This disease affects all age groups, both genders, and all races, and is rapidly spreading worldwide.[4] Obesity has proven itself to be remarkably recalcitrant to treatment. Lifestyle changes, behavior modification, and dieting, either singly or in combination, are mostly ineffectual. Results of pharmacologic management of morbid obesity have been limited. The combination of the amphetamines phentermine and fenfluramine suppresses appetite but was removed from the market by the United States Food and Drug Administration because of its association with significant pulmonary and cardiac complications. In contrast, surgery for obesity has proven itself successful in the long-term management of morbid obesity, but it has not been without its failures, such as the jejunoileal bypass.[5] In the evolution of treatments and our assessment of failures, it has become evident that an understanding of the mechanisms of obesity is necessary; knowledge of the causes of obesity will eventually facilitate targeted, successful therapy.

It is interesting that some studies suggest that comorbid conditions improve or even resolve long before the targeted weight loss has been achieved. Data show that some of the improvements in diabetic patients may not be due simply to food restriction but to the rerouting of intestinal pathways, as is the case after gastric bypass.[6] It is likely that elevations of the signaling hormone glucagonlike peptide-1 following surgery are responsible for this. Glucagonlike peptide-1 is an anorexigenic hormone that improves glucose sensitivity and contributes to the postprandial incretin effect in healthy patients.[7,8] An understanding of why bariatric surgery works will give us an understanding of why morbid obesity occurs. Metabolic balancing of food intake and energy expenditure facilitates weight homeostasis in nonobese individuals, whereas inadequate or faulty regulation of key hormones (e.g., leptin, resistin, cholecystokinin, ghrelin) inhibits appropriate selection of food type and quantity by the obese and impairs their efforts to engage in energy-expending activity. Bariatric surgical procedures provide an excellent model for the study of extreme weight loss as they employ anatomic rearrangements ranging from simple restriction to bypass of the foregut to malabsorptive procedures.

▶ ENERGY METABOLISM

It appears that energy regulation is controlled via a homeostatic system involving both the brain and the periphery. The central nervous system component of this system is the hypothalamus, which is modulated by peripheral and central peptides to create changes in behavior. There exists a balance between anabolic peptides (orexigenic), which stimulate feeding behavior, and catabolic peptides (anorexigenic), which attenuate food intake. The equilibrium between these neuropeptides is dynamic in nature, shifting across the day-night cycle and from day to day and also in response to dietary challenges and peripheral energy stores. These shifts occur in close relationship with circulating levels of the hormones leptin, insulin, ghrelin, and corticosterone and also with the nutrients glucose and lipids. These circulating factors together with neural processes are primary signals that relay information regarding the availability of fuels needed for current cellular demand in addition to information about the level of stored fuels needed for long-term use. Together, these signals have profound impact on the expression and production of neuropeptides that, in turn, initiate the appropriate anabolic or catabolic responses for restoring equilibrium.[9,10]

There are more than 250 genetic associations with morbid obesity. In rare cases there are single-gene, or monogenic, causes of obesity. These include the leptin gene and leptin receptor mutations, the genes involved in the production of melanocortin, and the SIM 1 gene, which is involved in the formation of the parventricular nuclei. Both are important regulators of eating behavior and metabolism.[11]

It is important to realize that the fat cell is not an innocent bystander in the pathogenesis of obesity. It is now known that the numbers of fat cells can increase with an increase in weight, and decrease in number with weight loss.[12] This is significant in that the fat cells secrete cytokines and other hormones (e.g., tumor necrosis factor-α, α-c protein, resistin, and leptin) that act in the hypothalamus to influence eating behavior. Triglycerides stored in the fat cells store most of the caloric reserves in the body. The duration of survival is dependent on the amount of adipose tissue in the body. It is known that obese persons can survive much longer than the nonobese, given appropriate water, vitamin, and mineral intake.[11]

In specific ways, obesity is a disease of energy metabolism or, rather, of energy imbalance. In obesity, the total energy consumed is less than the total energy expended. The regulation of these two opposing forces and, therefore, of energy balance is complicated by the common misapprehension that total energy expenditure is a function of weight.

Individuals whose weight is within normal ranges metabolize energy in the following manner: 40% to 44% of food is destined for the production of adenosine triphosphate (ATP) through oxidative processes; the remaining 56% to 60% is used to produce heat. Total body metabolism can be expressed as total energy expenditure (TEE).

TEE is equivalent to the basal metabolic rate (BMR), plus activity, plus the thermal effect of food (TEF), plus adaptive thermogenesis (AT) (TEE = BMR + activity + TEF + AT). The BMR is the lowest level of energy needed to maintain life, whereas activity represents the additional energy needed for daily activities. The TEF is the body heat produced; the AT is the fluctuation in TEF due to environmental temperature and humidity.[13]

Leibel and colleagues reported the effect on TEE in patients who were fed to increase their body weight by 20%.[14] In these patients, the body became "inefficient," using more calories with respect to those taken in, as compared with baseline energy expenditure. When these patients subsequently fasted, the converse was observed: less energy was consumed with respect to intake. In obese individuals, normal homeostatic mechanisms are blunted, and there is a decrease in the TEF and a subsequent decrease in the TEE.

Metabolic studies of obese patients suggest, ironically, that energy expenditure increases in weight-stable obese individuals compared with nonobese individuals. This increase is likely related to an increase in fat-free mass (lean body mass). If energy expenditure is normalized, based on fat-free mass, there is no difference in energy expenditure in obese versus nonobese individuals. It is possible that the adipocyte mass is the mediator of this weight "set point." Energy is obtained from ingested food. As food is consumed, energy is expended, and ATP is captured at the expense of body heat. This is a thermodynamically favorable process, going from a high-energy state to a low-energy state.

Thermodynamic processes are tightly coupled to electron transport. For each molecule of ATP consumed or produced, there is a flux of electrons in and out of the mitochondria. In studies of brown adipose tissue in obese rodents, these metabolic processes undergo an uncoupling, with a disturbance in electron flux. The result is heat production out of proportion to metabolic activity. This increased energy expenditure may correlate with decreased energy conservation. This uncoupling of electrons and energy production is likely regulated by uncoupling proteins that exist in the mitochondrial membrane. A state of energy conservation or impairment appears to exist as an individual becomes obese. Once a certain weight is attained, energy consumption normalizes. When this weight is exceeded, energy expenditure increases. These fluctuations in energy expenditure support the concept of a set point for weight and the notion that obese patients are obese because that outcome is predicted by a complex of competing metabolic forces set in motion, in particular, by fluctuations in their weight.[13]

The nature of energy metabolism after obesity surgery is not well understood. Flancbaum and colleagues identified a variable preoperative TEE in patients selected for gastric bypass.[15] They compared resting TEE, using indirect calorimetry, to that calculated by the Harris-Benedict equation. They identified some patients who had lower-than-predicted preoperative TEEs. The preoperative BMIs in those patients was no different from the BMIs in patients whose measured resting TEEs equaled the calculated TEE. Patients who had normal TEEs preoperatively experienced no change in TEE postoperatively.

However, patients who were hypometabolic preoperatively experienced normalization of the TEE postoperatively. This study suggests that after gastric bypass, there is less energy conservation in some patients, a finding not seen in morbidly obese patients who diet. A recent paper by Bobbioni-Harsch and colleagues showed that the degree to which energy economy is preserved correlates negatively with the amount of weight loss after gastric bypass.[16]

Das and colleagues reported on the effect of bariatric surgery on metabolism.[17] The objectives of the study were to determine the changes in energy expenditure and body composition with weight loss induced by gastric bypass surgery and to identify presurgery predictors of weight loss. Thirty extremely obese women and men with the mean age (± SD) of 39.0 (± 9.6) years and BMIs (in kg/m^2) of 50.1 (± 9.3) were tested longitudinally under weight-stable conditions before surgery and after weight loss and stabilization (14 ± 2 mo). Resting energy expenditure (REE), TEE, body composition, and fasting leptin were measured. Subjects lost 53.2 (± 22.2) kg body weight and had significant decreases in REE (2400 ± 1000 RJ/d $P<0.001$) and TEE (3.6 ± 2.5 MJ/d; $P<0.001$). Changes in REE were predicted by changes in fat-free mass and fat mass. The average physical activity level (TEE/REE) was 1.61 at both baseline and follow-up ($P = 0.98$). Weight loss was predicted by baseline fat mass and BMI, but not by any energy expenditure variable or leptin. Measured REE at follow-up was not significantly different from predicted REE. TEE and REE decreased by 25% on average after massive weight loss induced by gastric bypass surgery. REE changes were predicted by loss of body tissue; thus, there was no significant long-term change in energy efficiency that would independently promote weight regain, as is seen with short-term weight loss.

NEURAL PATHWAYS

Many brain areas are involved in the regulation of eating, but the hypothalamus appears to be the key center in obesity. The median hypothalamus deserves particular attention. It is composed of several areas that act on each other through hormonal and neuropeptide regulation. Galanin-containing cells bridge the medial preoptic area to the periventricular nucleus and from there, on to the median eminence. This pathway is involved in fat consumption and fat oxidation. Neuropeptide Y neurons project from the arcuate nucleus (ARC), another center of the median hypothalamus, onto the periventricular nucleus. This circuit regulates carbohydrate ingestion and metabolism. Growth hormone releasing hormone neurons from the ARC project to both the medial preoptic area and the suprachiasmatic nucleus to control protein ingestion. All of these areas are influenced by a variety of gut hormones, hypothalamically derived hormones, and other peptides.[10]

In the ARC of the brain there are two types of neurons whose effects are opposite. These are the AgRP/NPY and the Pro-opiomelanocortin/cocaine-amphetamine related transcript (POMC/CART) neurons. Activation of the former increases both appetite and metabolism, whereas activation of the latter results in the opposite. These neurons project to second-order neurons which, in turn, project signals to the nucleus tractus solitarius satiety center. Some of these hormones have direct action on the nucleus tractus solitarius, which also receives afferent signals from the vagus nerve.[9]

BIOCHEMISTRY

This section provides a brief review of the key elements currently known about the biochemistry of obesity.

Leptin

An important paradigm shift has occurred in our understanding of the role of adipose tissues in the regulation of metabolic processes. For many decades, the adipocyte was thought of only as a repository of fat. Recent evidence, however, shows that fat can function as endocrine tissue as well. The discovery of leptin in 1994 was significant in many ways. It was the first link of the adipocyte to the central nervous system as a pathway for the regulation of weight.

Leptin is derived from the Greek word *leptos*, which means *thin*. Leptin is a protein hormone that functions in the metabolic regulation of body weight. The genetic message for this protein is encoded in the mouse gene, which has been isolated by cloning genetically obese mice. Mutation of either the obesity gene itself (ob/ob) or its receptor (db/db) can cause mice to be massively obese. Leptin is expressed primarily by the adipocytes; it can also be expressed by the stomach and the placenta. Leptin affects the hypothalamus, where it counteracts the effect of neuropeptide Y and a-melanocyte-stimulating hormone.[9,11]

These observations are derived from animal experiments and have not been replicated in human studies. Human mutations of the ob/ob gene are exceedingly rare; however, in the vast majority of obese patients, leptin levels are elevated. Leptin levels in the morbidly obese seem to correlate with the degree of energy conservation capacity. After gastric bypass, leptin levels are known to fall. It is now believed that leptin may play a role in energy adaptation during negative nitrogen balance.[18,19]

Resistin

The relationship between obesity and type 2 diabetes is well known; as many as 80% of patients with type 2 diabetes are overweight or obese. We know that insulin resistance correlates with the BMI, up to a BMI of 30 kg per m^2. Resistin, a recently described peptide hormone, may be key to this relationship. Almost solely derived from white adipose tissue, resistin is involved in the regulation of insulin resistance and of diet-induced obesity. Though some of the human data are controversial, an increased BMI appears to be associated with increased resistin levels; namely, the waist to hip circumference seems to be inversely correlated with resistin levels.[20]

Unfortunately, the precise role of resistin has been difficult to define in humans and difficult to study in animal models. The number of resistin isoforms identified in rodents and in humans differ. The cellular sources of resistin also differ significantly between humans and rodents.

Some evidence suggests that obesity is an inflammatory state. The resistin family of molecules was first identified in models of inflammation such as asthma. This peptide may, in fact, represent a new class of cytokines. Elevations of both C-reactive protein and interleukin-6 have been demonstrated in obese patients. Elevations of C-reactive protein have also been associated with the number of obesity-related comorbid conditions that an obese patient exhibits.[21]

Acylation-Stimulating Protein

Adipose tissue synthesizes and secretes a number of cytokine hormones that are involved in the regulation of energy homeostasis. Acylation-stimulating protein is a lipogenic cytokine that is linked to the pathogenesis of obesity. Its primary effect on the pathogenesis of obesity is to enhance triglyceride synthesis and storage in the adipocyte. It increases insulin-dependent glucose uptake and fatty-acid esterification. Acylation-stimulating protein levels are increased in obesity, type 2 diabetes, and coronary artery disease. Weight loss, through dieting or surgery, lowers the levels of acylation-stimulating protein.[18,22]

Adiponectin

Adiponectin is a common adipose tissue factor. Low levels of adiponectin are associated with a decrease in the ability of insulin to phosphorylate insulin receptor tyrosine residues. Adiponectin levels are low in the morbidly obese. Preoperative adiponectin levels may indicate the extent of weight loss after gastric bypass.[18]

Enteroglucagon

We know that the mechanisms of obesity are related to a disturbance in the gut-brain axis. In rat studies, it has been demonstrated that obesity is induced by damaging the ventromedial hypothalamus. By transposing a segment of the terminal ileum to the duodenum, a similar weight-loss effect is seen. In these operations, as well as in patients with a jejunoileal bypass, a sustained reduction in food intake has been observed. A large increase in enteroglucagon, which arises from a common gene for the production of a 160-amino acid proglucagon, also occurs. Enteroglucagon is composed of 78 to 107 amino acids. Some of the effects of enteroglucagon include pancreatic glucagon inhibition, insulin secretion inhibition, decreased insulin resistance, prolonged gastric emptying, and decreased intestinal motility.[7,8,23]

Cholecystokinin

Many non-adipose-derived hormones deserve attention in the discussion of obesity. In fact, the discovery and characterization of gastrointestinal tract hormones has led many to regard the foregut as an endocrine organ. Cholecystokinin is a well-known, short-acting, satiety-producing peptide. It can function both as a paracrine hormone and as a neurotransmitter. In its hormonal role, it delays gastric emptying; centrally, it inhibits a feeding response to food incentives.[24]

Ghrelin

Ghrelin, a recently described hormone, is found in the fundus of the stomach and the proximal duodenum. It has been identified in other areas of the body as well, including the pancreas. It acts primarily to increase growth hormone secretion by the pituitary. In normal-weight subjects, ghrelin levels are lowered by the ingestion of glucose and increased by fasting. Diet-induced weight loss increases serum ghrelin levels. Results after a gastric bypass are mixed. In the short term, there appears to be a profound drop in serum ghrelin levels; however, data from a recent study with 15 months of mean follow-up showed no change or a slight rise in the serum ghrelin levels.

Several opposing pathways in the hypothalamus regulate eating behavior and satiety. These sites are influenced by the interplay of hormones such as ghrelin and leptin. Recent evidence has shown that obesity surgery, in particular gastric bypass, can create profound changes in the levels of these hormones. Within the ARC of the brain, there are two separate receptors for satiety mediation. These neurons have reciprocal effects: one set of neurons contains receptors for substances that increase appetite and the other set has receptors for hormones with the opposite effect.[25-28]

Insulin

Insulin, secreted by the β islet cells of the pancreas, is perhaps the hormone that we know the most about. Receptors for insulin are located throughout the brain. Insulin works through neuropeptide Y mechanisms to suppress appetite. As long as insulin sensitivity is appropriate, an increase in central insulin levels results in diminished appetite and weight loss.

▶ CONCLUSION

Overweight (body mass index [BMI]$\geq$25 kg/m^2) is correlated with a variety of health problems, and obesity (BMI$\geq$30 kg/m^2) is a clear and powerful detriment to good health. Although many still do not view obesity as more than a behavioral problem of inadequate self-control, obesity is characterized by energy metabolism anomalies and is responsible for multiple comorbid conditions. Morbid obesity (BMI$\geq$40 kg/m^2 or BMI$\geq$35 kg/m^2 in the presence of obesity comorbidities), like atherosclerosis, is most definitely a life-shortening, malignant disease of multifactorial origins that can be identified and treated independently. Today, obesity is epidemic, affecting all age groups, both genders, and all races worldwide.

Obesity is a disease whose mechanisms arise in the pathways between the gut, the adipocyte mass, and the brain axis. These areas act on one another via hormonal and neuropeptide interchanges that influence fat consumption and fat oxidation and that regulate carbohydrate ingestion and metabolism. Hormonal input from the ARC projects to the medial preoptic area and the suprachiasmatic nucleus to control protein ingestion. All of these areas are influenced by a variety of gut hormones, hypothalamically derived hormones, and other peptides.

The central mediator of the complex mechanism of weight may prove to be fat, an endocrine organ itself. A number of hormones secreted by adipocytes can alter energy metabolism distinctly in various tissues, which eventually may explain the apparent differences in the way obese and nonobese individuals gain, maintain, and lose weight. Further investigation of the types and metabolic functions of adipose tissue in obese and nonobese subjects, in addition to ongoing study of the results of bariatric surgery, will deepen our knowledge of energy metabolism and the biochemistry of obesity.

▶ REFERENCES

1. Brechner RJ, Farris C, Harrison S, et al: Summary of Evidence: Bariatric Surgery. http://www.cms.hhs.gov/mcac/id137c.pdf. Accessed May 31, 2006.
2. NCA Tracking Sheet for Obesity as an Illness (CAG-00108N). http://www.cms.hhs.gov/med/viewtrackingsheet.asp?id=57. Accessed May 22, 2006.
3. Hill JO, Wyatt HR, Reed GW, et al: Obesity and the environment: where do we go from here? Science 2003;299:853-855.
4. Kelner K, Helmuth L: Obesity—what is to be done? Science 2003;299:845.
5. Steinbrook R: Surgery for severe obesity. N Engl J Med 2004;350:1075-1079.
6. Pories WJ, Swanson MS, MacDonald KG, et al: Who would have thought it? an operation proves to be the most effective therapy for adult-onset diabetes mellitus. Ann Surg 1995;222:339-350.
7. Greenway SE, Greenway FL III, Klein S: Effects of obesity surgery on non-insulin-dependent diabetes mellitus. Arch Surg 2002;137:1109-1117.
8. Chelikani PK, Haver AC, Reidelberger RD: Intravenous infusion of ghrelin increases meal frequency and attenuates anorexigenic responses to peptide YY (3-36), glucagons-like peptides, and CCK in rats. SSIB 2005;(abstract).
9. Marx J: Cellular warriors at the battle of the bulge. Science 2003;299:846-849.
10. Leibowitz SF, Wortley KE: Hypothalamic control of energy balance: different peptides, different functions. Peptides 2004;25:473-504.
11. Klein S, Romijn JA: Obesity. In Larsen PR, Kronenberg HM, Melmed S, et al (eds): Williams Textbook of Endocrinology, ed 10, pp. 1619-1641. Philadelphia, W.B. Saunders, 2002.
12. Hoffstedt J, Näslund E, Arner P: Calpain-10 gene polymorphism is associated with reduced β_3-adrenoceptor function in human fat cells. J Clin Endocrinol Metab 2002;87:3362-3367.
13. Wildman R, Center for Nutrition, Metabolism & Performance, University of Louisiana at Lafayette: Energy metabolism, body composition, and obesity. http://www.ucs.louisiana.edu/~rew5073/energymet.html. Accessed Sept. 25, 2003.
14. Leibel RL, Rosenbaum M, Hirsch J: Changes in energy expenditure resulting from altered body weight. N Engl J Med 1995;332:621-628.
15. Flancbaum L, Choban PS, Bradley LR, et al: Changes in measured resting energy expenditure after Roux-en-Y gastric bypass for clinically severe obesity. Surgery 1997;122:943-949.
16. Bobbioni-Harsch E, Morel P, Huber O et al: Energy economy hampers body weight loss after gastric bypass. J Clin Endocrinol Metab 2000;85:4695-4700.
17. Das SK, Roberts SB, McCrory MA, et al: Long-term changes in energy expenditure and body composition after massive weight loss induced by gastric bypass surgery. Am J Clin Nutr 2003;78:22-30.
18. Faraj M, Havel PJ, Phelis S, et al: Plasma acylation-stimulating protein, adiponectin, leptin, and ghrelin before and after weight loss induced by gastric bypass surgery in morbidly obese subjects. J Clin Endocrinol Metab 2003;88:1594-1602.
19. Rubino F, Michel G, Gentileschi P, et al: The early effect of the Roux-en-Y gastric bypass on hormones involved in body weight regulation and glucose metabolism. Ann Surg 2004;240:236-242.
20. Steppan CM, Bailey ST, Bhat S, et al: The hormone resistin links obesity to diabetes. Nature 2001;409:307-312.
21. Holcomb IN, Kabakoff RC, Chan B, et al: FIZZ1, a novel cysteine-rich secreted protein associated with pulmonary inflammation, defines a new gene family. EMBO J 2000;19:4046-4055.
22. Brun RP, Spiegelman BM: Obesity and the adipocyte: PPARγ and the molecular control of adipogenesis. J Endocrinol 1997;155:217-218.
23. Verdich C, Flint A, Gutzwiller J-P, et al: A meta-analysis of the effect of glucagons-like peptide-1 (7-36) amide on ad libitum energy intake in humans. J Clin Endocrinol Metab 2001;86:4382-4389.
24. Leibowitz SF, Hoebel BG: Behavioral neuroscience of obesity. In Bray GA, Bouchard C, James WPT (eds): Handbook of Obesity, pp. 313-359. New York, Marcel Dekker, 1998.
25. Cummings DE, Wiegle DS, Frayo RS, et al: Plasma ghrelin levels after diet-induced weight loss or gastric bypass surgery. N Engl J Med 2002;346:1623-1630.
26. le Roux CW, Bloom SR: Why do patients lose weight after Roux-en-Y gastric bypass? J Clin Endocrinol Metab 2005;90:591-592.
27. Korner J, Bessler M, Cirilo LJ, et al: Effects of Roux-en-Y gastric bypass surgery on fasting and postprandial concentrations of plasma ghrelin, peptide YY, and insulin. J Clin Endocrinol Metab 2005;90:359-365.
28. Leonetti F, Silecchia G, Iacobellis G, et al: Different plasma ghrelin levels after laparoscopic gastric bypass and adjustable gastric banding in morbid obese subjects. J Clin Endocrinol Metab 2003;88:4227-4232.

section II

CONSEQUENCES

5

Obesity Comorbidities

Henry Buchwald, M.D., Ph.D.

Overweight (body mass index [BMI] ≥25 kg/m²) may not be healthy; obesity (BMI ≥30 kg/m²) is definitely detrimental to good health; and morbid obesity (BMI ≥40 kg/m² or BMI ≥35 kg/m² in the presence of obesity comorbidities) is a disease.[1,2] Certainly, there are multifactorial origins of morbid obesity. But once the BMI values defining morbid obesity are reached, we are addressing a disease—a life-shortening, incapacitating, malignant disease.[3-6] Yet, for society, and even for the medical community, to accept morbid obesity as the progenitor of certain comorbid diseases may be easier than to define morbid obesity per se as a disease. After all, coronary heart disease and peripheral arterial occlusive disease were recognized clinical disease entities for decades before their causative mechanism—atherosclerosis—was regarded as a disease. Nevertheless, atherosclerosis is itself a disease of multifactorial origins that can be identified and independently treated.

The comorbidites of morbid obesity affect essentially every organ system[7,8]: cardiovascular (hypertension, atherosclerotic heart and peripheral vascular disease with myocardial infarction and cerebral vascular accidents, peripheral venous insufficiency); respiratory (asthma, obstructive sleep apnea, obesity-hypoventilation syndrome); metabolic (type 2 diabetes, impaired glucose tolerance, dyslipidemia); musculoskeletal (back strain, disk disease, weight-bearing osteoarthritis of the hips, knees, ankles, and feet); gastrointestinal (cholelithiasis, gastroesophageal reflux disease, fatty metamorphosis of the liver [steatohepatitis], cirrhosis of the liver, hepatic carcinoma, colorectal carcinoma); urinary (stress incontinence); endocrine and reproductive (polycystic ovary syndrome, increased risk for pregnancy and fetal abnormalities, male hypogonadism, and cancer of the endometrium, breast, ovary, prostate, and pancreas); dermatologic (intertriginous dermatitis); neurologic (pseudotumor cerebri, carpal tunnel syndrome); and psychological (depression).

▶ INDIVIDUAL COMORBIDITIES

Hypertension

Approximately 50% of obese adults (BMI ≥30 kg/m²) are hypertensive, many of the cases undiagnosed. About 75% of all cases of essential hypertension can be attributed to obesity.[3,4] Even individuals who are only 20% above ideal weight have an eightfold increase in the risk for hypertension. As early as the 1960s, the Framingham Study demonstrated that a 15% increase in weight resulted in an 18% increase in systolic blood pressure.[9] Obesity, by far, is the strongest predictor of high blood pressure in both men and women, at all ages and in all races.[3,4] Hypertension together with dyslipidemia and cigarette smoking are the three primary risk factors for atherosclerotic cardiovascular disease.[10]

Dyslipidemia

Some form of dyslipidemia is associated with obesity in approximately 40% to 50% of individuals with a BMI of 30 kg per m² or more.[3,4] The Framingham Study determined that, for every 10% increase in weight, plasma cholesterol levels increased about 12 mg per dl.[9] The dyslipidemia of obesity is characterized by hypercholesterolemia, elevated low-density lipoprotein (LDL) cholesterol, reduced high-density lipoprotein (HDL) cholesterol, and hypertriglyceridemia. The HDL-LDL ratio is reduced and the total cholesterol-HDL ratio is elevated. This lipid profile is markedly atherogenic and, again, a primary risk factor for atherosclerotic cardiovascular disease.[10,11]

Diabetes and Impaired Glucose Tolerance

The prevalence of diabetes in any population is a function of the prevalence of obesity. Obesity is the primary risk factor for type 2 diabetes, and 90% of all type 2 diabetics are obese.[3,4] The National Health and Nutrition Examination Survey III (1988-1994) data showed that the relative risk for chemical diabetes at a BMI of 30 kg per m² or higher is about 50%, and at a BMI of 40 kg per m² or higher, it is more than 90%.[12] The Nurses' Health Study of 84,941 women (1980-1996) showed that the relative risk of diabetes increased nearly fortyfold as the BMI increased from below 23 kg per m² to above 35 kg per m².[13,14] Virtually all morbidly obese adults have a measurable impaired glucose tolerance[15]; 36% of individuals with impaired glucose tolerance will progress to frank type 2 diabetes within 10 years.

Enlarged visceral fat stores produce a rapid release of free fatty acids and glucose, leading to a block in insulin binding by the liver, gluconeogenesis, and functional insulin resistance. This results in concurrent hyperinsulinemia and hyperglycemia. Obese patients have an increased prevalence of impaired glucose control, elevated fasting insulin levels, elevated fasting glucose levels, suppressed metabolic glucose clearance rates, and insensitivity to insulin concentrations.

Diabetes is the fourth-ranked independent risk factor for atherosclerosis. Hypertension, hypercholesterolemia, cigarette smoking, and diabetes are the four cardinal obesity risk factors for atherosclerotic cardiac and peripheral vascular disease, myocardial infarction, and cerebrovascular accidents.[16] Diabetics have four times the prevalence of coronary heart disease and twice the prevalence of cerebrovascular accidents as compared with nondiabetics. In addition, diabetes is associated with blindness, renal failure, neuropathy, gastroenteropathy, and lower-extremity amputations.

In a study of volunteers with no history of diabetes, coronary heart disease, or hypertension, insulin resistance was quantified by determining the steady-state plasma glucose concentration during the last 30 minutes of an 180-minute infusion of octreotide, glucose, and insulin.[17] The BMI and the steady-state plasma glucose concentration in that study were significantly related (r = 0.465, $P<0.001$). The BMI and the steady-state plasma glucose concentration were independently associated with each of nine coronary heart-disease risk factors: age, systolic blood pressure, diastolic blood pressure, total cholesterol, triglycerides, HDL cholesterol, LDL cholesterol, and the glucose and insulin responses to a 75-g oral glucose load. Further, by multiple regression analysis, the steady-state plasma glucose concentration added modest to substantial power to the BMI as a predictor of five of these nine coronary heart-disease risk factors. It is evident, therefore, that even in the preclinical state, body weight and certainly obesity are strongly linked to diabetes, and that obesity and diabetes combined predict lethal health consequences.

Cardiac and Peripheral Vascular Disease

Obesity is an independent primary risk factor, as well as a secondary risk factor, for atherosclerotic cardiac and peripheral vascular disease.[16-19] The secondary influence is mediated by obesity's induction of hypertension and dyslipidemia. This summary cannot attempt to encompass even a review of the ravages of atherosclerotic coronary heart disease, cerebrovascular accidents, carotid occlusive disease, subclavian steal syndromes, aneurysmal disease, peripheral arterial occlusive disease, and visceral angina and occlusive disease. Such problems occur in relatively large-vessel arteries. To these manifestations in the obese diabetic must be added the independent and synergistic effects of diabetic small-vessel arterial disease. As a result of these cumulative risk factors, cardiac and peripheral vascular disease occurs in obese individuals at an earlier age, and often more dramatically, than in the nonobese population.

Peripheral Venous Insufficiency

Because peripheral venous insufficiency is rarely life threatening, it has not realized the data acquisition of many of the other comorbidities of obesity. For those who take care of the obese, however, the prevalence of superficial varicosities and pain on standing are quite evident. In addition, obese patients often have stasis dermatitis and stasis ulcers. For some patients, never-relenting, open, foul-smelling sores of the legs below the knees dominate their lives. In addition, the obese may have an increased incidence of deep vein thrombophlebitis and pulmonary embolization, especially after trauma, surgery, and immobilization.

Asthma

Asthma is characterized by paroxysmal dyspnea, a wheezing cough, and a sense of thoracic constriction. It is caused by spasmodic bronchial constriction, which is attributed to a reflux irritation usually linked to an allergen. Asthma is also a prevalent comorbidity of obesity.[20] It is conjectured that the decreased lung volumes resulting from increasing abdominal girth sensitize the respiratory tree to the asthma phenomenon. Further, sleep apnea and respiratory stasis as well as gastroesophageal reflux and aspiration may be contributory factors. Whatever the specific mechanisms, obese children have a threefold likelihood of experiencing asthma, with an incidence of about 30%; obese adults have a doubling of the prevalence, with an incidence of about 25%.[3,4]

Sleep Apnea

As much as 50% of the morbidly obese suffer from sleep apnea, an incidence of more than 10 times that of the community norm of 2% to 4%.[3,4] Early sleep apnea with heavy snoring may progress to severe sleep apnea, with frequent and prolonged periods of apnea, requiring continuous positive airway pressure support. Abdominal girth is the most significant risk factor for the development of sleep apnea.[21,22] Because abdominal girth, or central obesity, is more prevalent in men than in women, sleep apnea is more prevalent in obese men than in obese women. Nocturnal apnea has been associated with death. More commonly, the effects of episodic nocturnal apnea carry over to daytime hours, leading to drowsiness, inattentiveness, impaired job performance, and cognitive dysfunction. The incidence of car accidents is several times higher in individuals with sleep apnea than in the general population.[23]

Sleep apnea is characterized as central, oropharyngeal obstructive, or combined. Procedures to relieve oropharyngeal obstructive sleep apnea, such as uvulectomy, have had minimal to moderate success in obese patients.[24] Tracheotomies have been performed to improve nocturnal ventilation, again, with some success. Bariatric surgery with marked weight loss in the morbidly obese has been nearly 100% effective in managing sleep apnea.

Obesity-Hypoventilation Syndrome

Less common but more pathogenic than sleep apnea is obesity-hypoventilation syndrome. The obese have decreased lung volumes because of increased intraabdominal pressure and elevated diaphragms as well as increased pulmonary blood volume and cardiac output. The decreased lung volumes result in chronic shortness of breath, decreased expiratory reserve volume, increased oxygen consumption rates, and increased circulating carbon dioxide.

The long-term cumulative effects of these respiratory changes can cause pulmonary hypertension, right heart failure, and death.

Back and Disk Disease

The orthopedic problems caused by obesity are obvious. None are more prevalent than chronic back pain and lumbosacral disk disease. With increasing age, back problems in the obese will reach an incidence of 100%. Osteoarthritis is accelerated at BMI values higher than 25 kg per m².[3,4] The morbidly obese, therefore, commonly have not only back strain, but also osteoarthritic spurring, sciatic root pain, and collapsed disks and vertebrae. It is not uncommon to see the morbidly obese using canes, walkers, or wheelchairs for mobility.

Peripheral Osteoarthritis

Weight-bearing osteoarthritis of the hips, knees, ankles, and feet is accelerated in the obese and often complicates congenital or traumatic lower-extremity bony abnormalities.[25] Foot pain, especially Sever disease, which is characterized by heel pain, is closely associated with obesity. At the very least, peripheral osteoarthritis in the obese inhibits ambulation and the ability of the obese to exercise and, thereby, to burn calories. Most orthopedic surgeons prefer to defer hip and knee replacement surgery in the morbidly obese and first refer them for preliminary bariatric surgery.[26]

Cholelithiasis

Obesity, with its increased prevalence of dyslipidemia, is a predictor of cholelithiasis. It is part of the so-called Five Fs medical-school mnemonic of fat, fair, female, fertile, and forty. For accuracy, this memory tool needs only to be modified by the addition of Native American. The obese are three times more likely to have cholelithiasis than the nonobese, and this predictor holds true for men as well as women.[3,4] The occurrence of cholelithiasis in the obese after bariatric surgery has motivated some bariatric surgeons to perform routine cholecystectomies at the time of the bariatric operation. Certain bariatric surgeons routinely perform preoperative gallbladder ultrasonography in order to select patients for intraoperative cholecystectomy. Certainly, the gallbladder warrants careful palpation during open bariatric surgery and warrants removal if cholelithiasis is present. Laparoscopic bariatric surgery makes the intraoperative diagnosis of cholelithiasis more difficult.

Gastroesophageal Reflux Disease

Gastroesophageal reflux disease (GERD), usually with an associated hiatus hernia, is a common problem; the estimated incidence in the general population is 20%.[27] In approximately 7% of individuals, the disease is severe enough to require medication, usually with a proton-pump blocker. GERD is a precursor of Barrett esophagitis, which carries an increased likelihood that esophageal carcinoma will occur. The frequency of occurrence of GERD in the obese may rise to about 50%, with half of these patients requiring medication.[3,4,28,29] These clinical data are substantiated by

24-hour pH monitoring and esophageal manometry. More than likely, the increased intraabdominal pressure of obesity is a major causative factor in the development of obesity-related GERD.[6]

Fatty Metamorphosis, Cirrhosis, and Carcinoma of the Liver

Fatty hepatic metamorphosis, or nonalcoholic steatohepatitis, is present in nearly 100% of the morbidly obese, as ascertained by intraoperative biopsy during bariatric surgery.[30,31] Its severity seems to increase in a linear fashion with increases in the BMI. Over time, fatty metamorphosis can progress to pericentral fibrosis, bridging fibrosis and, finally, cirrhosis. In turn, cirrhosis is a progenitor of hepatocellular carcinoma.

Pseudotumor Cerebri and Carpal Tunnel Syndrome

The increased intraabdominal pressure in the obese can cause an increase in cerebrospinal fluid and, subsequently, intracranial hypertension.[6] When clinically manifest, this condition is known as pseudotumor cerebri. It is responsible for severe headaches, pulsatile tinnitus, and visual disturbances.[32]

The obese have been reported to have four times the incidence of peripheral median nerve neuritis or carpal tunnel syndrome than the nonobese.[33] In fact, obesity is a stronger risk factor for carpal tunnel syndrome than are repetitive occupational tasks involving the finger tendons' passing through the carpal tunnel.

Intertriginous Dermatitis

Although not life-threatening, the cutaneous manifestations of obesity are socially and sexually inhibiting and, at best, unpleasant. The morbidly obese commonly suffer from various forms of intertriginous dermatitis, including chronic fungus infections, boils, and macerated, weeping, foul-smelling lesions. These cutaneous problems are located primarily under abdominal, breast, groin, and armpit folds.

Stress Incontinence

The increased intraabdominal pressure in the obese creates pelvic floor stress and neuromuscular impairment of the urinary tract, possibly resulting in stress incontinence. Obesity-related stress incontinence is more common in women than in men and is accentuated during pregnancy and the postnatal period.

Female Endocrine and Reproductive Disorders

Estrogen is secreted by fat cells, and the obese have increased levels of circulating estrogens. This increase in estrogen levels is continuous in obese females, rather than showing the physiologic cyclical pattern of the normal premenopausal estrogen-progesterone secretion cycle. In addition, sex-hormone-binding globulin production is suppressed in the obese, which further increases serum estrogen levels as well as circulating levels of free androgens.

These hormonal abnormalities can induce erratic menstruation, amenorrhea, dysfunctional uterine bleeding, early menopause, and infertility. Further, polycystic ovary syndrome is three-times more prevalent in obese than in lean women.[34] During pregnancy, obese women have an increased prevalence of preeclampsia, urinary infections, gestational diabetes, hypertension, overdue births, prolonged labor, blood loss during delivery, and cesarean delivery. Fetal growth may also be impaired and neural tube defects in the newborn are more common.

In women with markedly increased androgen levels, hirsutism and android manifestations are present. They are far more prone to develop atherosclerotic cardiovascular disease than are pear-shaped women.

The continuous abnormal hormonal milieu of obesity, in particular the continuous estrogen bombardment of the reproductive organs, increases the incidence of endometrial (three- to fourfold), ovarian (three- to fourfold), and breast (at least twofold) carcinomas.[35] Obese women who develop breast carcinoma prior to menopause have a decreased survival probability as compared with normal-weight controls.

Male Endocrine and Reproductive Disorders

Obese men also may suffer from increased estrogen bombardment and, contrary to the increased androgen levels in certain obese women, a decrease in testosterone production. These hormonal changes can manifest clinically as infertility, impotence, hypogonadism, and decreased libido. Also, obese men have an increased prevalence of prostate cancer.

Other Carcinomas

Obesity carries a statistically increased risk of malignancies other than those of the female and male endocrine and reproductive systems, including those of the colon and rectum, gallbladder, esophagus, stomach, and pancreas.[36]

Depression

In addition to the social and economic implications of obesity and the obvious daily psychosocial burden the obese undergo, the prevalence of clinical depression is high, particularly in obese women (chapters 7 and 8).[3,4] Adolescent and young females are particularly sensitive to severe depression. More than 50% of women seeking bariatric surgery have been placed on antidepressants.

▶ METABOLIC SYNDROME CLUSTER

Certain of the individual comorbidities of obesity have been clustered and characterized as the metabolic syndrome of obesity (syndrome x). This syndrome includes essential hypertension, dyslipidemia, peripheral insulin resistance, hyperinsulinemia, type 2 diabetes, and an increased incidence of cardiovascular events.[37] The syndrome is associated with, and possibly causes, polycystic ovary syndrome and nonalcoholic steatohepatitis, with all of their manifestations and complications. The metabolic syndrome is found more often in patients with central obesity than in those with peripheral obesity.

▶ COMORBIDITIES AFTER BARIATRIC SURGERY

Bariatric surgery is performed to improve the quality of life of the morbidly obese and to make them more physically attractive, thereby enhancing their societal and economic opportunities but, for the most part, bariatric surgery is performed to ameliorate the myriad of obesity comorbidities, increase global health, and prolong life expectancy. One of the only metaanalyses performed in the field of bariatric surgery is a metaanalysis of outcomes with respect to weight, 30-day mortality, and resolution of or improvement in type 2 diabetes, hyperlipidemia, hypertension, and obstructive sleep apnea.[38] This report showed: (1) that weight loss, as a percentage of excess-body-weight loss, varied as a function of the procedure performed—from 47.5% in patients who underwent laparoscopic adjustable gastric banding to 61.6% for gastric bypass, 68.2% for gastroplasty, and 70.1% for biliopancreatic diversion/duodenal switch, with an average weight loss of 61.2%; (2) that the 30-day operative mortality was 0.1% for the restrictive operations (laparoscopic adjustable gastric banding and gastroplasty), 0.5% for Roux-en-Y gastric bypass, and 1.1% for the predominantly malabsorptive operations of biliopancreatic diversion/duodenal switch; and (3) that there was marked resolution of or improvement in the four comorbidities analyzed. Specifically, diabetes completely resolved in 76.8% of patients and resolved or improved in 86.0%; hyperlipidemia improved in 70% or more of patients; hypertension resolved in 61.7% of patients and resolved or improved in 78.5%; and obstructive sleep apnea resolved in 85.7% of patients and resolved or improved in (separate cohort) 83.6% of patients.

The outcomes of bariatric surgery with respect to nutrition, diabetes, hypertension, obstructive sleep apnea, and orthopedic conditions are so important as to warrant their own chapters in this book. The effects of bariatric surgery on some of the other comorbidities of morbid obesity are briefly reviewed in this chapter.

Dyslipidemia

The historic epoch of proving the lipid-atherosclerosis hypothesis came to an end in the last decade of the 20th century. In the 1990s, after years of suggestive but negative medical studies, a surgical randomized, controlled, clinical trial—the Program on the Surgical Control of the Hyperlipidemias (POSCH)—was the first statistically significant study to demonstrate that marked reductions in total (23%) and LDL cholesterol (38%), in association with an increase in HDL cholesterol (4%), caused beneficial cardiovascular outcomes.[39-41] These outcomes included reductions in overall mortality ($P = 0.05$); in mortality resulting from atherosclerotic coronary heart disease ($P = 0.03$); in mortality resulting from atherosclerotic coronary heart disease plus confirmed nonfatal myocardial infarction ($P<0.001$); in confirmed nonfatal myocardial infarction ($P<0.001$); in the incidence of coronary artery bypass grafting or percutaneous transluminal coronary angioplasty ($P< 0.001$); and in the onset of clinical peripheral vascular disease ($P = 0.02$). These clinical outcomes were confirmed in POSCH by sequential coronary arteriograms at baseline and then at 3, 5, 7, and 10 years of follow-up.

The arteriograms demonstrated decreased progression (P<0.001) and increased regression (P = 0.02) of plaque lesions. The intervention modality in POSCH was partial ileal bypass, which bypassed the distal 200 cm of the small intestine, resulting in minimal weight loss but demonstrable cholesterol and bile acid malabsorption.

The literature pertaining to nonbariatric surgery provides ample evidence that plasma lipids are normalized after weight reduction. As a rule, for every kg of weight lost, there is a 1% decrease in total and LDL cholesterol, a 1% increase in HDL cholesterol, a 3% decrease in the ratio of total to HDL cholesterol, and about a 1% decrease in triglycerides.

The literature pertaining to bariatric surgery confirms and dramatically emphasizes these findings. At least 30 studies describe favorable changes in plasma lipids after bariatric surgery.[11,38,42-44] These changes are independent of the procedure performed or the technique utilized. It is the degree of weight loss achieved that determines the degree of normalization of plasma lipids. The favorable changes after bariatric surgery, after about 12 months of follow-up, include a more than 20% decrease in total cholesterol, as much as a 70% decrease in LDL cholesterol, about a 40% decrease in triglycerides, and a variable increase in HDL cholesterol.

Considerable attention recently has focused on the Swedish Obese Subjects (SOS) study, in which 2010 patients underwent bariatric surgery (gastric bypass, gastroplasty, or gastric banding) and 2037 matched-pair controls underwent conventional nonoperative treatment.[10] After 2 years, the incidence of hyperlipidemia was lower by tenfold in the surgical-weight-loss group than in the control group.

Cardiac and Peripheral Vascular Disease

Many studies, including the POSCH trial, have now demonstrated the benefits of risk-factor modification in preventing, arresting, and even reversing atherosclerotic cardiac and peripheral vascular disease.[39-41] Bariatric surgery has been specifically demonstrated to benefit cardiovascular health. Schauer and colleagues showed a 25% resolution of, and a 75% decrease in, coronary artery disease symptoms as well as improvement in 67% of patients in coronary heart failure.[45] Other studies have shown similar findings.[46,47] The SOS study showed a one-third rate of progression of atherosclerotic disease in the surgical weight-loss group as compared with the control group, including a decrease in left ventricular mass, a decrease in the left ventricular stroke index and the cardiac output, and a decrease in left ventricular end-diastolic pressure.[48,49]

Peripheral Venous Insufficiency

There is no vast literature on improvement in peripheral venous insufficiency after weight loss induced by bariatric surgery. Nevertheless, this improvement is a common observation of bariatric surgeons and, most certainly, a much appreciated outcome in bariatric patients. Varicosities, pain on standing, stasis dermatitis, and stasis ulcers, as well as the incidence of deep-vein thrombophlebitis and pulmonary embolization, are all decreased after successful bariatric surgery.

Asthma

Obese children have a 30% incidence of asthma, and obese adults a 25% incidence. At least eight bariatric studies have shown that the rates of postoperative resolution of asthma ranged from 25% to 83%.[20]

Cholelithiasis

Obviously, if a cholecystectomy is performed at the same time as, or prior to, a bariatric procedure, the problem of cholelithiasis is avoided postoperatively. However, many bariatric surgeons elect not to remove an asymptomatic gallbladder free of stones by ultrasonography or palpation at the time of the bariatric procedure. What is the outcome of such a decision? Certainly, the patient remains subject to the normal rate of developing cholelithiasis, which may be accentuated by the risk factor of obesity, even after successful bariatric surgery. There is also excellent evidence for an increase in the incidence of cholelithiasis after weight loss per se and, possibly even more so, after the marked weight loss engendered by bariatric surgery.[50,51] This accentuated risk has been associated with an incidence of over 35% in some series at 12 months postoperatively, with a diminishing risk thereafter. To decrease cholelithiasis induced by bariatric surgery, some bariatric surgeons routinely prescribe ursodeoxycholic acid for their patients.[52]

Gastroesophageal Reflux Disease

The amelioration of GERD after bariatric surgery is one of the most gratifying outcomes in this field. More than any other favorable outcome, this effect is operation-dependent. Roux gastric bypass or long-limb Roux gastric bypass "cures" GERD.[53] After these procedures, very little acid is produced in the upper gastric pouch, and no bile can normally reflux up a Roux limb of adequate length (about 75 cm or longer). No acid, no bile—no reflux. Patients, after a properly performed Roux gastric bypass, walk out of the hospital free of GERD symptoms, without any further need for nocturnal bed elevation or anti-GERD medications such as proton pump inhibitors. If not for the weight loss it induces, gastric bypass with closure of the esophageal crura would become the operation of choice for the treatment of GERD and hiatus hernia in the normal-weight population.[54]

The same laudatory statements with respect to GERD cannot be made for vertical banded gastroplasty or laparoscopic adjustable gastric banding which, in certain patients, may actually increase the incidence of GERD symptoms postoperatively.[55] The persistence or new occurrence of GERD after biliopancreatic diversion and duodenal switch seems not to be influenced by those procedures.

Fatty Metamorphosis, Cirrhosis, and Carcinoma of the Liver

In some patients, unchecked morbid obesity is associated with a progression from fatty metamorphosis of the liver to cirrhosis and possibly to carcinoma. In the morbidly obese, the incidence of fatty metamorphosis is nearly 100%; the incidence of cirrhosis and carcinoma is quite low yet is higher than in the general population.[30] Several studies have shown a reversal, or at least a diminution, of fatty metamorphosis after bariatric surgery. Though there are no controlled series data to substantiate this assumption, it stands to reason that the incidence of cirrhosis and carcinoma of the liver would also be reduced after successful bariatric surgery.

Pseudotumor Cerebri

Idiopathic intracranial hypertension, or pseudotumor cerebri, is markedly alleviated after successful bariatric surgery.[32] This finding has been demonstrated in several series and is particularly gratifying in young bariatric patients.[56] Symptomatic improvement has been shown to be associated with a decrease in cerebrospinal fluid pressure after surgery.

Carpal Tunnel Syndrome

It is difficult to find specific references for the amelioration of carpal tunnel syndrome after bariatric surgery. Yet this affirmative outcome has been observed by most bariatric surgeons.

Intertriginous Dermatitis

The problem of intertriginous dermatitis, so commonly associated with morbid obesity, also is rarely mentioned in outcome assessments. Nevertheless, relief from this condition can be ascertained by careful questioning of patients after bariatric surgery. This difference in cutaneous pathology may be a relatively minor health gain, but it often elicits a major improvement in quality of life.

Stress Incontinence

Bariatric surgery is more successful in treating stress incontinence than are most other operative interventions.[57] By reversing the increased intraabdominal pressure present preoperatively, pelvic floor stress is relieved, and neuromuscular impairment of the urinary bladder is alleviated.[58]

Female Endocrine and Reproductive Disorders

Dysmenorrhea and polycystic ovaries syndrome routinely dissipate after bariatric surgery, with a return to normal menstrual activity.[34] Successful bariatric surgery reduces the risks of pregnancy for both the mother and the child. The incidence of preeclampsia, gestational diabetes, and gestational hypertension is reduced, and the baby's birth weight is normalized. Fertility may be enhanced after bariatric surgery.

The incidence of endometrial, ovarian, and breast carcinoma is greater in the morbidly obese. There are currently no prospective data to show a decrease in these problems after bariatric surgery.

Male Endocrine and Reproductive Disorders

There are currently no series reporting positive changes in infertility, impotence, hypogonadism, decreased libido, or the incidence of prostate cancer after bariatric surgery in males. There are data, however, that demonstrate the need for near-normal weight achievement to normalize sex hormone-binding globulin in massively obese men.[59]

Other Carcinomas

There are no current series reporting a reversal after bariatric surgery of the increased incidence of the colon, rectum, gallbladder, esophagus, stomach, and pancreas carcinomas associated with morbid obesity.

Depression

It is the impression of all bariatric surgeons that, if bariatric surgery has caused a significant weight loss, the great majority of patients are happier individuals postoperatively.[60,61] This change in outlook is manifested in both women and men. The prospective evaluation of clinical depression is a fertile area for exploration by the allied health teams involved in bariatric surgery.[62]

Beyond clinical depression, there is quality of life—a subject with considerable affirmative-outcome data.[63-66] General well-being scores tend to double, or show 100% improvement, postoperatively. The same trend is seen for social function, including body self-image, self-confidence, ability to interact with others, and time spent in recreational activities. Sexual activity often increases and is found to be more satisfying. These changes, as well as other perceptions of obese peoples' identity, may improve or be detrimental to a marriage. Bariatric surgery improves overall physical function, including mobility, energy, and vitality; more time is spent exercising and participating in physical activities. Further, productivity and economic opportunities are increased, including new employment and more lucrative employment.

Traditionally, the physician's perspective and definition of success focused on weight-loss statistics and, more recently, on the amelioration of obesity comorbidities. However, the patient's perspective and definition of success almost always focused—and still does—on improved quality of life and on decreased discrimination.[67] Thus, the assessment tool of Oria and Moorehead (the Bariatric Analysis and Reporting Outcome System [BAROS]) is gaining popularity.[68] This tool includes a quality-of-life assessment that is scored in association with the amount of weight lost and the improvement in comorbid conditions related to obesity. It comes close to testing the World Health Organization's definition of quality of life—a state of complete physical, mental, and social well-being—and not merely the absence of disease and infirmity.

SUMMARY

Obesity, in particular morbid obesity, is associated with medical comorbidities that affect essentially every organ system and, thereby, longevity (see chapter 6), as well as societal and economic comorbidities (see chapters 7 and 8). An exposition of the medical comorbidities and their response to bariatric surgery has been presented. It would seem that the single therapy of bariatric surgery not only ameliorates the primary disease process but concurrently has a favorable impact on the comorbid conditions associated with morbid obesity.

▶ REFERENCES

1. Jung RT: Obesity as a disease. Br Med Bull 1997;53:307-321.
2. Bray GA: Obesity, a time bomb to be defused. Lancet 1998;352:160-261.
3. North American Association for the Study of Obesity (NAASO) and the National Heart, Lung, and Blood Institute (NHLBI): Clinical Guidelines on the Identification, Evaluation, and Treatment of Overweight and Obesity in Adults: The Evidence Report, National Institutes of Health Pub #98-4083. Bethesda, MD, National Institutes of Health, Sept 1998.
4. North American Association for the Study of Obesity (NAASO) and the National Heart, Lung, and Blood Institute (NHLBI); The Practical Guide: Identification, Evaluation, and Treatment of Overweight and Obesity in Adults. National Institutes of Health Pub #00-4084. Bethesda, MD, National Institutes of Health, Oct 2000.
5. O'Brien PE, Dixon JB: Obesity—the extent of the problem: section 1: issues in obesity and treatment. Am J Surg 2002;184(6B):4S-8S.
6. Sugerman H: Pathophysiology of severe obesity. Probl Gen Sur 2000;17:7-12.
7. Herrara MF, Lozano-Salazar RR, Gonzalez-Barranco J, et al: Diseases and problems secondary to massive obesity. Eur J Gastroenterol Hepatol 1999;11:63-67.
8. Pi-Sunyer FX: Medical hazards of obesity. Ann Intern Med 1993;199:655-660.
9. Kannel WB, Brand N, Skinner JJ Jr, Dawber TR, et al: The relation of adiposity to blood pressure and the development of hypertension: the Framingham Study. Ann Intern Med 1967;67:48-59.
10. Sjostrom CD, Lissner L, Wedel H, et al: Reduction in incidence of diabetes, hypertension and lipid disturbances after intentional weight loss induced by bariatric surgery: the SOS Intervention Study. Obes Res 1999;7:477-484.
11. Gleysteen JJ: Results of surgery: long-term effects on hyperlipidemia. Am J Clin Nutr. 1992;55(suppl):591S-593S.
12. U.S. Department of Health and Human Services, National Center for Health Statistics: Third National Health and Nutrition Examination Survey, 1988-1994. NHANES III Laboratory Data File (CD-ROM), Public Use Data File Documentation #76200. Hyattsville, MD, Centers for Disease Control and Prevention, 1996. (Available from National Technical Information Service (NTIS), Springfield, VA.)
13. Hu FB, Manson JE, Stampfer MJ, et al: Diet, lifestyle, and the risk of type 2 diabetes mellitus in women. N Engl J Med 2001;345:790-797.
14. Manson JE, Willett WC, Stampfer MJ, et al: Body weight and mortality among women. N Engl J Med 1995;333:677-685.
15. Burstein R, Epstein Y, Charuzi I, et al: Glucose utilization in morbidly obese subjects before and after weight loss by gastric bypass operation. Int J Obes Relat Metab Disord 1995;19:558-561.
16. Hollander P: Confronting obesity: toward prevention of diabetes and cardiovascular disease. Cardiol Rev 2000;17:41-48.
17. Abbasi F, Brown BW Jr, Lamendola C, et al: Relationship between obesity, insulin resistance, and coronary heart disease risk. J Am Coll Cardiol 2002;40:937-943.
18. Alpert MA: Obesity cardiomyopathy: pathophysiology and evolution of the clinical syndrome. Am J Med Sci 2001;321:225-236.
19. Krauss RM, Winston M, Fletcher RN, et al: Obesity: impact on cardiovascular disease. Circulation 1998;98:1472-1476.
20. Dixon JB, Chapman L, O'Brien P: Marked improvement in asthma after LAP-BAND surgery for morbid obesity. Obes Surg 1999;9:385-389.
21. Kyzer S, Charuzi I: Obstructive sleep apnea in the obese. World J Surg 1998;22:998-1001.
22. Van Kralinger KW, de Kanter W, de Groot GH, et al: Assessment of sleep complaints and sleep-disordered breathing in a consecutive series of obese patients. Respiration, 1999;66:312-316.
23. Haraldsson PO, Akerstedt T: Drowsiness—greater traffic hazard than alcohol: causes, risks and treatment. Lakartidningen 2001;98:3018-3023.
24. Li KK, Powell NB, Riley RW, et al: Morbidly obese patients with severe obstructive sleep apnea: is airway reconstructive surgery a viable treatment option? Laryngoscope 2000;110:982-987.
25. Deitel M: Commentary: joint pains after various intestinal bypasses and secondary to obesity. Obes Surg 1998;8:265.
26. Parzivi J, Trousdale RT, Sarr MG: Total joint arthroplasty in patients surgically treated for morbid obesity. J Arthroplasty 2000;15:1003-1008.
27. Kahrilas PJ: Gastroesophageal reflux disease. JAMA 1996;276:983-988.
28. Lundell L, Ruth M, Sandberg N, et al: Does massive obesity promote abnormal gastroesophageal reflux? Dig Dis Sci 1995;40:1632-1635.
29. Rigaud D, Merrouche M, Le Moel G, et al: Factors of gastroesophageal acid reflux in severe obesity. Gastroenterol Clin Biol 1995;19:818-825.
30. Marubbio AT, Buchwald H, Schwartz MZ, et al: Hepatic lesions of central peri-cellular fibrosis in morbid obesity and after jejunoileal bypass. Am J Clin Pathol 1976;66:684-691.
31. Luyckx FH, Desaive C, Thiry A, et al: Liver abnormalities in severely obese subjects: effect of drastic weight loss after gastroplasty. Int J Obes 1998;22:222-226.
32. Kupersmith MJ, Garnell L, Turbin R, et al: Effects of weight loss on the course of idiopathic intracranial hypertension in women. Neurology 1998;50:1094-1098.
33. Kouyoumdjian JA, Morita MD, Roche PR, et al: Body mass index and carpal tunnel syndrome. Arq Neuro-Psiquiatr 2000;58:252-256.
34. Hoeger K: Obesity and weight loss in polycystic ovary syndrome. Obstet Gynecol Clin North Am 2001;28:85-97.
35. Ballard-Barbash R, Swanson CA: Body weight: estimation of risk for breast and endometrial cancers. Am J Clin Nutr 1996;63(suppl):437S-41S.
36. Carroll KK: Obesity as a risk factor for certain types of cancer. Lipids 1998;33:1055-1059.
37. Reaven GM: Role of insulin resistance in human disease (syndrome X): an expanded definition. Annu Rev Med 1993;44:121-131.
38. Buchwald H, Avidor Y, Braunwald E, et al: Surgery: a systematic review and meta-analysis. JAMA 2004;292:1724-1737.
39. Buchwald H, Varco RL, Matts JP, et al: Effect of partial ileal bypass surgery on mortality and morbidity from coronary heart disease in patients with hypercholesterolemia. Report of the Program on the Surgical Control of the Hyperlipidemias (POSCH). N Engl J Med 1990;323:946-955.
40. Buchwald H, Matts JP, Fitch LL, et al: Changes in sequential coronary arteriograms and subsequent coronary events. JAMA 1992;268:1429-1433.
41. Buchwald H, Williams SE, Matts JP, et al: Overall mortality in the Program on the Surgical Control of the Hyperlipidemias. J Am Coll Surg 2002;195:327-331.
42. Brolin RE, Kenler HA, Wilson AC, et al: Serum lipids after gastric bypass surgery for morbid obesity. Int J Obes 1990;14:939-950.
43. Buffington CK, Cowan GSM, Hughes TA, et al: Significant changes in the lipid-lipoprotein status of premenopausal morbidly obese females following gastric bypass surgery. Obes Surg 1994;4:328-335.
44. Cowan GSM Jr, Buffington CK: Significant changes in blood pressure, glucose, and lipids with gastric bypass surgery. World J Surg 1998;232:987-992.
45. Schauer PR, Ikramuddin S, Gourash W, et al: Outcomes after laparoscopic Roux-en-Y gastric bypass for morbid obesity. Ann Surg 2000;232:515-529.
46. Alpert AM, Lambert CR, Terry BE, et al: Effect of weight loss on left ventricular mass in nonhypertensive morbidly obese patients. Am J Cardiol 1994;73:918.
47. Reisen E, Frohlich ED, Messerli FH, et al: Cardiovascular changes after weight reduction in obesity hypertension. Ann Intern Med 1983;98:315-319.
48. Karason K, Wallentin I, Larsson B, et al: Effects of obesity and weight loss on left ventricular mass and relative wall thickness: survey and intervention study. BMJ 1997;315:912-916.
49. Karason K, Wallentin I, Larsson B, et al: Effects of obesity and weight loss on cardiac function and valvular performance. Obes Res 1998;6:422-429.
50. Shiffman ML, Sugerman HJ, Kellum JM, et al: Gallstone formation following rapid weight loss. I. Incidence of gallstone formation and relation to gallbladder (GB) bile lipid composition. Gastroenterology 1990:90:A262 (abstract).
51. Shiffman ML, Sugerman HJ, Kellum JM, et al: Gallstone formation after rapid weight loss: a prospective study in patients undergoing gastric bypass surgery for treatment of morbid obesity. Am J Gastroenterol 1991;86:1000-1005.
52. Worobetz LJ, Inglis FG, Shaffer EA: The effect of ursodeoxycholic acid therapy on gallstone formation in the morbidly obese during rapid weight loss. Am J Gastroenterol 1993;88:1705-1710.
53. Smith SC, Edwards CB, Goodman GN: Symptomatic and clinical improvement in morbidly obese patients with gastroesophageal

reflux disease following Roux-en-Y gastric bypass. Obes Surg 1997;7:479-484.

54. Jones KB: Roux-en-Y gastric bypass: an effective anti-reflux procedure in the less than morbidly obese. Obes Surg 1998;8:35-38.

55. Balsiger BM, Murr MM, Mai J, et al: Gastroesophageal reflux after intact vertical banded gastroplasty: correction by conversion to Roux-en-Y gastric bypass. J Gastrointest Surg 2000;4:276-281.

56. Sugerman HJ, Felton WL 3rd, Sismanis A, et al: Gastric surgery for pseudotumor cerebri associated with severe obesity. Ann Surg 1999;229:634-640.

57. Bump RC, Sugerman HJ, Fanti JA, et al: Obesity and lower urinary tract function in women: effect of surgically induced weight loss. Am J Obstet Gynecol 1992;167:392-397.

58. Sugerman H, Windsor A, Bessos M: Effects of surgically induced weight loss on urinary bladder pressure, sagittal abdominal diameter and obesity co-morbidity. Int J Obes Relat Metab Disord 1998;22:230-235.

59. Pasquali R, Vicennati V, Scopinaro N, et al: Achievement of near-normal body weight as the prerequisite to normalize sex hormone-binding globulin concentrations in massively obese men. Int J Obes 1997;21:1-5.

60. Bull RH, Legorreta G: Outcome of gastric surgery for morbid obesity: weight changes and personality traits. Psychother Psychosom 1991;56:146-156.

61. Larsen F: Psychosocial function before and after gastric banding surgery for morbid obesity: a prospective psychiatric study. Acta Psychiatr Scand 1990; 359(suppl):1-57.

62. Wadden TA, Sarwer DB, Arnold ME, et al: Psychosocial status of severely obese patients before and after bariatric surgery. Probl Gen Surg 2000;13-22.

63. Isacsson A, Frederiksen SG, Nilsson P, et al: Quality of life after gastroplasty is normal: a controlled study. Eur J Surg 1997;163:181-186.

64. Karlsson J, Sjostrom L, Sullivan M: Swedish Obese Subjects (SOS)—an intervention study of obesity: two-year follow-up of health-related quality of life HRQL and eating behavior after gastric surgery for severe obesity. Int J Obes Relat Metab Disord 1998;22:113-126.

65. Van Gemert WG, Adang EM, Greve JW, et al: Quality of life assessment of morbidly obese patients: effect of weight-reducing surgery. Am J Clin Nutr 1998;67:197-201.

66. Dymek MP, Le Grange D, Neven K, et al: Quality of life and psychosocial adjustment in patients after Roux-en-Y gastric bypass: a brief report. Obes Surg 2001;11:32-39.

67. Dixon JB, O'Brien PE: Changes in comorbidities and improvements in quality of life after LAP-BAND placement. Am J Surg 2002;184:51S-54S.

68. Oria HE, Moorehead MK: Bariatric analysis and reporting outcome system (BAROS). Obes Surg 1998;8:487-499 (comment).

6

Longevity and Obesity

Jarl S. Torgerson, M.D., Ph.D. and Erik Näslund, M.D., Ph.D.

The mortality issue is so central in the field of obesity that the World Health Organization's body mass index (BMI) classification is based primarily on the association of obesity with mortality.[1] This does not imply, however, that there are no mortality-related controversies or scientific problems still to be solved. In this chapter, we discuss total- and specific-cause mortality in the obese, as well as the ambiguous effects of weight loss on obesity-related mortality.

▶ MORTALITY IN THE OBESE

Hippocrates stated that the obese suffer a greater risk of sudden death than the lean. In contemporary medicine, insurance statistics and actuarial data were the first to indicate that obesity is associated with a higher level of early mortality.[2] Several large prospective epidemiologic studies confirmed this and have repeatedly shown an increased total early mortality rate in the obese, as well as a greater number of deaths resulting from diabetes, cardiovascular disease, and cancer.[1-3] Typically, a BMI of 35 kg per m^2 is associated with approximately a doubling of all-cause mortality, which was illustrated by American Cancer Society data on 750,000 men and women (Fig. 6-1). Coronary heart disease was the major killer in both overweight and obese subjects. Mortality due to cancer and diabetes was also significantly more common.[4,5]

Another way of quantifying the effects of obesity on mortality is to calculate the expected number of years of life lost (YLL). YLL refers to the difference between the number of years an individual would be expected to live if not obese and the number of years he or she would be expected to live if obese. Figure 6-2 demonstrates YLL in white men and women in various BMI and age groups as compared to those with a BMI of 24 kg per m^2. There is a gradual buildup in YLL with increasing BMI in both men and women. In men, there seems to be a substantial age-related variability (i.e., young men have more YLL than do older men in the same BMI range). This is especially evident among the severely obese.[6]

The number of deaths attributable to overweight and obesity can be estimated also at the societal level.

Allison and colleagues used data from six U.S. studies and estimated that approximately 280,000 deaths per year of U.S. adults were related to overweight and obesity. More than 80% of the obesity-attributable deaths were seen in subjects with BMIs of 30 kg per m^2 or higher.[7] Recently it has been estimated that each year at least 1 in 13 deaths in the European Union is likely to be related to obesity.[8]

Although the association between being overweight or obese and increased mortality rates is unequivocal, the nature of the relationship in the lower BMI range has been much debated. The question is whether the overall relationship between BMI and mortality is J-shaped (as in Fig. 6-1), U-shaped, or linear. In short, is low BMI associated with increasing or monotonically decreasing mortality rates? Several investigators have addressed this issue and discussed in great detail the methodologic aspects and possible confounding factors. Important elements include sample size, length of follow-up, excluding or not excluding early mortality, controlling for smoking, inappropriately controlling for intermediate risk factors (e.g., hypertension and diabetes), as well as the importance of body-fat distribution. A detailed discussion of these aspects goes beyond the scope of this chapter; the interested reader is referred to comprehensive reviews.[2,9-11] However, a recent summary of available data concluded that a vast majority of studies showed a J- or U-shaped relationship between BMI and mortality.[11]

Age has been found to have an effect on excess mortality rates in the obese. In general, the relatively higher mortality rates seen with increasing BMIs are attenuated with increasing age.[6,11,12] Ethnic backgrounds other than Caucasian have also been found to modify the general relationship between obesity and mortality. It seems that increasing BMI is less detrimental in African-Americans than in European-Americans.[11] Figure 6-2 shows YLL in whites. The pattern found in black Americans differed somewhat; the life expectancy was not reduced until the BMI exceeded 37 kg per m^2 in women and 32 kg per m^2 in men. Whether this ethnic distinction is related to differing effects of BMI on mortality or to differences in other mortality-related factors, such as general health or socioeconomic status, is not known.[6]

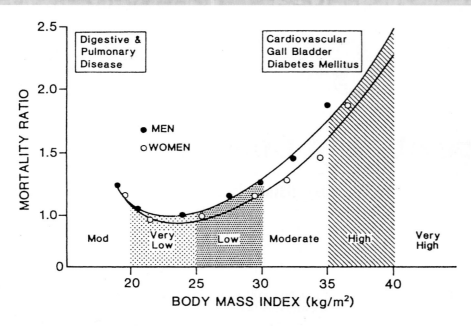

Figure 6-1. Mortality ratios for men and women at different levels of BMI. (From Lew EA, Garfinkel L: Variations in mortality by weight among 750,000 men and women. J Chron Dis 1979;32:563-576.)

Actuarial data from the late 19th century showed an increased mortality rate in men with abdominal obesity.[13] Swedish population studies have since demonstrated that increasing waist-to-hip ratio is associated with increasing total mortality rates as well as with increased risk for cardio-vascular disease in both men and women.[14,15] Data from the Iowa Women's Health Study have also shown a positive association between waist-to-hip ratio and total mortality rates.[16]

A recent analysis of data from the Lipid Research Clinics Study looked at fitness and fatness as predictors of mortality in middle-aged men and women. Using the "fit, not-fat" groups as references, the adjusted hazard ratios for all-cause mortality were highest in the "unfit, fat" groups (1.57 and 1.49 in women and men, respectively). The corresponding figures were 1.32 and 1.44 in the fit but fat groups and 1.30 and 1.25 in the unfit but not-fat groups, respectively. It is interesting to note that women who were

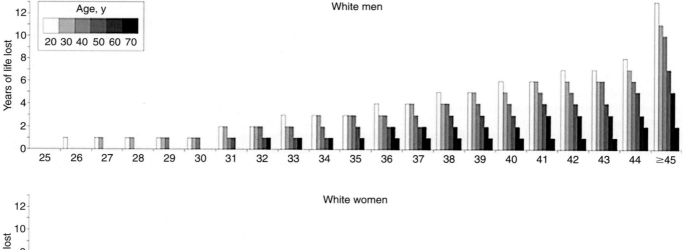

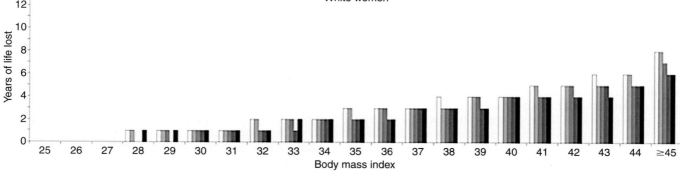

Figure 6-2. Years of life lost among white U.S. men and women. (Reprinted with permission from Fontaine KR, Redden DT, Wang C, et al: Years of life lost due to obesity. JAMA 2003;289:187-193.)

fit and fat seemed to have a mortality risk equal to that of unfit but not-fat women.[17]

Weight Loss and Mortality

Not only obesity but also weight gain during adulthood is related to an increase in mortality rates. Data from the Nurses' Health Study showed that women experiencing a weight gain of 10 to 20 kg had a relative risk (adjusted for age and baseline BMI) of having coronary heart disease (fatal and nonfatal) of 1.7 compared to women who gained less than 3 kg. The corresponding relative risk for women gaining 20 to 35 kg was 2.5.[18] More puzzling is that several epidemiologic studies indicate that weight loss is also associated with an increased risk for mortality.[19] Data from the first National Health and Nutrition Examination Survey (NHANES I) showed an increased mortality rate following weight loss, especially in women and also in subjects that were overweight or obese at baseline.[20,21]

From the perspective of mortality, there are data in the literature indicating that obesity, weight gain, and also weight loss are associated with an increased risk for mortality. This is paradoxical because it is well known that weight loss decreases risk factors for cardiovascular disease (e.g., blood pressure, blood glucose, and lipid levels). Furthermore, reduced energy intake, which is a cornerstone of obesity treatment, extends life span in all investigated species.[22] There are, however, some clinical trials indicating that dietary change and weight reduction might reduce cardiovascular risk factors and decrease mortality after myocardial infarction.[23]

Several explanations for the obesity-weight change-mortality paradox have been brought forward. Most observational studies have not paid any attention to whether the observed weight loss was intentional or unintentional. This is problematic because intentional and unintentional weight loss occur at a similar frequency and because unintentional weight loss is related to known risk factors such as age, poor health status, and smoking.[24,25] The relationship between mortality and intentional and unintentional weight loss has been analyzed separately in some studies. Data from the Iowa Women's Health Study showed that unintentional weight loss increases both total and cardiovascular mortality, especially in women with preexisting disease. Intentional weight loss, on the other hand, did not affect the total mortality risk negatively.[26] Results from the Cancer Prevention Study I showed a reduction in mortality (total, cardiovascular, and diabetic) following intentional weight loss in women with obesity-related disorders, whereas the findings in women without preexisting illness were more equivocal.[27] Corresponding data in men showed that intentional weight loss in healthy men generally did not affect mortality. In men with preexisting nondiabetic illness, intentional weight loss did not affect total or cardiovascular mortality, whereas diabetes-related mortality was substantially reduced.[28]

Data on overweight and obese subjects with diabetes have shown that intentional weight loss reduces total mortality by 25%. An intentional weight reduction of 10 to 15 kg was associated with the largest mortality reduction (33%).[29] Recent U.S. data from the National Health Interview Survey on 6391 individuals with BMIs of 25 kg per m[2] or more found a lower mortality rate in subjects intentionally losing weight than in weight-stable subjects not trying to lose any weight. Furthermore, unintentional weight loss was associated with a substantial increase in the likelihood of mortality.[30]

Another explanation for the paradox could be that the beneficial effects of weight loss on cardiovascular risk factors are generally reported in short-term clinical trials (less than 2 years), whereas studying the effects on mortality rates and other hard end points requires much longer observation periods. This is especially important because some obesity-related risk factors and disorders tend to relapse over time in spite of weight-loss maintenance. Data from the Swedish Obese Subjects (SOS) study showed highly significant reductions in the incidence of diabetes 2 and 8 years after bariatric surgery, but the 2-year reduction in hypertension was not maintained after 8 years, in spite of sustained weight losses of 16.5% (20 ± 16 kg).[31] It could also be that weight loss, or loss of lean body mass, is related to an increased likelihood of mortality, whereas loss of body fat reduces the mortality risk.[32] There are also reports indicating inadequate nutrient intake during weight reduction, which in turn could increase cardiovascular risk factors.[33]

In an attempt to shed light on the enigmatic relationship between weight loss and mortality, the SOS study was initiated in 1987. SOS consists of a registry study of 6328 individuals and an intervention study of 4047 individuals. The registry study is in essence a cross-sectional health examination focusing on medical history, cardiovascular risk factors, anthropometry, diet, health-related quality of life, health economy, and genetics. The registry study also serves as a requirement base for the subsequent intervention. In the intervention study, 2010 obese patients underwent surgery (gastric banding, vertical bandedgastroplasty, or gastric bypass), and 2037 subjects receive conventional nonsurgical treatment in primary health care. All patients will be followed for 20 years. The main question of the intervention study is whether intentional weight loss reduces total mortality rates. Secondary aims include determining the effects of weight loss on specific morbidity and mortality rates, on cardiovascular risk factors, on health-related quality of life, and on health economy. The details and results of the SOS study have been summarized elsewhere.[34,35]

Cardiovascular Disease and Mortality

Obesity is a major contributor to the global prevalence of cardiovascular disease. In terms of disability-adjusted life years, ischemic heart disease is indeed thought to become the leading cause of the global disease burden in 2020.[36]

A 26-year follow-up of participants in the Framingham Heart Study found that obesity was a significant predictor of cardiovascular disease, independent of age, serum cholesterol levels, glucose intolerance, systolic blood pressure, smoking, and left ventricular hypertrophy.[37] Being obese, but not overweight, is significantly associated with myocardial infarction and fatal coronary events. The obese are also more likely to have additional risk factors, such as hypertension, high cholesterol levels, type 2 diabetes, and left ventricular hypertrophy, and are smokers.

Obesity is thus related to a cluster of risk factors influencing cardiovascular morbidity and mortality.[38] There is ample evidence suggesting that the presence of central obesity is an independent predictor of cardiovascular disease because these patients have disturbances in insulin and glucose homeostasis, elevated triglycerides, low high-density lipoprotein cholesterol levels, and increased low-density lipoprotein cholesterol. This risk factor profile is also associated with a prothrombotic and inflammatory state. Thus, the abdominally obese patient is characterized by an atherogenic, prothrombotic, and inflammatory profile that increases the risk for acute coronary syndrome and subsequent death.[39] Obesity is often associated with advanced atherosclerosis. A postmortem examination of coronary arteries of individuals 15 to 34 years of age who had died of accidental injury, suicide, or homicide showed that the degree of atherosclerosis in the right coronary artery was associated with obesity, especially in cases of central body-fat distribution.[40] Indeed, at one cardiac catheterization unit, the number of obese patients increased from 20% to 33% over a 10-year period.[41]

Recently, data from the National Health Interview Survey was used to study the relationship between obesity and overall mortality as well as to study mortality resulting from circulatory disease and diabetes among U.S. adults.[42] The study included 647,015 individuals who were followed for 8 years. A more U-shaped relationship was found between overall mortality and obesity, whereas a J-shaped relationship was observed between mortality due to circulatory disease and obesity, with an increased risk of fatal circulatory disease for all categories of BMI above 30 kg per m[2] (Table 6-1).

Diabetes and Mortality

Patients with type 2 diabetes have an increased risk for cardiovascular morbidity, renal failure, blindness, and death. There is a twofold to fivefold increase in the risk for coronary heart disease and stroke. In the United States, diabetes is the seventh underlying cause of death.[43]

The risk for developing type 2 diabetes increases with increasing BMI, and 90% of patients with type 2 diabetes are either overweight or obese. The global prevalence of diabetes among adults was 143 million in 1997. The number of afflicted is estimated to have been 154 million in 2000 and to become 300 million in 2025.[36] A recent telephone survey in the United States found that the prevalence of obesity had increased by 5.6% between 2000 and 2001. The corresponding increase in the prevalence of diabetes was 8.2%.[44] Against this background, an increasing number of diabetes-related deaths might be expected. A recent publication by Rogers and colleagues demonstrated that a patient with a BMI of 40 kg per m[2] had an almost nine times higher risk of dying of diabetes than did subjects of normal weight (see Table 6-1).[42]

Obstructive Sleep Apnea and Mortality

Obstructive sleep apnea (OSA) is an underrecognized disorder in the obese. Patients with OSA have impaired performance in tasks requiring divided attention as well as in cognitive function. Increasing severity of OSA results in

| Table 6-1 | **HAZARD RATIOS FOR OVERALL MORTALITY, MORTALITY CAUSED BY CIRCULATORY DISEASE AND BY DIABETES, BY BMI IN THE UNITED STATES** |

	OVERALL MORTALITY	CIRCULATORY DISEASE MORTALITY	DIABETES MORTALITY
BMI ≥40	1.77*	2.37*	8.97*
BMI 35.0 - ≤40	1.34*	1.78*	4.70*
BMI 30.0 - ≤35	1.01	1.27*	2.82*
BMI 25 - ≤30	0.87*	0.99	1.65*
BMI 18.5 - ≤25	Reference	Reference	Reference
BMI ≤18.5	1.91*	1.57*	1.02

(Based on Rogers RC, Hummer RA, Krueger PM: The effect of diabetes on overall circulatory disease and diabetes-specific mortality. J Biosoc Sci 2003; 35:107-129. By permission.)

*$P \leq 0.01$; n = 647,015; overall mortality, n = 47,271; circulatory disease mortality, n = 19,929; diabetes mortality, n = 1209.

higher blood pressure, independent of age and obesity. In addition, OSA is associated with a reduced nocturnal drop in blood pressure and this "nondipping" is associated with stroke and left ventricular hypertrophy, independent of daytime blood pressure.[45] OSA carries an increased risk for cardiovascular disease and an increased likelihood of mortality.[46]

Cancer and Mortality

There is a well-established relationship between obesity and cancer. The 1979 American Cancer Society data on 750,000 individuals who were followed for 12 years revealed that men and women who were at least 40% overweight were 33% and 55% more likely, respectively, to die from cancer than their lean counterparts.[4] Similarly, the Nurses' Health Study demonstrated that cancer mortality rose with increasing BMI. The death rate from cancer for women with BMIs of at least 32 kg per m[2] was twice that for women with BMIs of less than 19 kg per m[2].[10] Further evidence for an association between obesity and cancer mortality was recently presented in a prospective study of more than 900,000 U.S. adults. In this cohort, subjects with BMIs greater than 40 kg per m[2] had death rates from all cancers combined that were 52% and 62% higher for men and women, respectively, as compared to normal-weight men and women. In both men and women, BMI was significantly associated with increased death rates due to cancer of the colon and rectum, liver, gallbladder, lung, pancreas, and kidney. In men, an increased risk for death from stomach and prostate cancer was observed as was a higher risk for breast, uterine, cervical, and ovarian cancer in women (Table 6-2). Based on these data and the foregoing data, it is estimated that obesity accounts for 14% and 20% of all deaths in men and women, respectively, in the United States. This indicates that more than 90,000 deaths per year from cancer might be avoided if everyone in the adult population could maintain a BMI of less than 25 kg per m[2] throughout his or her lifetime.[47]

Table 6-2 — RELATIVE RISKS FOR MORTALITY DUE TO SELECTED FORMS OF CANCER ACCORDING TO BMI AMONG MEN AND WOMEN IN THE CANCER PREVENTION STUDY II, 1982-1998

TYPE OF CANCER	MEN						WOMEN					
BMI	18.5-24.9	25-29.9	30-34.9	35-39.9	≥40	P OF TREND	18.5-24.9	25-29.9	30-34.9	35-29.9	≥40	P OF TREND
All	1.00	0.97 (0.94-0.99)	1.09 (1.05-1.14)	1.20 (1.08-1.34)	1.52 (1.13-2.05)	0.001	1.00	1.08 (1.05-1.11)	1.23 (1.18-1.29)	1.32 (1.20-1.44)	1.62 (1.40-1.87)	<0.001
Esophageal	1.00	1.15 (0.99-1.32)	1.28 (1.00-1.63)	1.63 (0.95-2.80)		0.008	1.00	1.20 (0.86-1.66)	1.39 (0.86-2.25)			0.13
Stomach	1.00	1.01 (0.88-1.16)	1.20 (0.94-1.52)	1.94 (1.21-3.13)		0.03	1.00	0.89 (0.72-1.09)	1.30 (0.97-1.74)	1.08 (0.61-1.89)		0.46
Colorectal	1.00	1.20 (1.12-1.30)	1.47 (1.30-1.66)	1.84 (1.39-2.41)		<0.001	1.00	1.10 (1.01-1.19)	1.33 (1.17-1.51)	1.36 (1.06-1.74)	1.46 (0.95-2-24)	<0.001
Liver	1.00	1.13 (0.94-1.34)	1.90 (1.46-2.47)	4.52 (2.94-6.94)		<0.001	1.00	1.02 (0.80-1.31)	1.40 (0.97-1.20)	1.68 (0.93-3.05)		0.04
Gallbladder	1.00	1.34 (0.97-1.84)	1.76 (1.06-2.94)			0.02	1.00	1.12 (0.86-1.47)	2.13 (1.56-2.90)			<0.001
Pancreatic	1.00	1.13 (1.03-1.25)	1.41 (1.19-1.66)	1.49 (0.99-2.22)		<0.001	1.00	1.11 (1.00-1.24)	1.28 (1.07-1.52)	1.41 (1.01-1.99)	2.76 (1.74-4.36)	<0.001
Lung	1.00	0.78 (0.75-0.82)	0.79 (0.73-0.86)	0.67 (0.54-0.84)		<0.001	1.00	0.88 (0.83-0.94)	0.82 (0.72-0.92)	0.66 (0.50-0.86)	0.81 (0.52-1.28)	<0.001
Kidney	1.00	1.18 (1.02-1.37)	1.36 (1.06-1.74)	1.70 (0.99-2.92)		0.002	1.00	1.33 (1.08-1.63)	1.66 (1.23-2.24)	1.70 (0.94-3.05)	4.75 (2.50-9.04)	<0.001
Prostate	1.00	1.08 (1.01-1.15)	1.20 (1.06-1.36)	1.34 (0.98-1.83)		<0.001						
Breast							1.00	1.34 (1.23-1.46)	1.63 (1.44-1.85)	1.70 (1.33-2.17)	2.12 (1.41-3.19)	<0.001
Uterus							1.00	1.50 (1.26-1.78)	2.53 (2.02-3.18)	2.77 (1.83-4.18)	6.25 (3.75-10.42)	<0.001
Cervical							1.00	1.38 (0.97-1.96)	1.23 (0.71-2.13)	3.20 (1.77-5.78)		0.001
Ovarian							1.00	1.15 (1.02-1.29)	1.16 (0.96-1.40)	1.51 (1.12-2.02)		0.001

(Based on data from Calle EE, Rodriguez C, Walker-Thurmond K, et al: Overweight, obesity and mortality from cancer in a prospectively studied cohort of U.S. adults. N Engl J Med 2003;348:1625-1638.) Relative risk (95% CI)

Mortality and Obesity in the Young

During the past decades, the number of overweight children has increased rapidly in the United States. In 1983, 18.6% of preschool children were overweight, and 8.5% obese; whereas, in the year 2000, 22% of preschool children were overweight and 10% were obese.[48] In the wake of this increase in childhood obesity, obesity-related disorders such as type 2 diabetes and hypertension are also increasing in the young. It has been estimated that the annual obesity-related hospital costs in 6- to 17-year-olds in the United States has reached $127 million per year.[49]

Few studies have examined the effect of childhood obesity on mortality. In one study of 508 lean or overweight adolescents (13 to 18 years old) followed for 55 years, it was shown that overweight during adolescence was associated with an increased risk for mortality from all causes as well as increased disease-specific mortality among men, but not women. The relative risk for death was 1.8 (CI = 1.2-2.7, $P = 0.004$) for mortality from all causes and 2.3 (CI = 1.4-4.1, $P = 0.002$) for mortality from coronary heart disease in men. No comparable association was found in women.[50] In addition, it seems that even a moderately increased body weight during adolescence is associated with a higher mortality rate in adulthood. Men 18 years old with BMIs of more than 25 kg per m² who were followed for 32 years had increased mortality rates from all causes and from coronary heart disease.[51] In a Swedish study of 504 obese children, a 40-year follow-up demonstrated a higher rate of mortality and morbidity than in reference subjects. The average age was 41.3 years in the 55 subjects who died.[52]

▶ REFERENCES

1. World Health Organization: Obesity: Preventing and Managing the Global Epidemic. WHO Technical Report Series 894. Geneva, WHO, 2000.
2. Sjöström LV: Mortality of severely obese subjects. Am J Clin Nutr 1992;55:516S-523S.
3. Solomon CG, Manson JE: Obesity and mortality: a review of the epidemiologic data. Am J Clin Nutr 1997;66:1044S-1050S.
4. Lew EA, Garfinkel L: Variations in mortality by weight among 750 000 men and women. J Chron Dis 1979;32:563-576.
5. Gray DS: Diagnosis and prevalence of obesity. In Bray GA (ed): The Medical Clinics of North America, pp. 1-13. Philadelphia, W.B. Saunders, 1989.
6. Fontaine KR, Redden DT, Wang C, et al: Years of life lost due to obesity. JAMA 2003;289:187-193.
7. Allison DB, Fontaine KR, Manson JE, et al: Annual deaths attributable to obesity in the United States. JAMA 1999;282:1530-1538.
8. Banegas JR, Lopez-Garcia E, Gutierrez-Fisac JL, et al: A simple estimate of mortality attributable to excess weight in the European Union. Eur J Clin Nutr 2003;57:201-208.
9. Troiano RP, Frongillo Jr EA, Sobal J, et al: The relationship between body weight and mortality: a quantitative analysis of combined information from existing studies. Int J Obes 1996;20:63-75.
10. Manson JE, Willett WC, Stampfer MJ, et al: Body weight and mortality among women. N Engl J Med 1995;333:677-685.
11. Allison DB, Heo M, Fontaine KR, et al: Body weight, body composition and longevity. In Björntorp P (ed): International Textbook of Obesity, pp. 31-48. Chichester, UK, John Wiley, 2001.
12. Bender R, Jöckel KH, Trautner C, et al: Effect of age on excess mortality in obesity. JAMA 1999;281:1498-1504.
13. Kahn HS, Williamson DF: Abdominal obesity and mortality risk among men in nineteenth-century North America. Int J Obes 1994;18:686-691.
14. Lapidus L, Bengtsson C, Larsson B, et al: Distribution of adipose tissue and risk of cardiovascular disease and death: a 12-year follow-up of participants in the population study of women in Gothenburg, Sweden. BMJ 1984;289:1257-1261.
15. Larsson B, Svärdsudd K, Welin L, et al: Abdominal adipose tissue distribution, obesity, and risk of cardiovascular disease and death: 13 year follow up of participants in the study of men born 1913. BMJ 1984;288:1401-1404.
16. Folsom AR, Kaye SA, Sellers TA, et al: Body fat distribution and 5-year risk of death in older women. JAMA 1993;269:483-487.
17. Stevens J, Cai J, Evenson KR, et al: Fitness and fatness as predictors of mortality from all causes and from cardiovascular disease in men and women in the Lipid Research Clinics Study. Am J Epidemiol 2002;156:832-841.
18. Manson JE, Colditz GA, Stampfer MJ, et al: A prospective study of obesity and risk of coronary disease in women. N Engl J Med 1990;322:882-889.
19. Khaodhiar L, Blackburn GL: Health benefits and risks of weight loss. In Björntorp P (ed): International Textbook of Obesity, pp. 413-439. Chichester, UK, John Wiley, 2001.
20. Pamuk ER, Williamson DF, Madans J, et al: Weight loss and mortality in a national cohort of adults 1971-1987. Am J Epidemiol 1992;136:686-697.
21. Pamuk ER, Williamson DF, Serdula MK, et al: Weight loss and subsequent death in a cohort of U.S. adults. Ann Intern Med 1993;119:744-748.
22. Walford RL, Harris SB, Weindruch R: Dietary restriction and aging: historical phases, mechanisms and current directions. J Nutr 1987;117:1650-1654.
23. Singh RB, Rastogi SS, Verma R, et al: Randomised controlled trail of cardioprotective diet in patients with recent myocardial infarction: results of one year follow up. BMJ 1992;304:1015-1019.
24. Meltzer AA, Everhart JE: Unintentional weight loss in the United States. Am J Epidemiol 1995;142:1039-1046.
25. Williamson DF: Intentional weight loss: patterns in the general population and its association with morbidity and mortality. Int J Obes 1997;21 (suppl 1):S14-S19.
26. French SA, Folsom AR, Jeffery RW, et al: Prospective study of intentionality of weight loss and mortality in older women: the Iowa women's health study. Am J Epidemiol 1999;149:504-514.
27. Williamson DF, Pamuk ER, Thun M, et al: Prospective study of intentional weight loss and mortality in never-smoking overweight US white women aged 40-64 years. Am J Epidemiol 1995;141:1128-1141.
28. Williamson DF, Pamuk ER, Thun M, et al: Prospective study of intentional weight loss and mortality in overweight white men aged 40-64 years. Am J Epidemiol 1999;149:491-503.
29. Williamson DF, Thompson TJ, Thun M, et al: Intentional weight loss and mortality among overweight individuals with diabetes. Diabetes Care 2000;23:1499-1504.
30. Gregg EW, Gerzoff RB, Thompson TJ, et al: Intentional weight loss and death in overweight and obese U.S. adults 35 years of age and older. Ann Intern Med 2003;138:383-389.
31. Sjöström CD, Peltonen M, Wedel H, et al: Differentiated long-term effects of intentional weight loss on diabetes and hypertension. Hypertension 2000;36:20-25.
32. Allison DB, Zannolli R, Faith MS, et al: Weight loss increases and fat loss decreases all-cause mortality rates: results from two independent cohort studies. Int J Obes 1999;23:603-611.
33. Borson-Chazot F, Harthe C, Teboul F, et al: Occurrence of hyperhomocysteinemia 1 year after gastroplasty for severe obesity. J Clin Endocrinol Metab 1999;84:541-545.
34. Sjöström L, Larsson B, Backman L, et al: Swedish Obese Subjects (SOS): recruitment for an intervention study and selected description of the obese state. Int J Obes 1992;16:465-479.
35. Sjöström L: Surgical intervention as a strategy for treatment of obesity. Endocrine 2000;13:213-230.
36. Kumanyika S, Jeffery RW, Morabia A, et al: Obesity prevention: the case for action. Int J Obes 2002;26:425-436.
37. Hubert HB, Feinleib M, McNamara PM, et al: Obesity as an independent risk factor for cardiovascular disease: a 26-year follow-up of participants in the Framingham Heart Study. Circulation 1983;67:968-977.
38. Kannel WB, Wilson PWF, Nam B, et al: Risk stratification of obesity as a coronary risk factor. Am J Cardiol 2002;90:697-701.
39. Grundy SM: Obesity, metabolic syndrome, and coronary atherosclerosis. Circulation 2002;105:2696-2698.

40. McGill HCJ, McMahan CA, Herderick EE, et al: Obesity accelerates the progression of coronary atherosclerosis in young men. Circulation 2002;105:2696-2698.
41. Eisenstein EL, Shaw LK, Nelson CL, et al: Obesity and long-term clinical and economic outcomes in coronary artery disease patients. Obes Res 2002;10:83-91.
42. Rogers RC, Hummer RA, Krueger PM: The effect of obesity on overall, circulatory disease- and diabetes-specific mortality. J Biosoc Sci 2003;35:107-129.
43. Harris MI, Eastman RC: Early detection of undiagnosed diabetes mellitus: a US perspective. Diabetes Metab Res Rev 2000;16:230-236.
44. Mokdad AH, Ford ES, Bowman BA, et al: Prevalence of obesity, diabetes, and obesity-related health factors, 2001. JAMA 2003;289:76-79.
45. Pankow W, Nabe B, Lies A, et al: Influence of sleep apnea on 24-hour blood pressure. Chest 1997;112:1253-1258.
46. He J, Kryger MH, Zorick FJ, et al: Mortality and apnea index in obstructive sleep apnea: experience in 385 male patients. Chest 1988;97:27-32.
47. Calle EE, Rodriguez C, Walker-Thurmond K, et al: Overweight, obesity, and mortality from cancer in a prospectively studied cohort of U.S. adults. N Engl J Med 2003;348:1625-1638.
48. Deckelbaum RJ, Williams CL: Childhood obesity: the health issue. Obes Res 2001;9:239S-243S.
49. Goran MI, Ball GDC, Cruz ML: Cardiovascular endocrinology 2: obesity and risk of type 2 diabetes and cardiovascular disease in children and adolescents. J Clin Endocrinol Metab 2003;88:1417-1427.
50. Must A, Jacques PF, Dallal GE, et al: Long-term morbidity and mortality of overweight adolescents: a follow-up of the Harvard Growth Study of 1922-1935. N Engl J Med 1992;327:1350-1355.
51. Hoffmans MDAF, Kromhout D, de Lezenne Coulander C: The impact of body mass index of 78612 Dutch men on 32-year mortality. J Clin Epidemiol 1988;41:749-756.
52. Mossberg H-O: 40-year follow-up of overweight children. Lancet 1989;2:491-493.

7

Social Implications of Obesity

Emanuel Hell, M.D., and Karl Miller, M.D.

Corpulence has been viewed in various ways during the past millennium. It was considered to be an expression of prosperity and a symbol of fertility in women. This concept has survived until the present day in some cultures. However, until the middle of the last century, only a small number of individuals were able to consume a hypercaloric diet over the long term. For approximately the past two generations, affordable food has been readily available to large segments of the population. The result has been a marked and, in part, extreme weight increase in many populations, not only in industrialized society but also in developing countries (e.g., Latin America, Asia, and Africa). Obesity, thus, has become a global problem with health-related economic and social implications.[1,2]

We are living in an age during which the anorexic model is stylized as an ideal of beauty, which necessarily excludes the obese from experiencing a sense of public acceptance. Ironically, the food industry makes every effort to promote the consumption of food, a lure to which children, apparently, are most susceptible. The incidence of obesity among North American children has more than doubled over the past 25 years; 20% of children are now obese.[3-6]

In addition, video games, computers, and a reduced level of commitment to physical education and sports in many schools have diminished the level of physical activity of the current generation of children. Children have come to rely on vehicular transportation to an increasing extent. Adolescents and adults are exposed to greater availability of high-fat and high-carbohydrate low-nutrient foods, fast-food restaurants, and supersized portions. Ubiquitous temptations are major contributors to this new disease. Genetic factors are important, but the rapid increase in obesity has occurred in too short a time to be explained adequately by a significant genetic change.

Many physicians today consider obesity a purely self-incurred disease arising from overindulgence due to moral weakness. This disrespectful, inaccurate and, thus, untenable viewpoint renders their treatment efforts meaningless. Physicians are also products of our culture, and they share in the responsibility for nurturing an obesity paradigm. Obese persons are regularly confronted with these prejudices, the social implications of which are manifold. To better understand these interactions it is important to be familiar with the social characteristics surrounding obesity.

▶ SELF-PERCEIVED CHARACTERISTICS OF MORBIDLY OBESE INDIVIDUALS

Body Perception in Morbid Obesity

We interviewed and tested 410 persons (338 female, 72 male) within a body mass index (BMI) range of 19 to 40 kg per m^2. We asked the following questions: How do you feel about yourself? How would you like yourself to be? How do you feel others look at you? Who feels most comfortable about himself/herself? On a body-perception scale showing human figures of varying corpulence, the test persons marked their personal impressions.[7] It was found that with reference to the questions How do you feel about yourself? and How do you feel others look at you? the size of the corpulent figures was highly significantly correlated with the BMI. In other words, the objective BMI value is perceived in a very realistic way by obese individuals. The relatively large perceived difference between normal weight and overweight was remarkable. This finding reflects the social ideal of slimness.

In response to the question Who feels most comfortable about himself/herself? there was no correlation with the BMI, but there were significant differences in the distribution of BMI in the five groups of normal weight, overweight, and grade 1 to grade 3 obesity. This finding is of practical interest. It would be incorrect to assume that persons with obesity problems entertain desires and expectations in keeping with their current figures, or even that they share the mental concepts of persons of normal weight or pursue a homogeneous ideal. The responses to the question How would you like yourself to be? revealed no significant differences. There was uniform agreement among persons of all weight categories in respect to the general ideal of slimness.

Stigmatization

The type and intensity of perceived stigmatization were questioned during the interview. In addition, on a three-point scale, the test persons were asked to rate the extent to which they felt they were victims of discrimination. The degree of discrimination revealed the expected significant association with BMI after the persons had been divided into five groups, as mentioned under body perception. The individual results confirm previous studies of prejudice. The only significant differences were those between persons of normal weight and all other groups. With increasing weight, no major quantitative differences were perceived.

In this study we also observed that the extent of stigmatization correlated with the occurrence of depression. It may be assumed that a mutual amplification process occurs here as well: the greater the weight, the more depression and the more stigmatization. Based on the literature[8] and our own study in the United States, comprising about 100 persons who had undergone surgery, we found that stigmatization originates from the habitual environment of the individual and also very strongly from medical staff.

Self-Confidence

Self-confidence was investigated in the areas of work, social contact during leisure time, and the personal sector of intimate relationships and the family.[7] In all fields, self-confidence is related to BMI. At work, the association is moderate; in all other fields it is remarkably high. The first three BMI groups experience no major problems at work. Such problems start at a BMI of 35 kg per m[2]. After this point, the individual's mobility and physical capacity are reduced and those limitations become perceptible in the person's professional life.

In the area of social contact during leisure time and in intimate personal relationships, the progress is nearly continuous. The significant turning point of the overweight limit is a reflection of our (stressful) leisure-oriented society. These results could easily be elaborated on by citing the long stories of suffering that were narrated during the interviews.

A qualitative content analysis developed by Mayring revealed five main categories in the following sequence of feeling stigmatized[9]:

1. Exercise (sports in the company of acquaintances, especially swimming),
2. Going out (walking through a restaurant, etc.),
3. Going shopping, especially for clothes,
4. Invitations from acquaintances (including their observation of, and comments on, eating behavior) and, regrettably,
5. Visiting the doctor.

Some women had not visited a gynecologist for 15 years because of comments like, "Watch out, don't damage the chair!" or their own sense of shame about their "mass of fat in the chair." The health risks of failing to undergo preventive examinations need no elaboration, and the women were aware of these risks. The results clearly illustrate that the psychological aspect of obesity is related to the problems of an environment that nurtures a specific ideal of beauty. It is interesting to note that persons engaged in professions in which overweight is more or less a part of the profession are much more self-confident than others. A cook, a restaurant owner, a happy mother and housewife, or a strong sportsman reported a much easier life than did a secretary, a hairdresser, or a traveling salesman (whose managers demanded a specific external appearance of them). This leads us to the question of how quality of life is associated with weight in various areas of living.

Quality of Life

In a study currently in progress, more than 1000 obese individuals were evaluated using the Moorehead-Ardelt quality-of-life questionnaire.[10] This instrument consists of a single page. It uses drawings as a visual aid and a categorical scale for the response options. The questions concern five areas of quality of life: well-being, physical activity, social life, working conditions, and sexual activity. Overall, it was found that quality of life was linearly and conversely proportionally correlated with the BMI. The study showed that subjective general well-being can be improved in about 90% of cases once the morbidly obese person achieves an adequate weight reduction. This would signify a reduction of at least one half of the person's excess weight. Simultaneously, the individual's physical and psychological well-being can be improved in 80% of cases, and social contact and the pleasure of work can be improved or strongly improved in more than 60% of cases. Such studies are now being performed throughout the world. All of them demonstrate a dramatic improvement in the subjective quality of life after weight reduction.

Personality

The question of whether the problems of obesity are associated with typical personalities that deviate from those of the normal population was negated in the literature as well as in our own studies performed thus far. The data obtained from the previously mentioned 410 test persons also showed no significant correlations between the scales of the Giessen test and the BMI. The Giessen test was selected because it contains subscales that measure the social area and depression. These two areas have the highest theoretical probability of causing changes in the personality structure that result from stigmatization and the subsequent impairment of self-confidence, including withdrawal and other elements. The assessment of one's popularity is a factor that distinguishes persons of normal weight and, in fact, even overweight individuals, from all persons who have BMIs of more than 30 kg per m[2]. The ability and willingness to be open toward others is, in principle, characterized by the same tendency, with the difference that morbidly adipose individuals do not differ from persons of normal weight with regard to openness.

The results conclusively supplement the data concerning perceived stigmatization and self-confidence in the area of "social contacts during leisure time." These could be interpreted to mean that self-confidence starts to fall in the overweight range. With increasing weight, along with defamation and mockery in specific social situations, the personality values in the social area are eventually altered; the morbidly obese possibly reconcile themselves to the situation and are at least able to return to a more open way of dealing with others.

Eating Behavior

The results of a questionnaire focusing on eating behavior, which was presented to the previously mentioned 410 probands, are in conformity with the data reported by Pudel and Westenhöfer.[11] It was found that an individual's control more or less collapses from a BMI of 40 kg per m^2 upward; thus it does not fall consistently. However, the individual's "susceptibility" starts to become volatile from the overweight limit upward; the same is true for hunger pangs. The latter show a further significant rise from a BMI of 40 kg per m^2 upward. In practice, this would mean that training the individual to overcome external "temptations" as well as working on one's hunger pangs should be started much earlier than is usually done. According to these results, in the overweight range of a BMI of 25 kg per m^2 upward, there are significantly more individuals at risk who should learn better control of external and internal stimuli. We believe that these results underscore the immense importance of prevention. From a psychological point of view, they also raise the question of whether it is appropriate to treat a BMI of 35 or 40 kg per m^2 as a rigid marker for bariatric surgery.

▶ SELF-PERCEPTION OF OBESE INDIVIDUALS FOLLOWING SURGERY

Surgery for weight reduction is controversial in discussions in the public setting. The general belief that weight reduction can be achieved without "the risk of an operation" is widespread. One element of the spectrum of prejudices toward obese individuals[12,13] is that they are weak-willed. It is believed that they could reduce their weight if they really wanted to, if they "simply ate less" or "exercised a little more."[12,13] Regrettably, these prejudices are accepted by obese individuals as well, who then despise themselves for their alleged weaknesses, despair over their unfashionably fleshy bodies and, also, their own supposed "incapability."

The delusion of the "simplicity" and "ease" of weight loss is proffered in numerous costly and irresponsible offers made by various agencies and individuals. Even persons engaged in counseling professions, such as psychologists and psychotherapists, often believe that one only has to reach "the root of the problem," the place "where the protective armor has been built," and "work" at this armor to achieve weight reduction. However, the existing evaluations of therapy contradict this point of view.[14] According to current knowledge, the so-called roots—that is, old patterns—certainly should be identified and worked on, but such work must necessarily be followed by the painstaking process of acquiring and practicing new, appropriate behavior.

Based on carefully conducted studies, research groups have identified variables in eating behavior that are able validly to predict weight reduction and weight increase. High rigid or very low cognitive "control" coupled with "susceptibility" (to external stimuli such as odor, the sight of food, etc.) and strong hunger pangs are significantly more common in overweight individuals.[15] In an earlier study, we were able to show that these data are also true for individuals who have undergone obesity operations.[16]

Weight reduction can be optimized by programs developed on the basis of the previously mentioned research, programs that work on the altering of control, susceptibility, and hunger pangs. Such programs are based on behavior therapy. They can be effective to the extent required by international standards, namely, a weight reduction of more than 5 kg achieved over a period of more than 48 months.

This is an excellent figure in the overweight range, especially if one considers the fact that obesity is a progressive disease. However, the success statistics show that the mean weight loss usually does not exceed 5 kg.[17] The question that then arises is which therapy one should offer the obese and, especially, the morbidly obese.

Bariatric surgery has made dramatic advancements since it was started in the middle of the last century. It is the only therapy proven to achieve a sustained weight reduction. Concurrently, it results in an exceptional improvement of physical and psychological well-being over the preoperative baseline condition.

To assess the results of surgical treatment of grade 3 obesity, we used the procedure developed by H. E. Oria and M. Moorehead (bariatric analysis and presentation of the results of obesity treatment)[18] and achieved results similar to those of other investigators,[19] namely, that patients who underwent surgery lost about 80% of their physical comorbidities after 10 years, and 90% of patients achieved an improvement or a major improvement in their quality of life (general well-being, physical activity, social contact, work, and sexuality). In other words, the 200,000 operations being performed annually throughout the world at the present time are a significant contribution to reducing the detrimental social effects of discrimination against the obese individual.

▶ OBESITY AND A DIAGNOSIS OF ADDICTION

Addiction has been warily mentioned now and then in obesity analyses. It has been either denied or superficially reported in the published literature on obesity. This is best exemplified by the following statement made by Ellis: "Obesity is also wrongly considered to be evidence of mental disease and addiction."[19] In contrast, there are statements made by obese individuals themselves[20]:

"Being overweight makes me feel worthless, subhuman, but I can't control my eating."
"I can't stand frustration and pain, I can't bear being deprived."
"I need immediate gratification."
"Life is too boring without sweets. I must have them."
"If I just think about stopping, I'll get so upset, I'll have to eat more."
"I feel hunger pangs, deprivation from food, nervousness and irritability, depression due to deprivation...."
"If there is a celebration I must eat to fully enjoy the day."
"It is too hard to control my eating. I can't stand the discomfort of fighting my urge to eat."

Each of these sentences expresses an urge, a craving, an inability to control. "Craving" is considered to be a feature of most dependent individuals.[21]

The relevant literature on dependence also contains the points mentioned in the previously cited statements. These include having an urge or craving; the outbreak of impulses; irrational beliefs concerning the intake of a specific substance (an exceptionally strong desire for relaxation, an exceptionally strong desire to experience as much pleasure as possible) and inadequate control techniques;

a controlled habit of consuming a specific substance; an unbalanced ratio between control and urge; a genetic predisposition that is frequently enhanced by the reaction of the environment.[22-24]

Of course, it is problematic to introduce the concept of addiction into a discussion of obese individuals, who are victims of strong discrimination to start with. However, addiction delineates the drama of obesity in a particularly lucid manner. One cannot abstain from eating or from sugar, which releases endorphins; one cannot abstain from fat, one cannot abstain from food. The obese individual is no more able to resist the overwhelming offer of surplus food than the nicotine- or alcohol-dependent individual is able to resist the objects of his or her addiction. The same is true for the social aspect of food ingestion; it is difficult to remain abstinent from drink or to refrain from smoking on certain occasions; refusing food one is offered is interpreted as gross impoliteness.

More than any other substance in the world, food is linked with emotions. The physiologic and psychological aspects of food cannot be strictly separated from each other. The first relationships established by human beings are all associated with food.

We believe that the consideration of addiction makes sense because we have a number of scientifically tested addiction therapies that enrich the existing range of offered treatments.

At first glance it appears absurd to speak of food dependence; one cannot remain "dry" as far as food is concerned because food is required by all living organisms to sustain life. However, food dependence is relative. Studies published so far have been concerned primarily with eating-behavior disorders[25] and less with the aspects of obesity related to addiction. Most of all, remarkably little has been written about a fact known for more than 10 years, namely, that a substantial percentage of obese individuals suffer from attacks of so-called binge eating. The cited figures vary, but the majority report about 25%.[26,27] Several studies have shown that the number of attacks of binge eating significantly increases with the grade of obesity.[28]

Binge eating is a phenomenon of addiction. When psychological associations between obesity problems and addiction are discussed, it is usually done in a generalized way, such as, "Food is a means of dealing with one's feelings of reluctance or escaping from problems and conflicts."[29,30] These approaches are certainly justified. Yet the question of whether the quest for substitute gratification differentiates obese individuals from persons of normal weight needs to be investigated. Possibly, all individuals indulge in substitute gratification to a similar extent, but with less severe consequences. Obesity cannot be explained by psychological problems alone. Only a small number of obese individuals use food as substitute gratification.[25,31]

Therefore, merely discovering the feeling that lies behind it cannot be the solution. We are probably dealing with a multifactorial, inhomogeneous disease whose individual factors amplify each other. Aliabadi and Daub[31] were able to prove that obesity and the stigmatization associated with it drive a person further into addiction. Unfortunately, we have found no carefully conducted empirical studies dealing with the associations between addiction and obesity.

Interviews and contact with individuals who have obesity problems during the course of therapy led us to examine the extent to which obese individuals reveal addictive traits.[7] From the existing addiction questionnaires, we constructed a questionnaire to measure the specific urge related to dependence, namely the uncontrollable craving for excessive food. In addition, we adapted Breitkopf's helplessness questionnaire[32] for situations in which one is confronted with a tempting offer of food.[22]

Although 20% of normal-weight individuals agree with the concept of urge, about 45% of overweight individuals and about 60% of morbidly obese individuals do so. In the range of the scale measuring the use of food as a substitute (in the presence of frustration, etc.), the ratios are similar. However, the values are much lower, starting with about 5% of normal-weight individuals and ranging to 35% of the morbidly obese. The last percentage is remarkably similar to the 30% conflict drinkers have reported in the literature.[23,24]

One further result at the item level is noteworthy. If one looks at the percentage distribution of answers for the item "Eating is better than everything else," the percentages are reversed: 30% of normal-weight individuals agree, as opposed to 5% of overweight individuals and none of the morbidly obese. The last group experiences eating as a problem, not as a pleasure!

The results facilitate an interesting observation. According to the data we have obtained so far, an urge is not something that all persons with obesity problems experience to the same extent. The addiction factor of urge is highly correlated with susceptibility and hunger, but it differs strongly among categories of BMI.

It may be said that the craving mentioned in the relevant literature as well as the other variables of addiction distinguish among overweight individuals of various BMI categories and also distinguish them from normal-weight individuals.

▶ SUMMARY

Obesity, morbid obesity or, more precisely, an excessively high proportion of body fat and its associated risks has been termed the epidemic of the third millennium by the World Health Organization (WHO). Altered living habits are responsible for this global epidemic. The disproportion between the lowered energy consumption resulting from reduced physical activity and the increasing energy supply through the ingestion of high-energy, high-sugar, and high-fat foods has led to the current problem. The Western lifestyle and its surpluses as well as its preference for fast food, snacks, and high-sugar beverages in particular bear significant responsibility for the situation. This lifestyle is willingly emulated in developing countries. The advancing urbanization and the population shift from rural areas into cities are commonly associated with a similar adoption of unhealthful habits in developing countries. The figures cited by the WHO plainly show that the highest rates of obesity no longer exist in industrialized countries alone. The most extreme example is Samoa, an island in the South Sea, where 56% of men and 74% of women are obese.

The public health costs resulting from the secondary diseases associated with obesity are enormous. Of equal magnitude is the human suffering that accompanies obesity because it is not considered by the general public to be a chronic disease. The layperson and many medical specialists prefer to believe in the simple feasibility of weight reduction. At least this is proffered in a number of expensive and irresponsible offers. In fact, individuals with BMIs of more than 40 kg per m^2 have no more than a 3% chance of achieving a sustained weight reduction by means of conservative methods. It is surprising to note, as reported in the studies mentioned earlier, that individuals in the overweight range, those with BMIs of 25 to 30 kg per m^2, already feel massively discriminated against, are less self-confident than others, and perceive their bodies to be much fatter than they actually are. The anorectic ideal of beauty is extremely harmful. The belief by society that obesity is a purely self-incurred disease that could be easily avoided creates significant tension and unfair discrimination.

To offset these conceptions, the public must be made aware that obesity is a genetically induced disease that manifests itself when the susceptible individual is faced with facilitating environmental conditions.

Although the WHO has presented a new report on the subject of obesity, according to which 1.1 billion persons fall in the category of overweight or obese, reactions by the public in terms of counter-strategies are meager. Most governments of the world have ignored the problem of obesity. It is extremely difficult to influence the food industry. The industry must learn to become part of the solution rather than part of the problem. Along with the development of therapeutic facilities, long-term prevention strategies will be the most important measures in the struggle against obesity. Individual measures such as removing soft-drink machines from schools are clearly not sufficient. Rather, we will have to develop national strategies that will be borne by political institutions and will encompass schools, business organizations, and the mass media. Prevention programs should be started in kindergarten, where children can be taught to handle food properly and consciously and where suitable exercise programs can be offered on a regular basis.

The social effects of obesity are manifold. Eventually, they lead to a degree of discrimination unparalleled by that shown toward any other minority group. We need to make effective changes in the negative social attitudes toward obesity.

▶ REFERENCES

1. World Health Organization: Obesity: Preventing and Managing the Global Epidemic. Technical report series no. 894. Geneva, World Health Organization, 2000.
2. Kopelman PG: Obesity as a medical problem. Nature 2000;404:635-643.
3. Katzmarzyk PT: The Canadian obesity epidemic, 1985-1998. CMAJ 2002;166:1039-1040.
4. International Obesity Task Force, 2002:.www.iotf.org. Accessed.
5. Tremblay MS, Willms JD: Secular trends in the body mass index of Canadian children. CMAJ 2000;163:1429-1433; www.cmaj.ca/cgi/content/full/163/11/1429. Accessed 2000.
6. National Center for Health Statistics: Using the Body Mass Index-for-Age (Children) growth charts. www.cdc.gov/nccdphp/dnpa/growthcharts. Accessed May 30, 2000.
7. Ardelt-Gattinger E, Lechner H, Weger P, et al: BMI 40: the point of no return. In Hell E, Miller K (eds): Morbide Adipositas. Ecomed Verlag 2000;S194-S217.
8. Maroney D, Golub S: Nurses' attitudes toward obese persons and certain ethnic groups. Percept Mot Skills 1992;75:387-391.
9. Mayring P: Qualitative Inhaltsanalyse, p. 45. Weinheim: Deutscher Studienverlag, 1992.
10. Ardelt E, Moorehead M: The validation of the Moorehead-Ardelt quality of life questionnaire. Obes Surg 1999; 9:132 (abstract).
11. Pudel V, Westenhöfer J: Ernährungspsychologie, pp. 76-78. Göttingen: Hogrefe, 1996.
12. Stunkard A, Wadden T: Psychological aspects of severe obesity. Am J Clin Nutr 1992;55:524-532.
13. Wardle J, Volz C, Golding J: Social variation in attitudes to obesity in children. Int J Obes 1992;19:562-569.
14. Rand C, Stunkard A: Obesity and psychoanalysis. Am J Psychiatry 1978;135:547-551.
15. Rossner S: Defining success in obesity management. Int J Obes 1997; 21(suppl 1):S2-S4.
16. Hell E, Miller KA, Moorehead MK, et al: Evaluation of health status and quality of life after bariatric surgery: comparison of standard Roux-en-Y gastric bypass, vertical banded gastroplasty and laparoscopic adjustable silicone gastric banding. Obes Surg 2000;10:214-219.
17. Hell E, Miller K: Morbide Adipositas. Chirurgische Behandlung der Morbiden Adipositas. Ergebnisse 2000;237-267.
18. Oria HE: Reporting results in obesity surgery: evaluation of a limited survey. Obes Surg 1996;6:361-368.
19. Ellis A, Abrams M, Dengelegi L: Rational Eating. New York: Barricade Books, 1992.
20. Saß H, Wittchen H, Zaudig M, et al: Diagnostische Kriterien DSM IV, pp. 79-81. Göttingen, Hogrefe, 1998.
21. Birch L, Fisher J: Development of eating behaviors among children and adolescents. Pediatrics 1997;539-546.
22. Feuerlein W: Kognitive Therapie der Sucht, pp. 231-232. Weinheim: Psychologie Verlags Union, 1997.
23. Klicpera C, Gasteiger-Klicpera B: Klinische Psychologie. Wien, WUV, 1996.
24. Schaef A: Im Zeitalter der Sucht. Munich, DTB, 1991.
25. Fairburn C: Overcoming Binge Eating, pp. 74-76. New York, Guilford, 1995.
26. Marcu M: Binge eating and obesity. In Brownell K, Fairburn C (eds): Eating Disorders and Obesity, pp. 441-444. New York, Guilford, 1995.
27. Telch C, Agras W, Rossiter H: Binge eating increases with increasing adiposity. Int J Eat Disord 1998;7:115-119.
28. Ardelt-Gattinger E, Lechner H: Psychological aspects of bariatric surgery. Zentralbl Chir. 2002;127(12):1057-1063.
29. Bruch H: Essstörungen, pp. 21–22. Frankfurt, Fischer, 1991.
30. Gross W: Was ist das Süchtige an der Sucht? pp. 51-55. Guesthacht, Neuland, 1993.
31. Aliabadi C, Daub M: Der unstill-bare Hunger. In C. Merfert – Diete, R. Soltau (Hrsg) Frauen und Sucht, S 171-178. Hamburg. Rowohlt, 1984.
32. Breitkopf L: Die Hilflosigkeitsskala. Diagnostica 1985;31:221-233.

8

Economic Implications of Obesity

Louis F. Martin, M.D., F.A.C.S., F.C.C.M.

The prevalence of obesity in the populations of the United States and of most developed countries has increased to such an extent that obesity has finally gained status as a disease. Public health officials, the National Institutes of Health (NIH), and the World Health Organization (WHO) have all recognized that there is an obesity epidemic, that our attempts to prevent and treat it are inadequate, and that it is one of the most important public health problems of this century.[1-4]

Previous chapters in this book have outlined evidence demonstrating that obesity shortens life expectancy, is directly associated with and largely responsible for numerous comorbid conditions, and decreases quality of life. This evidence has led public health officials to the inevitable conclusion that the health care and the social security and disability systems will accumulate direct medical costs and indirect societal costs related to obesity that will be more substantial than those for any other primary disease for the next 20 years. As this reality diffuses into our political, business, and media environments, it will evoke a number of uncoordinated responses that will gradually reshape public policy within this generation. This chapter examines the evidence and the speculations that have fueled interest in controlling the major public health problem of obesity, and it considers society's response from an economic perspective.

▶ EVOLUTION OF OBESITY AS A DISEASE

Prior chapters have presented a wealth of information documenting how increasing degrees of obesity are directly related to increased rates of premature mortality; to the development of serious comorbid medical conditions, including hypertension, diabetes, elevated lipid levels, atherosclerosis, osteoarthritis, and respiratory disease, such as sleep apnea and obesity hypoventilation syndrome; and to the increased likelihood that obese individuals will be victims of discrimination, limiting their educational, employment, and relationship opportunities and increasing their incidence of depression and other symptoms associated with decreased quality of life. Although it may

seem obvious to most physicians and even to the public that these associations between obesity and significant life issues should exist, their documentation is relatively recent.

Dr. George Bray, an endocrinologist at the University of California Los Angeles School of Medicine, has devoted his career to the study of obesity. Dr. Bray was instrumental in getting the NIH to examine obesity as a public health problem in the 1970s and thereafter. The consensus of the early NIH reviews and expert panels was that a cause-and-effect relationship between obesity and "illness" was lacking.[5,6] These public forums, however, attracted the attention of a generation of investigators who began to document the links between obesity and other medical conditions.

By 1985, when the NIH held its next Consensus Conference on the health implications of obesity, a substantial body of research had been completed, and it allowed this panel to identify obesity as a health risk and to acknowledge the importance of both the prevention and the treatment of obesity.[7] The NIH awarded several grants to investigators (e.g., Harvard University, Policy Analysis, Inc.) to develop the first estimates of how much obesity impacted the direct costs of providing medical care in the United States. In 1992, Colditz[8] presented his arguments that the total cost of all medical treatments in the United States could be reduced by 5.5% if obesity were eliminated—obviously an impossible task, then and now. Governments of developed nations commissioned similar estimates using data from their health care systems which, in the socialized medical systems, had more centralized data. Estimates from France, the Netherlands, Australia, and Canada, where obesity was not as prevalent as it was in the United States in the 1980s and early 1990s, also suggested that somewhere between 2% and 4% of the direct costs of medical care in these countries would be eliminated if obesity could be eliminated.[9-12] This attracted the attention of public health officials and policy makers everywhere. These estimates continue to be updated and have gained authority because the figures and assumptions behind them have remained stable over time.[13]

Simultaneously, public health experts documented the increasing prevalence of obesity in all age and ethnicity groups, and they attempted to validate the number of premature deaths attributable to obesity. Using survey data in populations in which mortality was documented, McGinnis and Foege concluded in 1993 that 300,000 to 500,000 "preventable deaths" or premature deaths occurred annually in the United States as the result of "poor diet and inactivity."[14] Former surgeon general Dr. C. Everett Koop and others began warning the public that 300,000 deaths per year in the United States were due to obesity.[1] Allison and a team of obesity experts published a report in 1997 presenting solid methodology for the figure of 300,000 premature deaths per year in the United States due to obesity, making it the second leading cause of premature death behind tobacco-related illnesses.[15] Obesity had arrived as a disease and loomed as a threatening public health problem.

COSTS ASSOCIATED WITH FAILING TO TREATING OBESITY

The costs associated with a disease include the direct medical care costs of treating the symptoms, complications, and comorbid conditions associated with the disease plus the often more expensive indirect costs to our gross national product index caused by sick days, early retirement and disability payments, and lost productivity by those with impaired work efficiency. Individuals and society suffer from diseases in similar fashion. Obesity is associated with lower-than-average household income and, more important, with lost opportunities.

When a society chooses not to treat or to expend resources to help prevent a given disease from developing, whether it is obesity, AIDS, mental illness, or cancer, it establishes a value judgment that can lead to social injustice. Sometimes the socioeconomic profile, class, ethnicity, leisure time, or other characteristics of the people who develop a disease identity are such that this group can band together to achieve a political action group to fight effectively for their rights and their portion of the dollars spent on health care. For example, senior citizens, who have more leisure time than the parents of young children, lobby effectively to obtain money to treat diseases that affect their age group (e.g., cancer, atherosclerosis, Alzheimer disease). The obese have not been able to gather as a political group and, therefore, suffer levels of discrimination that most other groups would not tolerate.[16] Not only does the public feel free to discriminate against them, but politicians,[17] the press,[18] and even members of other groups that suffer from societal intolerance[19] feel free to attack the disease of obesity as not being worthy of serious study or society's resources.

Within the public health community, however, there is a strong sense of need to provide objective measures of the relative importance of various diseases to the overall expenditure of resources on health care and social security. Cost-of-illness studies[8-13] provide limited information and do not provide information concerning the availability of treatments or preventions, their costs, or the effectiveness of these options. An illness can have a very high cost merely because there are no effective treatments, even though social pressures cause an illness to be aggressively treated (e.g., incurable cancer). Alternatively, the chronicity of an illness can make it expensive to society even if it is not immediately virulent (e.g., osteoarthritis).

It is equally important to determine what portion of the population is susceptible to the disease. Unless an illness affects a sufficiently adequate number of people to justify the allocation of research dollars by government agencies and industry, the likelihood of determining the mechanisms of the disease's activation and the products or treatments that can be used to treat or prevent it is diminished. Also, if a disease affects a significant portion of the population (e.g., obesity or morbid obesity) and the treatments are either expensive (surgery) or ineffective (diet, behavior modification, exercise, medications), a society may try to restrict access to treatments or allow reimbursement only for effective treatments by developing a system to evaluate outcomes. If the frequency and severity of a disease are increasing, and inadequate resources have been devoted to preventing, controlling, or curing it, eventually society must recognize that ignoring the problem has not worked and must acknowledge that an undertreated illness can bankrupt the system if left unchecked. Obesity has reached this stage, and governments are scrambling to find solutions to the medical and social problems obesity causes before it bankrupts the system.

In addition to all of the studies documenting that increased body mass index (BMI) is associated with a higher incidence of hypertension, diabetes, osteoarthritis, and other illnesses, studies began to appear in the 1980s documenting that the obese, and especially the morbidly obese, cost the health care system significantly more to treat, even while therapies that could improve or resolve their obesity were being denied. Epstein and colleagues, for example, reported that morbidly obese patients had a significantly longer length of stay after joint-replacement surgery, which caused the average cost of surgery to be 35% above that of normal-weight patients.[20]

Quesenberry, Caan, and Jacobson examined the costs associated with treating three different weight levels of participants (more than 17,000 people) in a health maintenance organization in northern California.[21] They reported that the morbidly obese (BMI = 35 kg/m^2) had average expenses for medical treatments that were 44% higher than those of participants in the normal weight range (BMI = 25 kg/m^2). The morbidly obese had significantly higher overall costs and more laboratory services than did normal-weight participants. Most of these increased costs were associated with the added expenses of treating the three most expensive comorbid diseases associated with morbid obesity: diabetes, hypertension, and coronary artery disease.

There are no studies that compare the rates at which members of the heaviest sector (the morbidly obese) of the societies of developed nations are granted early retirement and disability pensions compared to those who are just overweight or obese. There are data, however, from both Finland and Sweden that compare relatively normal-weight citizens to those either overweight or obese.[22] Unfortunately, these studies are not directly comparable because definitions of overweight, obesity, and morbid obesity have varied over the years. In 1985, the NIH Consensus Conference recommended using the BMI to evaluate patients for obesity rather than using charts to discuss ideal body weight.[7]

The panel defined morbid obesity somewhat differently in men and women: it designated those with BMIs of 28 kg per m² as mildly obese, those with BMIs of 30 as obese, and those with BMIs of 35 as severely obese. Morbid obesity evolved as a medical insurance term used by bariatric surgeons in the early 1970s to describe the patients they felt would die prematurely due to their extreme obesity if they did not receive surgical therapy. The term was validated by its inclusion in the ninth revision of the International Classification of Diseases (ICD-9) in 1994.[22]

Initially, morbid obesity was identified as being 200% of ideal body weight, using the Metropolitan Life Insurance actuarial tables. During a 1991 NIH Consensus Panel addressing the use of gastrointestinal surgery for severe obesity, the definition of morbid or severe obesity was broadened to include a BMI of 40 kg per m² without comorbid conditions or a BMI of 35 kg per m² with comorbid conditions.[23]

The NIH avoided use of the term *morbid*, as it was considered politically incorrect. This is unfortunate because we need to promote the use of the definitions used in the ICD-9 coding system so that clinicians will use them and not make up new definitions that cannot be assimilated into coding terminology for several decades. The WHO had different definitions for overweight; these discrepancies were somewhat resolved with a modified class of definitions in the 1998 guideline books published by the NIH[3] and WHO.[4] *Extreme obesity*, as opposed to *severe obesity* is another term used by the NIH in the 1980s and 1990s, and it has a different meaning in the surgical literature, where severe obesity refers to a BMI of 50, 55, or 60 kg per m², depending on the author and text.

The WHO owns the copyrights to the ICD-9 system[22] and needs to address this proliferation of definitions and encourage clinicians to code for obesity and morbid obesity and to use new obesity codes as they develop so as to allow for the tracking of the expenses of obesity's comorbid conditions using the proper weight code so this financial information is available for the Medicare and Medicaid insurance programs.

In Sweden, an extensive study of the association between obesity and disability, including sick leave, was published in 1996 on the basis of the initial data collected for patients entered in the registry of the Swedish Obese Subjects (SOS) study, for which patients were required to have a BMI of 38 kg per m² to qualify; it was supplemented by data collected from an outpatient obesity center at Sahlgrenska Hospital, where patients were required to have a BMI of 28 kg per m² to qualify.[24] The study compared the data from 1298 obese women, ages 30 to 59 years (mean 46 years), who had BMIs of 28 to 68 kg per m² (mean 39 kg per m²) with data for all Swedish women in this age range, obtaining the data from the Swedish National Insurance Board. The study calculated the indirect costs of lost productivity due to absence from work by using the mean annual income for Swedish women aged 30 to 59 years divided by the number of working days in the year, adjusted to 1994 price and wage levels, including social service overhead costs.

The study showed that obese women took fewer short-term sick days (defined as 1 to 5 days per year) than the rest of the population (16.5% for obese women as opposed to 22.1% for nonobese women, $P<0.001$). This might be explained by the discrimination obese women feel at a job where they have to work harder to receive similar levels of recognition for their work. However, when long-term disability (when women took off 6 months to 1 year) was compared, obese women had more than twice the sick-leave rate (10.0% vs. 4.0%, $P<0.0001$). Combining all disability days, short-term and long-term, obese women had 1.9 times the number of sick-leave days than nonoverweight women had in the general population. This increased with each decade of life; obese women ages 30 to 39 averaged 40 sick-leave days per year as opposed to 26 days for nonoverweight women; obese women ages 40 to 49 averaged 52 sick-leave days per year as opposed to 26 days for nonoverweight women; and obese women 50 to 59 years averaged 70 sick-leave days per year as opposed to 26 days for nonoverweight women.[24]

Similarly, the percentage of the population that was on disability pension after retiring from work due to disability was higher for obese women in all age classes and at all BMI levels. In 50- to 59-year-old women with BMIs of 40 kg per m², 22% were disabled, a rate 3.9 times higher than that of the Swedish population as a whole. The authors calculated that approximately 10% of the total cost of loss of productivity due to lost work days is the result of obesity and obesity-related diseases in Swedish women. Using Swedish mean annual wage figures for women, this amounts to $300 million (in 1994 U.S. dollars) in lost wages per million adult women per year due to obesity, making it an extremely expensive illness for society.

A follow-on study, which compared 369 morbidly obese Swedish citizens who had bariatric surgery between 1987 and 1990 to a matched group of 371 morbidly obese Swedish citizens who did not want surgical therapy, concluded that surgical treatment resulted in the reduction of sick leave and disability pension in the 4 years following surgery or initiation of observation, particularly in subjects aged 47 to 60 years.[25] This is a study, however, that does not translate well into the current state of bariatric surgery in the United States because none of the surgery in the Swedish study was performed laparoscopically (the most common form of bariatric surgery in the United States), and Swedish rules governing sick days allowed after surgery are much more lenient than those in the United States. A study in the United States would be expected to show far greater differences than the limited differences reported in the Swedish study.

A study examining the relationship of obesity and disability in Finland demonstrated similar significant associations and emphasized the importance of obesity-caused osteoarthritis of the knees as a major component of the morbidity associated with early retirement.[26] The Mini-Finland Health Survey followed 5625 men and women, aged 30 to 64 years when initially interviewed between 1978 and 1980, for 15 years, until 1995. Disability was defined as receiving a work disability during the follow-up period before retirement at age 65 years. This study used the more current definitions of overweight (a BMI of 25.0 kg per m² and less than 30.0 kg per m²) and obesity (a BMI of 30.0 kg per m²).

More than half the men and women were either overweight or obese at the start of the study: 44.9% of men were overweight and 11.3% were obese; 32.5% of women were overweight and 16.4% were obese. Overall, 3% of men and 10% of women had osteoarthritis of the knees, the highest rates in any of the joints surveyed, including back disease. Both obesity and osteoarthritis were independently and significantly related to early disability pensions. When both obesity and osteoarthritis were present, the relative risk for developing work disability requiring early retirement during the 15-year follow-up period was 2.4 (95%, CI,1.3-4.3). Compared to normal-weight subjects without osteoarthritis, these individuals were 7.9 times more likely to report difficulties in performing activities of daily living (quality-of-life indexes). These data supplement National Health Survey data that document that increasing weight is directly related to increases in the number of days spent being sick or bedridden.[27]

▶ EVIDENCE THAT SURGICAL THERAPY IS COST-EFFECTIVE

It has been difficult to document circumstances that prevent these huge indirect costs in government social services programs. No program to prevent obesity has proven itself to be effective anywhere in the world. Only a few weight-loss programs have been able to show an economic impact.

The most direct evaluation of a treatment—gastric bypass to treat morbid obesity—was completed in Quebec Province in Canada.[28] In a 4-year study using government figures for health care expenses, 1035 morbidly obese patients who underwent open gastric bypass in one hospital using a standard technique were compared to 5746 morbidly obese patients who did not seek surgical treatment in the same province. The population was 65% female and had a mean age of 46 years; treated patients lost a mean of 92 lb, which was a mean of 74% of their excess body weight. The patients receiving surgical treatment had 28% fewer hospital stays (2.5 vs. 3.2), a significantly lower number of hospital days (21.1 vs. 36.6 hospital days), and fewer physician visits (9.6 vs. 17.1 visits), which translated into a significant reduction in the mean 4-year cost of surgically treated patients, even though the cost of surgery was included in the 4-year total.

Another method of calibrating whether a treatment is cost-effective has been developed by public health officials and has been standardized by a commission paid by the U.S. Public Health Service to develop rules by consensus. Two recent reviews have outlined the process developed over the past 3 decades to develop cost-effectiveness analyses (CEAs) for health care decisions.[22,29] The standards created by the commission were published in 1996 as a book, *Cost-Effectiveness in Health and Medicine*.[30] The four basic outcomes of a CEA are outlined in Table 8-1, although the entire book is needed to explain what is allowed in the numerator of the equation (the costs to society, which include direct medical care costs and indirect societal costs) and what units should be used to count the benefits of an outcome. The Public Health Service and Center for Medicare and Medicaid Services (CMMS) wants the health benefits of a treatment to be measured in differences in years of life produced by different therapies.[20,30] When this is not possible due to lack of data, a measure of

Table 8-1	COST EVALUATION OF NEW TREATMENT vs. NO TREATMENT OR PRIOR TREATMENT	
	HIGHER COST	LOWER COST
Better Quality of life	Too Expensive (willingness to pay line) OK Treatment	Best treatment (least often achieved)
Poorer Quality of life	Easily eliminated as a choice	Society saves money at the individual's expense

quality-adjusted life-years (QALYs)[22,30] is calculated by asking a group of citizens to rate subjectively the quality of life and the quantity of time they want to have by answering this question: Taking into account your age, pain and suffering, immobility, and lost earnings, what fraction of a year would you be willing to give up to be completely healthy for the remaining fraction of a year instead of your present level of health status for a full year?[31]

This question can be difficult to answer, and it leads to vastly different results if differences in years of life are compared to QALYs. The removal of bilateral cataracts and the insertion of artificial lenses may vastly improve QALYs (being able to see rather than being blind) but has no impact on length of life. The choice between accepting angioplasty over coronary artery bypass grafting for treatment of a blocked coronary artery causing congestive heart failure carries twice the risk of immediate death in the perioperative period but produces almost no pain, which may be a significant factor in a QALYs score. Several testing instruments have been identified to measure these quality-of-life variables and have been validated so that a QALYs score can be obtained.[22]

In spite of these limitations, the four basic scenarios that can occur when two therapies are compared for the treatment of the same problem by a CEA are fairly obvious and are outlined in Table 8-1. If a new treatment costs less than the standard current treatment and produces a better quality of life (or a longer life), it is obvious that it should be embraced. If a new treatment costs more than the standard therapy and produces a poorer quality of life or a shorter life, it should be discontinued. The other two scenarios are much more value-influenced. If a new therapy costs more than the current therapy but produces a better quality of life, then society has to examine how much it is willing to "pay" for this improvement. If a new cancer treatment costs a million dollars but produces only 1 additional month of life or decreases the pain of having the cancer only by an amount that most people would not be willing to give up more than an extra month of life to achieve, it is going to be too expensive to replace a standard, much less expensive therapy. However, it is easy to imagine that a patient with cancer might expect society to pay more for some incremental increase in the length of his or her life than an individual without cancer who is answering a quality-of-life survey would be willing to think was a fair price for society to pay for that same increase in life expectancy.

When CEA is used as a test of how beneficial a given therapy is, bariatric surgery appears to be a bargain.

The only study published to date that meets most criteria for a valid CEA is from Denmark. It involved 21 patients undergoing an operation, vertical banded gastroplasty, that is diminishing in popularity in favor of another restrictive operation, the adjustable gastric band.[32,33] Zhang and his colleagues at the U.S. Centers for Disease Control and Prevention, however, felt it was a study that had merit and compared it to the only other two studies in the literature reporting creditable CEAs of obesity treatments in the literature as of July 2002.[29] The Diabetes Prevention Program (DPP) study was a multicenter clinical trial among 3234 Americans with BMIs of more than 25 kg per m^2 and impaired glucose tolerance. It examined whether a program of one-on-one behavioral modification counseling; the teaching of a low-calorie, low-fat diet; and moderate-intensity physical activity (brisk walking) for more than 150 minutes per week over a 3-year period could improve weight loss and inhibit the development of type 2 diabetes. The control group underwent a placebo intervention that provided a study manual, yearly visits to a counselor, and metformin (850 mg twice daily).[34,35] The other CEA examined a 2-year intervention that compared sibutramine (Orlistat) treatment (120 mg three times a day) plus a hypocaloric diet to a hypocaloric diet alone.[36]

The CEA of bariatric surgery produced by this group of federal economists suggested that the vertical banded gastroplasty improved quality of life and lowered costs over the 2 years of the study; it was the best of the treatments reviewed, and it produced a level of results that is rarely achieved.[29] The major mechanism by which surgical therapy saved money was by producing a gain in productivity. The percentage of the 21 patients who worked increased from 19% (4 patients) to 48% (10 patients). This was similar to results reported by our group at Pennsylvania State College of Medicine: more than 42% of the 40 morbidly obese patients who were dependent on public welfare because they could not obtain employment (n = 26) or were disabled before the age of 65 years (n = 14) were able to obtain either full-time employment (n = 9) or part-time employment (n = 8) after gastric bypass, thereby decreasing their levels of need for public assistance.[37] Three disabled people returned to full-time employment, paying taxes into the Social Security system rather than absorbing resources from it, a double benefit to society.

The behavior-modification treatments and the drug treatments, with or without behavior modification,[34-36] are expensive to society because the effort produces relatively little weight loss (1.9-5.5 kg) and relatively minor changes in QALYs.[29] Even though these treatments increased costs while minimally improving quality of life, Zhang and colleagues noted that their CEA values were within the ranges of the cost-effectiveness of many health care treatments for diseases that are routinely covered by health insurance.[29] The authors could not understand why health insurance companies often refused to pay for obesity treatments but paid for many other therapies in the same range of cost-effectiveness. They suggested that it was only the lack of long-term studies (beyond the 2 to 3 years in these studies) that influenced the insurance carriers to refuse to pay for medical obesity treatments. It seems highly unlikely, however, that health insurance companies will change policies unless they are forced to do so.

Another method of determining how important obesity treatments are to the obese is to ask them how much they would be willing to pay for a successful obesity treatment. Narbro and Sjostrom received responses from 3579 patients who entered the SOS study with a mean age of 47 years and a mean BMI of 40 kg per m^2.[38] They found a wide range of responses, from nothing to very large sums of money. Most people were willing to pay twice their monthly salaries which, in this population, were approximately $3280 in 2000. People with higher BMIs and those who perceived their health as being poorer were willing to pay even more and were willing to consider obtaining a loan to pay for such treatment. Obese and even nonobese people already spend hundreds of dollars per year of their own discretionary money on diet products and medical treatments[39]; however, this is the first time a population has placed and recorded a price on medical treatment.

▶ PREDICTING FUTURE FUNDING FOR OBESITY TREATMENTS

Medical insurance companies have successfully prevented the majority of consumer groups seeking insurance contracts in small numbers (fewer than several thousand people) from obtaining coverage for surgical treatment in the United States.[33] As more information accumulates about the relative benefits of surgical obesity treatments and the consequences of being morbidly obese, this level of discrimination will become problematic for medical insurance companies and the businesses that contract with them. Already, state legislators, the U.S. Circuit Court of Appeals, and the U.S. Supreme Court have attacked insurance laws that protect both the insurance companies and the businesses that contract with them from providing "beneficial care" or "life-saving" care at their discretion.[40] In February 2003, the Second Circuit Court of Appeals stated that insurance plans could be sued for failing to cover needed care. It may take years or decades to determine who will define what "needed" care is and how this will affect the insurance industry.

In Louisiana, the major insurance agency that provides medical insurance for state employees, the Office of Group Benefits, believed that by 2004 it would have to cover bariatric surgery. The problem the agency faces is that more than 1000 of its 240,000 members that meet qualification requirements for bariatric surgery responded to a survey in December of 2002 by applying for the surgical therapy. This therapy had been unavailable for more than 10 years. Determining how to obtain qualified surgeons to perform this quantity of surgeries and a way to ration it so that all the expenses of satisfying the number of patients desiring surgery are spread out, so as to prevent the plans from experiencing financial ruin, are problems that must be faced now. The agency is attempting to set criteria that surgeons will be expected to meet (number of bariatric cases performed per year, mortality and morbidity rates for these procedures, standards for levels of hospital support, etc.) before being "credentialed" to perform bariatric surgery on its members. How these criteria will be enforced and whether this type of restriction is legal under state law are unanswered questions.

In addition, media attention now has focused on the number of obese children and how public schools and their financing are contributing to the "passive" development of obesity (a term used to recall "passive" consumption of cigarette smoke) because of food advertising and subsequent consumption of high-calorie food and beverages in the schools. The Surgeon General's 2001 Call to Action to Prevent and Decrease Overweight and Obesity[2] spent a considerable portion of its message addressing the alarming increase in the prevalence of obesity among children and the dire effect this will have on health care cost increases as obese children become adults.

An examination of the ways in which elementary and secondary schools partner with food and beverage companies to find new sources of discretionary funds was first presented in Dr. Marion Nestlé's book *Food Politics*.[41] Changes in public school funding have left many school systems searching for nontax dollars to provide essential books, equipment, and personnel. Dr. Nestlé argues that partnering with soft-drink (sweetened carbonated beverage) companies to obtain funding in exchange for allowing advertising and vending machine access is unacceptable. It is analogous to the companies that provide televisions and computers to schools in exchange for the commitment to expose school children to viewing commercials for several minutes a day during classes. Both are mechanisms that legitimize these advertisements and make children marketing targets so as to instill brand loyalty at an early age.

School administrators also frequently ignored their responsibility to provide good nutrition by relying on high-fat, low-cost meals in federally subsidized school lunch programs or by allowing fast-food companies to operate school food services. Also, many school districts with poor funding have eliminated or reduced physical education and activity programs to save money. Instead of helping children to learn about good nutrition, teaching them physical activity skills they can use to stay healthy throughout life, and providing them with appropriate meals based on the recommendations of the Food Guide Pyramid, many schools facilitate childhood obesity.[42] A 1997 report documented that only 1% of American children ate diets conforming to the Food Guide Pyramid recommendations, whereas 45% of children met none of the recommendations.[43] Furthermore, U.S. children consumed diets in which at least 50% of their calories were from fat (35%) or sugar (15%) in the form of soft drinks and snack foods.

Between 2001 and 2002, 60% of U.S. middle and high schools sold soft drinks in vending machines and more than 240 U.S. school districts had exclusive contracts with soft drink companies and received funding based on the number of beverages sold and the extent of the marketing allowed (advertisements in hallways, on book covers, and in auditoriums, gymnasiums, and school athletic fields).[44] This aggressive advertising has produced a backlash in which parent groups force school districts to terminate these types of contracts, sometimes using litigation to claim unfair marketing practices by the companies involved.[44,45] Voters also have asked for referendums on city and state ballots to eliminate soft drinks from school vending machines and to demand more healthful school meals.

Consumer response has also caused some larger food companies to reevaluate their products and activities.

Kraft Foods, Inc., the largest food manufacturer in the United States, has pledged to examine its products (including Oreo cookies and Kraft Macaroni and Cheese) and attempt to decrease their fat and sugar content.[46,47] The easiest solution would be to decrease portion size, but they are also examining how to maintain taste using fat and sugar substitutes. They have also pledged to stop in-school marketing and are considering eliminating some products from their vending machine businesses. Cynics suggest that this strategy arises from their parent companies' fear of lawsuits rather than from true altruistic policies.[46,47] Either way, this approach is laudable and will probably force other large corporations to copy the example.

Public and government bodies are becoming concerned about the passive development of obesity in children in the United States and in other developed nations. In the 107th Congress, the U.S. Senate considered a bill titled the Improved Nutrition and Physical Activity Act (IMPACT). The bill did not have sufficient political support to become a law in 2003, but its introduction demonstrates political support for finding ways to prevent and treat childhood obesity that did not exist 2 or 3 years ago. The majority of the $280 million of funding outlined in the bill was directed at developing a Youth Media Campaign to prevent obesity and to demonstrate projects that treat or prevent obesity through community- or school-sponsored programs. Also, when Aetna insurance company settled a class-action suit filed by physicians claiming unfair payment practices in 2003, it created a $300 million research fund that could be accessed only to study three issues in health care; one was childhood obesity.

After years of no media attention or unfavorable media attention, 2003 became the year that the television industry discovered obesity, morbid obesity, bariatric operations, and childhood obesity. Newspapers, weekly news magazines, and monthly magazines directed at women have all increased their coverage of obesity-related issues by several orders of magnitude. Society's response to this epidemic is evolving.[48]

Dr. Kelly Brownell, a psychologist at Yale University, is another established bariatric research scientist who is actively trying to shape this response by offering suggestions about how to manage the obesity epidemic in a book directed to the public and published in August 2003. The book is titled *Food Fight: The Inside Story of the Food Industry, America's Obesity Crisis, and What We Can Do About It*.[49] He outlines many of the points made in the preceding paragraphs but emphasizes that the fast food, soft drink, candy, and sugared-cereal companies have produced a "toxic food environment" for children through the 10,000 food advertisements a year the average child watches on television shows aimed at children. He suggests we limit this type of advertising directed at children in ways similar to those defined by laws established in Belgium, Greece, Norway, and Sweden so as to prevent children from being conditioned to prefer these products and to recognize the brands when they shop with their parents. He has also been an advocate for taxing foods that have little or no nutritional value and that contain sugar, fat or both.[49] His colorful quotes, willingness to fight the food and beverage industry, and proximity to the New York City media outlets have enhanced his ability to serve as a spokesperson for obesity experts and public health officials working to decrease the continuing rise in the prevalence of childhood obesity.

There is clear movement in the business community to recognize the economic consequences of obesity. In June 2003, the 175 member companies of the Washington Business Group on Health (whose companies provide health coverage for more than 40 million U.S. citizens) established a new think tank, the Institute on the Costs and Health Effects of Obesity.[50] It is important to note that 19 Fortune 500 companies, including Ford Motor Company, IBM, Pepsi Company, Aetna, and Honeywell, have joined the Director's Board of the institute. The institute recommends to companies strategies to help their employees increase exercise time and make more nutritious food choices and ways of providing access to exercise classes on-site and improving the nutritional content of foods offered in company cafeterias and vending machines.

The 2003 survey by the Society for Human Resource Management of several hundred employee-benefit managers showed an increase in the percentage of companies that are providing on-site fitness centers and on-site weight-loss programs and nutritional counseling and are reimbursing or subsidizing employee gymnasium membership fees. Increases ranged from 1% to 10 % of businesses (which range from 10% to 30% of the industries providing each incentive) in the entire survey, but many specific businesses have started to show an understanding of their employees' expectations. For example, almost 50% of insurance companies provide on-site weight-loss programs for their employees; almost 55% of educational services businesses have on-site fitness centers; and 50% of high-technology companies subsidize gymnasium memberships.[50] Individual businesses are tracking their own rates of sick days and disability leave and are trying to use monitored exercise and dieting as a means of obtaining more favorable health insurance contracts.

A change that is probably more significant is that two recent publications in the business literature attempt to define the costs to businesses of their obese (BMI > 30 kg/m^2) employees using the techniques developed by Colditz[8,13] (in which data from secondary sources are used to estimate costs).[51,52] In one publication from Policy Analysis, Inc., the costs of paid sick leave as well as for life and disability insurance for U.S. businesses were estimated at $2.4 billion, $1.8 billion, and $800 million, respectively, for the obese segment of employees.[50] The other publication is from the Centers for Disease Control and Prevention and is coauthored by one of the same authors who performed the CEA of obesity treatments.[29] They used data from the 1998 Medical Expenditure Panel Survey and the 1996 and 1997 National Health Interview Surveys to calculate that total health care spending for the overweight (BMI > 25 kg/m^2) and the obese (BMI > 30 kg/m^2) in 2002 dollars was $92.6 billion.[51] They separated out these costs to private insurance, Medicaid, and Medicare programs.[52] The assumptions used in these studies need to be confirmed by prospective data, but this type of information is very worrisome to the U.S. business community and to CMMS.

The cost of any proposed response will be a key component of what actually evolves. Prevention of obesity is obviously one of the most important long-term goals for society. Until successful preventive strategies are developed, however, we will be evaluating whether it is cheaper to treat obesity or the numerous diseases associated with it. To date, only bariatric surgery has been shown to treat any form of obesity in a truly cost-effective manner. The first two credible studies examining costs suggest that the bariatric procedures decrease the costs of treating the morbidly obese over the short term (5 years or less) while increasing quality of life.[28,32] Additional long-term studies that demonstrate the economic consequences of treating obesity are obviously needed.

▶ REFERENCES

1. Shape Up America! Foundation and American Obesity Association: Guidance for Treatment of Adult Obesity. Washington, D.C., Shape Up America!, 1996.
2. Deitel M: The Surgeons General's call to action to prevent an increase in overweight and obesity. Obes Surg 2002;12:3-4.
3. National Heart, Lung, and Blood Institute: Clinical Guidelines on the Identification, Evaluation, and Treatment of Overweight and Obesity in Adults: The Evidence Report, National Institutes of Health, Publication No. 98-4083. Washington, D.C., Department of Health and Human Services, 1998.
4. World Health Organization: Obesity: Preventing and Managing the Global Epidemic. Geneva, World Health Organization, 1998.
5. Bray GA: Obesity in Perspective: A Conference. John E. Fogarty International Center for Advanced Study in the Health Sciences, Department of Health, Education and Welfare, National Institutes of Health, Publication No. 75-708. Washington, D.C., Government Printing Office, 1975.
6. Bray GA: Obesity in America: an overview of the Second Fogarty International Center for Advanced Study in the Health Sciences Conference on Obesity. Int J Obes 1979;3:363-375.
7. National Institutes of Health: Health implications of obesity. National Institutes of Health Consensus Development Conference Statement. Ann Intern Med 1985;103:1073-1077.
8. Colditz GA: Economic costs of obesity. Am J Clin Nutr 1992;55: 5503-5507.
9. Levy E, Levy F, Le Pen C, et al: The economic costs of obesity: the French situation. Int J Obes Relat Metab Disord 1995;19:788-792.
10. Seidell JC, Deerenberg I: Obesity in Europe: prevalence and consequences for use of medical care. Pharmacoeconomics 1994;5:38-44.
11. Segal CI, Carter R, Zimmet P: The cost of obesity: the Australian perspective. Pharmacoeconomics 1994;5:45-52.
12. Birmingham CL, Muller JL, Palepu A, et al: The cost of obesity in Canada. CMAJ 1999;160:483-488.
13. Wolf AM, Colditz GA: Current estimates of the economic cost of obesity in the United States. Obes Res 1998;6:97-106.
14. McGinnis JM, Foege WH: Actual causes of death in the United States. JAMA 1993;270(18):2207-2212.
15. Allison DB, Fontaine KR, Manson JE, et al: Annual deaths attributable to obesity in the United States. JAMA 1999;282:1530-1538.
16. Coleman JA: Discrimination at large. Newsweek 1993;1:9.
17. Jindel B: Choice-sensitive health costs. J La State Med Soc 1997;149:62-67.
18. Gill J: The fatness racket. The Times-Picayune 1999;Sept 19:B-5.
19. Vincent N: The politics of obesity. The Times-Picayune 2003;July 13:B-7.
20. Epstein AM, Read JL, Hoefer M: The relation of body weight to length of stay and charges for hospital services for patients undergoing elective surgery: a study of two procedures. Am J Public Health 1987;77:993-997.
21. Quesenberry CP, Caan B, Jacobson A: Obesity, health service use, and healthcare costs among members of a home maintenance organization. Arch Int Med 1998;158:466-472.
22. Martin LF, White S, Lindstrom W Jr: Cost-benefit analysis for treatment of severe obesity. World J Surg 1998;22:1008-1017.
23. National Institutes of Health: Gastrointestinal surgery for severe obesity, National Institutes of Health consensus development

conference draft statement on gastrointestinal surgery for severe obesity, March 25-27, 1991. Am J Clin Nutr 1992;55:615S-619S.

24. Narbro K, Jonsson E, Larsson B, et al: Economic consequences of sick-leave and early retirement in obese Swedish women. Int J Obes 1996;20:895-903.

25. Narbro K, Agren G, Jonsson E, et al: Sick leave and disability pension before and after treatment for obesity: a report from the Swedish Obese Subjects (SOS) study. Int J Obes 1999;23:619-624.

26. Visscher TLS: The Public Health Impact of Obesity, pp. 1-76. Wageningen, The Netherlands, Wageningen University, 2001.

27. Blaxter M: Evidence on inequality in health from a national survey. Lancet 1987;2:30-33.

28. Sampalis JS, Liberman M, Auger S, et al: The impact of weight reduction surgery on health-care costs in morbidly obese patients. Obes Surg 2004;14:939-947.

29. Zhang P, Wang G, Narayan KMV: Cost-effectiveness of interventions for reducing body weight. In Medeiros-Neto G, Halpern A, Bouchard C (eds): Progress in Obesity Research 9, pp. 579-584. Eastleigh, UK, John Libbey, 2003.

30. Gold MR, Siegel IE, Russell LB, et al (eds). Cost-effectiveness in Health and Medicine. New York, Oxford University Press, 1966.

31. Weinstein MC, Stason WB: Foundations of cost-effectiveness analysis for health and medical practices. N Engl J Med 1977;296: 716-721.

32. Van Gemert MG, Adang EMM, Kop M, et al: A prospective cost-effectiveness analysis of vertical banded gastroplasty for the treatment of morbid obesity. Obes Surg 1999;9:484-491.

33. Martin LF, Robinson A, Moore BJ: Socioeconomic issues affecting the treatment of obesity in the millennium. Pharmacoeconomics 2000;18:335-353.

34. Diabetes Prevention Program (DPP) Research Group: The cost-effectiveness of DPP to delay or prevent type 2 diabetes. Diabetes 2002;51:A74 (abstract).

35. Diabetes Prevention Program Research Group: Reduction in the incidence of type 2 diabetes with lifestyle modification or metformin. N Engl J Med 2002;346:393-403.

36. Lamotte M, Annemans L, Lefever A, et al: A health economic model to assess the long-term effects and cost-effectiveness of Orlistat in obese type 2 diabetic patients. Diabetes Care 2002;25:303-308.

37. Martin LF, Tan TL, Holmes P, et al: Preoperative insurance status influences postoperative complication rates for gastric bypass. Am J Surg 1991;161:625-634.

38. Narbro K, Sjostrom L: Willingness to pay for obesity treatment. Int J Technol Assess Health Care 2000;16:50-59.

39. Horm J, Anderson K: Who in America is trying to lose weight? Ann Intern Med 1993;119:672-676.

40. Bloche MG: Managed care no longer containing costs. The Times-Picayune 2003;May 6:B-5.

41. Nestlé M: Food Politics: How the Food Industry Influences Nutrition and Health. Berkley, University of California Press, 2002.

42. Carter RC: The impact of public schools on childhood obesity. JAMA 2002;288:2180.

43. Munoz KA, Krebs-Smith SM, Ballard-Barbash R, et al: Food intakes of U.S. children and adolescents compared with recommendations. Pediatrics 1997;100:323-329.

44. Fried EJ, Nestlé M: The growing political movement against soft drinks in schools. JAMA 2002;288:2181.

45. Daynard RA, Hash LE, Robbins A: Food litigation: lessons from the tobacco wars. JAMA 2002;288:2179.

46. A healthy customer base. The Times-Picayune 2003;July 5:B-6 (editorial).

47. Goodman E: Obesity is in the air. The Times-Picayune 2003;July 27:B-8.

48. Martin LF, Rum WJ: What will society's response be to the obesity epidemic? In Medeiros-Neto G, Halpern A, Bouchard C (eds): Progress in Obesity Research 9, pp. 591-595. Eastleigh, UK, John Libbey, 2003.

49. Brownell KD, Horgan KB: Food Fight: The Inside Story of the Food Industry, America's Obesity Crisis, and What We Can Do About It. New York, McGraw-Hill, 2003.

50. Johnson L: Going for a leaner work force. The Times-Picayune 2003;Sept5:C1-C4.

51. Thompson D, Edelsberg J, Kinsey LK, et al: Estimated economic costs of obesity to U.S. businesses. Am J Health Promot 1998;13: 120-127.

52. Finkelstein EA, Fiebelkorn IC, Wang G: National medical expenditures attributable to overweight and obesity: how much and who's paying? Health Aff 2003;22:219-226.

NONOPERATIVE MANAGEMENT

9

Dietary Management of Obesity

Jeanne D. Blankenship, M.S., R.D., and Bruce M. Wolfe, M.D.

The efficacy of long-term, sustainable weight loss has continued to elude researchers and clinical practitioners. The reasonable doubt of efficacy has left many to question the provision of weight management services in the context of medical management. It is important, however, to distinguish true evidence-based practice from hearsay and unproven popular regimens and also from poorly designed and misinterpreted clinical studies. The complexity of weight management makes the evaluation of interventions difficult despite their large number because few studies have been randomized and most have multiple confounding variables that make the interpretations indefinite. This chapter reviews current research with regard to dietary management of obesity and its expected outcomes.

▶ ENERGY BALANCE

In the simplest context, weight gain and eventual obesity result from a net positive energy balance. Even minor changes in energy intake and physical activity can impact the prevalence of obesity. Hill and colleagues have proposed that a net 100-kcal reduction in energy intake per day would stop weight gain in the population of the United States.[1] Although this minor change would theoretically prevent additional weight gain, it has not been proven to facilitate long-term weight loss or a reduction in comorbidities. Extrapolating data from the National Health and Nutrition Examination Survey and assuming a linear rate of gain, Hill proposed that the average American adult gains approximately 1 kg of body weight per year because energy intake exceeds energy requirements. If it is standard to gain weight, it should also be routine to address impending gain and, whenever possible, thwart the gain by manipulating the energy equation.

Energy needs are influenced by both controllable and noncontrollable factors. Those that can be controlled include physical activity and food intake. Noncontrollable factors include genetics (sex, habitus), age, and the presence of certain disease states. Ultimately, weight loss occurs when energy intake is less than energy expended. Greater energy deficits result in greater weight loss. Therefore, the overall goal of diet therapy is to control food intake while maximizing physical activity, thereby creating a negative energy balance. This concept is simple in theory, but it is less simple in practice. The idea that macronutrient distribution (such as restricting carbohydrate to 10% to 15% of calories) rather than energy intake promotes weight loss warrants direct comment and is discussed in a later section.

▶ DIET THERAPY

Dietary intake has been described by some as the most important component in the treatment of obesity.[2] Ironically, one study showed that two thirds of subjects who were attempting to lose weight reported no attempts to restrict food and energy intake, but rather focused on restricting fat, sugars, snacks, and the amount eaten at meals.[3] Compliance with prescribed regimens can be challenging; therefore, individualization of the program to suit the lifestyle of the individual is imperative. In addition, successful treatment depends largely on matching the level of information and treatment goals to the stage of change in which the individual is currently categorized. Finally, when individualizing treatment plans, the use of structured meal plans, including prepackaged foods and meal replacement products, must be considered along with variable distributions in macronutrient composition and energy density.

Energy Content

Energy requirements can be estimated using predictive equations for resting metabolic rate (RMR), such as the Harris Benedict Formula or the Mifflin-St. Jeor Formula. The Harris Benedict equation tends to overestimate RMR in both men and women. In weight-adjusted obese subjects, the Harris Benedict equation underestimates RMR and the underestimation becomes more severe as higher body weight values are used. Recent evidence comparing the validity of these equations to values derived using indirect calorimetry suggests that the Mifflin-St. Jeor equation more accurately represents the energy needs of obese individuals.[4] Common equations for estimating energy requirements based on sex, age, height, and weight are listed in Box 9-1.

BOX 9-1 • PREDICTIVE EQUATIONS FOR ENERGY EXPENDITURE

1. Harris Benedict (Basal Energy Expenditure, BEE)
   Women:
   $$BEE = 65.5 + 9.56 \text{ (weight kg)} + 1.85 \text{ (height cm)} - 4.68 \text{ (age)}$$
   Men:
   $$BEE = 66.5 + 13.75 \text{ (weight kg)} + 5 \text{ (height cm)} - 6.78 \text{ (age)}$$

   BEE × activity factor (AF) = (total energy expenditure, TEE)
   Activity factors:
   1.2: confined to bed
   1.3: ambulatory
   1.5: normally active person
   2.0 extremely active person
   If BMI <40, use actual weight
   If BMI >40, use ideal body weight

2. Mifflin-St. Jeor (Resting Energy Expenditure, REE)
   Women:
   $$REE = 10 \text{ (weight kg)} + 6.25 \text{ (height cm)} - 5 \text{ (age)} - 161$$
   Men:
   $$REE = 10 \text{ (weight kg)} + 6.25 \text{ (height cm)} - 5 \text{ (age)} + 5$$

   REE × activity factor (AF) = (total energy expenditure, TEE)

3. Macronutrient Panel of the Institute of Medicine (TEE)
   Men >19 years:
   $$TEE = 864 - 9.72 \times age (y) + PA \times [14.2 \times wt (kg) + 503 \times ht (m)]$$
   Women ≥19 years:
   $$TEE = 387 - 7.31 \times age (y) + PA [10.9 \times wt (kg) + 660.7 \times ht (m)]$$

   Where PA = physical activity coefficient
   Sedentary (>1.0 to <1.4)
   Low active (>1.4 to <1.6)
   Active (>1.6 to <1.9)
   Very active (>1.9 to <2.5)

Age adjustment: For women, ± 7, for men ± 10 for each year above or below age 30 years

---

An alternative measure of energy requirements can be made using the MedGem device recently approved by the Food and Drug Administration. This noninvasive and cost-efficient medical device measures oxygen consumption and metabolic rate with greater accuracy than predictive equations.[5]

LOW-CALORIE DIETS

For the morbidly obese, those who have a body mass index of 35 kg per m², an energy restriction of 500 to 1000 calories per day will result in a 1- to 2-lb per week weight loss if the regimen is complied with. In order to establish the usual energy intake of the individual, a registered dietitian can evaluate 24-hour recall records or periodic self-recorded diet records. Because dietary intake by individuals is often underreported by 30% to 50% and daily activity is often overestimated, the use of preestablished energy-restricted regimens is useful until the individual can be coached in reading food labels, measuring portion sizes, and recording and planning food intake.[6] In practice, obese

individuals without previous failed weight-loss attempts should be prescribed a daily caloric restriction of 1000 to 1600 calories per day. The national Heart, Lung, and Blood Institute/North American Association for the Study of Obesity guide recommends 1000 to 1200 kcal per day for most overweight women and 1200 to 1600 kcal per day for overweight men.[7] Women who do not exercise regularly or weigh more than 75 kg should also be prescribed the higher energy restriction.

Adherence to a low-calorie diet (LCD) can result in an approximate loss of 8% of body weight after 4 to 6 months of treatment.[7] The first 2 weeks of the diet produce the largest weekly weight change. During this time, the patient loses water due to a decrease in sodium consumption and as glycogen is mobilized for gluconeogenesis during the induced energy deficit. A weight loss of 1 to 2 lb per week or 1% of initial weight is desirable so as to promote loss of fat rather than lean tissue and additional water loss. The caloric level of the diet should be increased by increments of 200 cal per day until a 1- to 2-lb, or 1%, loss is maintained, thereby promoting the loss of adipose tissue.[7] Frequent monitoring of weight loss and compliance is essential. Adjustments of energy restriction should be made incrementally to ensure that weight loss continues.

Very-Low-Calorie Diets

Very-low-calorie diets (VLCDs) are typically recommended for individuals with body mass indexes greater than 30 kg per m² who have failed to lose weight following an LCD. VLCDs provide 200 to 800 kcal per day, with a substantial number of calories coming from protein in order to preserve lean body mass. Protein recommendations are from 70 to 100 g per day. VLCDs require medical supervision because of the increased risk for medical complications, including electrolyte imbalance, dehydration, gallstones, and other abnormalities. Although there is increased medical risk, VLCDs produce greater short-term weight changes than do LCDs. Weight losses of 15% to 25% in 8 to 16 weeks have been reported in the literature[3]; however, long-term maintenance of losses through VLCDs was no more effective than that resulting from LCDs after 1 year of treatment.[8–10] Instances in which rapid weight loss is medically indicated might make the cost of administration ($3000 for a 6-month program) of a VLCD a worthwhile expense. For example, weight loss required to decrease surgical risk associated with organ transplantation or orthopedic surgery might warrant consideration of a VLCD. However, for those with less critical weight-loss needs, the cost of administration must be weighed against the unlikelihood of long-term weight loss and maintenance.

The most common VLCDs consist of medical-grade formulas designed to contain adequate protein, carbohydrate, and fat along with the appropriate micronutrients. In addition to providing 70 to 90 g per day of high-biological-value protein, the formulas contain enough carbohydrate to prevent ketosis. Between 50% and 60% of calories are typically derived from carbohydrate in the form of maltodextrins and sucrose. Most contain very little fiber and are sweetened by aspartame, sucralose, or saccharine. The formulas typically contain enough fat to prevent deficiency of essential fatty acids and to meet the recommended dietary allowances of vitamins and minerals, with the exception of calcium. Supplementation of vitamins and minerals should be reviewed and evaluated during VLCD administration.[11]

VLCDs are typically administered for 12 to 16 weeks, at which time careful assistance with a reentry diet is required. Calories are gradually increased by 100 to 150 kcal per day to a goal of 1200 to 1500 kcal per day; this process can take 4 to 6 weeks. Close monitoring by the physician is needed, and especially close attention must be paid during the early phases of the diet, until the goal of 1000 to 1200 kcal per day is achieved. The combination of a VLCD and behavioral modification in the treatment of obesity was studied by Atkinson and colleagues.[12] They found that although weight loss was similar in two groups that received VLCDs and behavioral therapy, the timing of the intervention (either before or simultaneously) may influence long-term weight maintenance.

Structure versus Self-Selected Diets

Wing and colleagues randomized women to one of four weight-loss groups with varying levels of structure and found that the provision of structure induced greater weight loss than did a self-selected diet.[13] The study found that there were no differences in weight loss between structured groups that were given both behavior therapy and prescribed menus and groups that were given behavior therapy and were provided with prescribed food. However, the structured groups lost significantly more weight after 6 months than did those who received behavior therapy and self-selected their meals. Moreover, the structured groups maintained greater losses at 18 months than did those with self-selected diets. The findings of this study and that of Jeffrey and colleagues[14] suggest that detailed menus may provide adequate structure to promote adherence and facilitate weight loss.

Heymsfield and colleagues compared six studies of LCDs that consisted of partial meal-replacement plans and found that there was significantly greater weight loss in subjects who received a partial meal replacement (7% to 8% loss) than in those who followed a conventional reduced-calorie diet (3% to 7% loss).[15] One randomized, controlled, long-term trial supported by industry looked at the use of meal replacements for weight loss and open continuation of a single meal replacement daily over a 4-year period. The initial weight loss in subjects using meal replacements was greater than in those following an isocaloric conventional diet, and 75% of those who used a meal replacement were successful in maintaining the loss after 4 years.[16]

Macronutrient Composition

Perhaps no debate in the history of weight loss has received greater attention than that of dietary macronutrient composition. Recent reviews of the literature have concluded that the primary reason that individuals lose weight is decreased energy intake rather than the distribution of macronutrients.[17] Freedman and colleagues reviewed more than 200 dietary studies conducted over the past 60 years and found that a reduction in calories results in weight loss independent of the distribution of macronutrients.[18] The review found that most prescribed diet plans resulted in an energy intake of 1200 to 1600 calories. This energy level, as previously described, would result in an energy deficiency and subsequent weight loss in most overweight and obese individuals. Three classes of dietary approaches to macronutrient composition are shown in Table 9-1.

Data from the National Weight Control Registry (NWCR), which is composed of individuals who have maintained a weight loss of 30 lbs for more than 1 year, indicates that individuals lose weight following a variety of dietary modification programs, but that they follow a similar program to maintain weight loss. Weight-loss maintenance is further described in chapter 11.

Some authors of popular diets have hypothesized that there may be a metabolic advantage to following a high-protein, low-carbohydrate diet, and that weight loss is attainable without regard to energy intake. Although numerous studies exist that attempt to evaluate the impact of macronutrient manipulation in the diet, study design has been poor or inconsistent, and the results cannot be applied or generalized. The use of high-protein, low-carbohydrate diets has been popular in varying degrees since first described by Banting in 1863.[19] Advocates insist that these diets promote the metabolism of adipose tissue in the absence of carbohydrate and that weight loss occurs rapidly.[20] There have been no published scientific studies that confirm this hypothesis.

Table 9-1	THREE CLASSES OF DIETARY APPROACH TO MACRONUTRIENT COMPOSITION		
TYPE	DISTRIBUTION	EXAMPLE	COMMENT
Low-carbohydrate, high-fat diet	<20% energy from carbohydrate or <100 g total carbohydrate	• Atkins Diet • Protein Power	
Very-low-fat, high-carbohydrate diet	<10% of total energy from fat and >55% of energy from carbohydrate	• Dean Ornish's Reversing Heart Disease Program • The Pritikin Program	Originally used for heart disease; diet is high in complex carbohydrates and fiber and low in energy density.
Moderate-fat, high-carbohydrate diet	20%-30% of total energy from fat and >55% of energy from carbohydrate	• Weight Watchers • Jenny Craig • The American Heart Association's Shape-Up America Program	Typical American diet contains 35%-40% of energy from fat.

Bravata and colleagues conducted a systematic review of 94 dietary intervention studies published between 1966 and 2003 to evaluate the relationship of low carbohydrate diets to specific outcome measures, including cardiovascular risk markers and weight.[21] The authors concluded that among these published studies, weight loss was associated primarily with an overall decrease in energy intake and the length of the imposed caloric deficit. They did not find that a reduction in carbohydrate intake per se was responsible for the weight loss.

Two recent randomized studies related to low-carbohydrate diets are noteworthy. A 1-year multicenter study conducted by Foster and colleagues found that low-carbohydrate diet subjects had significantly more weight loss than low-fat dieters at 6 months but not at 1 year.[22] The low-carbohydrate diet was associated with greater improvement in some coronary heart-disease risk factors. It is unknown whether the risk reduction was attributable to the type of dietary fat (monounsaturated, polyunsaturated, or saturated) consumed by the low-carbohydrate group. Because the study did not include dietary intake data, the actual carbohydrate intake of the subjects was not measured. Thus, although individuals may have been assigned to the low-carbohydrate group, it is unknown if they actually consumed this type of diet. The study is further limited by the attrition rate, small sample size, and gender bias.

A study by Samaha and Iqbal compared a low-carbohydrate diet to a low-fat diet in 79 randomly assigned subjects.[23] The low-carbohydrate group had lost significantly more weight at 6 months; however, the authors concluded that the difference was attributable to a greater reduction in energy intake compared to the low-fat diet group rather than to macronutrient distribution. An important consideration in the review of this study is the actual carbohydrate intake of study participants. Extrapolating from the data provided, the low-carbohydrate group reported a mean intake of 163 g of carbohydrate. This amount is 20% more than the minimum level of 135 g per day recommended by the American Diabetes Association and others to support normal brain function. The intake of the group is consistent with the daily required intake of 175 g per day; thus, one must question whether this group can truly be called a low-carbohydrate group.

Given that individuals who follow low-carbohydrate programs do achieve significant weight loss, this approach cannot be discounted as an appreciable method of decreasing energy intake. There may be a greater degree of satiety when individuals follow diets that promote higher levels of protein and fat intake. Furthermore, as described by Samaha and Iqbal, the simplicity of the diet and its novelty make it popular with the general population.[23] Additional studies of the long-term nutrition status and weight-loss maintenance of those who follow such regimens are warranted.

PHYSICAL ACTIVITY

Popular belief that increasing energy expenditure will result in weight loss has been unproven in the medical literature. The importance of physical activity, however, is thought to play a key role in weight-loss maintenance. Evidence from the NWCR suggests that among successful subjects, physical activity is the number-one predictor of long-term success.[24]

Among sedentary overweight and obese individuals, the limitation for early exercise efforts is that the intensity of exercise required to facilitate meaningful caloric expenditure is nearly impossible. The issue of the appropriate amount of physical activity to prescribe with regard to weight loss has been complex. Three studies, by Klem,[25] Schoeller,[26] and Jakicic[27] and their colleagues collectively suggest that an energy expenditure of 2200 to 2800 kcal per week is associated with improved weight-loss maintenance. Despite the agreement of these studies, none prospectively tested the efficacy of a prescription of that amount of physical activity for long-term weight loss. A review of a large body of literature comparing short-term weight loss by dietary restriction with and without exercise found no significant difference in total weight loss between groups. Only metaanalyses reveal the fact that added physical activity does indeed lead to a fat loss that is significantly greater by approximately 1 kg, although weight differences are small or not significant.[28,29]

LONG-TERM RESULTS OF MEDICAL THERAPY

The short-term weight loss associated with drug therapy, diet and behavioral diet therapy, behavior modification, and exercise, conducted as sole interventions or in various combinations, has been the subject of countless studies and reports. Virtually all studies show that at least some weight loss in comparison to untreated controls can be achieved. Individual cases of patients with morbid obesity in whom 100 or more lbs of weight are lost, although not common, clearly occur. Few studies have provided meaningful long-term longitudinal follow-up data. In recent years, however, several studies with follow-up to 1 year and a small number of studies with 5-year follow-up have been published.

A classic study defining the problem of long-term recurrence of obesity following successful weight reduction was published by Drenick and Johnson in 1978.[30] A total of 207 morbidly obese patients were hospitalized for weight reduction via prolonged fasting and subsequent semistarvation. Under such circumstances, virtually all patients can and do accomplish weight loss. Following accomplishment of weight reduction, 121 of the patients were followed for a mean of 7.3 years. The percentage of patients remaining in the program fell gradually over the first 5 years, so that at 5 years of follow-up, obesity had recurred in more than 90%. The authors concluded that although major weight loss could be accomplished in a supervised environment with fasting followed by semistarvation, such intervention is rarely justifiable because of the nearly uniform recurrence of obesity.

More recent reviews and metaanalyses of long-term results of weight loss confirm the findings of Drenick and Johnson.[30] Specifically, although weight may be lost in the short term, long-term maintenance of weight loss is rarely achieved. A consistent observation is that whatever the intervention (diet, pharmacotherapy, behavior modification, or exercise), when active intervention or participation of the patient in the specific therapeutic environment ceases, the weight is regained. Thus, for any intervention, including pharmacotherapy, to be successful, permanent intervention and active participation are required. The lack of feasibility and practicality of such permanent participation in these therapeutic modalities accounts, in large part, for the ultimate failure of these interventions.[31-35] A common theme among these many studies is the observation that a common, if not uniform, characteristic of those few patients who do achieve long-term successful maintenance of weight reduction is continued active participation in a vigorous exercise program. Thus, even though exercise alone has proved disappointing as a primary modality for accomplishing weight reduction, it appears to be a critical component of the maintenance of weight reduction among those patients who also achieve lasting dietary restriction.[24] This population of patients is documented in a national Web-based registry established by Wing and Hill and colleagues.[1]

The most extensively studied population of patients over an interval of several years appears to be the Swedish Obese Subjects trial. In this trial, patients who underwent surgical intervention for morbid obesity were matched with patients in a national database who did not undergo surgery. Weight loss after 8 years was 20 plus or minus 16 kg (16.5%) in the surgical group, whereas the controls had gained 0.7 plus or minus 12 kg.[36] The controls were reported to show modest initial weight loss but a slight weight gain prevailed at the 8-year mark.

▶ IMPLICATIONS FOR BARIATRIC SURGERY

Epidemiologic data have clearly defined obesity as a major risk factor for premature mortality[37] and for the development of certain comorbidities, including cancer, diabetes, and many others, as noted elsewhere in this volume. Effective weight loss is therefore clearly indicated. Bariatric surgical intervention has often been criticized in the past and continues to be criticized as an extreme intervention with unacceptable risk, considering the availability of alternative treatments—diet, pharmacotherapy, exercise, behavior modification, and combinations of these modalities, as discussed earlier. Yet it is the failure of medical therapy and its modifications to accomplish durable weight loss in the obese population in general and in individual cases that justifies surgical intervention, despite the potential for postoperative complications. As in many other situations in which surgical therapy is performed, surgical procedures represent a practical solution to a life-threatening disease.

The issue of the specifics required to declare that all efforts in medical therapy have been tried and have failed before a given patient should proceed to surgery is a matter on which there is little agreement. Various requirements have been imposed by surgeons, insurance companies, referring physicians, and others to satisfy the criterion of failure of medical therapy. These requirements include variable intervals of active intervention; a certain amount of weight loss, even if that has been transient in the past; demonstration of the understanding of nutrition principles;

active participation in an exercise program; and others. At this time, there are no definitive data demonstrating the long-term efficacy of any of these measures, although a clear understanding of nutrition and the patient's requirement of a successful outcome of surgery are certainly reasonable. Patients who seek surgery are, by definition, a subgroup of the severely obese population because they have determined that, for themselves, further medical therapy is not warranted and surgical intervention is required if they are to achieve durable weight loss. The great majority of such patients have achieved transient weight loss on many occasions prior to seeking surgical consultation. The authors believe that there is no useful purpose in requiring patients to participate in further diet therapy and other components of a weight-reduction program prior to proceeding with surgery if the individual patient has determined that, in his or her case, medical therapy has failed.

Medical therapy for patients with morbid obesity is a dismal failure for the entire population at large and is even less likely to be successful in those patients who honestly believe they have exhausted all efforts to accomplish medical therapy. An exception might be a patient with such severe obesity and associated comorbidities that operative risk is judged to be excessive. Patients with heart failure and anasarca are such possible examples. Routine mandatory preoperative weight loss has been advocated for all surgical candidates, but it is not supported by the published literature. Delay of surgical intervention for a year or more may, in fact, be deleterious because of the continued exposure of the patient to the adverse health effects of severe obesity.

▶ SUMMARY

Successful weight management using nonsurgical approaches in the obese patient continues to elude researchers and clinicians. Progression and expansion of targeted research in the field of obesity are necessary to identify optimal dietary and behavioral strategies as alternative therapies or as adjuncts to surgical intervention. Energy-restricted eating patterns, along with physical activity and behavioral modification, result in significant weight loss in some individuals. The noninvasive aspect of dietary management makes it a worthwhile consideration for all overweight individuals who are committed to a lifestyle change. Although the long-term likelihood of weight maintenance after significant weight loss is questionable, data from the NWCR suggest that certain lifestyle characteristics and commonalities can be associated with long-term success and should, therefore, be encouraged and monitored.

▶ REFERENCES

1. Hill JO, Wyatt HR, Reed GW, et al: Obesity and the environment: Where do we go from here? Science 2003; 299:853-855.
2. Klein S: Medical management of obesity. Obes Surg 2001;81(5): 1025-1038.
3. Wadden TA, Osei S: The treatment of obesity: an overview. In Wadden TA, Stunkard AF (eds): Handbook of Obesity Treatment, pp. 229-248. New York, Guilford Press, 2002.

4. Frankenfield DC, Rowe WA, Smith S, et al: Validation of several established equations for resting metabolic rate in obese and nonobese people. J Am Diet Assoc 2003;103(9):1152-1159.

5. Nieman DC, Trone GA, Austin MD: A new handheld device for measuring resting metabolic rate and oxygen consumption. J Am Diet Assoc 2003;103(5):588-592.

6. Lichtman SW, Pisarka K, Berman ER, et al: Discrepancy between self-reported and actual caloric intake and exercise in obese subjects. N Engl J Med 1992;327:1893-1898.

7. National Institutes of Health/National Heart Lung and Blood Institute, North American Association for the Study of Obesity: Practical Guide to the Identification, Evaluation and Treatment of Overweight and Obesity in Adults. Bethesda, MD, National Institutes of Health, 2000.

8. Wing RR, Blair E, Marcus MD, et al: Year-long weight loss treatment for obese patients with type II diabetes: does inclusion of intermittent very low calorie diet improve outcome? Am J Med 1994;97:354-362.

9. Wing RR, Marcus MD, Salata R, et al: Effects of a very-low-calorie diet on long-term glycemic control in obese type II diabetic subjects. Arch Intern Med 1991;151:1334-1340.

10. Wadden TA, Foster GD, Letizia KA: One-year behavioral treatment of obesity: comparison of moderate and severe caloric restrictions and the effects of weight maintenance therapy. J Consult Clin Psychol 1994;62:165-171.

11. Reeves R, Bolton MP, Gee M: Dietary approaches in managing obesity. In Foster GD, Nonas CA (eds): Managing Obesity: A Clinical Guide. American Dietetic Association, 2003.

12. Atkinson RL, Fuchs A, Pastors JG, et al: Combination of very low-calorie diet and behavioral modification in the treatment of obesity. Am J Clin Nutr 1992;56(1 suppl):199-202S.

13. Wing RR, Jeffrey RW, Burton LR, et al: Food provisions vs. structured meal plans in the behavioral treatment of obesity. J Consult Clin Psychol 1996;20:56-62.

14. Jeffery RW, Wing RR, Thomson C, et al: Strengthening behavioral interventions for weight loss: a randomized trial of food provision and monetary incentives. J Consult Clin Psychol 1993;61:1038-1095.

15. Heymsfield SB, Van Mierlo CA, van der Knaap HC, et al: Weight management using a meal replacement strategy: meta and pooling analysis from six studies. Int J Obes Relat Metab Disord 2003;27(5):537-549.

16. Flechtner-Mors M, Ditschuneit HH, Johnson TD, et al: Metabolic and weight loss effects of long-term dietary intervention in obese patients: four-year results. Obes Res 2000;8(5):399-402.

17. Kennedy ET, Bowman SA, Spence JT, et al: Popular diets: correlation to health, nutrition and obesity. J Am Diet Assoc 2001;101(4):411-420.

18. Freedman MR, King J, Kennedy E: Popular diets: a scientific review. Obes Res 2001;9(1 suppl):1-40S.

19. Bray GA: Low carbohydrate diets and realities of weight loss. JAMA 2003;289:1853-1855.

20. Atkins RC: Dr. Atkins' New Diet Revolution. New York, Avon Books, 1998.

21. Bravata DM: Efficacy and safety of low carbohydrate diets: a systematic review. JAMA 2003;289:1837-1850.

22. Foster GD, Wyatt HR: A randomized trial of a low carbohydrate diet for obesity. N Engl J Med 2003;348:2082-2090.

23. Samaha FF, Iqbal N. A low-carbohydrate as compared with a low-fat diet in severe obesity. N Engl J Med 2003;348:2031-2074.

24. Wing RR, Hill JD. Successful weight loss maintenance. Annual Rev Nutr 2001;21:323-341.

25. Klem ML, Wing RR, McGuire MT, et al: A descriptive study of individuals successful at long-term maintenance of substantial weight loss. Am J Clin Nutr 1997;66:239-246.

26. Schoeller DA, Shay K, Kushner RF. How much physical activity is needed to minimize weight gain in previously obese women? Am J Clin Nutr 1997;66:551-556.

27. Jakicic JM, Winter C, Wing RR. Effects of intermittent exercise and use of home exercise equipment on adherence, weight loss and fitness in overweight women: a randomized trial. JAMA 1999;282:1554-1560.

28. Ballor DL, Pochlman ET. Exercise training enhances fat-free mass preservation during diet-induced weight loss: a meta-analysis finding. Int J Obes Relat Metab Disord 1994;18:35-40.

29. Saris WHM, Blair SN, van Baak MA, et al: How much physical activity is enough to prevent unhealthy weight gain? Outcome of the IASO 1st Stock Conference and Consensus Statement. Obes Rev 2003;4:101-114.

30. Drenick EJ, Johnson D. Weight reduction by fasting and semistarvation in morbid obesity: long-term follow-up. Int Obes 1978;2:123-132.

31. Giusti V, Suter M, Heraief E, et al: Rising role of obesity surgery caused by increase of morbid obesity, failure of conventional treatments and unrealistic expectations: trends from 1997 to 2001. Obes Surg 2003; 13:693-698.

32. Anderson JW, Konz EC, Frederich RC, et al: Long-term weight-loss maintenance: a meta-analysis of US studies. Am J Clin Nutr 2001; 74:579-584.

33. Glenny AM, O'Meara S, Melville A, et al: The treatment and prevention of obesity: a systemic review of the literature. Int J Obes 1997;21:715-737.

34. McTigue KM, Harris R, Hemphill B, et al: Screening and interventions for obesity in adults: summary of the evidence for the U.S. Preventive Services Task Force. Ann Intern Med 2003;139:933-949.

35. Glazer G: Long-term pharmacotherapy of obesity 2000: a review of efficacy and safety. Arch Intern Med 2001;161:1814-1824.

36. Torgerson JS, Sjostrom L: The Swedish Obese Subjects (SOS) Study—rationale and results. Int J Obes 2001;25(1 suppl):S2-54.

37. Calle EE, Thun MJ, Petrelli JM et al: Body-mass index and mortality in a prospective cohort of U.S. adults. N Engl J Med 1999;341(15):1097-1105.

10

Drug Management in Obesity

George A. Bray, M.D.

Surgical treatment of obesity is appropriate for individuals with substantial degrees of excess weight, usually a body mass index (BMI) greater than 40 kg per m^2. Before reaching this stage of obesity, however, many overweight individuals will have tried other ways of losing weight, including diet, exercise, commercial weight-loss programs, lifestyle changes, and medications. This chapter focuses on the use and abuse of medications in treating obesity.

A report from the Heart, Lung, and Blood Institute of the National Institutes of Health titled *Clinical Guidelines on the Identification, Evaluation, and Treatment of Overweight and Obesity in Adults: The Evidence Report* emphasizes the need for physicians to address obesity in their patients.[1] This report sanctions the clinical recommendation of weight-loss drugs approved by the Food and Drug Administration (FDA) for long-term use as part of a concomitant lifestyle-modification program. Appropriate patients are those who have been unsuccessful in previous weight-loss attempts and whose BMIs exceed 27 kg per m^2; those who have associated conditions, such as diabetes, hypertension, or dyslipidemia; and those whose BMIs exceed 30 kg per m^2.

The management of obesity by the use of drugs has been tarnished by a number of problems.[2] Since the introduction of thyroid hormone to treat obesity in 1893, almost every drug used to treat obesity has led to undesirable outcomes that have resulted in injury and death and, ultimately, withdrawal of the drug. Thus, caution must be used in accepting any new drug for the treatment of obesity unless the safety profile makes it acceptable for almost everyone.

An additional seriously negative aspect of using drug treatment for obesity is the negative halo surrounding the fact that the first pharmaceutical drug to be used, amphetamine, is addictive.[3] Amphetamine stands for alpha-methyl-phenethylamine. It is indicated for narcolepsy and attention deficit disorder, but it is also addictive. It reduces food intake, but it is not recommended for obesity management. The addictive nature of amphetamine is probably related to its effects on dopaminergic neurotransmission. On the other hand, its anorectic effects appear to result from modulation of noradrenergic neurotransmission. Drugs such as phentermine, diethylpropion, fenfluramine, sibutramine, and the antidepressant venlafaxine are all β-phenethylamines. Phentermine and diethylpropion are sympathomimetic amines, like amphetamine, but they differ from amphetamine in having little or no effect on dopamine release or reuptake at the synapse. Abuse of either phentermine or diethylpropion is rare.[2] Fenfluramine is also a β-phenethylamine, but it has no effect on reuptake or release of either norepinephrine or dopamine in the brain. Fenfluramine is a potent serotonin releaser and it inhibits monoamine reuptake; its effect on dopamine is minimal and it partially inhibits serotonin reuptake. There have been no reports of addiction to fenfluramine. Sibutramine has no evident abuse potential.[4] Thus, derivatives of β-phenethylamine have a wide range of pharmacologic effects and a highly variable potential for abuse. However, if examined uncritically, they could all be lumped with amphetamine and carry its negative history. It is thus misleading to use the term *amphetamine-like* in reference to appetite-suppressant β-phenethylamine drugs other than amphetamine and methamphetamine because of the negative images that arise and because of its inaccuracy.

A third issue surrounding drug treatment in obesity is the negative attitude that results when patients relapse after successful treatment. The perception arises that the drugs are ineffective because weight regain occurs when drug treatment is stopped.[5] Cure for obesity is rare, and treatment is thus aimed at palliation. As clinicians, we do not expect to cure such diseases as hypertension or hypercholesterolemia with medications. Rather, we expect to palliate them. When the medications for any of these diseases are discontinued, we expect the disease to recur. This means that medications work only when used. The same arguments are applicable to medications used to treat overweight. It is a chronic, incurable disease for which drugs work only when used.

Reports of valvular heart disease associated with the use of fenfluramine, dexfenfluramine, and phentermine have provided the most recent ammunition for those who disapprove of treating obesity with medications.[6-8] This is an example of the law of unintended consequences. The reports of valvulopathy in patients treated with fenfluramine or dexfenfluramine were totally unexpected. Thankfully, the extent of the problem has not proven to be as great as first suspected.[8] It is now recognized that risk for valvulopathy associated with fenfluramine is associated with duration of exposure to the medication[8] and that the lesions are likely to remit once the patient has stopped taking the medication.[9,10] This finding of toxicity, however, will elicit caution when any future drugs are marketed to treat obesity and will provide support to those who believe that drug treatment of obesity is inappropriate and risky.

The final preliminary issue to address is the plateau of weight that occurs with all treatments for obesity.[11-17] At the beginning of treatment, a weight loss of less than 15% would be considered unsatisfactory by most obese patients.[18] There is a discrepancy in the amount of weight loss that is cosmetically desired and the amount of weight loss that produces health benefits. Yet the reality is that none of the treatments, except bariatric surgery,[17] produce a consistent weight loss of more than 15%. When weight plateaus at a level above the desired cosmetic goal, patients usually blame the treatment. This perceived loss of effectiveness often leads patients to terminate treatment, which results in the inevitable slow regain of the weight that had been lost.

In weighing the options regarding treatments for obesity, physicians must be cognizant of these barriers to success. It is against these limitations that we will review currently available medications. Drugs to treat obesity can be divided into three groups: those that reduce food intake, those that alter metabolism, and those that increase thermogenesis. Monoamines acting on noradrenergic receptors, serotonin receptors, dopamine receptors, and histamine receptors can reduce food intake. A number of peptides also modulate food intake. The noradrenergic drugs phentermine, diethylpropion, benzphetamine, and phendimetrazine are approved only for short-term use. Sibutramine, a norepinephrine-serotonin reuptake inhibitor, is approved for long-term use. Also approved for long-term use is orlistat, an antimetabolic agent that inhibits pancreatic lipase and can block hydrolysis of 30% of the dietary triglyceride in subjects eating a 30% fat diet. The thermogenic combination of ephedrine and caffeine has not been approved by regulatory agencies.

Table 10-1 summarizes the effects of a number of drugs that are currently available in the United States to treat obesity.[2,19,20] They are discussed in more detail subsequently.

Table 10-1	**DRUGS APPROVED BY THE FDA TO TREAT OBESITY**			
DRUG NAME	TRADE NAME	DOSAGE	DEA SCHEDULE	SIDE EFFECTS AND COMMENTS
		Pancreatic lipase inhibitor		
Orlistat	Xenical	120 mg tid before meals	None	Daily vitamin pill in the evening; may interact with cyclosporine
		Serotonin-norepinephrine reuptake inhibitor		
Sibutramine	Meridia Reductil	5-15 mg/d	IV	Raises blood pressure slightly; do not use with monoamine oxidase inhibitors, selective serotonin reuptake inhibitors, sumatriptan, dihydroergotamine, merperidine, methadone, pentazocine, fentanyl, lithium, tryptophan
		Sympathomimetic drugs		
Diethylpropion	Tenuate Dospan Tepanil	25 mg tid 25 mg tid 75 mg in am	IV	All sympathomimetic drugs are similar; do not use with monoamine oxidase inhibitors, guanethidine, alcohol, sibutramine, tricyclic antidepressants
Phentermine	Standard release: Adipex-P Fastin Obenix Oby-Cap Oby-Trim Zantryl Slow release: Ionamin	18.75 to 37.5 mg/d tid 15-30 mg/d in am	IV	See above
Benzphetamine	Didrex	25-50 mg 1-3 times/d	III	See above
Phendimetrazine	Standard release: Bontril PDM Plegine X-trozine Slow release: Bontril Prelu-2 X-Trozine	35 mg tid before meals 105 mg/d in am	III	See above

tid, three times a day

▶ SYMPATHOMIMETIC DRUGS THAT REDUCE FOOD INTAKE

Pharmacology

The sympathomimetic drugs are grouped together because they can increase blood pressure and, in part, act like norepinephrine (NE). Drugs in this group work by a variety of mechanisms, including the release of NE from synaptic granules (benzphetamine, phendimetrazine, phentermine, and diethylpropion); the blockade of NE reuptake (mazindol); or the blockade of reuptake of both NE and serotonin (5-hydroxytryptomine, 5-HT; i.e., sibutramine).

All of these drugs are absorbed orally and reach peak blood concentrations within a short time. The half-life in blood is also short for all except the two pharmacologically active metabolites of sibutramine, which have a long half-life.[2] Although the two metabolites of sibutramine are active, this is not true for the metabolites of other drugs in this group. Liver metabolism inactivates a large fraction of these drugs before excretion. Side effects include dry mouth, constipation, and insomnia. Food intake is suppressed either by delaying the onset of a meal or by producing early satiety. Sibutramine and mazindol have both been shown to increase thermogenesis as well.[21-25]

Efficacy

The criteria used by the FDA for the efficacy of appetite-suppressing drugs is the demonstration in randomized, double-blind, placebo-controlled clinical trials of statistically significant weight loss that is 5% below that in the placebo group.[2] A decrease in weight that is 10% below baseline and significantly greater than that in the placebo group is the major criterion for the European Committee on Proprietary Medicinal Products. Clinical trials of sympathomimetic drugs that were run before 1975 were generally short term because it was widely believed that short-term treatment would "cure obesity."[26] This was unfounded optimism, and because the trials were of short duration and often crossed over in design, they provided few long-term data. In this review, we focus on long-term trials lasting 24 weeks or more and on only those trials in which there were adequate control groups.

PHENTERMINE, DIETHYLPROPION, BENZPHETAMINE, AND PHENDIMETRAZINE

Only a few long-term clinical trials have been conducted of the first generation of sympathomimetic drugs.[2,14,19,27-32] The best and one of the longest of these clinical trials lasted 36 weeks and compared placebo treatment against continuous use of phentermine and intermittent use of phentermine.[14] Both continuous and intermittent phentermine therapy produced more weight loss than did the placebo. In the drug-free periods the patients treated intermittently slowed their weight loss, only to lose more rapidly when the drug was reinstituted.

Phentermine and diethylpropion are classified by the U.S. Drug Enforcement Agency as schedule IV drugs, and benzphetamine and phendimetrazine as schedule III drugs. This regulatory classification indicates the government's belief that they have the potential for abuse, although this potential appears to be very low. Phentermine and diethylpropion are approved for use for only "a few weeks," which is usually interpreted to mean up to 12 weeks. Weight loss with phentermine and diethylpropion persists for the duration of treatment, suggesting that tolerance to these drugs does not develop. If tolerance were to develop, the drugs would be expected to lose their effectiveness, or increased amounts of drug would be required for patients to maintain weight loss. This does not occur. Of the agents in this group, phentermine is prescribed most frequently in the United States, probably because it is inexpensive, no longer being protected by patents. Phentermine is not available in Europe. A recent review in a prestigious journal recommends obtaining written informed consent if phentermine is prescribed for longer than 12 weeks,[33] because this is off-label usage and there are not a sufficient number of published reports concerning the use of phentermine over the long term.

SIBUTRAMINE

In contrast to the older sympathomimetic drugs, sibutramine has been extensively evaluated in several multicenter trials lasting 6 to 24 months.[11,34-46] In a clinical trial lasting 8 weeks, sibutramine produced a dose-dependent weight loss with doses of 5 and 20 mg per day.[47] Several long-term, randomized, placebo-controlled, double-blind clinical trials have been conducted in men and women of all ethnic groups with ages ranging from 18 to 65 years and with BMIs between 27 kg per m² and 40 kg per m². In a 6-month dose-ranging study of 1047 patients, 67% achieved a 5% weight loss and 35% lost 10% or more.[35] There is a clear dose response in this 24-week trial, and regain of weight occurred when the drug was stopped, indicating that the drug remained effective when used. Nearly two thirds of the patients treated with sibutramine lost more than 5% of their body weight from baseline and nearly one third lost more than 10%. In an interesting study by virtue of the magnitude of weight lost, patients who initially lost weight eating a very-low-calorie diet were randomized to sibutramine 10 mg per day or placebo and a behavioral program.[36] Sibutramine produced additional weight loss (16% from baseline at 1 year), whereas the placebo-treated patients regained weight.

A number of observations about sibutramine can be drawn from the Sibutramine Trial of Obesity Reduction and Maintenance (STORM), but the effects of sibutramine in aiding weight maintenance are most persuasive.[38] Seven centers participated in this trial in which patients were initially enrolled in an open-label fashion and treated with 10 mg per day of sibutramine for 6 months (Fig. 10-1). The patients who lost more than 5% (and 77% of enrolled patients met this goal) were then randomized, two thirds to sibutramine and one third to placebo. During the 18-month double-blind portion of the trial, the placebo-treated patients steadily regained weight, maintaining only 20% of their weight loss at the end of the trial. In contrast, the subjects treated with sibutramine maintained their weight for 12 months and then regained an average of only 2 kg, thus maintaining 80% of their initial weight loss after 2 years. In spite of this difference in weight at the end of the 18 months of controlled observation, the mean blood

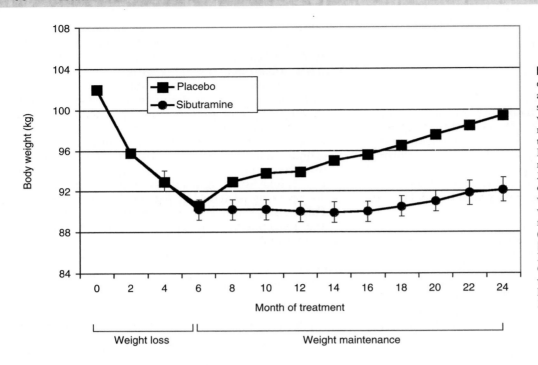

Figure 10-1. Patients were initially enrolled in an open-label fashion and treated with 10 mg per day of sibutramine for 6 months. Those who lost more than 5% were then randomized, two thirds to sibutramine and one third to placebo. Placebo-treated patients steadily regained weight, maintaining only 20% of their weight loss at the end of the trial, whereas subjects treated with sibutramine maintained their weight for 12 months and then regained an average of only 2 kg. (From James WPT for the STORM [Sibutramine Trial of Obesity Reduction and Maintenance] Study Group: Effect of sibutramine on weight maintenance after weight loss: a randomize trial. Lancet 2000; 356:2119-2125.)

pressure of the sibutramine-treated patients was still higher than that of the patients treated with placebo, even though they had a weight difference of several kilograms.

Sibutramine given continuously for 1 year has been compared to placebo and sibutramine given intermittently.[42] In this study, patients who had lost 2% or 2 kg after 4 weeks of treatment with sibutramine (15 mg/day) were randomized to placebo; to continued sibutramine; or to sibutramine prescribed intermittently (weeks 1-12, 19-30, and 37-48). Both sibutramine treatment regimens produced equivalent results, and they were significantly better than the results with the placebo regimen. The stopping of sibutramine caused small increases in weight, which were then reversed when the medication was restarted.

Four clinical trials document sibutramine use in patients with diabetes. One lasted for 12 weeks[48] and the other three for 24 weeks.[42-44] In the 12-week trial, diabetic patients treated with sibutramine (15 mg/d) lost 2.4 kg (2.8%) compared to 0.1 kg (0.12%) in the placebo group.[48] In this study, hemoglobin A_{1c} (HbA$_{1c}$) fell -0.3% in the drug-treated group and remained stable in the placebo-treated group. In the study by Gockel and colleagues, 60 female patients who had poorly controlled glucose levels (HbA$_{1c}$ >8%) on maximal doses of sulfonylureas and metformin were randomly assigned to 10 mg sibutramine twice daily or placebo.[44] The weight loss at 24 weeks was 9.6 kg in the sibutramine-treated patients and 0.9 kg in those on placebo. The improvements in glycemic control were equally striking. In the sibutramine-treated patients, HbA$_{1c}$ fell 2.73% compared to 0.53% with the placebo. Insulin levels fell 5.66 U per ml compared to 0.68 for placebo, and fasting glucose fell 124.88 mg per ml compared to 15.76 mg per ml for placebo. Although in most of the studies of patients with diabetes, their weight loss does not appear to be as great as it is in nondiabetic patients, in all of the studies the percentage of patients who achieved

weight loss of more than 5% from baseline was significantly greater than it was in those in the placebo group. In all studies, the degree of weight loss corresponded to the degree of improvement in glycemic control.

Two trials have been reported in which sibutramine was used to treat hypertensive patients over 1 year,[11,46] and two additional studies provide data on 12 weeks of treatment.[49,50] In all instances, the weight-loss pattern favors sibutramine. However, except for one study, mean weight loss, though favorable, was associated with mean blood pressure increases.[50] In a 3-month trial all patients were receiving β-blockers with or without thiazides for their hypertension.[49] The sibutramine-treated patients lost 4.2 kg (4.5%) compared to a loss of 0.3 kg (0.3%) in the placebo-treated group. Mean supine and standing diastolic and systolic blood pressure were not significantly different between drug-treated and placebo-treated patients. Heart rate, however, increased 5.6 ± 8.25 beats per minute (M ± SD) in the sibutramine-treated patients as compared to an increase in heart rate of 2.2 ± 6.43 beats per minute (M ± SD) in the placebo-treated group. McMahon and colleagues reported a 52-week trial in hypertensive patients whose blood pressure was controlled by calcium channel blockers with or without β-blockers or thiazides.[11] Sibutramine doses were increased from 5 to 20 mg per day during the first 6 weeks. Weight loss was significantly greater in the sibutramine-treated patients, averaging 4.4 kg (4.7%), as compared to 0.5 kg (0.7%) in the placebo-treated group. Diastolic blood pressure decreased 1.3 mmHg in the placebo-treated group and increased by 2.0 mmHg in the sibutramine-treated group. The systolic blood pressure increased 1.5 mmHg in the placebo-treated group and 2.7 mmHg in the sibutramine-treated group. Heart rate was unchanged in the placebo-treated patients but increased 4.9 beats per minute in the sibutramine-treated patients.[11] One small study in eight obese men demonstrated that an aerobic exercise program mitigated the adverse blood pressure effects of sibutramine.[51]

Because the dose of sibutramine influences the amount of weight loss with the drug, the intensity of the behavioral component is also likely to have an effect.[34,35] This is readily demonstrated in a study by Wadden and colleagues.[52] With minimal behavioral intervention, the weight loss in that study was about 5 kg during 12 months. When group counseling to produce behavior modification was added to sibutramine, the weight loss increased to 10 kg, and when a structured meal plan using meal replacements was added to the medication and behavior plan, the weight loss increased further to 15 kg. This indicates that the amount of weight loss observed during pharmacotherapy is due in part to the intensity of the behavioral approach.

Sibutramine is available in 5-, 10-, and 15-mg pills; 10 mg per day as a single daily dose is the recommended starting level, with titration upward or downward based on response. Doses above 15 mg per day are not recommended by the FDA. The chance of achieving meaningful weight loss can be determined by the response to treatment in the first 4 weeks. In one large trial, of the patients who lost 2 kg (4 lb) in the first 4 weeks of treatment, 60% achieved a weight loss of more than 5%, compared to less than 10% of those who did not lose 2 kg (4 lb) in 4 weeks.[35] Except for blood pressure, weight loss with sibutramine is associated with improvement in profiles of cardiovascular risk factors. Combining data from the total of 11 studies of sibutramine showed a weight-related reduction in triglyceride, total cholesterol, and low-density lipoprotein (LDL) cholesterol and a weight-loss-related rise in high-density lipoprotein (HDL) cholesterol that was associated with the magnitude of the weight loss.[53]

Safety

The side-effect profiles for sympathomimetic drugs are similar.[2] They produce insomnia, dry mouth, asthenia, and constipation. The sympathomimetic drugs phentermine, diethylpropion, benzphetamine, and phendimetrazine have very little abuse potential as assessed by the low rate of reinforcement when the drugs are self-injected intravenously to test animals.[2] In this same paradigm, neither phenylpropanolamine (PPA) nor fenfluramine showed any reinforcing effects and no clinical data show any abuse potential for either of these drugs. Sibutramine, likewise, has no abuse potential,[4] but it is nonetheless a schedule IV drug.

Phenylpropanolamine can increase blood pressure and, at doses of 75 mg or more, PPA has been associated with hemorrhagic stroke in women.[54] In December 2000, the FDA removed PPA from cold remedies and weight-loss products because of the alleged relationship to the development of hemorrhagic strokes. PPA has also been reported in association with cardiomyopathy.

There are two issues to consider regarding blood pressure management and sibutramine use. The first is the development of clinically significant blood pressure elevations. Individual blood pressure responses to sibutramine are quite variable. In the studies reviewed, withdrawals for clinically significant blood pressure increase were usually

2% to 5% of the participants in the trial. Higher doses tend to produce higher withdrawal rates,[35] so lower doses are preferred. The other issue concerning blood pressure increases is the small mean increase of 2 to 4 mmHg in systolic and diastolic blood pressure that occurs in sibutramine-treated patients but not in controls. Weight loss is usually associated with improvement in risk factors for cardiovascular disease (blood pressure, lipids, measures of glycemic control). If sibutramine has mixed effects on risk factors, with improvement in some (lipids, glycemic control) but slight worsening of others, then the prescribing physician must use judgment in the decision to continue sibutramine.

Managing potential increases in blood pressure should be a part of the sibutramine treatment plan. Evaluation of blood pressure 2 to 4 weeks after starting sibutramine is recommended. The initial dose is usually 10 mg per day. About 5% of patients who take sibutramine will have unacceptable increases in blood pressure so for them, the medication should be stopped. If the blood pressure is less than 135/80 and there has been a rise from baseline of less than 10 mmHg systolic and 5 mmHg diastolic, continued use of the medication is acceptable. If patients have acceptable weight loss in the first month of treatment (4 pounds in 4 weeks), the blood pressure response should then be a part of the decision to continue treatment.

Sibutramine should not be used in patients with a history of coronary artery disease, congestive heart failure, cardiac arrhythmias, or stroke. There should be a 2-week interval between the termination of monoamine oxidase inhibitors and the start of sibutramine. Sibutramine should not be used with selective serotonin reuptake inhibitors. Because sibutramine is metabolized by the cytochrome P_{450} enzyme system (isozyme CYP3A4), when drugs like erythromycin and ketoconazole are taken, there may be competition for this enzymatic pathway, and prolonged drug metabolism can result.

▶ ORLISTAT: A DRUG THAT ALTERS METABOLISM

Pharmacology

Orlistat is a potent selective inhibitor of pancreatic lipase that reduces intestinal digestion of fat. The drug has a dose-dependent effect on fecal fat loss, increasing it to about 30% of ingested fat in a diet that has 30% of energy as fat.[55] Orlistat has little effect in subjects eating low-fat diets, as might be anticipated on the basis of the mechanism by which this drug works.

Efficacy

A number of long-term clinical trials of orlistat, lasting 6 months to 2 years, have been published.[12,56-66] In a 2-year trial, patients received a hypocaloric diet calculated to be 500 kcal per day below the patient's requirements.[58] During the second year, the diet was calculated to maintain weight. By the end of year 1, the placebo-treated patients had lost between 4% and 6 % of their initial body weight and the drug-treated patients had lost between 8% and 10%.

In one study, the patients were rerandomized at the end of year 1. Those switched from orlistat to placebo gained weight from 10% to 6% below baseline. Those switched from placebo to orlistat lost from 6% to 8.1%, which was essentially identical to the 7.9% in the patients treated with orlistat for the full 2 years.

In a second 2-year trial, 892 patients were randomized.[59] One group remained on placebo throughout the 2 years (n = 97 completers) and a second group remained on orlistat (120 mg 3 times/d) for 2 years (n = 109 completers). At the end of 1 year, two thirds of the group treated with orlistat for 1 year were changed to orlistat 60 mg three times a day (n = 102 completers), and the others to placebo (n = 95 completers).[59] After 1 year, the weight loss was 8.67 kg in the orlistat-treated group and 5.81 kg in the placebo-treated group (P<0.001). During the second year, those switched to placebo after 1 year reached the same weight as those treated with placebo for 2 years (4.5% in those with placebo for 2 years and 4.2% in those switched from orlistat to placebo during year 2).

In a third 2-year trial, 783 patients remained for 2 years in the placebo group or one of two orlistat-treated groups at 60 or 120 mg three times a day.[62] After 1 year on a weight-loss diet, the completers in the placebo group lost 7.0 kg, which was significantly less than the 9.6 kg in the completers treated with 60 mg of orlistat thrice daily or the 9.8 kg in the completers treated with 120 mg of orlistat thrice daily. During the second year, when the diet was liberalized to a weight-maintenance diet, all three groups regained some weight. At the end of 2 years, the completers in the placebo group were 4.3 kg below baseline; the completers treated with 60 mg orlistat three times daily were 6.8 kg below baseline; and the completers treated with 120 mg orlistat three times daily were 7.6 kg below baseline.

Yet another 2-year trial that has been published was carried out in 796 subjects in a general-practice setting.[61]

After 1 year of treatment with 120 mg per day of orlistat, completers (n = 117) had lost 8.8 kg compared to 4.3 kg in the completers in the placebo-treated group (n = 91). During the second year, when the diet was liberalized to "maintain body weight," both groups regained some weight. At the end of 2 years, the orlistat group receiving 120 mg three times daily were 5.2 kg below their baseline weights compared to 1.5 kg below baseline in the group treated with placebo (Figure 10-2).

Weight maintenance with orlistat was evaluated in a 1-year study.[60] The patients who were enrolled had lost more than 8% of their body weight over 6 months while on a 1000-kcal per day diet. The 729 patients were one of four groups randomized to receive either placebo or 30 mg, 60 mg, or 120 mg of orlistat three times a day for 12 months. At the end of this period, the placebo-treated patients had regained 56% of their weight loss, compared to 32.4% in the group treated three times a day with 120 mg of orlistat. The other two doses of orlistat were not statistically different from placebo in preventing the regain of weight.

Effects of Orlistat on Lipids and Lipoproteins

The modest weight reduction observed with orlistat treatment may have a beneficial effect on lipids and lipoproteins.[22] Orlistat seems to have an independent effect on LDL cholesterol. A metaanalysis of the data relating orlistat to lipids showed that orlistat-treated subjects had almost twice as much reduction in LDL cholesterol as their placebo-treated counterparts for the same weight-loss category reached after 1 year.[67]

One study is representative of the effects of orlistat on weight loss and on cardiovascular risk factors, particularly serum lipids, in obese patients with hypercholesterolemia.[68] The main findings were that orlistat promoted clinically significant weight loss and reduced LDL cholesterol in obese patients with elevated cholesterol levels more than

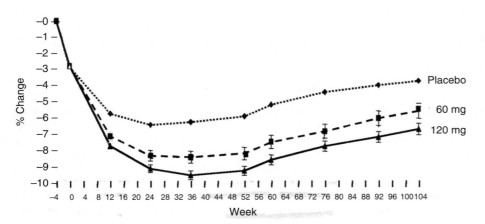

PERCENT CHANGE FROM INITIAL BODY
WEIGHT OVER 2 YEARS:
INTEGRATED DATABASE

Figure 10-2. The percent change in body weight over 2 years of orlistat at 60 mg and 120 mg. At the end of 2 years, the orlistat group receiving 120 mg three times daily were 5.2 kg below their baseline weight compared to 1.5 kg for the group treated with placebo. (From Hauptmann J for the Orlistat Primary Care Study Group: Orlistat in the long-term treatment of obesity in primary care settings. Arch Fam Med 2000;9:160-167.)

could be attributed to weight loss alone. The ObelHyx study demonstrates an additional lowering of 10% of LDL cholesterol in obese subjects with baseline elevated LDL cholesterol levels when compared to placebo.[69] These data indicate that the difference in mean percentage change in LDL cholesterol between orlistat and placebo is roughly 10% to 12% in all studies, whether this difference is computed as change from the start of the single-blind placebo dietary run-in or from the start of double-blind treatment. It is noteworthy that LDL cholesterol levels continued to decline after the start of double-blind treatment in orlistat-treated subjects in all trials, but that LDL cholesterol remained largely unchanged or increased during double-blind therapy in placebo-treated recipients, despite further weight loss. This independent cholesterol-lowering effect probably reflects a reduction in intestinal absorption of cholesterol. Because lipase inhibition by orlistat prevents the absorption of approximately 30% of dietary fat, the prescribed diet of 30% of energy from fat would thus become in effect 20% to 24% of available fat in the diet when associated with orlistat treatment.

It has been hypothesized that inhibition of gastrointestinal lipase activity may lead to retention of cholesterol in the gut through a reduction in the amount of fatty acids and monoglycerides absorbed from the gut or may lead to sequestration of cholesterol within a more persistent oil phase in the intestine or both. Partial inhibition of intestinal fat and cholesterol absorption probably leads to decreased hepatic cholesterol and saturated fatty acid concentration, upregulation of hepatic LDL receptors, and decreased LDL cholesterol levels. The decrease in LDL cholesterol observed in the study with hypercholesterolemic subjects[69] is comparable to the 14% LDL cholesterol reduction that was previously achieved with a plant stanol ester-containing margarine but is of a lesser magnitude than the LDL cholesterol-lowering effects that are commonly observed with fibrate or statin drugs.[70,71]

Effects of Orlistat on Glucose Tolerance, Diabetes, and Metabolic Syndrome

The orlistat-treated subjects in trials lasting for at least 1 year were analyzed by Heymsfield and co-workers, who found that orlistat reduced the conversion of impaired glucose tolerance (IGT) to diabetes and that the transition from normal to IGT was also reduced in subjects treated with orlistat for 1 year.[72] In orlistat-treated subjects the conversion from normal glucose tolerance to diabetes occurred in 6.6% of patients, whereas approximately 11% of placebo-treated patients had a similar worsening of glucose tolerance. Conversion from IGT to diabetes was less common in orlistat-treated patients than in placebo-treated obese subjects by 3.0% and 7.6%, respectively. Although these data are based on a retrospective analysis of 1-year trials in which data on glucose tolerance was available, it shows that modest weight reduction with pharmacotherapy may lead to an important risk reduction for the development of type 2 diabetes.

One study randomized 550 insulin-treated patients to receive either placebo or 120 mg of orlistat three times a day for 1 year.[65] Weight loss in the orlistat-treated group was 3.9 + 0.3% compared to 1.3 + 0.3% in the placebo-treated group. HbA$_{1c}$ was reduced 0.62% in the orlistat-treated group but only 0.27% in the placebo-treated group. The required dose of insulin decreased more in the orlistat group, as did plasma cholesterol.

In a study in patients with diabetes, orlistat improved metabolic control with a reduction of up to 0.53% in HbA$_{1c}$ and a decrease in the concomitant ongoing antidiabetic therapy, despite limited weight loss.[64] Independent effects of orlistat on lipids were also shown in this study. Orlistat also has an acute effect on postprandial lipemia in overweight patients with type 2 diabetes.[73] By lowering both remnant-like particle cholesterol and free fatty acids in the postprandial period, orlistat may contribute to a reduction in atherogenic risk.[74]

The longest clinical trial with orlistat is the Xenical Diabetes Outcome Study (XENDOS).[75] In this 4-year, randomized, placebo-controlled clinical trial 1640 patients were assigned to receive 120 mg of orlistat three times daily plus lifestyle counseling, and 1637 patients were assigned to receive matching placebos plus lifestyle counseling. The study enrolled Swedish patients who had BMIs higher than 30 kg per m^2 and normal or impaired glucose tolerance (21%). More than 52% of the orlistat-treated patients and 34% of the placebo-treated patients continued to adhere to the clinical protocol. The patients receiving orlistat were 6.9 kg below their baseline weight by the end of year 4, as opposed to 4.1 kg for the placebo-treated group ($P<0.001$). Cumulative incidence of diabetes was 9.0% in the placebo group and 6.2% in the orlistat group, a 37% reduction in relative risk.

In an analysis of orlistat's effect on patients with syndrome X, or metabolic syndrome, Reaven and colleagues subdivided patients who had participated in previously reported studies into those in the highest and lowest quintile for triglycerides (TGs) and HDL cholesterol.[76] Those with high TGs and low HDL were labeled Syndrome X, and those with the lowest TGs and the highest HDL were in the non-Syndrome X controls. In this analysis, there were almost no males in the non-Syndrome X group, whereas there was an equal gender breakdown in the Syndrome X group. The other differences between these two groups were the slightly higher systolic and diastolic blood pressures in those with Syndrome X and the nearly twofold higher level of fasting insulin. With weight loss, the only difference between placebo- and orlistat-treated patients along with weight was the drop in LDL cholesterol. However, the Syndrome X subgroups showed a significantly greater decrease in TGs and insulin than those without Syndrome X. HDL cholesterol rose more in the Syndrome X subgroup, but LDL cholesterol showed a smaller decrease than in the non-Syndrome X control group.

Safety

Orlistat is not absorbed to any significant degree and its side effects are thus related to the blockade of TG digestion in the intestine.[55] Fecal fat loss and related gastrointestinal symptoms are common initially but subside as patients learn to use the drug.[58,59] During treatment, small but significant decreases in fat-soluble vitamins can occur, although these almost always remain within the normal range.[77] However, a few patients may need supplementation with

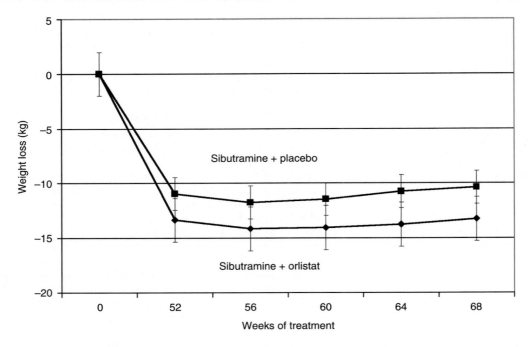

Figure 10-3. Addition of orlistat or placebo for 4 months following 1 year of treatment with sibutramine. Patients were randomly assigned to orlistat or placebo in addition to sibutramine following 1 year of treatment with sibutramine alone. During the additional 4 months of combination treatment there was no further weight loss. (From Wadden TA, Berkowitz RI, Womble LG, et al: Effects of sibutramine plus orlistat in obese women following 1 year of treatment by sibutramine alone: a placebo-controlled trial. Obes Res 2000; 8:431-437.)

fat-soluble vitamins. It is impossible to tell a priori which patients need vitamins, so we routinely provide a multivitamin with instructions to take it before bedtime. Absorption of other drugs does not seem to be significantly affected by orlistat.

Combining Orlistat and Sibutramine

Because orlistat works peripherally to reduce TG digestion in the gastrointestinal track, and sibutramine works on noradrenergic and serotonergic reuptake mechanisms in the brain, their mechanisms do not overlap at all, and combining them might provide additional weight loss. To test this possibility, Wadden and his colleagues[78] randomly assigned patients to orlistat or placebo following a year of treatment with sibutramine, as depicted in Figure 10-3. During the additional 4 months of treatment there was no further weight loss. This result was a disappointment, but additional studies are obviously needed before firm conclusions can be made about combining therapies.

▶ RIMONABANT: A CANNABAINOID RECEPTOR ANTAGONIST

Pharmacology

Rimonabant (Acomplia) is an antagonist to the cannabinoid-1 (CB-1) receptors of the endocannabinoid system that is widely represented in the central nervous system and peripherally. It acts on the presynaptic receptors to prevent the naturally occurring endocannabinoids (anadamide and arachadonyl-2-glycerol) from working. In animals that became obese from eating a high-fat diet, rimonabant produced weight loss, but it had little effect on normal animals. Animals with genetic deletion of the receptor

have a lean phenotype with resistance to diet-induced obesity and dyslipidemia.

Clinical Trials

Rimonabant, a cannabinoid receptor antagonist, has been investigated as a potential treatment for obesity in one 2-year trial. In all trials there was a hypocaloric diet (600 kcal/d deficit) and a 6-week, run-in period in which weight loss averaged about 2 kg. This was followed by 52 or 104 weeks of treatment with placebo or rimonabant at 5 or 20 mg/d. In a 1-year trial of 1507 patients with BMI >30 kg/m² (or > 27 kg/m²) with dyslipidemia hypertension, or both) the mean weight loss ($\pm$SD) at 1 year was −3.4 kg $\pm$ 5.7, −6.6 kg $\pm$ 7.2, and −1.8 kg $\pm$ 6.4 in the rimonabant 5 mg, 20 mg, and placebo groups, respectively.[79] More patients in the rimonabant 20 mg group than in the placebo group, achieved weight loss of greater than 5% (51 versus 19%) or 10% (27 versus 7%).

At the higher dose of 20 mg/d, rimonabant produced significantly greater than placebo in waist circumference, HDL, triglycerides, insulin resistance, and prevalence of the metabolic syndrome. Side effects including mood changes nausea and vomiting, diarrhea, headache, dizziness, and anxiety, were more frequent in the rimonabant 20 mg group than in the 5 mg or placebo groups. Dropout rates were similar in all three groups.

Similar results were seen in the second 1-year trial of 1036 overweight subject with untreated dyslipidemia.[80] Significantly greater declines in body weight, waist circumference, and serum triglyceride concentration, as well as a greater increase in mean serum HDL concentrations were observed in subject treated with rimonabant 20 mg compared with rimonabant 5 mg or placebo.

Data from one 2-year trial with 3045 obese or overweight patients have also been reported. After the 6 week run-in with diet and exercise, they were randomly assigned in year 1 to rimonabant 5 mg/day, 20 mg/day, or placebo, after which rimonabant-treated patients were reran-domized to receive placebo or continue on the same rimonabant dose. The placebo group continued with placebo.[81] Weight losses at 1 year were nearly identical to those in the 1-year studies. In the second year, patients who continued to take rimonabant (20 mg/day) main-tained their weight loss, whereas those randomized to placebo regained their weight at almost exactly the rate that they had lost it in the first year. The dropout rate was high whereas (about 50%), and there were some modest psychiatric symptoms. Patients in the 5 mg group gained some weight, but not back to baseline. Blood pressure and lipids improved significantly in the patients treated with 20 mg/d of rimonabant as they had in the previous trials. Thus rimonabant, in conjunction with diet and exer-cise, resulted in modest but sustained weight loss, as well as favorable changes in waist circumference and cardiac and metabolic risk factors. The trial was limited by a very high dropout rate (approximately 50% in all groups by the end of year 1).

▶ SUMMARY

Medications for obesity treatment should be viewed as useful adjuncts to the prescription of diet and physical activity and may help selected patients achieve and main-tain weight loss. Thus, physicians must be knowledgeable regarding the efficacy and safety profiles of currently avail-able medications.

▶ REFERENCES

1. National Institutes of Health, National Heart, Lung, and Blood Institute: Clinical guidelines on the identification, evaluation, and treatment of overweight and obesity in adults—the evidence report. Obes Res 1998;6:51S-210S.
2. Bray GA, Greenway FL: Current and potential drugs for treatment of obesity. Endocr Rev 1999;20:805-875.
3. Weintraub M, Bray GA: Drug treatment of obesity. Med Clin North Am 1989;73:237-249.
4. Cole JO, Levin A, Beake B, et al: Sibutramine: a new weight-loss agent without evidence of the abuse potential associated with amphetamines. J Clin Psychopharmacol 1998;18:231-236.
5. Bray GA: Obesity: a time-bomb to be defused. Lancet 1998;352:160-161.
6. Connolly HM, Crary JL, McGoon MD, et al: Valvular heart disease associated with fenfluramine-phentermine. N Engl J Med 1997;337:581-588.
7. Ryan DH, Bray GA, Helmcke F, et al: Serial echocardiographic and clinical evaluation of valvular regurgitation before, during, and after treatment with fenfluramine or dexfenfluramine and mazindol or phentermine. Obes Res 1999;7:313-322.
8. Jick H: Heart valve disorders and appetite-suppressant drugs. JAMA 2000;283:1738-1740.
9. Hensrud DD, Connolly HM, Grogan M, Miller FA et al: Echocardiographic improvement over time after cessation of use of fenfluramine and phentermine. Mayo Clin Proc 1999;74:1191-1197.
10. Mast ST, Jollis JG, Ryan T, et al: The progression of fenfluramine-associated valvular heart disease assessed by echocardiography. Ann Intern Med 2001;134:261-266.
11. McMahon FG, Fujioka K, Singh, BN, et al: Efficacy and safety of sibutramine in obese white and African-American patients with hypertension. Arch Intern Med 2000;160:2185-2191.
12. Finer N, James WP, Kopelman PG, et al: One-year treatment of obesity: a randomized, double-blind, placebo-controlled, multicentre study of orlistat, a gastrointestinal lipase inhibitor. Int J Obes Relat Metab Disord 2000;24:306-313.
13. Flechtner-Mors M, Ditschuneit HH, Johnson TD, et al: Metabolic and weight-loss effects of long-term dietary intervention in obese patients: four-year results. Obes Res 2000;8:399-402.
14. Munro JF, MacCuish AC, Wilson EM, et al: Comparison of contin-uous and intermittent anorectic therapy in obesity. Br Med J 1968;1:352-354.
15. Greenway FL, Ryan Greenway FL, Ryan DH, et al: Pharmaceutical cost savings of treating obesity with weight-loss medications. Obes Res 1999;7:523-531.
16. Astrup A, Breum L, Tourbro S, et al: The effect and satiety of an ephedrine/caffeine compound compared to ephedrine, caffeine and placebo in obese subjects on an energy-restricted diet: a double blind trial. Int J Obes 1992;16:260-277.
17. Sjostrom CD, Lissner L, Wedel H, et al: Reduction in incidence of diabetes, hypertension and lipid disturbances after intentional weight loss induced by bariatric surgery: the SOS Intervention Study. Obes Res 1999;7:477-484.
18. Foster GD, Wadden TA, Vogt RA, et al: What is a reasonable weight loss? Patients' expectations and evaluations of obesity treatment outcomes. J Consult Clin Psychol 1997;65:79-85.
19. Bray GA: Evaluation of drugs for treating obesity. Obes Res 1995;3(suppl 4):425S-434S (review).
20. Bray GA, Tartaglia LA: Medicinal strategies in the treatment of obesity. Nature 2000;404(6778):672-677 (review).
21. National Task Force on the Prevention and Treatment of Obesity: Long-term pharmacotherapy in the management of obesity. JAMA 1996;276:1907-1915 (review).
22. Astrup A, Hansen DL, Lundsgaard C, et al: Sibutramine and energy balance. Int J Obes Relat Metab Disord 1998;22(suppl 1):S30-S42.
23. Hansen DL, Toubro S, Stock MJ, et al: Thermogenic effects of sibu-tramine in humans. Am J Clin Nutr 1998;68:1180-1186.
24. Sykas SL, Danforth Jr E, Lien EL: Anorectic drugs which stimulate thermogenesis. Life Sci 1983;33:1269-1275.
25. Lupien JR, Bray GB: Effect of mazindol, d-amphetamine and diethylpropion on purine nucleotide binding to brown adipose tissue. Pharmacol Biochem Behav 1986;25:733-738.
26. Scoville B: Review of amphetamine-like drugs by the Food and Drug Administration: clinical data and value judgments. In Obesity in Perspective, Publication no. 75-708, pp. 441-443. Washington, D.C., Department of Health, Education, and Welfare, 1975.
27. Silverstone JJ, Solomon T: The long-term management of obesity in general practice. Br J Clin Pract 1965;19:395-398.
28. McKay RHG: Long-term use of diethylpropion in obesity. Curr Med Res Opin 1973;1:489-493.
29. Langlois KJ, Forbes JA, Bell GW, et al: A double-blind clinical eval-uation of the safety and efficacy of phentermine hydrochloride (Fastin) in the treatment of exogenous obesity. Curr Ther Res 1974;16:289-296.
30. Gershberg H, Kane R, Hulse M, et al: Effects of diet and an anorectic drug (phentermine resin) in obese diabetics. Curr Ther Res 1977;22:814-820.
31. Campbell CJ, Bhalla IP, Steel JM, et al: A controlled trial of phenter-mine in obese diabetic patients. Practitioner 1977;218:851-855.
32. Williams RA, Foulsham BM: Weight reduction in osteoarthritis using phentermine. Practitioner 1981;225:231-232.
33. Yanovski SZ, Yanovski JA: Drug Obesity. N Engl J Med 2002;346:591-602.
34. Bray GA, Ryan DH, Gordon D, et al: A double-blind randomized placebo-controlled trial of sibutramine. Obes Res 1996;4:263-270.
35. Bray GA, Blackburn GL, Ferguson JM, et al: Sibutramine produces dose-related weight loss. Obes Res 1999;7:189-198.
36. Apfelbaum M, Vague P, Ziegler O, et al: Long-term maintenance of weight loss after a very-low-calorie diet: A randomized blinded trial of the efficacy and tolerability of sibutramine. Am J Med 1999;106:179-184.
37. Fanghanel G, Cortinas L, Sanchez-Reyes L, et al: A clinical trial of the use of sibutramine for the treatment of patients suffering essential obesity. Int J Obes 2000;24:144-150.
38. James WPT for the STORM study group: Effect of sibutramine on weight maintenance after weight loss: a randomized trial. Lancet 2000;356:2119-2125.

39. Cuellar GEM, Ruiz AM, Monsalve MCR, et al: Six-month treatment of obesity with sibutramine 15 mg: a double-blind, placebo-controlled monocenter clinical trial in a Hispanic population. Obes Res 2000; 8(1):71-82.

40. Smith IG, Goulder MA: Randomized placebo-controlled trial of long-term treatment with sibutramine in mild to moderate obesity. J Fam Pract 2001;50(6):505-512.

41. Dujovne CA, Zavoral JH, Rowe E, et al: Effects of sibutramine on body weight and serum lipids: a double-blind, randomized, placebo-controlled study in 322 overweight and obese patients with dyslipidemia. Am Heart J 2001;142(3):489-497.

42. Wirth A, Krause J: Long-term weight loss with sibutramine. JAMA 2001;286(11):1331-1339.

43. Fujioka K for the Sibutramine/Diabetes clinical study group: Weight loss with sibutramine improves glycemic control and other metabolic parameters in obese type 2 diabetes mellitus. Diabetes Obes Metab 2000;2:1-13.

44. Gockel A, Karakose H, Ertorer EM, et al: Effects of sibutramine in obese female subjects with type 2 diabetes and poor blood glucose control. Diabetes Care 2001;24:1957-1960.

45. Serrano-Rios M, Melchionda N, Moreno-Carretero E, Spanish Investigators: Role of sibutramine in the treatment of obese type 2 diabetic patients receiving sulphonylurea therapy. Diabetes Med 2002;19(2):119-124.

46. McMahon FG, Weinstein SP, Rowe E, et al: Sibutramine is safe and effective for weight loss in obese patients whose hypertension is well controlled with angiotensin-converting enzyme inhibitors. J Hum Hypertens 2002;16:5-11.

47. Weintraub M, Rubio A, Golik A, Byrne L, et al: Sibutramine in weight control: a dose-ranging, efficacy study. Clin Pharmacol Ther 1991;50:330-337.

48. Finer N, Bloom SR, Frost GS, et al: Sibutramine is effective for weight loss and diabetic control in obesity with type 2 diabetes: a randomised, double-blind placebo-controlled study. Diabetes Obes Metab 2000;2:105-112.

49. Hazenberg BP: Randomized, double-blind, placebo-controlled, multicenter study of sibutramine in obese hypertensive patients. Cardiology 2000;94:152-158.

50. Sramek, JJ, Seiowitz MT, Weinstein SP, et al: Efficacy and safety of sibutramine for weight loss in obese patients with hypertension well controlled by β-adrenergic blocking agents: a placebo-controlled, double-blind, randomized trial. Am J Hypertens 2002;16:13-19.

51. Berube-Parent S, Prudhomme D, St-Pierre S, et al: Obesity treatment with a progressive clinical tri-therapy combining sibutramine and a supervised diet-exercise intervention. Int J Obes Relat Metab Disord 2001;25(8):1144-1153.

52. Wadden RA, Berkowitz RI, Sarwer DB, et al: Benefits of lifestyle modification in the pharmacologic treatment of obesity: a randomized trial. Arch Intern Med 2001; 161:218-227.

53. Van Gaal LF, Wauters M, De Leeuw IH: The beneficial effects of modest weight loss on cardiovascular risk factors. Int J Obes 1997; 21(suppl. 1): S5-S9.

54. Kernan WN, Viscoli CM, Brass LM, et al: Phenylpropanolamine and the risk of hemorrhagic stroke. N Engl J Med 2000;343(25): 1826-1832.

55. Hauptman J: Orlistat: selective inhibition of caloric absorption can affect long-term body weight. Endocrine 2000;13(2):201-206.

56. James WP, Avenell A, Broom J, et al: A one-year trial to assess the value of orlistat in the management of obesity. Int J Obes Relat Metab Disord 1997;21(suppl 3):S24-S30.

57. Van Gaal LF, Broom JI, Enzi G, et al: Efficacy and tolerability of orlistat in the treatment of obesity: a 6-month dose-ranging study. Eur J Clin Pharm 1998;54:125-132.

58. Sjostrom L, Rissanen A, Andersen T, et al, European Multicentre Orlistat Study Group: Randomised placebo-controlled trial of orlistat for weight loss and prevention of weight regain in obese patients. Lancet 1998;352:167-172.

59. Davidson MH, Hauptman J, DiGirolamo M, et al: Long-term weight control and risk factor reduction in obese subjects treated with orlistat, a lipase inhibitor. JAMA 1999;281:235-242.

60. Hill JO, Hauptmann J, Anderson JW, et al: Orlistat, a lipase inhibitor, for weight maintenance after conventional dieting: a 1-year study. Am J Clin Nutr 1999;69:1108-1116.

61. Hauptmann J, for the Orlistat Primary Care Study Group: Orlistat in the long-term treatment of obesity in primary care settings. Arch Fam Med 2000;9:160-167.

62. Rossner S, Sjostrom L, Noack R, et al, on behalf of the European Orlistat Obesity Study Group: Weight loss, weight maintenance, and improved cardiovascular risk factors after 2 years' treatment with orlistat for obesity. Obes Res 2000;8:49-61.

63. Lindgarde F, on behalf of the Orlistat Swedish Multimorbidity study group: The effect of orlistat on body weight and coronary heart disease risk profile in obese patients, The Swedish Multimorbidity study. J Intern Med 2000;248:245-254.

64. Hollander P, Elbein SC, Hirsch IB, et al: Role of orlistat in the treatment of obese patients with type 2 diabetes. Diab Care 1998;21: 1288-1294.

65. Kelley D, Bray G, Pi-Sunyer FX, et al: Clinical efficacy of orlistat therapy in overweight and obese patients with insulin-treated type 2 diabetes mellitus: a one-year, randomized, controlled trial. Diabetes Care 2002;25:1033-1041.

66. Miles JM, Leiter L, Hollander P, et al: Effect of orlistat in overweight and obese patients with type 2 diabetes treated with metformin. Diabetes Care 2002;25(7):1123-1128.

67. Zavoral JH: Treatment with orlistat reduces cardiovascular risk in obese patients. J Hypertens 1998; 16:2013-2017.

68. Muls E, Kolanowski J, Scheen A, et al: The effects of orlistat on weight and on serum lipids in obese patients with hypercholesterolemia: a randomized, double-blind, placebo-controlled, multicenter study. Int J Obes Relat Metab Disord 2001; 25:1713-1721.

69. Tonstad S, Pometta D, Erkelens DW, et al: The effects of gastrointestinal lipase inhibitor, orlistat, on serum lipids and lipoproteins in patients with primary hyperlipidaemia. Eur J Clin Pharmacol 1994; 46:405-410.

70. Linton MF, Fazio S: Re-emergence of fibrates in the management of dyslipidemia and cardiovascular risk. Curr Atheroscler Rep 2000; 2:29-35.

71. Maron DJ, Fazio S, Linton MF: Current perspectives on statins. Circulation 2000; 101:207-213.

72. Heymsfield SB, Segal KR, Hauptman J, et al: Effects of weight loss with orlistat on glucose tolerance and progression to type 2 diabetes in obese adults. Arch Intern Med 2000; 160:1321-1326.

73. Tan MH: Current treatment of insulin resistance in type 2 diabetes mellitus. Int J Clin Pract 2000;113 (suppl):54-62.

74. Ceriello A: The postprandial state and cardiovascular disease: relevance to diabetes mellitus. Diabetes Metab Res Rev 2000; 16:125-132.

75. Torgerson JS, Hauptman J, Boldrin MN, et al: Xenical in the prevention of diabetes in obese subjects (XENDOS) study: a randomized study of orlistat as an adjunct to lifestyle changes for the prevention of type 2 diabetes in obese patients. Diabetes Care 2004;27:155-161.

76. Reaven G, Segal K, Hauptman J, et al: Effect of orlistat-assisted weight loss in decreasing coronary heart disease risk in patients with Syndrome X. Am J Cardiol 2001;87:827-831.

77. Drent ML, van der Veen EA: First clinical studies with orlistat: a short review. Obes Res 1995;3:S623-S625.

78. Wadden TA, Berkowitz RI, Womble LG, et al: Effects of sibutramine plus orlistat in obese women following 1 year of treatment by sibutramine alone: a placebo-controlled trial. Obes Res 2000;8(6):431-437.

79. Van Gaal LF, Rissanen AM, Scheen AJ, et al: Effects of the cannabinoid-1 receptor blocker rimonabant on weight reduction and cardiovascular risk factors in overweight patients: 1-year experience from the RIO-Europe study. Lancet 2005;365:1389-1397.

80. Despres JP, Golay A, Sjostrom L: The Rimonabant in Obesity-Lipids Study Group. Effects of rimonabant on metabolic risk factors in overweight patients with dyslipidemia. N Engl J Med 2005;353: 2121-2134.

81. Pi-Sunyer FX, Aronne LJ, Heshmati HM, et al: RIO-North America Study Group. Effect of rimonabant, a cannabinoid-1 receptor blocker, on weight and cardiometabolic risk factors in overweight or obese patients: RIO-North America: A randomized controlled trial. JAMA 2006;295:761-775.

11

Nonsurgical Methods of Weight Loss

George S. M. Cowan, Jr., M.D.

Numerous weight-loss theories, plans, and programs have been developed and successfully promulgated through diet books, infomercials, other media, and meetings to assist those seeking help for their overweight or obesity. They employ variations of the four main approaches to the voluntary, nonsurgical management of excess weight: weight-loss diets, behavior modification, exercise, and medication. This chapter provides a brief overview and discussion of these methodologies upon which Americans are spending many billions of dollars a year.

▶ WEIGHT-LOSS DIETS

The basic goal of a weight-loss diet is to limit caloric intake to a level less than that which the dieter's body can burn per unit of time. This may also involve the use of particular foodstuffs or substitutes, such as grapefruit, nonabsorbable fat, sweeteners, or fiber. These materials are intended to produce weight loss by inducing the individual to consume fewer calories, excrete some of those consumed without intestinal absorption, increase the body's metabolic rate, or otherwise eliminate or metabolize excess fat from the body.

These methodologies had their origins in the 19th century when dietary weight-loss "principles" were initially propounded, often with questionable bases, by various medical and lay individuals. They have since been innovatively recycled in many different combinations and permutations. Millions of overweight, obese, and morbidly obese individuals continue to use many of them.

Bariatric surgeons and their staffs need to be familiar with at least some of these diets, dietary principles, and entities that patients mention on their lists of unsuccessful prior weight-loss attempts. It is important to note that they may be continuing to use one or more of them, even for some time after bariatric surgery. For this purpose, the chapter outlines some of the history of the weight-loss approaches used during the past 2 centuries and discusses certain principles, some highly questionable, as well as actual diets employed. Other materials, including biological extracts and other natural, albeit in some instances potentially harmful, substances used for weight loss are also listed (Table 11-1). The huge numbers involved allow only a representative sampling.

Origins

The first published modern diet was vegetarian. Laced with comments on the deadly sin of gluttony, it was propounded by the Rev. Sylvester Graham in *Graham Journal of Health and Longevity*, which began publication 1837.[1] Vegetarian weight-loss diets can be deficient in the amounts or combinations of high-biological-value protein or other nutrients. Vegetarian patients may therefore present with multiple nonclinically apparent nutrient deficiencies preoperatively and may exacerbate them for months or years after bariatric surgery; therefore, such patients require particularly careful preoperative workup and attentive postsurgical follow-up.

The first popular diet book, titled *Letter on Corpulence Addressed to the Public* and written by William Banting, an undertaker and coffin maker, appeared in 1862. It arose from, and describes in part, how he managed his own obesity by using a carbohydrate-restrictive, high-fat diet recommended by a physician, Dr. William Harvey; it lacked any caloric restriction. This diet later fell into disrepute but has recently regained some popularity (vide infra Dr. Atkins' diet). In 1879, the artificial sweetener saccharin was invented (Monsanto). In 1894, thyroid compounds were extracted from animal tissues, followed shortly thereafter by the prescription by physicians of thyroid pills for weight loss. The first public advertisements solely for weight loss appeared in 1896; the ingredients of some of the matter offered therein included laxatives, purgatives, arsenic, strychnine, washing soda, and Epsom salts.

Thorough mastication of food was espoused by the Englishman Horace Fletcher, the "Great Masticator," who reportedly lost 65 pounds by chewing his food 100 times per minute, until it was completely liquefied. This practice was influenced to some extent by British Prime Minister William Ewart Gladstone, who emphasized masticating 32 times per mouthful (once for each of the 32 adult teeth). Fletcher published *The A.B.-Z. of Our Own Nutrition* in 1898, a book that directed readers to masticate until their food was liquefied and to avoid all fiber. He advised,

Table 11-1	COMMERCIAL AND FAD WEIGHT-LOSS DIETS

1837: First modern weight loss diet (Rev. Sylvester Graham)
1850: American Vegetarian Society founded (Dr. John Kellogg)
1862: First weight loss diet book (William Banting)
1878: First sugar substitute (saccharin [benzosulfamide]) discovered (Johns Hopkins University)
1898: Masticate until food is liquefied; avoid all fiber (Horace Fletcher)
1907: Saccharin as sugar replacement in food for diabetics
1911: Eat proteins, fruits, and starches separately (William Howard Hay)
1913: Government dietary guides first issued (U.S. Department of Agriculture)
1918: Counting calories first introduced to the public for weight loss (Lulu Hunt Peters, M.D.)
1919: First domestic bathroom scale (Health-O-Meter, sold by the Continental Scale Co.)
1930: Very-low-calorie diet (Hollywood Diet, later known as Grapefruit Diet/Mayo Clinic Diet)
1930s: Seaweed diets
1943: Mineral oil as a dietary fat substitute (Marian White)
1963: First sugar-free soft drink (Tab)
1963: Weight-Loss Support Group founded (Weight Watchers, housewife Jean Nidetch)
1967: High-protein plus low-carbohydrate diet (Dr. Irwin Stillman)
1972: High-protein, high-fat, low-carbohydrate diet (Dr. Robert Atkins)
1974: Commercial Physician-Supervised Weight Loss Program (Optifast)
1977: Low-fat, high-fiber diet (Pritikin)
1977: The liquid protein diet and fasting (Robert Linn, D.O.)
1978: High-protein plus low-carbohydrates diet (Scarsdale Medical Diet, H. Tarnower)
1981: High-fruit diet (The Beverly Hills Diet, Judy Mazel)
1982: High-fiber diet <10%-fat, vegetarian, unrestricted intake diet (Dean Ornish, M.D.)
1983: High-fiber diet (The F-Plan Diet, Audrey Eyton)
1990: Anatomically selective weight loss by dieting (Rosemary Conley)
1995: Carbohydrate-fat-protein ratio goal 40-30-30 (The Zone Diet; Barry Sears)
2003: High-fat, low-glycemic index, unrestricted diet (South Beach Diet, A. Agatston, M.D.)

"Don't eat until you're truly hungry" and "Don't allow depressing or unpleasant feelings at meal times." Recommended foods, in any amount, were beans, cornbread, potatoes, and minimal use of eggs but no meat, alcohol, coffee, or tea.[2] Thorough mastication, or Fletcherism, as this practice was called, has resurfaced as a component of bariatric surgical patient education and is particularly important for those patients whose surgery involves gastric restriction.

The origin of Kellogg's Corn Flakes resulted from Dr. John Harvey Kellogg's (1852-1943) adherence to the mastication concept and disagreement with Fletcher's fiber-avoidance caveat. In addition, as a reflection of his Seventh-Day Adventist upbringing, which included a regimen of vegetarian diet and exercise, Kellogg cofounded the American Vegetarian Society (1886) and took charge of the Adventist Sanitarium, which featured this program. He and his brother, William Keith Kellogg, also founded the Sanitas Food Company to produce whole-grain cereals.[3] After a major disagreement over the addition of sugar to their cereals, William founded his own company, the Battle Creek Toasted Corn Flake Company, which eventually became the Kellogg Company that continues to produce the brothers' original product. Anecdotally, Dr. Kellogg reportedly would remove a small section of a patient's intestines when that patient was not cured of his or her ailment by a vegetarian diet; if reliable documentation of any of these procedures should be discovered, Kellogg could justifiably be known as the world's first bariatric surgeon.

The combining of protein, fruits and starches, and the eating of certain types of foods separately, was a dietary principle initially employed by William Howard Hay (1866-1940), a surgeon, to manage his own obesity and related cardiac problems. He first advocated this principle in 1911. It was based on the concept that the single basic cause of problems with health was "the wrong chemical condition in the body," namely, acidity caused by acid that accumulates as a result of digestion and metabolism to an extent greater than can be eliminated by the body. This acid lowers the body's alkaline reserve, leading to toxemia. He divided foods into three groups: alkali-forming (fruits and vegetables); concentrated proteins (meats, eggs, and dairy products); and acid-forming foods (bread, grains, and sucrose-containing foods). He formulated rules for which foods ought to be combined or consumed separately and when they should be eaten. He also advocated the ingestion of mostly fresh fruit, vegetables, and salads and the avoidance of processed food.[4] Although he correctly maintained that carbohydrates and proteins have different digestive requirements, his conclusion that they, therefore, needed to be ingested separately to enhance the manner in which the body handles them has little, if any, scientific validity.

Government dietary guides were first issued by the U.S. Department of Agriculture in 1913. They provided advice on daily servings from the various food groups, encouraging consumption of a wider range of foods, initially the most prominent among them from animal sources.[5]

Counting calories was first introduced to the public in 1918 by Lulu Hunt Peters, M.D., with her book *Diet and Health With a Key to the Calories*.[6] With its stress on self-discipline and self-control, it appears to be the earliest instance in which lack of adequate self-control was stressed as the main reason for failure to control one's excess weight.

The first domestic bathroom scale, the Health-O-Meter, was initially sold by the Continental Scale Company in 1919.

A very-low-calorie diet, the Hollywood Diet, appeared in about 1930, its originator unknown. It is also referred to as the Grapefruit Diet and the Mayo Clinic Diet, although the Mayo Clinic completely disavows it. Different versions involve eating between about 585 and 800 calories per day, including only grapefruit, hard-boiled eggs, green vegetables, coffee, and melba toast.[7] The diet provides much fiber and vitamin C, but it is deficient in many other nutrients, making it dangerous to follow for any extended period of time. The diet also makes the highly questionable claim that grapefruit contains a special fat-burning enzyme; none has been identified.

Seaweed diets of bladder wrack and kelp were used in the 1930s. Together with sushi bars, they have enjoyed a resurgence in popularity. However, some British scientists have recently found large amounts of arsenosugars or their metabolites within algae and seaweed.[8] Seaweed soap and various skin creams are also marketed with claims that they, incredibly, dissolve subcutaneous excess body fat.

Mineral oil as a dietary fat substitute first appeared in 1943, when Marion White published *Diet Without Despair*, advocating this nonabsorbable oil in place of olive oil as her diet's main source of fat.[9] This advocacy was a forerunner of today's synthetic, also nonabsorbable, fat molecules such as Olestra. Apart from this diet's minimal nutritive value, the liberal use of mineral oil was responsible for intestinal cramping, flatulence, bloating, and diarrhea.

Modern Era

The first sugar substitute, saccharin (benzosulfamide; Sweet'N Low), was discovered by accident in 1878 by two scientists at Johns Hopkins University who found a sweet substance in a toluene derivative. By 1907, it was used as a sugar replacement in foods for diabetics. In 1963, it was used by the makers of Tab in the first sugar-free soft drink; this was soon followed on a massive scale by others in the soft-drink industry. Later, other sugar substitutes were introduced. Aspartame (Nutrasweet) appeared in 1981, and acesulfame-k (Sunette, Sweet & Safe, Sweet One) was approved by the FDA in 1988 as a sugar substitute in packet or tablet form, in chewing gum, dry mixes for beverages, instant coffee and tea, gelatin desserts, puddings, and nondairy creamers but not for soft drinks and baked goods. Sucralose (Splenda) was FDA-approved in 1998 for use in multiple food and drink categories. Although these products have been approved by the FDA, consumer groups and others have expressed concerns about potential toxicity, carcinogenicity, and other issues.

Weight-loss support group and calorie-counting-centered Weight Watchers was founded in 1963 by Jean Nidetch, a Brooklyn-born and increasingly obese housewife, and her business partner, Al Lippert; it is now a publicly held company.[10] It arose from a successful support group of six overweight friends who had begun meeting 2 years earlier and used motivational support, self-help, group-leader-led discussions, and strict portion sizes and calorie control (1200 to 1600 kcal/day). These continue today, along with its relatively low entry cost. In 1996, it introduced a calorie-counting points system. Its short- and intermediate-term success record in weight loss has been as good as any other weight-loss diet program.

A book advocating a diet high in protein and low in carbohydrates appeared in 1967, titled *The Doctor's Quick Weight Loss Diet*, by Dr. Irwin Stillman.[11] Based on the established fact that protein is less thermally efficient to assimilate into the body than other nutrients, his diet allowed only fish, lean meat, cheese, skim milk, and water but no fat or carbohydrates. The author claimed total body-weight losses of up to 6 kg a week. Eleven years later, in 1978, his coauthor, Samm Sinclair Baker, also coauthored *The Complete Scarsdale Medical Diet*,[12] which follows essentially the same principles, including some serious nutrient deficiencies. Those using the diet have experienced, constipation, nausea, weakness, and halitosis due to ketosis. Dr. Stillman later died of a heart attack.

A high-fat (including saturated fat), high-protein, low-carbohydrate diet was introduced in 1972 by cardiologist Dr. Robert C. Atkins, a little more than a century after Banting popularized the first high-fat diet.[13] It was reintroduced several years ago and was condemned by most of the medical establishment, particularly for its unrestricted use of saturated fat, together with severe limitations on carbohydrate ingestion. Although it is extremely controversial, research has shown that low-carbohydrate diets produce, at least within the first 6 months, weight-loss results that are superior to those of low-fat diets while concomitantly reducing serum lipid levels. Dr. Atkins' diet has achieved enormous popularity and has spawned a whole new billion-dollar industry of "low-carb" products. The diet's popularity has waned since Dr. Atkins' death, and his commercial organization has recently gone into receivership, but research is ongoing and current recommendations are to wait until long-term results are available before even considering this diet for use by patients.

The liquid-protein diet plus fasting was developed by Robert Linn, D.O., in the 1970s, as described in his book *The Last-Chance Diet*.[14] The protein was made from a hydrolyzed collagen protein, called Prolinn, which was obtained from bovine hide, tendons, horns, and hooves, and included artificial flavoring and coloring. At under 400 kcal per day, it was effectively a semistarvation, incomplete, low-quality-protein diet. Dr. Linn advised using the protein several times a day to interrupt the fasting program. The so-called Cambridge Diet was a derivative of this diet.[15]

Optifast is a commercial, physician-supervised, supplemental fasting weight-loss program that was introduced in 1974. It has consistently claimed a large average weight loss for those who complete treatment which is, unfortunately, a relatively small percentage of the number who start the program. Combined with behavior-modification techniques and under medical supervision, supplemental fasting programs such as this can be a useful initial approach to managing obese patients.[16]

A low-fat, high-fiber diet described by Robert Pritikin, an electronic engineer, appeared in 1979, first as *The Pritikin Program for Diet and Exercise*.[17] It combines low fat (<10%) with high fiber and encourages the consumption of complex, fibrous carbohydrate foods such as fruits and vegetables. In some studies of cholesterol-lowering regimens, there has been a significant increase in the number of suicides by those with low blood cholesterol levels. Nathan Pritikin committed suicide in February 1985.

A high-fruit diet, the Beverly Hills Diet, in which only fruit is allowed for the first 10 days, appeared in 1981.[18] Its author, Judy Mazel, who was trained in drama, not nutrition, started the diet with a 35-day plan. For the first 10 days, food consumption is limited solely to fruit, after which carbohydrates and butter are added; protein is added on day 19. She claimed that papaya and pineapple have "fat-burning enzymes" that work on body fat in the fat cells. Additionally, she advised her readers to eat foods that do not fight each other, a concept reminiscent of Dr. William Howard Hay's questionable doctrine discussed earlier. Dangerously low in protein as well as in several vitamins and minerals, her dietary guidelines are not based on any scientific evidence.

A high-fiber, less-than-10%-fat, vegetarian diet with unrestricted intake of beans, legumes, fruits, grains, and vegetables, accompanied by moderate exercise, is the basis of the Dean Ornish, M.D., 1982 book, *Eat More, Weigh Less*.[19] It is adapted from the regimen he created to reverse heart disease.

The high-fiber, or F-Plan, diet was introduced in 1983 based on Audrey Eyton's theory that fiber fills the stomach and, thereby, reduces the desire to overeat. It promoted a high-fiber, low-fat, calorie-controlled eating plan.[20] Although useful in binding cholesterol and containing many other health benefits, very-high-fiber, whole-grain diets can lead to decreased absorption of magnesium, calcium, zinc, phosphorus, and other nutrients, to constipation if not accompanied by an increase in water ingestion, and to gastrointestinal upset if introduced too rapidly.[21]

Anatomically selective weight loss by dieting or, rather, the claim to produce it, was made in 1993 with Rosemary Conley's *The Complete Hip and Thigh Diet*. There is no known basis in this book or elsewhere for the support of this incredible claim.[22]

A carbohydrate-fat-protein ratio goal of 40-30-30 with avoidance of "bad carbohydrates," such as bread, pasta, carrots, cranberries, and corn, is the basis of the low-glycemic diet described by biochemist Barry Sears (b.1947) in his book *The Zone: A Dietary Road Map to Lose Weight Permanently, Reset Your Genetic Code, Prevent Disease, Achieve Maximum Physical Performance*, published in 1995.[23] He emphasizes the importance of eicosanoids and the benefits of his diet in reducing hyperinsulinemia and insulin production that adversely influence fat storage. More recently, he has criticized the new food pyramid recommendations as being weighted too heavily with "high-density, high-glycemic carbohydrates." The American Heart Association classifies the Zone Diet as high-protein and therefore does not recommend it for weight loss.

A diet high in monounsaturated fat and low in glycemic index that allowed unlimited portions was designed by cardiologist Dr. Arthur Agatston for his patients so they could reduce their hyperinsulinemia-producing hunger and fat storage. He published it as The South Beach Diet in 2003.[24] The first of three diet phases requires 2 weeks of severe carbohydrate restriction, emphasizing lean meat, chicken, fish, eggs, low-fat cheese, some nuts, and olive oil, and usually produces a weight loss of 8 to 13 lb. Low-glycemic-index carbohydrates are gradually added in phase two until a target weight loss of 1 to 2 lb per week is reached. Unlike the Atkins Diet, it is low in saturated fats, emphasizes monounsaturates, and does not severely restrict carbohydrates after the first 2 weeks. Cream and butter are not allowed at any time. Phase three allows a wider variety of foods for lifetime weight maintenance. Because the glycemic value of a meal changes when certain foods are eaten together, it does not seem logical to ban all high-glycemic foods.

▶ BEHAVIOR MODIFICATION AND WEIGHT LOSS

Many within the lay and medical communities have tended to view obesity as a largely behavior-based problem arising from "bad" eating habits and aided and abetted by a lack of self-control within the American food-toxic environment. Self-righteous, empty phrases, usually uttered by nonobese individuals, such as "They [the obese] just need to zip their lips" or "Just push away from the table" are often heard. The concept that obesity has a psychogenic cause that involves, *inter alia*, the unconscious meaning of food and eating that leads to overeating has persisted for decades.[25]

However, if behavior were so puissant and fundamental, behavior therapy ought to have shown itself to be considerably more effective in controlling weight in the majority of obese subjects than it has. Instead, obesity appears to be largely resistant to behaviorally based therapy. Nor has psychotherapy been demonstrated to be an effective obesity cure. The fundamental absence of an obesity-specific personality type or an intrinsic "obesity psychopathology" also mitigates against behavior as a core cause of obesity. And lacking persuasive, well-controlled, psychotherapeutic studies to the contrary, the basic cause of obesity appears most likely not to be behavioral in origin.

Behavior seems likely to be potentiating the development and successful maintenance of the obese state. It is probably contributing to the increasing global epidemic of obesity across the relatively short span of several decades because this epidemic cannot be attributed to genetic issues alone. A major causal element logically resides within our obesity-promoting environment and the culture of permissiveness and plenty that is force-fed by commercially driven purveyors of inexpensive, readily available, highly attractive, and calorie-dense foods of all kinds.

Although behavior is likely not the core cause of obesity, behavioral therapy targeting this condition appears to have a place within a broader approach. Brownell and Kramer express it realistically: "Behavior modification, therefore, is appropriately aimed at improving the obese person's eating habits rather than the etiology of these habits."[26] In the service of this cause, behavioral therapy aimed at modifying behavior with regard to calorie consumption has become a popular treatment modality that continues to be refined.

One of the main components of obesity management is behavior modification, also termed behavior therapy. A wide variety of educational topics reside under this rubric. Most programs include modular elements that may include such subjects as self-monitoring, stimulus (cue) control, self-control, cognitive-behavior modification, goal setting, social support, self-esteem, assertiveness training, relaxation exercises, changing behavior parameters, nutrition education, mental programming, relaxation techniques, body image, self-image, stress management, behavioral goal setting, maintenance support, and contingency management (rewards), among others. With time, programs winnow out the modular components that appear less successful and replace them with what appear to be more effective alternatives.

These subjects are often taught in weekly behavioral-modification, educational discussion groups as part of a comprehensive weight-loss program. They can involve audiovisual aids, weigh-ins, handouts, and homework assignments as well as, sometimes, group exercise, any of a variety of meditation techniques, and shopping expeditions to model healthful food choices. Instructors have varied from basic trainees to physicians to social workers and psychologists. This approach has also expanded to the Internet. Traditional individual therapy sessions are also used but are more expensive and less popular.

There are different predictors of successful, as opposed to unsuccessful, weight loss in programs that emphasize behavior modification. Weight regain is more likely to occur in association with emotional or binge eating patterns, small initial weight loss, life stress such as family dysfunction, and negative coping style. Successful weight loss is more likely with emphasis on realistic goal setting, social-support networking, sustained self-monitoring, effective problem solving, regular nonexcessive exercise maintenance, enhanced self-esteem, greater treatment length, and continued contact with therapists. This approach has shown success in helping the obese lose modest amounts of weight.[27]

Behavior modification is wisely offered to patients as part of an obesity treatment clinic that involves a team including a physician and a nutritionist. They are responsible for assessment and treatment planning (average 4 to 6 weeks), implementation of the treatment plan (up to 1 year), and long-term weight maintenance (1 to 5 or more years). Most effective programs combine behavior modification with exercise and dieting.

▶ EXERCISE

Poor Fitness Levels of the Morbidly Obese, Especially Males

Morbidly obese males appeared to be less physically and biochemically fit than morbidly obese females in a cross-sectional rest and exercise study that found females' maximal $\dot{V}O_2$ was significantly higher than that of males (119% vs. 92% of predicted). The females' anaerobic threshold was also significantly higher than males' (64% vs. 48% of predicted). The males' mean fat-free mass (FFM), FFM indexes, fasting blood glucose levels, and insulin levels were all significantly higher than those of the females.[28] The males' tendency to be more deconditioned and less healthy in general than females provides a rationale for greater emphasis on exercise for morbidly obese males. Because their lack of fitness is also likely to be associated with their known greater postoperative morbidity and mortality rates, perhaps preoperative exercise conditioning ought to be given consideration at least equal to that of preoperative weight loss, particularly in those with upper-body obesity where greater perioperative risk resides.

Exercise and Its Goals

Exercise is any skeletal-muscle-induced movement of the body that produces energy expenditure. It can occur in any environment and under a wide range of circumstances.

The goal of such exercise need not be cardiovascular fitness, an outcome that often requires a level of intensity that many morbidly obese patients, in particular, may not be able to achieve. However, any exercise represents an increase in energy expenditure above the resting level and that, in and of itself, contributes towards a negative balance relative to caloric intake. Starting somewhere is preferable to not starting at all; at least the start signals some prospect of benefit, particularly for those who are moderately to seriously unfit.

Exercise Alone Without Weight-loss Dieting Has Limited Effects

Obesity is commonly associated with low physical fitness as a result of inactivity. To address this, a regular increase in energy expenditure through exercise can create a negative energy balance that leads to a reduction in body fat. However, compared with diet alone, exercise alone would require treating 17 patients to successfully have 1 patient lose 10 lb. Exercise by itself, without dieting, is usually unsuccessful in reducing weight.[29]

Diet With Exercise Increases Weight Loss

The combination of diet and exercise results in more weight loss than is achievable with either diet or exercise alone. There also seems to be some evidence that, although diet alone will achieve greater weight loss than exercise can achieve by itself without dieting, physical activity alone is associated with maintaining weight loss better than diet alone over the long term. Ultimately, successful weight-loss maintenance is a matter of the magnitude of the additional energy expenditure regularly provided through exercise. In most instances, with the poor fitness level of the morbidly obese population, their energy expenditure with exercise is of a relatively low level, but less is required with weight maintenance than with active weight loss.

Exercise Helps Maintain Weight Loss While Improving Fitness

In addition to other benefits, regular long-term exercise appears to be important in the weight-maintenance phase following weight loss. Here the individual, at the completion of his or her weight-loss phase, is attempting to maintain the new set-point level already reached. Doing so requires fewer calories of extra energy expenditure than did the actual weight loss itself because no further weight is being lost. Maintenance becomes, therefore, a matter of sustaining the caloric output sufficient to balance the dietary intake. Given an individual in an otherwise steady weight state, if that individual were to exercise to expend an additional 100 kcal of energy by exercise each day for a year over and above that individual's steady state, the result will ordinarily be a weight loss of about 10 lb. However, given the typical dietary recidivism following the weight-loss phase, sometimes due to a lower resting energy expenditure resulting from loss of lean body mass, that same 100 kcal of energy expended on a daily basis through exercise also has the equivalent potential to prevent 10 lb of weight regain over the span of 1 year and for each year thereafter. In addition to sustaining maintenance of weight loss, exercise can also improve physical fitness as measured by the $\dot{V}O_{2max}$, which averaged 20% in one study.[29]

Preexercise Workup and Testing

Before patients are given an exercise prescription, it is wise to complete the necessary history and physical examination that detects and documents any musculoskeletal limitations, cardiovascular risk factors, or medications that may interfere with an exercise regimen. It is important to examine for and detect any symptoms or signs of pulmonary or cardiovascular disease.

Exercise testing is indicated in patients in whom histories and physical examination reveal possible or actual heart murmur; pulmonary disease, including asthma and chronic obstructive pulmonary disease; cardiovascular disease, including peripheral vascular disease; metabolic syndrome; shortness of breath with mild to moderate exertion; ankle edema; paroxysmal nocturnal dyspnea; unusual fatigue; or palpitations, tachycardia, intermittent claudication, cerebrovascular disease, or similar morbidity. Because most of the morbidly obese population suffers from one or more of these conditions, preexercise testing is important before prescribing an appropriate exercise program for members of this population.

Exercise Recommendations for Weight Loss

As discussed earlier, to fight the typical recidivism following successful weight loss, it is important to encourage patients to perform or reach a performance level at moderate intensity exercise at least 4 to 5 times a week for 30 minutes or more. If weight maintenance starts to slip, the exercise time will have to be lengthened and dietary counseling instituted. Realistically, patients may require an hour or even more for successful weight-loss maintenance in the long term.[30]

The type of exercise most successful over the long term, in our experience with thousands of morbidly obese patients, has been walking. The important considerations are to encourage patients to set aside religiously a given amount of time and insist upon it as a key, high-priority, lifestyle change. A walking companion is often a necessity for success so as to encourage compliance and combat the strong tendency toward recidivism in the morbidly obese.

Self-monitoring

Patients' willingness and ability to follow instructions to monitor themselves is an excellent prognostic indicator of success in weight loss. Therefore, it is wise to test patients by asking them to commence their own self-monitoring, including exercise, almost from the beginning of their weight-loss programs. The advantages are that by monitoring themselves, patients obtain a better grasp of their exercise and other patterns and find barriers they need or want to change. Self-monitoring is an effective tool to use to provide participants with their unique first-party, regular feedback loop.

To help sustain and confirm compliance with the self-monitoring process, patients should maintain logs of their intervisit exercise programs and take them to each clinic encounter. It is wise to have the office staff instruct them to clearly record the number of minutes of exercise, the particular exercise, and the number of steps (or miles) walked each day. It is also useful to have them record the perceived intensity of each exercise so that they can monitor their progress by means of this additional dimension.

Pedometer

Plain pedometers are useful in monitoring patients' activities for their own information and for that of the weight-loss program personnel. Studies have shown that patients who record 10,000 steps or more daily are likely meeting the physical activity requirements for successful weight loss and maintenance. First, patients should obtain baseline numbers, the steps taken during a typical day. With these data, program staff can better work with patients to set increasing weekly goals for exercise, for example, 200 to 500 steps more each day until reaching the target level.

▶ OFFICE POLICY AND PROCEDURE FOR OVERSEEING PATIENT SELF-MONITORING

In order to maximize the benefits of patients' efforts, it is important to develop a coordinated plan to carefully monitor and constructively motivate patients' progress, with the office staff's assistance. One or two staff members, together with the program's physicians, should develop a policy and procedure to accommodate the regular, sustained, careful monitoring and counseling needs of the patient exercise program. As part of this work, it is also useful to develop lists of local exercise programs and other local, catalog, or Internet resources as well as a small collection of handouts and other literature and audio or visual tapes for patient instruction and motivation. It is also important to stress, monitor, and educate patients in lay terms about their biochemical achievements (e.g., lipid levels), particularly those that they are making or sustaining through regular long-term exercise.

Insulin Resistance and Weight Loss

Skeletal muscle insulin resistance entails dysregulation of both glucose and fatty-acid metabolism. There appears to be a consensus that treatment of this dysregulation by weight loss reduces insulin resistance, with concomitant improvement in the skeletal muscle metabolism of fatty acids and glucose.[31] However, it is useful to clarify whether exercise achieves this effect by itself, independent of weight loss.

It has been shown that a single bout of exercise by itself can acutely improve insulin sensitivity, but this effect is not lasting. It dissipates over a period of several days or less and, of course, weight loss is not an issue in this brief time frame.[32] Long-term exercise in the obese also shows little sustained improvement in insulin sensitivity absent any weight change.[33] In stark contrast, exercise-trained, fit, nonobese individuals, also in a steady-weight state, generally exhibit low insulin resistance[34] and high fat oxidation by their skeletal muscles during exercise.[35]

The contrasting lower rates of fat oxidation in the obese predict, and appear related to, the cause of their weight gain.[36] The lower rates of fat oxidation in the obese also are logically predictive of poor weight-loss maintenance over the long term following successful short-term dieting.[37]

A study of weight loss alone without exercise in the obese demonstrated an improvement in their insulin-stimulated glucose utilization but no change in their fasting lipid oxidation rates.[38] This begged the obvious question of whether adding exercise to a dietary-restrictive weight-loss program would meaningfully improve fasting lipid oxidation patterns together with improved insulin resistance. A follow-on study clearly demonstrated that exercise combined with weight loss significantly enhanced postabsorptive fat oxidation and improved insulin sensitivity. It also showed that exercise, when combined with caloric restriction, significantly improved insulin sensitivity by 49% (±10%), a rate that was the same in men and women. Improvement in insulin sensitivity was due entirely to an improvement in nonoxidative glucose disposal, which increased by 159%. There was, however, no change in rates of insulin-stimulated glucose oxidation.[39]

An important consideration in insulin sensitivity is whether changes induced in total and regional body-fat volume are predictive of improved insulin sensitivity. Studies have found that loss of total body fat, subcutaneous abdominal fat, and subfascial thigh fat, but not the selective loss of visceral fat or subcutaneous thigh fat, was associated with improved insulin sensitivity.[39]

Changes in $\dot{V}O_{2max}$ and energy expenditure tended to be associated with the improved insulin sensitivity. However, the strongest simple correlate with improved insulin sensitivity was increased fasting rates of fat oxidation as reflected by the reduced fasting respiratory quotient (RQ), an indication of increased fat oxidation as opposed to carbohydrate substrate. Similar associations were observed with respect to the nonoxidative component of insulin sensitivity.[39] The addition of exercise to weight-loss dieting appears to be a key aspect of the improvement in insulin sensitivity in obesity. Logically, it ought to have a strong prophylactic effect on the development of these and other components of the metabolic syndrome. Clearly, long-term exercise as an accompaniment to weight-reduction programs in the obese is essential for maintaining more than purely weight loss.

▶ ANTIOBESITY MEDICATIONS

Currently available antiobesity prescription medications work by means of appetite suppression or reduction of gastrointestinal absorption. They are recommended for use only in persons with body mass indexes (BMIs) of 30 or higher, as well as in those with BMIs between 27 and 30 kg per m² who have two or more significant obesity comorbidities, such as hypertension, diabetes, or hyperlipidemia.

There are only two antiobesity medications that are currently approved for patient use for longer than 12 weeks. One, sibutramine (Meridia), is an appetite suppressant. The other, orlistat (Xenical), is a lipase inhibitor that acts by blocking absorption of approximately one third of ingested fat. They may be prescribed for patient use up to a maximum of 2 years. However, orlistat may be continued after 1 year in patients who demonstrate sustained weight loss and medication tolerance.[40] Treatment failure and the effects of fat malabsorption, including oily spotting, fecal urgency, fecal incontinence, flatulence, abdominal cramping, and diarrhea, caused 12.9% of volunteer subjects to drop out of a 104-week orlistat trial.[41] The consumer group Public Citizen recently submitted a request to the

U.S. Food and Drug Administration to have sibutramine withdrawn from the market due to issues with this medication's known hypertensive effects.

Reported effectiveness in a metaanalysis of these medications was less than 10 lb of net weight loss in excess of that lost with placebo.[42] This lack of effectiveness or, perhaps, the side effects may be responsible for the brief usage of sibutramine (102 days) and orlistat (110 days) in only 2.4% of adults under 65 years of age who had insurance coverage for antiobesity medication.[41,43]

Six other appetite suppressants have a sympathomimetic, amphetamine-like activity but are approved for maximum use of only 12 weeks. They are phentermine, mazindol, phenylpropanolamine, diethylpropion, benzphetamine, and phendimetrazine.[44]

Two other antiobesity medications are in phase-III development, with 19 more in earlier stages.[45] One of them, rimonabant (Acomplia, Sanofi-Aventis), appears to work by blocking a food-craving (cannabinoid) pathway in the brain; it reportedly produced weight loss of more than 10% in 1 year in nearly half (44%) of the volunteer subjects as compared with weight loss in only 10% of placebo subjects; an average of 16 lb of weight loss was reported in nonplacebo subjects who completed 2 years of the study.[46] A group of medications described as β-3 receptor stimulators are aimed at increasing metabolic activity.[47] Others are designed to block the appetite-stimulating effects of ghrelin.[48]

Approval of any of these medications by the Food and Drug Administration will probably increase antiobesity medication usage among the more than 60% of Americans who are overweight, perhaps even surpassing the $12 billion in sales of the statin medication Lipitor in 2004. This is particularly so, given the recent announcement by Medicare that it will reimburse for "effective" obesity treatments. Currently, drug usage has dramatically lessened following discontinuation of the popular Phen-Fen (dexfenfluramine and fenfluramine) combination due to reports of pulmonary hypertension and heart valve complications associated with their use.

Over-the-counter (OTC) medicines and herbal treatments for obesity have long been available. For example, amphetamines were widely used for weight loss more than 50 years ago, prior to the time when their addictive effects were properly recognized. OTC amphetamine-like products are currently available.

There is some reason for concern as to whether these or any other herbal or herbal-like supplements should continue to remain available in the OTC marketplace. This position is supported by a systematic review of data from double-blind, randomized, controlled trials of herbal supplements used for body-weight reduction that were recently conducted.[49] The herbal supplements evaluated included *Ephedra sinica, Paullinia cupana,* guar gum, *Plantago psyllium, Ilex paraguariensis,* and *Pausinystalia johimbe.* The reviewers uncovered reports of adverse events, including hepatic injury and death, that have occurred with the use of some of them. Increased risk for psychiatric, autonomic, or gastrointestinal adverse events and heart palpitation were reported specifically for ephedra and ephedrine-containing food supplements. Although the reviewers felt that the quality of the data did not justify definitive or uniform attribution of causality, they concluded that the reported risks in taking these herbal supplements are sufficient to shift the risk-benefit balance against the use of most of them.

Further, herbal treatments such as *Garcinia cambogia*, also commonly used in commercial weight-loss medicines, have not been found beneficial in the treatment of obesity. A randomized, double-blind, placebo-controlled trial at the Obesity Research Center, St Luke's-Roosevelt Hospital, concluded that *G. cambogia* failed to produce significant weight loss and fat-mass loss beyond that observed with placebo.[50]

▶ CONCLUSION

Dietary and pharmaceutical methods of weight loss are currently fairly ineffective, especially in the morbidly obese. In the absence of a dramatic but unanticipated breakthrough, it appears that this will remain the case for many years to come.

▶ REFERENCES

1. Graham S: The Graham journal of health and longevity 1837-1839, vols. 1-3.
2. Fletcher H: The A.B.-Z. of Our Own Nutrition. New York, F. A. Stokes, 1898.
3. Schwarz RW: John Harvey Kellogg: Father of the Health Food Industry. Berrien Springs, MI, Andrews University Press, 1970.
4. Habgood J: The Hay Diet Made Easy: A Practical Guide to Food Combining. London, Souvenir Press, 1997.
5. Nestle M, Porter DV: Evolution of federal dietary guidance policy: from food adequacy to chronic disease prevention. Caduceus 1990;6: 43-47.
6. Peters LH: Diet and Health With a Key to the Calories. Chicago, Reilly & Britton, 1918.
7. Rating the diets. Consumer Guide 1981;304:228.
8. Hansen HR, Pickford R, Thomas-Oates J, et al: 2-Dimethylarsinothioyl acetic acid identified in a biological sample: the first occurrence of a mammalian arsinothioyl metabolite. Angewandte Chemie 2004;43:337-340 (international ed).
9. White M: Diet Without Despair. New York, M.S. Mill, 1943.
10. Nidetch J: Weight Watchers Cook Book. New York, Hearthside Press, 1966.
11. Stillman I, Baker SS: The Doctor's Quick Weight-Loss Diet. Englewood Cliffs, N.J., Prentice-Hall, 1967.
12. Tarnower H, Baker SS: The Complete Scarsdale Medical Diet. New York, Bantam Books, 1978.
13. Akins RC: Dr. Atkins' Diet Revolution. New York, Literary Guild, 1972.
14. Linn R, Stuart SL: The Last-Chance Diet. New York, Bantam Books, 1977.
15. Drenick EJ: Risk of obesity and surgical indications. Int J Obes 1981;5(4):387-398.
16. Valenta LJ, Elias AN: Modified fasting in treatment of obesity: effects on serum lipids, electrolytes, liver enzymes, and blood pressure. Postgrad Med 1986;79(4):263-267.
17. Pritikin R: The Pritikin Program for Diet and Exercise. New York, Grosset & Dunlap, 1981.
18. Mazel J: The Beverly Hills Diet. New York, Macmillan, 1981.
19. Ornish D: Stress, Diet and Your Heart. New York, Holt, Rinehart Winston, 1982.
20. Eyton A: The F-Plan Diet: Lose Weight Fast and Live Longer. New York, Crown, 1983.
21. Reinhold JG, Faradji B, Abadi P, et al: Decreased absorption of calcium, magnesium, zinc and phosphorus by humans due to increased fiber and phosphorus consumption as wheat bread. J Nutr 1976;106(4):493-503.
22. Conley R: The Complete Hip and Thigh Diet. New York, Warner Books, 1990.
23. Sears B, Lawren B: The Zone: A Dietary Road Map to Lose Weight Permanently, Reset Your Genetic Code, Prevent Disease, Achieve Maximum Physical Performance. New York, Regan Books, 1995.
24. Agatston A: The South Beach Diet: The Delicious, Doctor-Designed, Foolproof Plan for Fast and Healthy Weight Loss. New York, Random House, 2003.
25. Kaplan HL, Kaplan HS: The psychosomatic concept of obesity. J Nerv Ment Dis 1957;125:181-201.
26. Brownell KD, Kramer FM: Behavioral management of obesity. Med Clin North Am 1989;73:185-201.
27. Goodrick GK, Foreyt JP: Why treatments for obesity don't last. J Am Diet Assoc 1991;91:1243-1247.
28. Dolfing JG, Dubois EF, Wolffenbuttel BHR, et al: Different cycle ergometer outcomes in severely obese men and women without documented cardiopulmonary morbidities before bariatric surgery. Chest 2005;127(7):256-262.
29. Orzano AJ, Scott JG: Diagnosis and treatment of obesity in adults: an applied evidence-based review. J Am Board Fam Pract 2004;17(5): 359-369.
30. Klem ML, Wing RR, McGuire MT, et al: A descriptive study of individuals successful at long-term maintenance of substantial weight loss. Am J Clin Nutr 1997;66:239-246.
31. Pi-Sunyer FX: Short-term medical benefits and adverse effects of weight loss. Ann Intern Med 1993;119:722-726.
32. Dela F, Larsen JJ, Mikines KJ, et al: Insulin-stimulated muscle glucose clearance in patients with NIDDM. Diabetes 1995;44:1010-1020.
33. Segal KR, Edano A, Abalos A, et al: Effect of exercise training on insulin sensitivity and glucose metabolism in lean, obese, and diabetic men. J Appl Physiol 1991;71:2402-2411.
34. Goodpaster BH, He J, Watkins S, et al: Skeletal muscle lipid content and insulin resistance: evidence for a paradox in endurance-trained athletes. J Clin Endocrinol Metab 2001;86:5755-5761.
35. Romijn JA, Coyle EF, Sidossis LS, et al: Regulation of endogenous fat and carbohydrate metabolism in relation to exercise intensity and duration. Am J Physiol 1993;265:E380-E391.
36. Zurlo F, Lillioja S, Esposito-DelPuente A, et al: Low ratio of fat to carbohydrate oxidation as a predictor of weight gain: a study of 24-h RQ. Am J Physiol 1990;259:E650-E657.
37. Ranneries C, Bulow J, Buemann B, et al: Fat metabolism in formerly obese women. Am J Physiol 1998;274:E155-E161.
38. Douketis JD, Feightner JW, Attia J, et al: Canadian Task Force on Preventive Health Care: Periodic health examination, 1999 update. 1. Detection, prevention and treatment of obesity. CMAJ 1999;160: 513-525.
39. Goodpaster BH, Katsiaras A, Kelley DE: Enhanced fat oxidation through physical activity is associated with improvements in insulin sensitivity in obesity. Diabetes 2003;52(9):2191-2197.
40. American Society of Health-System Pharmacists: Drug Information. Bethesda, Md., ASHSP, 2004.
41. Hauptman J, Lucas C, Boldrin MN, et al: Orlistat in the long-term treatment of obesity in primary care settings. Arch Fam Med 2000;9:160-167.
42. Shekelle P, Morton SC, Maglione M, et al: Southern California-RAND Evidence-based Practice Center, Santa Monica, Cal.: Pharmacological and Surgical Treatment of Obesity: Evidence Report, Technical Assessment No. 103, No. 04-E028-2. Rockville, Md., Agency for Healthcare Research and Quality, 2004.
43. Encinosa WE, Bernard DM, Steiner CA, et al: Use and costs of bariatric surgery and prescription weight-loss medications. Health Aff 2005;24(4):1039-1046.
44. Mosby's Drug Consult, ed 14. St. Louis, Mosby, 2004.
45. Datamonitor, Commercial and Pipeline Perspectives: Obesity. London, Datamonitor, June 2004.
46. Korner J, Aronne LJ: Pharmacological approaches to weight reduction: therapeutic targets. J Clin Endocrinol Metab 2004;89:2616-2621.
47. Vansal S: Beta-3 receptor agonists and other potential anti-obesity agents. Am J Pharmaceut Ed 2004;68:1-10.
48. Bays H, Dujovne C: Anti-obesity drug development. Expert Opin Invest Drugs 2002;11:1189-1204.
49. Pittler MH, Schmidt K, Ernst E: Adverse events of herbal food supplements for body weight reduction: systematic review. Obes Rev 2005;6:93-111.
50. Heymsfield SB, Allison DB, Vasselli JR, et al: Garcinia cambogia (hydroxycitric acid) as a potential antiobesity agent: a randomized controlled trial. JAMA 1998;280:1596-600.

PREOPERATIVE, PERIOPERATIVE, AND POSTOPERATIVE PATIENT CARE

12

Patient Selection for Bariatric Surgery

Heena Santry, M.D., John Alverdy, M.D., F.A.C.S., and Vivek Prachand, M.D., F.A.C.S.

The decision to operate on any patient is generally shaped by four variables—the seriousness of the underlying condition, the urgency with which the condition must be treated, the probability of a successful outcome, and the risks associated with the surgical procedure. Patient selection for bariatric surgery is uniquely challenging because of the broad continuum of values that these variables can take on.

In this chapter, we discuss how to approach the complex topic of patient selection in bariatric surgery. The rapid rise in the incidence of obesity has been accompanied by an increasing number of bariatric procedures, estimated by the American Society of Bariatric Surgery to be in excess of 140,000 in 2004. The issue of patient selection is critical to understand not only for practicing surgeons but also for insurance providers, referring physicians, risk management teams, policy makers, and patients, all of whom are keenly aware of the variability in patient selection.[1] In this chapter, we do not deal with issues of procedure selection.[2] For a formal decision-analysis model, we refer you to Patterson's Markov decision analysis model for bariatric surgery.[3] We do not focus on the broader issues of cost-benefit analysis in decision making in bariatric surgery. The costs to society of obesity and related illnesses are well established and data have proven that bariatric surgery can greatly reduce obesity's financial burden on the health care system.[4-11] This chapter focuses on decision making relative to an individual candidate in question.

▶ CHALLENGES OF PATIENT SELECTION

Patient selection in bariatric surgery is more challenging than in other areas of surgery because the underlying disorder, its treatment, and the outcomes of treatment are not easily understood. Dr. Atul Gawande describes bariatric surgery as "the most drastic treatment we have for obesity...[and as] among the strangest operations surgeons perform. It removes no disease, repairs no defect or injury. It is an operation that is intended to control a person's will—to manipulate his innards so that he does

not overeat...."[12] Yet the serious nature of morbid obesity is predicted not only by the patient's actual weight but also by the presence of comorbidities, the likelihood that other comorbidities may develop if the obesity remains, and the psychosocial and quality-of-life detriments associated with obesity.[13-16]

A major tenet of patient selection for bariatric surgery is that weight-reduction surgery is elective and almost never is associated with a comorbid condition requiring emergency surgery. Although obesity is a proven cause of early mortality, the imminence of death for a given patient is unknown.[13,17] Thus, although a practitioner has the ability to consider completely and contemplatively his or her decision to operate, there is a degree of urgency that guides the decision-making process when the patient's and the family's sense of doom is dramatized by the realization that morbid obesity takes a progressive daily toll on almost all organ systems and leads to increasing disability and premature mortality.

As in all surgery, patient selection for bariatric surgery is strongly linked to the surgeon's and the patient's perceptions of the risks and benefits of the surgery. Both patient and surgeon need to have a comprehensive, evidence-based understanding of the benefits of bariatric surgery. What constitutes a successful outcome for the patient, his or her family, and the surgeon should not be at variance with the accepted standard of success for bariatric surgery. Although a severely diabetic patient who uses more than 100 units of insulin per day may be completely cured of diabetes within 1 month of surgery, this degree of dramatic success after bariatric surgery is not universal. In most cases, weight loss and the benefits related to it occur over long periods after surgery. Patient selection, therefore, must also take into account how "success" is defined after bariatric surgery. Yet measuring success in terms of weight loss alone is complicated; the optimal means of measuring weight loss has not been universally agreed upon.

Weight loss can be construed as total body fat lost, percentage of excess body weight lost, or change in body mass index (BMI). Each of these measurements is limited in its ability to distinguish among loss of total fat mass, of lean body mass, and of total body water. Beyond absolute weight loss, the definition of success must also take into account amelioration or resolution of comorbidities and the presumed prevention of future comorbidities, as well as quality-of-life improvements. Furthermore, success may result not only from the technical skill of the surgeon but also from the ability of the patient to cope with the lifestyle effects of surgery and to comply with the behaviors required to sustain weight loss.

Bariatric surgery has been described as "behavioral surgery" in which a " 'satisfactory outcome' requires more pre- and postoperative patient education than most other surgery."[18] After many major surgical approaches to complex disease, the recurrence of the initiating disease process (e.g., reappearance of gastroesophageal reflux disease (GERD), detection of cancer following major resection, etc.), despite what was presumed to be a technically adequate operation, is considered both a treatment failure and a surgical failure.

If the success of bariatric surgery is defined only by percentage of excess weight lost, then indeed both treatment and surgical failure occur if patients regain a significant amount of their initial weight loss. Maintenance of at least 50% of excess weight lost is considered optimal for success. However, if improvement in medical comorbidities is considered the main end point for success, success is defined independent of weight loss alone. Patient selection, therefore, can change as the surgeon's notion of success changes. For these reasons, perhaps unlike other surgically treated disease, the risk-to-benefit ratio for bariatric surgery can vary.

Finally, in evaluating the risks and the benefits of bariatric surgery as guides in patient selection, the surgeon is left with the option of nonsurgical weight loss as a treatment option. In the case of morbid obesity, allowing a patient to attempt pharmacologic and behavioral treatments for obesity, even though these nonsurgical weight-loss methods have not been shown to result in durable long-term weight-loss, remains an alternative.[19,20] Allowing a patient to remain obese is also an option, despite the proven morbidity and mortality with which obesity is associated.

▶ INDICATIONS AND CONTRAINDICATIONS

Currently, the most widely accepted selection criteria for bariatric surgery, on the part of both clinicians and payers, are those of the National Institutes of Health (NIH) Consensus Development Conference Statement on Gastrointestinal Surgery for Severe Obesity (1991).[21] This conference was held in response to the increasing awareness of the medical and psychosocial implications of severe obesity, the ineffectiveness of medical and behavioral therapies, and the development of surgical alternatives safer than the jejeunoileal bypass. At the time, it was recognized that there were "insufficient data on which to base selection criteria using objective clinical features alone"[21] (as is still the case). Nonetheless, based on the available evidence, a series of recommendations was made, as summarized in Table 12-1. More recently, the NIH published an evidence-based guide for the identification, evaluation, and treatment of overweight and obesity in adults and prescribed surgery as a third-line therapy for

Table 12-1	SUMMARY OF PATIENT SELECTION CRITERIA, 1991 NIH CONSENSUS STATEMENT

The patient is an adult (specifically, not an adolescent)
The patient's BMI is:
1. Above 40
2. Between 35 and 40, with related medical comorbidities
3. Between 35 and 40, with functional limitations due to body size or joint disease

If, after evaluation by a multidisciplinary team, the patient is judged to:
1. Have a low probability of success with nonoperative weight-loss measures
2. Be well informed about the long- and short-term risks and benefits of surgery
3. Be highly motivated to lose weight through surgery
4. Have an acceptable operative risk
5. Be willing to undergo lifelong medical surveillance

obesity, again restricted to patients with BMIs greater than 35 kg per m[2].[22] The first recommended therapy in that document remained behavioral modifications, and the second therapy involved the addition of a pharmacologic agent to behavioral changes such as dieting and increasing exercise.

The recent publication of the 2004 Consensus Conference guidelines brings the recommendations for bariatric surgery up to the present and sets reasonable standards for patient selection.[23] "Ultimately, the best and final indicator for bariatric surgery is the well-informed, experienced bariatric surgeon's decision in any given case presentation."[24]

Age

The detrimental effects of obesity occur throughout the life course.[25,26] Anyone who meets all of the other medical and psychosocial criteria for surgery should not be denied surgery on the basis of age alone. We recommend that physiologic rather than chronologic age be the chief consideration, along with the other considerations discussed subsequently. There have been numerous reports demonstrating the safety and efficacy of bariatric surgery in older individuals.[27] If a patient's overall health status, regardless of chronologic age, does not confer a life expectancy of fewer than 5 years, then a patient should be considered for weight-reduction surgery.

Although we feel that the issue is clear in older individuals, we are not as certain when it comes to recommendations for weight-reduction surgery in adolescents. This remains a controversial area. We feel that prospective patients under 18 years of age are best treated with intensive diet and behavioral therapy, but there are a growing number of adolescents who meet all of the suggested NIH criteria except for age. Data show that surgery can be safely performed in patients between 11 and 18 years of age and have good outcomes.[28-33] Long-term outcome data are lacking, however, especially studies of the relationship between obesity and the rapid physiologic development that occurs in adolescence. Sugerman and colleagues published a series in which only 5 of 33 adolescent patients were considered treatment failures after 10 years.[33]

All studies have emphasized that strong familial support is requisite for successful treatment. Most have advocated a comprehensive multidisciplinary approach and treatment within a pediatric specialty center such as that described by Inge and colleagues in Cincinnati.[31]

Weight

The weight criteria can be divided into two categories: life-threatening obesity and clinically severe obesity. A patient with life-threatening obesity has surpassed the weight beyond which the probability of developing one or more weight-related illness and succumbing to a premature death becomes inevitable. Based on insurance life-table analyses using BMI as a measure of degree of obesity, the weight at which a patient is considered to have life-threatening obesity is 40 kg per m^2. Another common, but not the preferred, measure of life-threatening obesity is excess body weight. In absolute terms, this is generally 45 kg or 100 lb of excess body weight, or an actual weight 170% greater than ideal body weight. A patient with clinically severe obesity has a BMI of 35 to 39.9 kg per m^2 accompanied by major medical disorders, such as diabetes mellitus, obstructive sleep apnea, hypertension, disabling osteoarthritis, thromboembolic disorders, urinary stress incontinence, pseudotumor cerebri, cardiomyopathy of obesity with pulmonary hypertension, or intractable GERD.

Although theoretically, no maximum BMI is a contraindication to surgery, not all surgeons have the ability to treat all morbidly obese patients safely and effectively. Having decided that the patient's problem is severe enough for a surgical intervention, a surgeon must decide whether the patient is too overweight for the procedure offered. That is, a surgeon must establish a maximum BMI at which he or she feels adequately experienced to perform surgery safely. Safety considerations for patients with BMIs greater than 65 kg per m^2 should include not only the surgeon's technical skill but also the capability of the institution to handle super morbidly obese patients safely. The institution must have appropriate operative equipment for the extremely morbidly obese patient as well as the preparedness to perform indicated diagnostic procedures should a complication arise.

More difficult to assess than these absolute measures of weight is the degree to which the patient has struggled with his or her weight. Many patients report obesity from childhood or teenage years. Life-long struggle with obesity is certainly an indication for surgery, but any patient with a significantly long struggle with morbid obesity (at least 5 years) should be considered. Prior weight-loss attempts need to be considered not from the perspective of duration of successful weight loss and time to failure (weight regain) but from the perspective that the patient has previously exhibited the motivation to lose weight. Patients who have recently gained a significant amount of weight should be scrutinized carefully for a treatable medical cause such as hypercortisolism or hypothyroidism.

Another factor related to the overweight history that must be considered is a strong family history of obesity. The evidence is still emerging, and obesity is clearly a multifactorial disease, but there is undoubtedly a genetic component to obesity. Obesity could be considered to be the consequence of genotype as well as numerous other factors that play a role in the pathophysiology of obesity. Patients with first-order relatives who, similarly, have struggled with morbid obesity should be thought of as having a higher likelihood of being refractory to non-surgical intervention.

Absolute Medical Contraindications

There are few absolute contraindications for surgery. Some patients may not be candidates for general anesthesia. Under certain circumstances, an intervention prior to weight-reduction surgery (e.g., coronary artery stenting) will improve the operative risks involved in subsequent weight-loss surgery. The critical history and physical examination will indicate appropriate referral to pulmonologists or cardiologists. In the setting of morbid obesity, routine preoperative testing (pulmonary function testing, sleep evaluation, and electrocardiogram) may indicate the need for such a referral prior to surgery. We do not, however, believe that referral to these specialists is necessary for all patients. Suitability for general anesthesia also rests on the ability of the anesthesiologist to intubate the patient. We recommend that the anesthesiologist who will be present at the procedure thoroughly evaluate the airway of all prospective patients in advance of the planned procedure. In our experience, many patients have required fiberoptic intubation while awake because of their obesity.

Certain other physiologic or anatomic circumstances, though not prohibitive of general anesthesia, may be considered absolute contraindications to surgery because the operation cannot be performed safely. For example, the presence of gastric varices is a contraindication to surgery because of the risk of life-threatening hemorrhage. Similarly, even in the hands of the most technically gifted surgeon, it may not be possible to convert a prior gastrectomy into any kind of reasonable bariatric procedure. Active peptic ulcer disease should also be considered an absolute contraindication to surgery, as the proposed procedure will isolate a diseased organ that will then no longer be amenable to treatment. Suspected cases of peptic ulcer disease should be diagnosed by endoscopy. Confirmed cases should be appropriately treated with proton pump inhibitors and repeat endoscopy, and resolution of disease should be documented prior to reevaluation for weight-reduction surgery. Cases of *Helicobacter pylori* infection should be eradicated by an appropriate course of the recommended drug combinations prior to reevaluation.

Some absolute contraindications to surgery are present even when general anesthesia and the operation may be safely possible. For example, patients with conditions such as active malignancy or AIDS should not be considered for surgery because of their limited life expectancy and the fact that these conditions will not be improved by weight reduction. In other words, "the patient's prognosis, given weight reduction, should warrant the risk of the treatment."[24] In general, any non–weight-related condition that indicates an expected survival time of fewer than 5 years should be considered a contraindication to surgery.

Relative Medical Contraindications

Numerous disease processes have been suggested as relative contraindications and should be viewed individually in the context of the patient's full medical and psychosocial situation. These include HIV infection without signs or symptoms of AIDS and prior malignancy without evidence of recurrence, and other situations in which life expectancy cannot be predicted accurately. Cirrhosis of the liver due to nonalcoholic steatohepatitis may be a relative contraindication to surgery. There is considerable controversy in this area because many surgeons have performed both restrictive and malabsorptive procedures in the presence of nonalcoholic steatohepatitis with fibrosis and cirrhosis and have seen good outcomes. Again, patient selection must be tailored to the perception of risk and benefit which, in the case of cirrhosis, may be difficult to predict. In situations in which there is no clear medical reason not to operate, a patient's full medical history, including past and present conditions, must be carefully considered together with his or her age, history of overweight, psychiatric comorbidities, and ability to comply with the postsurgical lifestyle prior to making a final decision to operate. The final two considerations, psychiatric and behavioral issues, are discussed later.

Functional Status

In our experience, even appropriate candidates without any psychiatric or behavioral contraindications may not successfully adapt after surgery if they are not physically functional.

SPECIAL CASES OF THOSE WHO ARE SICKEST BECAUSE OF OBESITY

Some patients have several relative contraindications to surgery, the causes of which are obesity-related medical comorbidities themselves. The reasons these patients seek weight-loss surgery can often be the very factors that put them at high risk. Staging the course of care for these patients can convert many of them into good-risk candidates. Our approach to the problem of high-risk patients has been to set rigorous goals for the patients so as to shift their risk through preoperative weight loss, psychological counseling, physical therapy, better control of their medical disorders (hyperglycemia, hypertension, reversible heart disease, etc.), and resolution of all psychosocial issues. The entire team engages these patients to assist them in achieving their goals. Patients are seen every 3 months and evaluated for improvement in risk factors. In this manner, the patients are offered hope that they can become appropriate surgical candidates. Remaining within the program in which surgery can be performed offers patients both hope and motivation to comply and be successful.

Others have suggested an alternative surgical approach to high-risk patients that involves a staged weight-reduction procedure. First, they perform a less extensive, less invasive procedure, such as an adjustable gastric banding or a sleeve gastrectomy, that has been shown to be low in morbidity as a bridge to more extensive surgery. Others have advocated a more radical and definitive approach involving a fully malabsorptive bypass (a biliopancreatic diversion/ duodenal switch). Still others have suggested obtaining informed consent from the patient and family in accepting a high-morbidity and high-mortality possibility, as is done in the case of other high-risk situations, such as large thoracoabdominal aneurysms, multivessel heart disease, advanced cancer, and liver transplantation.

Our final recommendation in the cases of the highest risk candidates remains to minimize as much of the risk as possible through conservative measures prior to surgery and to offer the most appropriate surgery when the risk has been minimized. In cases in which perioperative risk remains high but there are no absolute contraindications to the procedure, the patient should be treated at a high-volume center where substantial experience minimizes risk even further.

▶ PSYCHOPATHOLOGIC CRITERIA

If a prospective patient is found to have satisfied all of the medical requirements for surgery, the ideal psychosocial candidate for surgery is someone with no history of major psychopathology, few stressors, good coping skills, high motivation, good appraisal of the surgical process, and high cognitive and social functioning. Psychiatric criteria for candidacy are more difficult to interpret than are the medical criteria discussed earlier. Most surgeons are generally well versed in the usual medical comorbidities that affect surgical outcomes, but they are usually not as familiar with the intricacies of psychiatric diagnosis and treatment. We strongly encourage independent psychological and psychiatric evaluation. At our institution, we have a group composed of a psychologist and several postdoctoral candidates who see each of our preoperative patients. Successful treatment of psychiatric conditions has been found to be a positive prognostic indicator.[34]

Axis I Disorders

Any newly diagnosed axis I disorder must be fully evaluated and successfully treated under the supervision of a psychiatrist for a period of at least 1 year prior to reevaluation for surgery. Anyone found to have suicidal ideation must be free of suicidal thoughts for at least 1 year prior to reconsideration. Well-controlled major depression, bipolar disorder, and schizophrenia do not preclude surgery. However, prospective patients must demonstrate both that they have been effectively treated and that they have the ability, in the form of personal commitment, psychiatric care, psychological counseling, and social support, to continue that treatment after weight-reduction surgery. We have not encountered patient inability to consume psychotropic medications and physiologic inability to absorb such medications postoperatively.

Substance Abuse

Active substance abuse or alcoholism diagnosed on psychological assessment should be considered an absolute contraindication to surgery. The behavioral manifestations of these disorders are not compatible with the postsurgical lifestyle that is mandated for patients. Patients with a history of any of these conditions should be carefully reassessed. A minimum of 1 year of being substance- or alcohol-free is mandatory prior to reconsideration. Interventions taken to achieve control of these addictive disorders in the past should be well documented, including letters from prior mental health providers who can attest to the likelihood of maintaining control of these disorders in the face of the dramatic physiologic and emotional stresses of weight-reduction surgery. As with the axis I disorders, patients should demonstrate a commitment to remain substance- and alcohol-free after surgery and have the necessary psychosocial mechanisms in place to do so.

Eating Disorders

Active anorexia (rare, though possible with a very high body weight) and bulimia should be considered absolute contraindications to surgery. Obviously, a major component of success after surgery involves controlling the types of food consumed and the portion sizes. Patients with active anorexia and bulimia cannot comply with these requirements. On the other hand, as with the major psychiatric and addictive disorders, a history of a major eating disorder should not absolutely preclude surgery. Once again, there should be thorough documentation by a psychiatrist or psychologist who has followed the patient, stating that the psychiatric and behavioral symptoms of anorexia and bulimia are well controlled. The patient should be judged to be able to satisfy the specific eating requirements of the surgical procedure in question.

Mild Psychiatric Conditions

Patients deemed to be suffering from milder psychiatric disorders, such as dysthymic disorder or binge-eating disorder, should be considered on an individual basis. These disorders generally do not require psychotropic medications or major intensive psychotherapy. In our experience, patients with these conditions, if equipped with adequate coping mechanisms and social support, can do quite well after surgery. They can comply with postsurgical lifestyle requirements and continued follow-up, and their symptoms often improve dramatically as a consequence of surgery. However, one should be particularly vigilant in observing such patients for signs that the disorders are evolving into major psychiatric disorders that require aggressive treatment.

Special Case of Prior Sexual or Physical Abuse

Data have shown that prior abuse, especially sexual abuse, is correlated with the development of obesity. All patients should be screened for history of abuse. The psychological sequelae of such abuse should be thoroughly evaluated and treated prior to any consideration for weight-reduction surgery.

▶ BEHAVIORAL CRITERIA

Success after surgery depends, in large measure, on the ability of a patient to comply with postoperative behavioral requirements. Compliance is not a medically definable entity, but inability to comply with the postoperative requirements of altered eating habits, life-long vitamin supplementation, and long-term follow-up should be viewed as an absolute contraindication to surgery. The ability to comply is multifactorial and, unlike other areas of surgical decision making, forces the surgeon to confront the complicated issues of the patient's intelligence, behavioral pathology, coping skills, functional status, socioeconomic status, and psychosocial support.

Brolin states that "the prospective patient's psychological stability should be evaluated, particularly in terms of his or her willingness to adjust to the permanent postoperative effects of gastric restriction and malabsorption."[35,36] Three of his suggested criteria for psychological stability are: (1) a basic understanding of how obesity surgery causes weight loss; (2) a realization that surgery itself does not guarantee weight loss; and (3) commitment to postoperative follow-up. (The fourth is that the patient be free of substance or alcohol abuse.)

Appraisal and Cognition

Appraisal refers to a patient's understanding of the surgical process, potential negative effects of the surgery, expected weight loss, and postsurgical diet and lifestyle. Some have suggested that persons of limited intellectual ability, such as those who are mentally retarded or illiterate, should not be considered for weight-reduction surgery because they cannot adequately appraise the process of and results of the surgery. Though formal intelligence-quotient testing is not required, a prospective patient should be able to demonstrate to the surgeon, the psychiatric team, and the social worker that he or she understands why he or she is a candidate for surgery and what surgery the entails before, during, and after the procedure.

In all circumstances, issues of ability to give informed consent should be considered. If a patient is able to give consent or meets the criteria that allow a legally defined proxy (such as next of kin) to give consent, then the decision to operate, if all medical criteria are met, should be based upon whether the patient has adequate social support to enable compliance with all postoperative lifestyle requirements. For example, a mentally retarded individual suffering from the detrimental physiologic consequences of obesity should not be denied surgery if he or she has a responsible care provider who demonstrates adequate appraisal of the surgery and who can function to guarantee that all of the postoperative behavioral requirements will be met. Unfortunately, in our experience, people from group-home environments for whom a caseworker may be that responsible party should not be considered for surgery because the responsible party has too many other obligations to other clients to be an effective guarantor of the patient's compliance.

Social Support

Isolated individuals are less likely to adjust successfully to postsurgical lifestyles. The support and encouragement provided by family and friends help to mitigate the patient's distorted postoperative role in the social phenomenon of eating. At our institution, a designated support person is mandatory for surgical clearance. The support person must show a commitment to assisting the patient in all practical matters associated with surgery, such as driving to and from appointments, preparing meals, and so forth, and to providing the patient with emotional support and encouragement throughout the process; this person may be a spouse, sibling, adult child, parent, or close friend. Social support must also be demonstrated in the form of a stable home environment that entails a safe and permanent physical structure free of emotional and physical threats to the patient's well being. Thus, situations of active abuse must be resolved and the patient must be in a safe environment prior to consideration for surgery.

Motivation

Patient motivation is the rigor with which a patient approaches surgery. A highly motivated patient is generally thought to be a better candidate. However, motivation is perhaps the most subjective criterion that must be met prior to selecting a patient for weight-reduction surgery. Ray has correlated "intrinsic motivation" with improved postsurgical weight loss.[37] Although there are certain psychometric instruments with which to gauge personal motivation, none has been proven necessary or sufficient to ensure success after surgery. Thus, experienced surgeons and the team of professionals they partner with in the decision-making process must individually evaluate each patient's motivation. A patient who seems hesitant or uncertain about surgery, who approaches surgery with a lack of seriousness, or who seems pressured to undergo surgery by outside forces, such as family members or a physician, should not be selected. A patient who is concerned enough that his or her obesity is imminently disabling or life-threatening, who believes that at least some element of the obesity is out of personal control, and who fully appraises the risk and benefits of surgery generally has the will to undergo a weight reduction procedure and take control of the lifestyle changes surgery imposes. However, one should cautiously approach any prospective patient who seems overzealous in his or her enthusiasm for surgery and who mistakenly views surgery as a rapid cure for obesity rather than a tool with which to take control of weight loss.[38] Such a patient tends to expect too much from surgery and therefore exert too little effort postoperatively to comply with the behavioral requirement of surgery. Motivation is, of course, cultivated in an environment of strong social support and adequate cognitive functioning.

Socioeconomic Status

Recent demographic analyses of potential candidates for bariatric surgery have demonstrated that among the over 20 million in the U.S. population who are potential candidates for weight-reduction surgery, the patients with the highest BMIs are the patients with the fewest socioeconomic resources.[39] In our experience, these candidates are also potentially at higher risk because of inadequate access to treatment for obesity-related comorbidities and psychiatric conditions; poorer cognitive functioning due to lack of education and educational resources; and higher personal stressors due to lack of employment, to neighborhood violence, to disrupted home environments and to less overall social support. We believe, however, that candidates from all socioeconomic backgrounds should be considered for surgery. To the extent that it is possible in today's complex society, all patients should be offered referrals to physicians, services, and agencies that can assist them in optimizing their psychosocial resources, regardless of their socioeconomic status.

Special Case of Pregnancy

A specific issue relating to compliance pertains to prospective female patients of childbearing age. In the 2 years immediately following surgery, rapid weight loss and metabolic adjustments significantly increase the risk to such patients for developing acute metabolic disorders and the risk to the developing fetus for growth retardation or severe electrolyte abnormalities.[40-43] Thus, all female patients who can become pregnant must be counseled about this risk and strongly encouraged to maintain or initiate contraception after undergoing surgery. Patients should be reassured that long-term outcomes in women of childbearing age who undergo weight-reduction surgery show an increase in fertility and in pregnancies that have fewer complications (such as pregnancy-induced hypertension and gestational diabetes) than the pregnancies of morbidly obese patients.[44-47]

▶ NUTRITION ASSESSMENT

Nutrition assessment is the final critical factor in patient selection. Complying with postoperative nutrition requirements is crucial for successful outcomes. At our center, all prospective patients are evaluated by a dietitian experienced with eating disorders and specifically bariatric surgery patients. Diagnosis of the eating disorders discussed earlier often occurs during this nutrition-assessment process. Patients are evaluated in multiple areas, including diet attempts, general nutrition knowledge, understanding of the diet after surgery, food logs, support, and motivation.

All prospective patients are sent a preoperative information packet that contains the basic explanation of the nutrition requirements for surgery. Patients are required to keep a detailed dietary log for the 7 days preceding the initial clinic visit. The initial clinic visit involves a detailed 30-minute nutrition assessment during which the dietitian first looks at the number and types of previous diet attempts as well as the successes, if any, of those attempts and the associated duration of success (Table 12-2). Patients are tested on their general nutrition knowledge and on aspects of the diet after surgery that they can recall based on their reading of the information that was previously mailed to them. They are asked to list various foods that contain protein and foods that are high in sugar and carbohydrates. If patients are unable to answer appropriately, nutrition knowledge is rated as poor. Detailed food logs, appropriate support, and motivation for surgery are other items the dietitian may use to assess appropriateness for weight-reduction surgery. An ideal candidate for surgery would meet the following criteria: numerous

Table 12-2	PRIOR NONSURGICAL WEIGHT-LOSS ATTEMPTS
Commercial	Diet Workshop
	Weight Watchers
	Jenny Craig
	LA Weight Loss
Pharmacologic	Xenical
	Meridia
	Tenuate
	Fen-Phen
Clinically supervised	Medifast
	Optifast
	New Direction
Self-directed	Low-fat
	Low-calorie
	Low-carbohydrate
Self-help programs	Overeaters Anonymous
	TOPS
Fad diets	Atkins Diet
	The Zone
	Grapefruit diet
	Peanut butter diet

previous diet attempts, including structured weight-loss programs; good general knowledge of nutrition; well-researched and informed awareness of the diet after surgery; 7 days of detailed food logs that are free of the suggestion of a major eating disorder; a display of good motivation; and adequate support from family and friends.

▶ MULTIDISCIPLINARY TEAM APPROACH TO PATIENT SELECTION

The dynamics, biases, and effectiveness of teams working as a group to solve a difficult problem have been the subject of intense research in the medical and social sciences, particularly in cognitive psychology.[48,49] "In general, teams create a synergy toward coordinated problem-solving efforts in areas of specialized knowledge, provide a competitive advantage to their organization, provide flexibility and speed, and provide for an outcome that is greater that the sum of its individual members."[50] In the case of bariatric surgery, the problem to be solved is Who are the most appropriate candidates? The outcomes of these decisions are positively influenced by a cohesive team within which a more thorough and thoughtful evaluation is developed than could be reached by a single individual.[11] Assembling and maintaining an effective team to screen patients for their suitability for bariatric surgery is essential for several reasons: (1) there is uniformity in the approach to the disease; (2) the sincerity of the patients' commitment to bariatric surgery is continually scrutinized, clarified, and maintained by the consensus of the team; and (3) refinements in patient selection and treatment protocols are continually made based on collective experience and periodic reviews of outcomes.

The foundation of an effective team is a cohesive working group in which each team member shares responsibility for planning, hypothesizing, intellectual direction, team development, and patient satisfaction.[51-53] Each member plays a meaningful role and shares credit for good outcomes and blame for bad outcomes. An effective team works in an open discussion forum in which opinions can be shared freely in an environment of respect for both individual opinions and the group consensus derived from those individual opinions. Each member must share responsibility for identifying and pursuing his or her area of expertise and for contributing that expertise to the group within the context of the goals of the project which, in the case of bariatric surgery, is a satisfied patient with successful weight loss and overall improvement in health. The development of an effective bariatric team requires governance, equality, open discussion, and responsibility among a group of diverse professionals, including the surgeon or surgeons, dietitians, psychologists, psychiatrists, physical therapists, physician extenders, internists, consultants from specialty fields, social workers, and administrative staff.

At our institution, patients are first seen in a 1-hour group forum of 4 to 5 prospective patients in which the clerical administrator and the clinical nurse specialist answer patients' preexisting questions about weight-loss surgery and address general concerns regarding the evaluation process. During this session, clinic staff also acquire general demographic information from prospective patients. Patients then undergo a full history and medical examination by the surgeon. In this first session, the interaction of the patient with the surgeon, nurse specialist, and dedicated clerical administrator provides significant insight to all providers about the pertinent medical issues, the extent of obesity, the social and cognitive issues, and the level of social support. On a separate day, usually the following week, the patient returns for a full examination by the team psychologist and dietitian. Following the psychiatric and nutritional assessments, the entire bariatric team meets in a conference room to discuss the individual patients. The decision as to whether a patient is an appropriate candidate is made by committee, with each member having a significant influence on the group decision.

Our team has generated a Candidacy Scale based on the formal and informal medical, psychological, and dietary assessments (Table 12-3). Each patient's ranking on that scale is generated at the group meeting. The ranking ranges from 1 to 10. Patients scoring 10 are ideal candidates. Patients scoring between 7 and 9 are acceptable candidates who may need further assessment, for example, a cardiac clearance or letter from a provider that alcoholism has indeed been quiescent for longer than a year. In our practice patients scoring between 3 and 6 will be advised on outstanding issues, encouraged to resolve those issues, and offered follow-up for repeat evaluation every 3 months for up to 1 year. Patients with a score of 1 or 2 generally fall into the categories of absolute contraindications and will be told that they are not appropriate candidates for surgery.

▶ CONCLUSION

Bariatric procedures can be technically challenging to the surgeon, but the greatest challenge a bariatric surgeon faces is selecting appropriate candidates. In this chapter, we have

Table 12-3	CANDIDACY SCALE
Medical issues	0: Absolute contraindication 1: Relative contraindications but judged acceptable 2: No medical contraindications
Psychopathology	0: Active psychiatric condition in need of treatment 1: Psychiatric condition well controlled 2: No psychiatric contraindications
Motivation	0: Poorly motivated 1: Highly motivated
Social functioning (coping skills, social skills)	0: Low functioning, high stress 1: High functioning (in cases of low cognitive ability, support person as proxy to enable social functioning)
Appraisal and cognition	0: Inadequate appraisal of surgery and its implications 1: Adequate appraisal of surgery and its implications (in cases of low cognitive ability, support person as proxy to enable appraisal)
Social support	0: Lacks adequate social support 1: Has strong support network (friends, family, etc.) and safe environment
Nutrition	0: Poor nutrition knowledge and understanding of postoperative dietary requirements 1: Good nutrition knowledge or adequate understanding of postoperative dietary requirements 2: Good nutrition knowledge and adequate understanding of postoperative dietary requirements

described the major criteria that we believe should be considered in evaluating prospective patients. These criteria are best understood and applied by a multidisciplinary team. A well-rounded and comprehensive approach to patient selection should enable the practitioner to select the patients who are most likely to reap the many physiologic, psychosocial, and quality-of-life benefits possible through safe and effective weight-reduction procedures.

▶ REFERENCES

1. Buchwald H; Overview of bariatric surgery. J Am Coll Surg 2002;194:367-375.
2. Buchwald H: A bariatric surgery algorithm. Obes Surg 2002;12:733-746.
3. Patterson EJ, Urbach DR, Swanstrom LL: A comparison of diet and exercise therapy versus laparoscopic Roux-en-Y gastric bypass surgery for morbid obesity: a decision analysis model. J Am Coll Surg 2003;196:379-384.
4. Agren G, Narbro K, Jonsson E, et al: Cost of in-patient care over 7 years among surgically and conventionally treated obese patients. Obes Res 2002;10:1276-1283.
5. Hauri P, Horber FF, Sendi P: Is bariatric surgery worth its costs? Obes Surg 1999;9:480-483.
6. Colditz GA: Economic costs of obesity. Am J Clin Nutr 1992;55:503S-507S.
7. Kortt MA, Langley PC, Cox ER: A review of cost-of-illness studies on obesity. Clin Ther1998;20:772-779.
8. Seidell JC: Societal and personal costs of obesity. Exp Clin Endocrinol Diabetes 1998;106:7-9.
9. Martin LF, Tan TL, Horn JR, et al: Comparison of the costs associated with medical and surgical treatment of obesity. Surgery 1995;118:599-606.
10. Wolf AM, Colditz GA: Social and economic effects of body weight in the United States. Am J Clin Nutr 1996;63:466S-469S.
11. Wolf AM, Colditz GA: The cost of obesity: the US perspective. Pharmacoeconomics 1994;5:34-37.
12. Gawande A: The man who couldn't stop eating. The New Yorker. July 19, 2001;66-73.
13. Allison DB, Fontaine KR, Manson JE, et al: Annual deaths attributable to obesity in the United States. JAMA 1999;282:1530-1538.
14. Herrara MF, Lozano-Salazar RR, Gonzalez-Barranco J, et al: Diseases and problems secondary to massive obesity. Eur J Gastroenterol Hepatol 1999;11:63-67.
15. Kral JG: Morbidity of severe obesity. Surg Clin North Am 2001;81:1039-1061.
16. Sullivan MB, Sullivan LG, Kral JG: Quality of life assessment in obesity: physical, psychological, and social function. Gastroenterol Clin North Am 1987;16:433-442.
17. Fontaine KR, Redden DT, Wang C, et al: Years of life lost due to obesity. JAMA 2003;289:187-193 (see comment).
18. Kral JG: Selection of patients for anti-obesity surgery. Int J Obes Relat Metab Disord 2001;21:S107-S112.
19. Fisher BL, Schauer P: Medical and surgical options in the treatment of severe obesity. Am J Surg 2002;184:9S-16S.
20. Sjostrom L: Surgical intervention as a strategy for treatment of obesity. Endocrine 2000;13:213-230.
21. National Institutes of Health: Gastrointestinal surgery for severe obesity, Consensus Development Conference statement. Am J Clin Nutr 1992;55:615S-619S.
22. National Institutes of Health: Clinical Guidelines on the Identification, Evaluation, and Treatment of Overweight and Obesity in Adults: The Evidence Report. Obes Res 1998;6(suppl 2):51S-209S.
23. Buchwald H: Consensus Conference Panel, Bariatric surgery for morbid obesity: health implications for patients, health professionals, and third-party payers. J Am Coll Surg 2005;200:593-604.
24. Cowan GS Jr, Hiler ML, Buffington C: Criteria for selection of patients for bariatric surgery. Eur J Gastroenterol Hepatol 1999;11:69-75.
25. Elia M: Obesity in the elderly: Obes Res 2001;9:244S-248S.
26. Kotz CM, Billington CJ, Levine AS: Obesity and aging. Clin Geriatr Med 1999;15:391-412.
27. Murr MM, Siadati MR, Sarr MG: Results of bariatric surgery for morbid obesity in patients older than 50 years. Obes Surg 1995;5:399-402.
28. Abu-Abeid S, Gavert N, Klausner JM, et al: Bariatric surgery in adolescence. J Pediatr Surg 2003;38:1379-1382.
29. Capella JF, Capella RF: Bariatric surgery in adolescence: is this the best age to operate? Obes Surg 2003;13:826-832.
30. Garcia VF, Langford L, Inge TH: Application of laparoscopy for bariatric surgery in adolescents. Curr Opin Pediatr 2003;15:248-255.
31. Inge TH, Garcia V, Daniels S, et al: A multidisciplinary approach to the adolescent bariatric surgical patient. J Pediatr Surg 2004;39:442-447.
32. Strauss RS, Bradley LJ, Brolin RE: Gastric bypass surgery in adolescents with morbid obesity. J Pediatr 2001;138:499-504.
33. Sugerman HJ, Sugerman EL, DeMaria EJ, et al: Bariatric surgery for severely obese adolescents. J Gastrointest Surg 2003;7:102-107.
34. Clark MM, Balsiger BM, Sletten CD, et al: Psychosocial factors and 2-year outcome following bariatric surgery for weight loss. Obes Surg 2003;13:739-745.
35. Brolin RE: Gastric bypass. Surg Clin North Am 2001;81:1077-1095.
36. Brolin RE: Bariatric surgery and long-term control of morbid obesity. JAMA 2002;288:2793-2796.
37. Ray EC, Nickels MW, Sayeed S, et al: Predicting success after gastric bypass: the role of psychosocial and behavioral factors. Surgery 2003;134:555-563.
38. Cowan GS Jr: What do patients, families and society expect from the bariatric surgeon? Obes Surg 1998;8:77-85.
39. Livingston EH, Ko CY: Socioeconomic characteristics of the population eligible for obesity surgery. Surgery 2004;135:288-296.
40. Weissman A, Hagay Z, Schachter M, et al: Severe maternal and fetal electrolyte imbalance in pregnancy after gastric surgery for morbid obesity: a case report. J Reprod Med 1995;40:813-816.

41. Granstrom L, Backman L: Fetal growth retardation after gastric banding. Acta Obstet Gynecol Scand 1990;69:533-536.

42. Gurewitsch ED, Smith-Levitin M, Mack J: Pregnancy following gastric bypass surgery for morbid obesity. Obstet Gynecol 1996; 88:658-661.

43. Printen KJ, Scott D: Pregnancy following gastric bypass for the treatment of morbid obesity. Am Surg 1982;48:363-365.

44. Brolin RE: Update: NIH consensus conference: gastrointestinal surgery for severe obesity. Nutrition 1996;12:403-404.

45. Friedman D, Cuneo S, Valenzano M, et al: Pregnancies in an 18-year follow-up after biliopancreatic diversion. Obes Surg 1995;5:308-313.

46. Richards DS, Miller DK, Goodman GN: Pregnancy after gastric bypass for morbid obesity. J Reprod Med 1987;32:172-176.

47. Wittgrove AC, Jester L, Wittgrove P, et al: Pregnancy following gastric bypass for morbid obesity. Obes Surg 1998;8:461-464.

48. Purtilo RB: Interdisciplinary health care teams and health care reform. J Law Med Ethics 1994;22:121-126.

49. Molyneux J: Interprofessional teamworking: what makes teams work well? J Interprofess Care 2001;15:29-35.

50. Feifer C, Nocella K, DeArtola I, et al: Self-managing teams: a strategy for quality improvement. Top Health Inform Man 2003; 24:21-28.

51. Donaldson MS, Mohr JJ: Improvement and Innovation in Health Care Microsystems: a technical report for the Institute of Medicine Committee on the Quality of Health Care in America. Princeton, NJ, Robert Wood Johnson Foundation, 2000.

52. Nelson E, Batalden P, Huber T, et al: Microsystems in health care, part 1: learning from high-performing front-line clinical units. Joint Commiss J Qual Safety 2002;28:472–493.

53. Mohr J, Batalden P: Improving safety at the front lines: the role of clinical microsystems. Qual Safety Health Care 2002;11:45-50.

13

Preoperative Preparation of the Bariatric Surgery Patient

Peter N. Benotti, M.D., F.A.C.S. and Hector Rodriguez, M.D.

Surgery for severe obesity is currently one of the most rapidly growing subspecialties in the field of surgery. Obesity has emerged as a major health problem in the United States, with the prevalence of obesity in the population rising from 15% in 1980 to 30% in 1990.[1] More than 5 million Americans are morbidly obese. During a 3-year period, 1999 to 2001, in Pennsylvania, gastric bypass surgical volume increased by 100% each year.[2] It was estimated that in 2002, 55,000 obesity operations were performed in the United States and that this figure rose to 140,000 in 2005. The recognition of the vital role of surgical treatment in the multidisciplinary management of severe obesity has been accelerated by several developments:

1. The acceptance of obesity as a chronic disease and not merely a social problem
2. The public awareness of the major health risks and impaired quality of life that accompany severe obesity
3. The documented improvement in health and quality of life that accompany surgical weight loss
4. The favorable reports in the lay press and the well-publicized life changes of several high-profile celebrities after bariatric surgery
5. The introduction of minimally invasive surgical options.

As a result of these developments, bariatric surgery has rapidly emerged as the treatment of choice for morbidly obese patients. Bariatric surgery is unique among gastrointestinal surgical procedures because it serves as a behavior-modification tool that, if used correctly, can be the catalyst for a complete life change for the patient. A prerequisite for the long-term success of surgical obesity treatment is full patient participation in the life-change process. The necessity of complete patient understanding and total participation in the postoperative weight-loss and weight-maintenance process requires a prolonged and labor-intense preoperative evaluation and preparation. The goals during the preoperative period involve patient education, informed consent, medical-risk assessment, and strategies for risk reduction.

▶ PATIENT EDUCATION AND INFORMED CONSENT

Surgical treatment for severe obesity is indicated in individuals who weigh 100 lb over or twice their desirable body weight, which corresponds to a body mass index (BMI) of 40 kg per m² or more.[3] Patients eligible for surgical treatment are those with BMIs between 35 and 40 kg per m² who have high-risk health problems like sleep apnea or diabetes and those who have physical disabilities affecting lifestyle (employment, mobility, or family function).[4] Contraindications to surgical obesity treatment include severe mental illness resulting in psychosis; substance abuse; and major organ failure refractory to treatment. Age is not a contraindication to bariatric surgery; there are many clinical reports of satisfactory surgical outcomes in both adolescents and patients 55 years and older.[5,6]

Patient education is an important aspect of the preoperative screening and evaluation process. The requirements of active lifestyle change and alteration in eating behavior imposed by bariatric surgery make it essential that candidates have a thorough understanding of all aspects of their surgery and the mechanisms of weight loss in order to avoid serious harm. During the past 5 years, there has been a marked increase in the availability of information for morbidly obese patients. Several celebrities and several bariatric surgeons have written books, and the television media provide educational programming on bariatric surgery on a regular basis. The Internet is a major resource for individuals seeking information about surgical treatment for morbid obesity.[7] The American Society for Bariatric Surgery has patient information booklets available and a very informative website (www.ASBS.org). Many established bariatric surgery programs conduct regular seminars and support groups for new-patient education and interaction with postoperative patients. Individuals who have changed their lives as a result of surgery for severe obesity are usually so grateful that they are more than willing to assist with the patient-education process.

Patients must be fully informed about the rationale for surgical treatment of severe obesity. The information should include an understanding of the significant health risks and poor quality of life associated with morbid obesity.[8,9] The low probability of long-term weight control using conventional weight-reduction treatments should be emphasized. The anticipated weight loss resulting from surgery, including failure rates, should be discussed in the context of the curative role of surgery in obesity treatment. The expanding body of evidence documenting the improved health risk and quality of life after surgical weight loss should also be emphasized.

Prospective candidates must understand the concepts of energy balance in the pathogenesis of obesity through discussions involving calories consumed as food versus calories utilized to support life and activity, as well as emphasis on the role of exercise in the control of energy expenditure and weight maintenance. The roles of energy intake and energy expenditure in weight gain and weight loss must be explained so that patients realize that there are no shortcuts to weight-loss success.

Surgical candidates need to understand the concepts of gastric restriction and malabsorption as they relate to weight loss. The accepted operations for obesity control should be reviewed, as should the risks and outcomes of laparoscopic and open procedures. The advantages and disadvantages of the various surgical procedures and the surgical risks of each procedure should be discussed. Late complications of surgical procedures must be explained and nutritional issues reviewed, with emphasis on the necessity of regular nutritional follow-up.[10,11]

The vital importance of multidisciplinary input in obesity management has been stressed for many years. Bariatric surgery programs should provide similar multidisciplinary capabilities to prepare patients for safe surgery, to care for them after surgery, and to ensure nutritional safety during[12] and after weight loss through surgery.[13]

▶ PREOPERATIVE RISK ASSESSMENT

The critical importance of a complete medical history and physical examination by the bariatric surgical team cannot be overemphasized. Many morbidly obese patients have had suboptimal health care for a variety of reasons, ranging from patient denial to lack of physician concern. Obesity was considered a social problem until 1985 when it was recognized as a chronic disease.[14] As a result, many health care professionals do not have an appreciation for all the major obesity-related health risks. The large number of comorbid medical conditions and the increased surgical risk associated with morbid obesity require that all significant medical conditions be carefully documented and fully treated in the preoperative phase. Bariatric surgeons are often the first to discover significant comorbid medical problems at the time of surgical consultation. The essential co-workers for multidisciplinary obesity care are medical specialists in pulmonary medicine, cardiology, gastroenterology, endocrinology, and anesthesiology, and they must be available for preoperative consultation for the evaluation and control of comorbid medical problems in order to optimize the condition of the patient.

Asymptomatic patients who remain active and productive with no impairment in physical performance despite their severe obesity are usually reasonable operative risks and will need limited study in preparation for surgery. At the other extreme, there are patients who cannot perform even four metabolic equivalents of work (i.e., climb one flight of stairs) without severe dyspnea. These patients will be at much greater risk and will need a more extensive preoperative workup.

Pulmonary

Changes in pulmonary function associated with obesity include reduction in lung and chest-wall compliance, increase in respiratory-system resistance, reduced lung volumes, and increased effort required in the work of breathing.[15] Reduction in lung volume is the physiologic parameter that has the greatest clinical significance because of its association with atelectasis, airway closure, and hypoxia. In addition, the magnitude of reduction in functional residual capacity is directly related to the rapidity of desaturation during apnea at anesthesia induction.

Preoperative pulmonary function studies should be obtained in severely obese patients with documented respiratory illness (asthma or sleep apnea) and in those whose performance status is limited by significant dyspnea with exertion. The preoperative pulmonary-function test results for 199 consecutive morbidly obese surgical patients are summarized in Table 13-1.[16] The most significant finding is a mean 30% reduction in functional residual capacity and a mean 63% reduction in expiratory reserve volume. Pulmonary function tests identify patients with major reductions in lung volumes or airflow rates as well as those who will improve with topical bronchodilators. Those patients with major abnormalities in pulmonary function may benefit from referral for instruction in the use of continuous positive airway pressure (CPAP) by nasal mask for administration of aerosolized inhalants to maximize bronchodilatation and for inspiratory muscle training to decrease the risks for pulmonary complications.

Table 13-1	MORBID OBESITY AND PULMONARY FUNCTION		
PARAMETER	MEAN ± SD	MINIMUM	MAXIMUM
Forced vital capacity (% predicted)	88.5 ± 19	40	204
Forced expiratory volume 1 sec (% predicted)	88.3 ± 27	28	384
Total lung capacity (% predicted)	89.6 ± 15	40	204
Functional residual capacity (% predicted)	70.1 ± 33	20	391
Residual volume (% predicted)	88.6 ± 36	5	269
Expiratory reserve volume (% predicted)	37.3 ± 22	4	137
PaO_2	85.5 ± 11	61	126

Preoperative pulmonary function studies were obtained for 199 consecutive patients undergoing surgical treatment for morbid obesity. The female to male ratio was 81.4% to 18.6%. The body mass index was 50.3 ± 9 kg/m². The results show consistent reductions in functional residual capacity, with a statistically significant ($P<0.05$) reduction in expiratory reserve volume. From Pereira B: Unpublished data.

Like all upper abdominal operations, surgery for morbid obesity is always associated with a major temporary reduction in pulmonary function.[17,18] In morbid obesity, the magnitude of this reduction in lung volumes, flow rates, and gas exchange approximates 50% to 60%.[19-21] This postoperative reduction is maximal for 48 to 72 hours after surgery and occurs with both open and laparoscopic bariatric surgery.[19] As a result of this postoperative reduction in lung function, patients with severely impaired lung function may be at risk for respiratory failure in the early postoperative period. Identification of these patients will dictate postoperative respiratory care and resource use. Preoperative arterial blood gas analysis is beneficial in patients whose performance status is impaired because of exertional dyspnea. A subset of these patients will be found to have previously undiagnosed hypercarbia, which is another risk factor for postoperative pulmonary complications.[17] Several recent clinical studies have confirmed the safety and beneficial results of CPAP after extubation in high-risk obesity surgery patients.[20-22] In two clinical trials, the use of CPAP by nasal mask during the first 24 hours after extubation resulted in improved oxygenation and pulmonary function in patients after bariatric surgery.[20,21] Instruction in the use of bilevel positive airway pressure by nasal mask begins in the preoperative period so as to optimize the postoperative use of this important resource.

Smoking is a proven risk factor for postoperative pulmonary complications. This risk declines with cessation of smoking for 8 weeks before surgery.[17,23] This has not been critically evaluated in bariatric surgery. However, because of past experience with the necessity for more prolonged postoperative mechanical ventilation in obese heavy smokers, the authors insist on this practice of smoking cessation. It is made clear to patients and families that this requirement will reduce the risk of severe respiratory complications and that failure to comply will result in unnecessary serious risks. Many patients who stop smoking in preparation for bariatric surgery do not return to smoking after surgery.

SLEEP APNEA

A detailed sleep history that searches for symptoms of obstructive sleep apnea (OSA) is an important aspect of the preoperative evaluation. Symptoms of OSA include heavy snoring, witnessed apnea by bed partner, excessive daytime somnolence, and lack of restful sleep. The incidence of moderate and severe OSA in morbidly obese patients is surprisingly high. Greene and colleagues studied 300 consecutive patients being prepared for obesity surgery and found a statistically significant direct relationship between the apnea and hypopnea index and BMI, especially in males. He found that all of his patients with BMIs above 55 kg per m^2 and 93% of his patients with BMIs of 50 to 55 kg per m^2 had moderate or severe OSA.[24] Central obesity, particularly when it involves the neck, carries the greatest risk of OSA.[25] Obesity is believed to influence the airway size by deposition of fat in the neck or by external compression.[26] Clinical consequences of OSA include hypoxemia, hypercapnia, pulmonary and systemic vasoconstriction, secondary polycythemia, and arrhythmia. Hypoxic pulmonary vasoconstriction can lead to right-heart failure.

The presence of sleep apnea results in additional risks of hypoxemia and mandates special attention to perioperative narcotic and airway management by the anesthesiologist and surgeon.[27] Untreated or inadequately treated OSA is associated with a higher incidence of perioperative complications. Patients suspected of having sleep apnea should be referred for preoperative sleep study and titration of CPAP. The preoperative use of CPAP will reduce severe hypoxemia and associated pulmonary vasoconstriction, resulting in improved right ventricular function. Patients with OSA are instructed to bring their CPAP machines to the hospital for use in the postoperative period. CPAP with supplemental oxygen is started immediately after extubation and is used continuously, with brief rest periods, until the first postoperative morning. It is subsequently used only during sleep until discharge.

AIRWAY

A careful and thorough assessment of a patient's airway is essential. Difficulty in securing the airway is the leading cause of anesthesia-related morbidity.[28] Severe obesity is not by itself a predictor of a difficult airway. The amount of body fat is much less important than the distribution of fat.[29] Morbidly obese patients can present significant challenges for mask ventilation, tracheal intubation and, in case of failed intubation, difficult cricothyroidotomy. Factors that contribute to airway problems in this population include a fat face and cheeks, large breasts, a short neck, a large tongue, redundant palatal and pharyngeal soft tissue, anterior larynx, restricted mouth opening, and limitation of cervical spine motion.[30]

The possibility of an awake look at the airway or awake intubation must be discussed with the patient and appropriate preparations made. Because obesity is a risk factor for aspiration of gastric contents, patients may benefit from aspiration prophylaxis.

Heart

Cardiac dysfunction of varying degrees is not uncommon in morbid obesity. Cardiovascular abnormalities associated with morbid obesity include cardiac hypertrophy, increased preload, diastolic dysfunction and, rarely, frank systolic dysfunction in association with cardiomyopathy.[31,32] Patients with super morbid obesity (BMI>50 kg/m^2) complicated by hypertension, those with sleep apnea in association with hypertension, and those with fluid retention complicating severe obesity should have detailed cardiac evaluations. The evaluation will allow for optimum control of systemic hypertension and for investigation of possible pulmonary hypertension, congestive heart failure, and ischemic heart disease. Cardiac work in severe obesity is increased because of the increase in total body oxygen consumption related to the large body mass. The increased incidence of sudden and unexplained death in morbid obesity may be a manifestation of occult cardiovascular disease in this population.[33]

Thromboembolism

Obesity is a well-known risk factor for postoperative thromboembolism.[34,35] The incidence of postoperative thromboembolic complications following surgery for severe obesity is 0.4% for lone deep venous thrombosis and 0.8% for pulmonary embolism. For experienced surgical teams that are able to minimize the risk of technical complications, thromboembolism is the leading cause of postoperative mortality. Additional risk factors for postoperative thromboembolism include a BMI of 60 kg per m² and chronic venous insufficiency.[36] High-risk patients and preoperative patients with previous histories or family histories of thromboembolism should be evaluated for hypercoagulable states.[37,38]

The optimal perioperative prophylactic regimen to prevent thromboembolism in obesity surgery has not been definitively established, but most experienced bariatric surgeons favor a combination of aggressive dosing of low-molecular-weight heparin and sequential leg-compression devices. Our experience with various prophylactic regimens over the past 10 years is summarized in Table 13-2. It is important to recognize that the dosing of heparin for thromboembolism treatment is weight-related, and that fixed dosing for prophylaxis can potentially result in underdosing.[39] This is particularly important in super morbid obesity (BMI>50 kg/m²), where higher doses of low-molecular-weight heparin are recommended. The optimal prophylaxis for patients with BMIs over 60 kg per m² and with prior histories of deep vein thrombosis and venous stasis disease remains controversial, with many holding the opinion that these patients are best served by preoperative placement of an inferior vena cava filter.

Endocrine

Approximately 15% to 25% of morbidly obese patients have type 2 diabetes. Glucose control in these patients is an important area of preoperative attention. The association between diabetes and surgical site infections is well known.[40] Hyperglycemia (>220 mg%) inhibits many important functions of polymorphonuclear leukocytes.[41] Recent evidence indicates that aggressive control of hyperglycemia during the perioperative period reduces this risk

for infection.[42] Bariatric surgery candidates and their families should be made aware of the importance of proper glucose control as a preoperative requirement. When glucose control is poorly responsive to adjustments in medication, a preoperative reduction in carbohydrate intake will be necessary to keep blood sugars under 200 to 220 mg%.

Postoperative hyperglycemia during the first 72 hours after surgery is common in morbidly obese patients. The authors have had excellent success by combining glucose-free intravenous fluid replacement with a sliding scale for intravenous insulin coverage (Table 13-3). Sliding-scale insulin coverage with subcutaneous insulin administration provides suboptimal glucose control.[43]

Rare endocrine causes of obesity include hypothyroidism and Cushing disease. Preoperative patients who have not had recent thyroid function evaluation should be tested. Adrenal function should be investigated if the patient demonstrates symptoms or signs of Cushing syndrome, which include hypertension, diabetes, central obesity, weakness, muscle atrophy, hirsutism, striae, osteoporosis, and acne.

Gastrointestinal

Gastroesophageal reflux symptoms occur in 20% of morbidly obese patients. Preoperative patients who complain of significant reflux symptoms should be referred for endoscopic foregut evaluation if this has not been done previously. Occasional cases of Barrett esophagus will be discovered, and *Helicobacter pylori* infestation should be treated if found. Documentation of a significant hiatal hernia is helpful in surgical planning. Obesity and weight cycling are risk factors for the development of cholelithiasis. Cholelithiasis is found in 15% to 20% of morbidly obese patients who are being prepared for obesity surgery. When cholelithiasis is documented preoperatively, cholecystectomy should be considered at the time of bariatric surgery because of the likelihood that biliary symptoms will develop during the postoperative period of weight loss. For patients without gallstones, the use of agents to increase cholesterol solubility in bile has been shown to reduce the incidence of gallstone formation during the postoperative period of rapid weight loss.[44,45] Mild abnormalities of liver function are common in morbid obesity. Elevation of alanine aminotransferase is

Table 13-2	**PROPHYLACTIC REGIMENS**				
YEAR	PROPHYLAXIS	N	DVT	PE	DEATH
1991-1995	Sequential leg compression and subcutaneous heparin	205	1(late)	1(late)	0
1995-1998	Calf compression and subcutaneous heparin	82	1	2	2
1998-2003	Sequential leg compression and low-molecular-weight heparin injection	626	2(late)**	1(late)**	0**

DVT, deep vein thrombosis; N, number of patients; PE, pulmonary embolism.
**P = 0.02 vs. calf compression and subcutaneous heparin injection.
Our experience with thromboembolism prophylaxis in 913 consecutive bariatric surgery patients treated between 1991 and 2003; the best prophylaxis was achieved with sequential leg compression and twice-daily low-molecular-weight heparin injections.

Table 13-3	**INSULIN AND FLUID REPLACEMENT**		
SCALE			
Glucose >250	Call MD		
Glucose 225-249	12 U IV regular bolus	+	5 U/hr infusion*
Glucose 200-224	7 U IV regular bolus	+	5 U /hr infusion*
Glucose 175-199	None	+	5 U/hr infusion*
Glucose 150-174	None	+	4 U/hr infusion*
Glucose 125-149	None	+	2 U/hr infusion*
Glucose <125	None		None

*Regular insulin infusion: 1U/ml
Protocol for intravenous insulin coverage begins in the recovery room. Glucose is measured hourly initially, and intravenous insulin is administered according to a sliding scale. When glucose levels stabilize at levels below 160 mg%, levels are measured every 4 hr, and treatment follows the sliding scale.

the most common finding. The major cause for this is varying degrees of hepatic steatosis and steatohepatitis.

Psychiatric

Preoperative psychiatric consultation and psychological testing should be utilized when indicated as part of the preoperative evaluation process. Consultation should be obtained for all patients receiving intensive psychiatric treatment in order to be certain that the changes in eating behavior necessitated by surgery are in the overall best interest of the patient's mental health. In addition, patients on high doses of major tranquilizers and those taking multiple mood-influencing medications should have preoperative consultation so as to provide optimum dosing and replacement of oral medications during the postoperative period when patients receive only parenteral medications.

Although preoperative psychiatric consultation has not been conclusively shown to have any definite outcome benefit, many have found it to be an important factor in assessing the appropriateness of surgical therapy for a given morbidly obese patient. Psychological screening is now required as necessary information by several insurance companies for insurance coverage of surgery. Recent evidence indicates that certain behavioral and psychosocial factors may be predictive of success after gastric bypass.[46] Additional related data must be obtained and analyzed by behavioral analysts familiar with outcomes after bariatric surgery to further improve the patient selection process.

ANESTHESIA

Preoperative consultation with the anesthesiologist is important for patients because morbid obesity is associated with significant anesthesia risks and challenges. Reduction in lung volume, sleep apnea, and difficulty in securing the airway increase the risk for hypoxia. At the time of induction of anesthesia, these patients will demonstrate accelerated desaturation, which mandates rapid control of the airway. The risk for hypoxia during the perioperative period is significant for these patients, especially for the super obese, those with major reductions in lung volumes, and those with severe OSA. The clinical significance of hypoxia as a potential risk factor in surgical wound healing and resistance to infection underscores the importance of respiratory management in the perioperative period.[47] In obese patients, intravenous access and the placement of intravascular monitoring devices may be difficult. Use of bedside ultrasound to determine vascular access is extremely helpful.

▶ SPECIAL MANAGEMENT OF HIGH-RISK PATIENTS

In a small subset of preoperative patients, the preoperative workup identifies major risk factors that, if not addressed, are associated with unacceptable risks for mortality and major complications. As an example, a 58-year-old man with a BMI of 60 kg per m^2, chronic venous insufficiency, fluid retention, hypoxemia, and obesity hypoventilation may be facing a significant surgical morbidity and mortality risk. The original indications for surgery established by the National Institutes of Health in 1991 require that the benefits of surgical weight loss outweigh the risks of surgical treatment. This risk-benefit analysis must be carefully evaluated in such high risk patients.

The mandate for preoperative weight reduction as a "bridge to safe surgery" is a viable treatment option for high-risk patients. Strategies to reduce caloric intake in these patients result in prompt lowering of blood pressure, spontaneous diuresis, improvement in glucose tolerance, improvement in hypercarbia, and reduction in thrombosis risk. These physiologic improvements can occur with as few as 20 lbs of weight loss. All of these changes contribute to reduced perioperative risks. Preoperative caloric restriction can be accomplished in these patients and does not adversely affect wound healing.[48] Although prospective trials supporting preoperative caloric restriction are lacking, the authors have found this to be valuable and worth the effort for many patients. Most patients are willing to cooperate with a preoperative weight-reduction plan if it will improve their chances for good surgical outcomes. A nutritionist, as part of the multidisciplinary bariatric team, can oversee this process.

▶ SUMMARY

The success of any bariatric surgery is measured by the results. Surgical outcomes are traditionally equated with 30-day mortality and morbidity data. In bariatric surgery, a good result includes an operation performed with a mortality of less than 1% and a life-threatening complication rate of less than 3%. A good surgical outcome also includes the appropriate nutrition counseling and surveillance to ensure nutritional safety and correct food choices during the weight loss. Finally, a good surgical outcome also requires prompt recognition and treatment of late surgical and nutritional complications. The preoperative evaluation process is a critical part of the foundation of a good surgical result. During this period, patients develop confidence in their providers as they meet the many professionals who are committed to assisting in this life change. The labor intensity that patients perceive during the busy preoperative preparation period establishes a trust that favorably affects patient understanding, satisfaction, learning, and participation in follow-up.

▶ REFERENCES

1. Kuczmarski R, Flegal K, Campbell S, et al: Increasing prevalence of overweight among adults: the National Health and Nutrition Examination Surveys, 1960 to 1991. JAMA1994;272:205-211.
2. Courcoulas A, Schuchert M, Gatti G: The relationship of surgeon and hospital volume to outcome after gastric bypass surgery in Pennsylvania: a 3-year summary. Surgery 2003;134:613-623.
3. Billewicz W, Kemsley W, Thomson A: Indices of obesity. Br J Prev Soc Med 1962;16:183-188.
4. Gastrointestinal Surgery for Severe Obesity Consensus Development Conference Panel: Ann Int Med 1991;115:956-960.

5. MacGregor A, Rand C: Gastric surgery in morbid obesity: outcome in patients aged 55 years and older. Arch Surg 1993;128:1153-1157.

6. Capella J, Capella R: Bariatric surgery in adolescence: is this the age to operate? Obes Surg 2003;13:826-832.

7. Allen J: Surgical Internet at a glance: bariatric surgery. Am J Surg 2000;179:33.

8. Pi-Sunyer FX: Medical hazards of obesity. Ann Int Med 1993;119:655-660.

9. Deitel M, Camillieri A: Overlooked problems in morbidly obese patients. Obes Surg 2000;10:125 (abstract 4).

10. Standards Committee, American Society of Bariatric Surgery: Surgery for severe obesity: information for patients. Obes Surg 1994;4: 66-72.

11. Mason E, Hesson W: Informed consent for obesity surgery. Obes Surg 1998;8:419-428.

12. Moize V, Geliebter A, Gluck M, et al: Obese patients have inadequate protein intake related to protein intolerance up to 1 year following Roux-en-Y gastric bypass. Obes Surg 2003;13:23-28.

13. Kushner R: Managing the obese patient after bariatric surgery: a case report and review of the literature. J Parent Ent Nutr 2000;24:126-132.

14. National Institutes of Health: Annual health implications of obesity. NIH Consensus Statement 1985;103:1073-1077.

15. Koenig S: Pulmonary complications of obesity. Am J Med Sci 2001;321:249-279.

16. Pereira B, unpublished data.

17. Smetana G: Preoperative pulmonary evaluation. N Engl J Med 1999;340: 937-944.

18. Meyers J, Lembeck L, O'Kane H, et al: Changes in functional residual capacity of the lung after operation. Arch Surg 1975;110:576-582.

19. Nguyen N, Lee S, Goldman C, et al: Comparison of pulmonary function and postoperative pain after laparoscopic versus open gastric bypass: a randomized trial. Am J Surg 2001;192:469-477.

20. Ebeo C, Benotti P, Elmagrhaby Z, et al: The effect of bi-level positive airway pressure (BIPAP) on postoperative pulmonary function after gastric surgery for severe obesity. Resp Med 2002; 96: 672-676.

21. Loris J, Sottiaux T, Chiche J, et al: Effect of bi-level positive airway pressure (BIPAP) nasal ventilation on the postoperative pulmonary restriction syndrome in obese patients undergoing gastroplasty. Chest 1997;111:665-670.

22. Huerta S, DeShields S, Shpiner R, et al: Safety and efficacy of postoperative continuous positive airway pressure to prevent pulmonary complications after Roux-en-Y gastric bypass. J Gastrointest Surg 2002;6:354-358.

23. Bluman L, Mosca L, Newman N, et al: Preoperative smoking habits and postoperative pulmonary complications. Chest 1998;113:883-889.

24. Greene B, Katebi P, Marcus W: Prevalence of occult sleep apnea in patients preparing to undergo morbid obesity surgery. Obes Surg 2003;13:203.

25. Dealberto M, Ferber C, Garma L, et al: Factors related to sleep apnea in sleep clinic patients. Chest 1994;105:1753-1758.

26. Mortimore I, Marshall I, Wraith P, et al: Neck and total body fat deposition in obese and non-obese patients with sleep apnea compared with that in control subjects. Am J Respir Crit Care Med 1998;157:280-283.

27. Benumof J: Obstructive sleep apnea in the adult obese patient: implications for airway management. J Clin Anesth 2001;13:144-156.

28. Caplan R, Posner K, Ward R, et al: Adverse respiratory events in anesthesia: a closed claims analysis. Anesthesiology 1990; 71: 828-833.

29. Brodsky J: Anesthetic management of the morbidly obese patient. Int Anesthesiol Clin 1986; 24:93-103.

30. Safar P, Escarraga L, Chang F, et al: Upper airway obstruction in the unconscious patient. J Appl Physiol 1959;14:760-764.

31. Thakur V, Richards R, Reisin E, et al: Obesity, hypertension and the heart. Am J Med Sci 2001;321:242-248.

32. Alpert M: Management of obese cardiomyopathy. Am J Med Sci 2001;321:237-241.

33. Drenick E, Fisler J: Sudden cardiac arrest in morbidly obese surgical patients unexplained after autopsy. Am J Surg 1988; 155:720-726.

34. Vague P, Juhan-Vague I, Aillaud M, et al: Correlation between blood fibrinolytic activity, plasminogen activator inhibitor level, plasma insulin level and relative body weight in normal and obese subjects. Metabolism 1986;35:250-253.

35. Batiste G, Bothe A, Bern M, et al: Low antithrombin III in morbid obesity: return to normal with weight reduction. J Parent Ent Nut 1983;7:447-449.

36. Sugerman H, Sugerman E, Wolfe L, et al: Risks and benefits of gastric bypass in morbidly obese patients with severe venous stasis disease. Ann Surg 2001;234:41-46.

37. Simoni P, Prandoni P, Lensing A, et al: The risk of recurrent venous thromboembolism in patients with an Arg[506] Gln mutation in the gene for factor V (factor V Leiden). New Eng J Med 1997; 336: 300-403.

38. Zoller B, Dahlback B: Linkage between inherited resistance to activated protein C and factor V gene mutation in venous thrombosis. Lancet 1994;343:1536-1538.

39. Scholten D, Hoedema R, Scholten S: A comparison of two different prophylactic dose regimens of low molecular weight heparin in bariatric surgery. Obes Surg 2002;12:19-24.

40. Golden S, Peart-Vigilance C, Kao W, et al: Perioperative glycemic control and the risk of infectious complications in a cohort of adults with diabetes. Diabetes Care 1999;22:1408-1414.

41. Rossini A: Why control blood glucose levels? Arch Surg 1976;111:229-233.

42. Van den Berghe G, Wouters P, Weekers P, et al: Intensive insulin therapy in critically ill patients. New Eng J Med 2001;345:1359-1367.

43. Queale W, Seidler A, Brancati F: Glycemic control and sliding scale insulin use in medical Inpatients with diabetes mellitus. Arch Intern Med 1997;157:545-552.

44. Sugerman H, Brewer W, Shiffman M, et al: A multicenter, placebo-controlled, randomized, double-blind, prospective trial of prophylactic ursodiol for the prevention of gallstone formation following gastric-bypass-induced rapid weight loss. Am J Surg 1995; 169:91-97.

45. Miller K, Hell E, Lang B, et al: Gallstone formation prophylaxis after gastric restrictive procedures for weight loss: a randomized double-blind placebo-controlled trial. Ann Surg 2003;238:697-702.

46. Ray E, Nickels M, Sayeed S, et al: Predicting success after gastric bypass: the role of psychological and behavioral factors. Surgery 2003;134:555-564.

47. Gordillo G, Sen C: Revisiting the essential role of oxygen in wound healing. Am J Surg 2003;186:259-263.

48. Martin L, Tan T, Holmes P, et al: Can morbidly obese patients lose weight preoperatively? Am J Surg 1995;169:245-253.

14

Anesthesia Considerations in the Obese

Lipi Ramchandani, M.B.B.S. and Kumar G. Belani, M.B.B.S., M.S.

Anesthesia providers must be familiar with the care of obese patients because obesity is a growing nutritional disorder in developed and developing nations.[1] In the year 1985, in developed nations, obesity rose to epidemic proportions.[2] Because bariatric surgery is commonplace, it is imperative that anesthesia care providers be knowledgeable about the pathophysiology of the morbidly obese and about the risks and difficulties encountered during their care. Problems include difficulties with intravenous access, tracheal intubation and extubation, and appropriate use of narcotics, muscle relaxants, and other drugs.[3] The Framingham Heart Study revealed that obese patients have thrice the risk for mortality than do nonobese humans.[4]

▶ CARDIOVASCULAR SYSTEM

With the onset and progression of obesity, patients develop hypertension, increased blood volume, and dyslipidemia. Even when they are normotensive, there is echocardiographic evidence of a significantly larger internal diameter of the ventricles and of thicker end diastolic septum and posterior wall of the left ventricle.[5] These changes are related to the increased amount of intraabdominal fat deposition. Hypertension is mild to moderate in the majority but severe in 5% to 10% of patients.[6] For every 10-kg gain in body weight, systolic blood pressure is reported to increase by 3 to 4 mmHg, with diastolic increases of 2 mmHg.[7] This occurs because of the increase in circulatory volume necessary for blood supply to the fat deposits, which also results in an increased cardiac output.[8] Weight gain also leads to metabolic alteration in insulin resistance. In addition, there is an effect on the sympathetic system by the arterial baroreceptors.[9] Because of the resulting hypertension, there is concentric hypertrophy and noncompliance of the left ventricle, which eventually leads to cardiac failure.[10]

Obesity is also associated with ischemic heart disease because obese patients are prone to hypercholesterolemia, a reduced density of lipoprotein levels, hypertension, and diabetes mellitus. The Framingham study noted a direct correlation among angina pectoris, sudden death, and obesity.[4] However, obesity did not increase the incidence of acute myocardial infarction. As mentioned earlier, there is an increase in cardiac output related to an increase in blood volume for blood supply to adipose tissue. This increment leads to an increase in oxygen consumption.

It has been noted that in response to exercise, cardiac output rises faster in the morbidly obese; when this occurs, there is an increase in the left ventricular pressure and pulmonary capillary wedge pressure. Although the total blood volume increases, the volume-weight base decreases, as compared to lean individuals (50 vs. 75 ml/kg body weight). Splanchnic blood flow is disproportionately increased when compared to the blood flow to the brain and kidneys. The approximate increase in splanchnic blood flow and blood volume is 20 to 30 ml per kg of excess body weight.[11] Ventricular hypertrophy and dysfunction worsen with increasing obesity; despite this, improvement has been noted to occur as a result of weight loss.[12] It has also been noted that during exercise by the obese, there is an increase in cardiac output that occurs as a result of an increase in heart rate without an increase in ejection fraction.

Obese patients are also prone to cardiac arrhythmias because of increased fat infiltration into the cardiac conduction system and because of the presence of cardiomyopathy and coronary artery disease. Extracardiac factors, such as obstructive sleep apnea with associated hypoxia, hypercapnia, and electrolyte imbalance, along with an increase in circulating catecholamines, increase this predisposition.

Many obese patients are asymptomatic, even though they have varying degrees of cardiovascular dysfunction. The primary reason for this is limitation of mobility. Thus, they may not complain of symptoms such as angina on exertion or exertional dyspnea. These symptoms, however, may be precipitated by minimal physical activity, such as walking, climbing stairs, and other regular day-to-day activities. These differences in obese patients warrant detailed and thorough cardiovascular examination. This should be performed irrespective of the type of surgical procedure to be done. History taking should include any history of hypertension, cardiac failure, myocardial insufficiency, or arrhythmias. It is vital to inquire about the various medications patients may be taking. Clinical examination should include taking blood pressure with appropriately sized cuffs (a 42-cm-wide bladder is recommended).[13,14] If an appropriate cuff is unavailable, blood pressure can be taken over the forearm using radial pulsations. Signs of cardiac failure, such as hepatomegaly, raised jugular venous pulse, additional audible sounds, pulmonary rales, or peripheral edema should be evaluated.

▶ RESPIRATORY SYSTEM

Obesity exerts profound effects on the respiratory system. The anatomic changes result in obstructive sleep apnea (OSA) and obstructive hypoventilation syndrome (OHS) because of a reduction in pharyngeal free space.[15-17] This is caused by deposition of adipose tissue into the pharyngeal walls, including the uvula, tonsils, tongue, and aryepiglottic folds. The compliance of the chest wall and the difference between extraluminal and intraluminal pressures along with oropharyngeal muscle tone determines airway patency. In obese individuals, collapse of the soft-walled oropharynx and obstruction of the airway occur easily because the pharyngeal free space is markedly diminished and extraluminal pressure is increased (due to deposition of adipose tissue in the neck).[17] As a single independent factor, obesity is responsible for OSA in 60% to 90% of the population with this disorder. OHS is different from OSA in that there is no cessation of airflow (Table 14-1).[15]

Both OSA and OHS repeatedly disrupt sleep because of arousal resulting from increased ventilatory effort; this causes daytime sleepiness and cardiopulmonary dysfunction. A properly performed study in a sleep laboratory helps to diagnose OSA and OHS. Agents that induce sleep and relaxation of the oropharyngeal and upper respiratory muscles (thiopental, narcotics, benzodiazepines, nitrous oxide, and neuromuscular relaxants) may result in airway obstruction in obese patients.[18-23]

Obesity also results in significant functional changes in breathing. Sharp and colleagues observed that in simple or uncomplicated obesity, chest wall and total respiratory compliance was 92% and 80% when compared to that of normal, nonobese individuals.[24] These values are even lower in obese patients suffering from OHS (chest wall and total respiratory compliance was 37% and 44% of that of normal, nonobese men). The decrease in chest wall compliance in obesity is caused by the mechanical and gravitational effects of adipose tissue that is pressing on the thoracic cage, diaphragm, and lungs.[25] The excess weight is an added inspiratory load that inspiratory muscles must overcome before inspiratory flow begins. Airway, chest wall, and respiratory resistance are all elevated in simple obesity, and they increase with increases in body mass index (BMI) and when OHS is present. Obese individuals have reduced functional residual capacity (FRC). Although specific airway conductance may be normal or reduced by 50%, the total respiratory resistance increases when obese patients shift from the upright to the supine position, probably due to further reductions in FRC. In this position, the FRC decreases even further, resulting in significant reductions in closing volume and affecting gas exchange. Respirations are typically rapid and shallow; the work of breathing is increased and inspiratory capacity becomes limited. This is particularly detrimental because obese patients have decreased respiratory muscle strength and endurance due to the overstretching of the diaphragm, especially in the supine position. It has been shown that there is significant improvement in the hypercapnic ventilatory response within 24 hours of initiating positive pressure ventilation in obese patients with OHS. There is rapid relief of respiratory muscle fatigue because of the reduced work of breathing.[25]

Spirometry and Lung Volumes

In obese patients, age, BMI, and type of fat distribution influence lung volumes. Displacement of the diaphragm into the chest by the obese abdomen results in a decrease in expiratory reserve volume. The forced expiratory volume in one second (FEV$_1$) to forced vital capacity ratio is also decreased. As discussed earlier, FRC is reduced and has been reported to be 75% to 80% of predicted value in obese individuals with OHS. These patients also show a 20% reduction in total lung capacity and a 40% reduction in maximum minute ventilatory volume and FEV$_1$. Even though obese patients have reduced lung volumes, their work of breathing is increased by 70%. When OHS is present the work may be increased to as much as 280%.

The respiratory rate is increased by 40% and tidal volumes are 50% to 80% of those of normal, nonobese individuals. These changes are related to the increase in BMI. Because the lung bases are well perfused but poorly ventilated due to secondary airway closure, leading to atelectasis or alveolar collapse, there is an increased mismatch of ventilation to perfusion, resulting in a widening of the alveolar-arterial difference for oxygen (A-aDO$_2$). As noted earlier, when OSA or OHS is present, hypoxia is a common occurrence in these patients. Several factors, namely, increased work of breathing, decreased endurance and respiratory muscle strength, and fatigue, contribute to elevations in resting partial pressure carbon dioxide (PaCO$_2$) in these patients. Relief of upper airway obstruction by the use of nasal continuous positive airway pressure (CPAP) or tracheostomy reverses hypercapnia but not the response to hypercapnia.[26-28]

Table 14-1	DIFFERENCES AND SIMILARITIES IN OBSTRUCTIVE SLEEP APNEA AND OBSTRUCTIVE HYPOVENTILATION SYNDROME	
CRITERION	OSA	OHS
Decrease in airflow >10s	100%	>50%
Times/hour	>5	>15
Ventilatory effort	Yes with obstruction	Yes with snoring
Decrease in O$_2$ saturation	≥4%	≥4%
Disrupted sleep	Yes	Yes
Daytime sleepiness	Yes	Yes
Sustained increase in PaCO$_2$	≥45 mmHg	≥45 mmHg

Modified from Benumof JL: Obstructive sleep apnea in the adult obese patient: implications for airway management. Anesth Clin North Am 2002;20:789-811 and Strollo PJ and Rogers RM: Obstructive sleep apnea. N Engl J Med 1996;334:99-104.

OHS, obstructive hypoventilation syndrome; OSA, obstructive sleep apnea.

Anesthesia Implications of Respiratory Aberration

Because of the significant changes seen in the physiology of the respiratory system, it becomes important for the anesthesia care team to carefully and completely assess the patient preoperatively. This will aid the anesthesia care team in deciding among the various modalities and options available so they can plan a successful anesthesia technique that is designed for the individual patient. Both general and regional anesthesia have been shown to have effects on the respiratory system.[29]

In patients who raise concern, preoperative assessment should include a complete blood count (to rule out polycythemia due to prolonged hypoxia), chest radiography, and arterial blood-gas analysis in both the supine and the upright position, lung function tests, and possibly overnight oximetry. It is important to elicit histories concerning OSA, OHS, and chronic daytime hypoventilation in these people. To confirm the diagnosis, a formal sleep study is helpful. Patients with OSA can receive treatment prior to surgery, such as nocturnal nasal CPAP or bilevel positive airway pressure (BiPAP).

▶ GASTROINTESTINAL SYSTEM

Obese people exhibit increases in intraabdominal pressure along with increases in gastric volume. Whether this predisposes them to aspiration and gastroesophageal reflux disease (GERD) is controversial. What is less controversial is that there is a higher incidence of hiatal hernia with GERD. Vaughan and associates suggest that obese patients should be treated like third-trimester obstetric patients who are at increased risk for aspiration.[30] This, however, was not borne out in the study by Harter and colleagues.[31] They studied the volume and pH of gastric contents in fasting obese and lean patients without gastrointestinal obstruction. Only 26.6% of obese patients had a high volume of gastric content with a low pH. This was in significant contrast to 42.05% of lean individuals who had a high volume with a low pH. Similar findings were suggested by a metaanalysis review by Kranke and associates.[32] On the other hand, Gomez and colleagues performed a cohort review to evaluate the relationship between obesity and GERD.[33] They also studied the impact of a hypocaloric diet and bariatric surgery on gastrointestinal reflux symptoms. They concluded that obesity as a condition predisposes to the development of GERD. Despite this report, no studies are available to correlate the degree of obesity with the symptoms of reflux. Hypotonic lower esophageal sphincter, ineffective esophageal motility, and hiatal hernia are pathophysiologic mechanisms that may be present in obesity. Obese patients with demonstrated large amounts of gastric fluid and slower gastric emptying time experience significant improvement in these indexes after achieving weight loss.[34,35]

Effects of Obesity on the Liver

Obesity predisposes patients to nonalcoholic steatohepatitis (NASH) and cholelithiasis. However, the metabolic function of the liver is not affected in the majority of obese patients. Diabetes mellitus also predisposes obese patients to NASH. Patients with NASH may have elevated liver enzymes, increases in triglycerides, hepatomegaly, and cirrhosis (10%).[36]

▶ HEMATOLOGIC SYSTEM

Both polycythemia and venous stasis predispose obese individuals to deep vein thrombosis (DVT). Venous stasis results from increased intraabdominal pressure and accompanying immobilization. Decreased fibrinolytic activity along with increased fibrinogen concentrations have been observed in obese individuals. Pivalizza and associates[37] evaluated 26 obese patients and compared them to lean patients undergoing operative procedures. With the help of the thromboelastograph, they found that obese patients demonstrated accelerated fibrin formation and improved platelet-fibrin interaction. However, fibrinolysis was similar in both groups.

Because of their enhanced tendency to form clots, the risk of DVT is doubled in obese individuals when compared to that of lean individuals (48% vs. 23%) during abdominal surgery performed for reasons other than malignancy.[38] This automatically increases the likelihood of pulmonary embolus, which is reported to be between 2.4% to 4.5% following bariatric surgery.[39,40] To reduce the risk of DVT and pulmonary embolism in obese patients, most surgical protocols favor the use of anticoagulant prophylaxis and pneumatic-compression lower-extremity stockings.

▶ RENAL SYSTEM

Obese patients have excessive adipose tissue around the kidney. This alters intrarenal physical forces due to medullary compression. In addition, because of increased abdominal pressure, obese patients have chronic renal vasodilatation with increased hydrostatic pressure and wall stress on the glomerulus. There is activation of the sympathetic and renin-angiotensin system, resulting in increases in tubular reabsorption. All this predisposes obese patients to chronic renal dysfunction, as noted by the presence of microalbuminuria. Associated hypertension, hyperglycemia (diabetes mellitus), hypercholesteremia, and hypertriglyceridemia accelerate chronic renal dysfunction in obesity.[41,42] The results of a study by Maddox and associates done in hyperphagic Zucker rats suggest that the development of renal damage (glomerular injury) secondary to obesity can be prevented by food restriction.[43]

▶ PREOPERATIVE ASSESSMENT

Intravenous Access

The presence of excessive subcutaneous tissue decreases the visibility of peripheral veins. Portable ultrasound equipment may be required for identification and cannulation of peripheral veins. In some patients it may be difficult to identify peripheral access, and central venous cannulation may be necessary. The presence of reliable venous access facilitates care in the postoperative period. In diabetic obese patients, the presence of a multiport central venous catheter facilitates blood glucose and other laboratory sampling.[44,45]

Cardiovascular System

A detailed history, physical examination, and focused investigations help to rule out the extent and severity of the cardiovascular physiologic changes reported in obese patients. The severity of hypertension and its control with medications, if any, should be noted. Ischemic heart disease, when present, must be stable and if extensive may require further preoperative assessment. Evaluation should also include an assessment for pulmonary hypertension and signs of right- or left-sided cardiac failure. Signs of cardiac failure include increased jugular pressure, additional heart sounds, pulmonary crackles, hepatomegaly, and peripheral edema. Symptoms of pulmonary hypertension include exertional dyspnea, fatigue, and syncope, which reflect the inability to increase cardiac output during activity. Identification of tricuspid regurgitation with echocardiography is most definitive confirmation of pulmonary hypertension. A chest radiograph must be done to rule out cardiomegaly. An electrocardiogram (ECG) helps (especially in the presence of advanced right ventricular failure) to demonstrate signs of right ventricular hypertrophy, such as tall precordial R waves, right axis deviation, and right ventricular strain. Special expertise is required in the interpretation of the ECG because of excessive overlying adipose tissue and epicardial fat that may interfere with the voltage of the QRS and other waves. The ECG also demonstrates the presence of arrhythmias and axis deviation.[29,46] Mild to moderate pulmonary hypertension warrants avoidance of hypoxemia, nitrous oxide, and other drugs that may further aggravate pulmonary vasoconstriction.[47,48]

Echocardiography helps to evaluate cardiac function in detail with respect to the ejection fraction, septal motility, valvular dysfunction, and any other functional problems. Thus, consultation with a cardiologist must be obtained when necessary for accurate diagnosis and institution of proper preoperative therapy. This may require postponing the procedure and also help in planning intraoperative invasive monitoring (e.g., transesophageal echocardiography with or without pulmonary artery catheterization).

Respiratory System

History taking must include evaluation for the presence of OSA, OHS, upper airway obstruction, and dyspnea. One should check for the presence of snoring, apnea during sleep, frequent arousals, daytime sleepiness, and fatigue. Results from a formal sleep study are useful to ascertain objectively the presence or absence of OSA or OHS.[15,49]

Pulmonary function tests may be necessary to note effects on lung capacities and airflow mechanics. Arterial blood gases indicate whether the patient is retaining carbon dioxide or has hypoxemia. The presence of polycythemia suggests long-standing hypoxemia. A chest radiograph evaluates the anatomic status of the lung and cardiac structures.

Other Pertinent Concerns

Certain patients who are scheduled for repeat bariatric surgery or have had bariatric surgery in the past may have some common long-term nutritional deficiencies that may include vitamin B_{12}, iron, calcium, thiamine, vitamin K, and zinc. Therefore, it becomes important prior to surgery to assess electrolyte and coagulation status. Chronic vitamin K deficiency (deficiency of clotting factors II, VII, IX, and X) can lead to an increase in prothrombin time with a normal partial thromboplastin time.[50] For elective surgery, vitamin K analogues such as phytonadione can be used to correct the coagulopathy within 6 to 24 hours. For emergency operations, fresh-frozen plasma may be required. As mentioned earlier, obese patients are at increased risk for developing DVT. For this reason, miniheparinization, elastic stockings, pneumoboots, and frequent leg lifts are advocated. Type 2 diabetes mellitus is common in obese patients and should be confirmed with a fasting blood glucose level and a check for the presence of ketones in blood and urine. Diabetes mellitus may worsen the risk of GERD.[51]

Perioperative Drug Use

Obese patients often are on medications to control their blood pressure and blood glucose levels. Antihypertensives should be continued preoperatively (with a sip of water). Oral hypoglycemic drugs should be withheld and blood glucose controlled with insulin, using a sliding scale. Some bariatric patients may be on weight-reducing medications including herbal remedies. These should be reviewed for possible unwanted systemic effects and drug interactions.

Two commonly used weight-loss drugs are sibutramine and orlistat. Sibutramine inhibits the reuptake of norepinephrine, serotonin, and dopamine, thereby causing anorexia. It causes transient dose-related increases in both systemic and diastolic blood pressure by a mean of 2 to 4 mmHg and induces a small increase in heart rate of 3 to 5 beats per minute. Orlistat is a product of *Streptomyces toxytricini*, which inhibits mammalian lipase. It blocks the digestion and absorption of dietary fat by binding lipases in the gastrointestinal tract. It causes fat malabsorption and decreases in serum concentration of fat-soluble vitamins (A, D, E, and K). In some cases, orlistat has been reported to result in aggravated hypertension.[52-54] Warfarin's anticoagulant effect may also be increased because orlistat decreases the absorption of vitamin K.

Perioperative antibiotic prophylaxis is important to minimize the risk of wound infection. The published rate of wound infection after gastric procedures in the morbidly obese is approximately twice that in lean patients. Nguyen and colleagues found that open Roux-en-Y gastric bypass has approximately a tenfold incidence of wound infection as compared to the laparoscopic approach.[55] However, practitioners recommend antibiotic prophylaxis for the laparoscopic approach as well.[56] Antibiotics should be administered no more than 45 minutes prior to the incision and repeated every 2 hours in protracted cases. Prophylaxis for DVT with haparin and compression devices is instituted just before surgery and continued until at least 12 hours postoperatively unless the patient has other significant medical problems that require prolonged anticoagulation.

Preoperative Airway Assessment

Obese patients are more difficult to mask, ventilate, and intubate. This is because of their size, the presence of a shorter neck that has a widened circumference, the presence of excessive pharyngeal tissue, and a tongue that has a large base.[15] It is imperative that every obese patient be carefully examined for the feasibility of mask ventilation and intubation, including aspiration risk. In the absence of significant reflux and hiatal hernia, most patients may be passively ventilated prior to intubation by mask, if required. This is important to know preoperatively because endotracheal intubation may take longer than anticipated, so mask ventilation becomes necessary. Although histories and reviews of medical records are necessary, one must remember that they may be misleading if the patient has gained significant amounts of weight. If the patient was difficult to ventilate by mask or difficult to intubate on a prior occasion, unless there has been a major weight loss with an improvement in the airway, the patient should be assumed to be difficult for airway care unless proven otherwise. Obese patients may have limited neck movement and mouth opening, making intubation difficult. Voyagis and colleagues looked at Mallampati class, mouth opening, and risks of intubation.[57] They found that a disproportionately large base of tongue predisposes a patient to difficult intubation. Those with a neck circumference of 42 cm are more likely to be difficult to intubate unless an increased mouth opening and tongue size compensate for this feature.[58,59] The presence of effortless breathing and patent nostrils should be noted. The presence of OSA and body size greater that 175% ideal body weight often suggests the possibility of a difficult airway. In two studies done in a series of morbidly obese patients undergoing abdominal surgery, the incidence of difficulty with the airway after general anesthesia was 13% and 24%, and the incidence of patients requiring awake intubation was 8%.[39,60] The authors felt that this was due to several factors: the presence of a short thick neck, the close relationship of a short neck and OSA, and excess pharyngeal tissue in the lateral walls of the larynx. Brodsky and associates[61] studied 100 morbidly obese patients to identify factors that complicate direct laryngoscopy and tracheal intubation. Preoperatively they recorded height, weight, neck circumference, width of mouth opening, sternomental distance, thyromental distance, and Mallampati score. They also scored the laryngoscopic view and the number of attempts at tracheal intubation. They found that neither obesity nor BMI was correlated with difficult intubation. Large neck and Mallampati score were the only two predictors of potential intubation problems. Patients with increased neck circumference required intervention by a fiberoptic bronchoscope to establish an airway. Also, patients with a Mallampati score greater than or equal to 3 had increased difficulty with tracheal intubation. Other routine assessments, such as jaw and neck mobility, dental status, patency of nostrils, and inspection of oropharynx, should be done prior to implementation of an anesthesia care plan for obese patients.

▶ DEVELOPMENT OF ANESTHESIA CARE PLAN

After completion of the preoperative assessment, either in a preoperative clinic or on the day of surgery in the preoperative area, the anesthesia care team must formulate an anesthesia care plan for the contemplated procedure. Most patients require general anesthesia, although some procedures could be done using a regional technique or using local infiltration of anesthetic combined with monitored anesthesia sedation. For all patients, adequate intravenous access must be established prior to intervention. This may require the use of a portable ultrasound device.[62] For blood pressure monitoring, one must have available an appropriately sized cuff (>42 cm). The cuff must occupy at least two thirds of the length of the upper arm and have a proportionately sized air bladder capacity. In patients with uncontrolled hypertension and in patients in whom excessive and sudden blood pressure shifts are expected, invasive monitoring with a radial artery catheter should be considered. A new method (the Vasotrac system) of measuring blood pressure noninvasively and continually over the radial artery has become available and has been shown to be useful and easy to use in the morbidly obese.[63] When extensive surgery is planned, a central venous catheter is useful for blood drawing and central venous pressure (CVP) monitoring. A pulmonary artery catheter to monitor pulmonary artery pressure, wedge pressure, and oxygen transport is recommended in patients with advanced cardiopulmonary disease.[51] We have found the use of portable ultrasound extremely useful in identifying the internal jugular veins for quick and safe access.

Depending upon their body weights, many obese patients must be transported on beds that can safely transfer their weight. Most operating tables are designed for patients 120 to 140 kg (maximum of 500 lbs) in weight. Exceeding this limit exposes the patient and staff to risk. Specially designed tables may be required for safe anesthesia. Operating tables capable of holding up to 455 kg (850 lbs) with little extra width to accommodate the extra girth are available. An electrically operated table helps to maneuver patients into surgically favorable positions. Patients undergoing bariatric surgery are prone to slipping off the table, so they must be securely strapped to the table. Beanbags as soft pads are available in various sizes and are useful for proper patient positioning.[51] As is true for other patients, but even more so for the obese, pressure areas must be protected to reduce the likelihood of pressure sores and nerve injuries (e.g., due to extreme abduction of arms).[64]

Some obese patients, as mentioned earlier, tolerate the supine position poorly. This must be tested preoperatively because when cardiac reserve is limited, assuming the supine position may be fatal. Assuming the supine position increases the preload in these patients and also increases the work of breathing and oxygen consumption.[65] Compression of the inferior vena cava may also occur and this can result in reduction in venous return with hypotension. This compression may be minimized by tilting the operating table to the left or by placing a wedge under the patient.[66,67] For these reasons, it is best to anesthetize the patient on the operating room table in the operating room.

For obese patients, an airway strategy must be decided on beforehand. Sometimes, a direct laryngeal examination on the operating table, with proper sedation and preoxygenation, helps to confirm whether intubation will be easy or difficult. If the airway strategy is deemed to be feasible, no special intervention is required. On the other hand, if airway difficulty is anticipated, then every effort should be made to establish endotracheal intubation before the patient is completely anesthetized. This will require patient education and preparation. In most instances, the use of a fiberscope in a properly prepared and optimally sedated, oxygenated, and ventilating patient is successful. One may also consider using an intubating laryngeal mask airway or other airway access devices for successful endotracheal tube placement into the larynx.[68]

During routine care of these patients, one must have available a portable difficult-airway unit. In addition to a fiberscope and laryngeal mask airway capability, the contents of this unit must include at least the availability of large sizes and types of laryngoscope blades, a Combitube, cricothyrotomy sets, and retrograde intubating kits. During conventional laryngoscopy, a set of towels or folded blankets placed behind the shoulders is helpful in compensating for the exaggerated flexed position that results from posterior cervical fat. This is known as "stacking"; the tip of the chin is at a higher level than the chest to facilitate laryngoscopy and intubation.[51,69]

Anesthetic Pharmacology

The physiologic changes associated with obesity lead to alterations in the distribution, binding, and elimination of many drugs. Highly lipophilic substances such as barbiturates and benzodiazepines show significant increase in volume of distribution (V_d) in the obese in comparison to normal-weight individuals.[70,71] Less lipophilic compounds have little or no change in distribution (V_d) with obesity. Certain exceptions to this rule include digoxin, procainamide, and remifentanil, highly lipophilic drugs that have no systemic relationship between their degree of lipophilicity and their distribution in the obese.[51] Their volume of distribution remains consistent, and doses have to be calculated according to the ideal body weight or, more accurately, according to the lean body mass. In 20% to 40% of obese individuals, ideal body weight and lean body mass are not identical. This is because increases in body weight may be due to increases in lean body mass. Therefore it has been suggested that in the case of lipophilic drugs, one may add 20% to the ideal body weight when calculating drug doses.[51]

Wada and colleagues performed a computer simulation of the effects of alterations in blood flows and body composition on thiopental pharmacokinetics in humans.[72] They found that increased body fat acts as a depot that retains thiopental in the body. This in turn leads to an increase in terminal half-life ($T_{1/2}$), from 7 hours in lean patients to 23 hours in obese patients, and in the volume of distribution (V_d), from 1.6 to 3.3 l per kg in lean versus obese patients. Thus, with thiopental and other lipophilic drugs (e.g., benzodiazepines) or potent inhalation agents, effects may persist for some time after discontinuation.[73]

Triglycerides, lipoproteins, cholesterol, and free fatty acids are increased in obesity and may inhibit the protein binding of some drugs and increase their unbound fractions. This is balanced by the increased concentration of α-1-acid glycoprotein, which increases the degree of protein binding of other drugs (e.g., local anesthetics); this reduces free plasma fractions.

Despite modest histologic abnormalities noted in obese patients, hepatic clearance and phase I reactions (oxidation, reduction, and hydrolysis) are unchanged or increased in the obese patient.[74] Also, the metabolism of drugs by phase II metabolism (e.g., lorazepam) is consistently increased. Cardiac failure and reduced liver blood flow may slow elimination of drugs by the liver (e.g., midazolam and lidocaine).[73]

Propofol is highly lipophilic and distributes rapidly from the blood, the initial V_d being 18 l. The large dose required for induction may lead to cardiovascular depression.[75] The kinetics of fentanyl, alfentanil, and sufentanil in the obese are somewhat unpredictable. Fentanyl kinetics are similar to those in the nonobese.[76] Alfentanil and sufentanil have longer elimination half-lives. In addition, the use of remifentanil can reduce emergence time in obese patients.[77,78]

With regard to inhalation anesthetics, the traditional view has been that emergence can be delayed because of a slow release from the excessive adipose tissue. Thus, desflurane is preferred because of its more rapid and consistent recovery profile.[79] Several studies compared sevoflurane to isoflurane for bariatric surgery.[80-82] They favored sevoflurane because of rapid recovery, good hemodynamic control, low incidence of nausea and vomiting, and prompt regaining of psychological and physical functioning, as well as early discharge from the hospital. Morbidly obese patients metabolize halothane and enflurane more than the nonobese. For this reason and because of preexisting hepatic changes, halothane is best avoided to decrease the likelihood of halothane-associated hepatitis.[83-85] Similarly, Higuchi and colleagues found that serum inorganic fluoride concentrations in the obese increased more rapidly and remained higher than in the nonobese during use of sevoflurane anesthesia.[86] However, fluoride levels after isoflurane are not increased significantly. Juvin and colleagues compared postoperative recovery after desflurane, propofol, and isoflurane anesthesia.[79] They found that postoperative immediate and intermediate recoveries after desflurane are more rapid and consistent after desflurane than after propofol or isoflurane anesthesia. Desflurane also has no hepatic metabolism nor does it have renal toxicity.

It has been suggested that the concentration and total dose exposure of volatile anesthetics can be reduced by supplementing general anesthesia with regional techniques such as continuous epidural blockade for abdominal and thoracic operations.

Muscle Relaxants

Obese patients recover more rapidly from succinylcholine because of an increase in pseudocholinesterase activity.[87,88] Thus, when used without pretreatment, a dose of 1.2 to 1.5 mg per kg is appropriate. Because obesity itself interferes with muscle relaxation during surgery, it is not uncommon to use higher doses of nondepolarizers. Because of this, Weinstein and associates[89] found that atracurium is superior to vecuronium and easier to antagonize[90] because it is independent of organ elimination. The recovery of neuromuscular blockade with vecuronium can be prolonged due to its hepatic elimination. On the other hand, in obese patients scheduled for gynecologic surgery, Puhringer and colleagues found that there was no alteration in the pharmacodynamics and pharmacokinetics of rocuronium.[91] Because maximal relaxation is commonly practiced, nondepolarizers must be reversed only when the patients have demonstrated significant recovery, as demonstrated by spontaneous regular breathing efforts and almost complete return of motor power. This is important so as to avoid inadequate reversal, which is characterized by thoracoabdominal uncoordination, hypoxemia, and increasing hypercarbia requiring postoperative reintubation and mechanical ventilation. In summary, a good rule of thumb is to administer general anesthetics based upon ideal body weight and titrate doses based upon patient response.

Tracheal Intubation and Extubation

All obese patients must be denitrogenated with oxygen prior to intubation and extubation. Their FRC is reduced and they desaturate very rapidly.[92] Denitrogenation is easily achieved by placing the patient in a 30-degree reversed Trendelenburg position with the shoulders stacked, as discussed earlier. The head and neck must be extended to ensure an open upper airway, and the face mask must be held so as to provide a complete seal. A 10-l-per-minute oxygen flow rate is recommended.[93,94] The patient should be instructed to take deep breaths with complete inhalations and exhalations. Denitrogenation of the lungs may take 5 to 10 minutes.

If the airway was deemed to be feasible for face-masking and intubation, after induction one may perform endotracheal intubation following succinylcholine or after relaxation with nondepolarizer relaxants. When using nondepolarizers, the onset of muscle relaxants can be increased by using the priming technique, followed by an intubating dose of nondepolarizing muscle relaxant. Using this approach, the authors have performed a large number of successful rapid-sequence inductions using cisatracurium. Because the likelihood of an unanticipated difficult airway is higher in obese patients, a portable difficult-airway unit must be available. In some instances, mask ventilation may be required, and this is usually successful with a significant jaw thrust and the use of an appropriately sized oral airway. Sometimes appropriate-length nasopharyngeal airways used individually or in combination may be necessary. One person holds the mask and another is quickly recruited to squeeze the ventilation bag with both hands to provide adequate ventilation.[15] If the intubation is difficult, one must resort to alternative pathways, as discussed in the American Society of Anesthesiologists Difficult Airway Algorithm.[69] In such instances one can achieve successful intubation by a change in blade or the use of an intubating laryngeal mask airway or a fiberscope.

In some patients one is unable to ascertain the feasibility of intubation during the preoperative examination. In such instances, direct laryngoscopy may be performed with the patient ready for induction but prepared only with a topical anesthetic and titrated sedation. If feasibility is confirmed, then one may proceed to intubation following induction. On the other hand, if it has been decided that it is too difficult or has been so ascertained during the preanesthetic assessment, one should establish endotracheal intubation using either the fiberscope approach, intubating laryngeal mask airway, or other "awake" techniques.

Obese patients must be extubated when they are fully awake and after they have return of motor power. It is less threatening to extubate patients who were not difficult to mask-ventilate and or intubate.[15] Factors that play a role in determining successful extubation include the severity of OSA and the duration and type of procedure. Using a retrospective cohort review of 135 patients, the risk of postextubation obstruction was found to be 5%.[95,96] These authors also suggested that obesity predisposes to the development of negative-pressure pulmonary edema when these patients attempt to ventilate spontaneously through an obstructed airway.

A conservative, safe approach must be implemented when difficulty is experienced during induction. The patient may require a brief period of postoperative ventilatory support. Extubation is done when inhalation anesthetics have been completely eliminated and the opioid levels, as determined clinically, are at levels that will sustain spontaneous ventilation following extubation. It is helpful for regional anesthesia, if given, to be operable at the time of extubation. The patient should be denitrogenated with oxygen and preferably should be in a 30-degree reverse Trendelenburg position prior to extubation, especially in patients whose airways might prove to be problematic. One may deflate the endotracheal tube cuff and see whether the patient is able to breathe around the tube when the tube is occluded. Another option is to extubate over a hollow airway-exchange catheter or fiberscope. The patient may then be easily reintubated if ventilation is inadequate. Nasal/oronasal CPAP should be readily available and may be required to splint the oropharynx, especially in those with severe OSA.[15]

Specialized Monitoring Needs

Apart from the use of routine monitoring and the difficulties with noninvasive blood pressure monitoring already discussed, some obese patients may need invasive monitoring; namely, a CVP or pulmonary artery catheter or an arterial line for direct blood pressure monitoring. In some patients, it may be necessary to place a transesophageal probe for echocardiography if the patient is suffering from cardiac failure or pulmonary hypertension.[51]

Fluid Replacement During Surgery

Clinical evaluation of hydration in obese patients is difficult. Although total blood volume is increased, calculation of blood volume is difficult and does not follow standard formulas. Total body water is reduced by 20% to 25% because fat itself contains little water.[65] Compounding these difficulties is the likelihood of increased duration of surgery, bowel preparation prior to surgery for bariatric operations, and the inability to accurately calculate insensible fluid loss. These factors may lead to hypovolemia in many patients. A steady urine output of approximately 1 ml per kg per hour, calculated using lean body mass, is a good predictor of adequate fluid replacement. Patients usually require 4 to 5 l of crystalloid for an average 2-hour operation.[51] This is approximately twice the amount of fluid, based upon standard calculations, used in lean individuals. In some patients, it may be necessary to place a CVP line or a pulmonary artery catheter to help guide fluid-replacement needs.[65]

Regional Anesthesia

The benefits of regional analgesia in lean patients are also applicable in the obese.[97] Thus, thoracic epidural analgesia used in conjunction with general anesthesia improves postoperative pulmonary function following abdominal surgery.[98] This allows rapid recovery because of the reduction in postoperative pulmonary complications. There may be difficulty in delineating anatomic landmarks in obese individuals for performance of regional block procedures. Special equipment may be required, such as longer needles for spinal and epidural space identification and access; the use of electrically active needles to identify peripheral motor nerves; and the use of fluoroscopy to help identify the epidural space. The epidural space in obese people has greater fat content and because of increased intraabdominal pressure, the epidural veins are larger. This decreases significantly the capacity of the epidural and intrathecal spaces. The volume of local anesthetic must be appropriately reduced by about 20% to 25% of doses normally used in lean patients.[99,100] Thus, one must carefully monitor epidural and subarachnoid blocks because rostral spread beyond the T-5 vertebra can occur easily and induce respiratory compromise. When used intraoperatively, continuous epidural blockade has been shown to reduce the dose requirements of inhalation agents, opioids, and other analgesics.[51,101]

Emergence From Anesthesia and Immediate Postoperative Care

Factors that determine emergence and extubation depend upon the type of surgery and whether the patient was easy or difficult to mask, ventilate, and intubate. In most instances of bariatric surgery, an obese patient with a feasible airway may be allowed to emerge from anesthesia at the end of surgery and be extubated. Spontaneous regular, steady breathing with adequate tidal volumes (6-8 ml/kg of ideal body weight), the presence of adequate muscle strength, and hemodynamic stability are requirements prior to extubation. In addition, the patient should be able to respond appropriately to verbal commands, demonstrate mouth opening and the ability to cough during extubation. A patient with a difficult airway and a strong history of OSA is allowed to recover more gradually. The patient is transferred to the postanesthesia care unit (PACU) and awakened with the head elevated (to approximately 45 degrees).[3] He or she is placed on respiratory support for a brief period while a more quantitative analysis of ability to breathe is conducted. Prior to extubation, the ability to breathe independently with only pressure

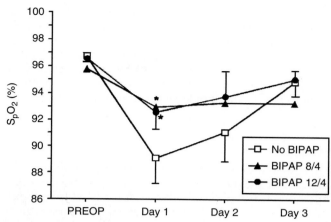

Figure 14-1. Effect of BiPAP on pulse oximetry following bariatric surgery. A BiPAP of 8/4 and 12/4 were both effective in preventing desaturation. *$P < 0.05$ for BiPAP 8/4 and 12/4 vs. no BiPAP. (From: Joris JL, Sottiaux TM, Chiche JD, et al: Effect of bi-level positive airway pressure (BiPAP) nasal ventilation on the postoperative pulmonary restrictive syndrome in obese patients undergoing gastroplasty. Chest 1997; 111:665-670.)

support is assessed, as is adequacy of pain control and the presence of stable vital signs, including normothermia. Either face-mask, nasal CPAP, or BiPAP support with oxygen may be required in some patients following extubation.[102] This is usually the case in a patient with a history of sleep apnea and in a patient who has used CPAP before surgery. Joris and associates were able to demonstrate the beneficial effects of positive airway pressure following gastroplasty (Fig. 14-1).[103]

Obese patients must be monitored continuously for sleep apnea, and oxygen pulse oximetry is recommended. Abdominal binders may promote the effects of incentive spirometry, pain-control measures, and early ambulation. Adequate pain control may be achieved through continuously administered thoracic epidural analgesics or by using a multimodal approach employing systemic drug combinations (nonsteroidal analgesics and acetaminophen plus opioids administered via patient-controlled devices). With the use of a carefully titrated epidural opioid and a low-concentration local anesthetic mixture, the risk of DVT is reduced and there is earlier recovery of intestinal motility. The following problems require special attention during recovery from anesthesia:

HEMODYNAMIC PROBLEMS

In some patients, left ventricular contractility immediately after the postoperative period is decreased. This may require inotropic support.

RESPIRATORY PROBLEMS

Morbidly obese patients are more prone to developing atelectasis than are nonobese patients. This is particularly true during the first 24 hours after surgery.[104] Following abdominal surgery, the incidence has been reported to be as high as 45%.[105] CPAP/BiPAP is the treatment of choice, and it should be started immediately in the PACU and continued overnight to prevent any airway obstruction. Many patients avoid taking deep breaths because of pain. Proper analgesia and good elastic abdominal binders for abdominal support may encourage patients to cooperate with early ambulation, spirometry, and other physiotherapeutic measures. These patients should be observed overnight in a special monitored care unit because they may have nocturnal nasal obstruction, apnea, and other respiratory discomfort. Supplemental oxygen should be used even during transport of the patient from operating room to PACU and should be continued for at least 3 days after surgery.[106]

COMMON INTRAOPERATIVE AND POSTOPERATIVE PROBLEMS

There is always a chance that the endotracheal tube will migrate into the trachea or move up into the larynx. Because intubation may have been difficult, it is advisable to secure the endotracheal tube properly to avoid unwanted extubation during surgery or transport to the PACU or intensive care unit. Similarly, because of their size and the unwanted effects of gravity, patients must be strapped to the operating table securely, with all four extremities well padded to avoid pressure sores or nerve compression. Pneumoboots should be applied to reduce the likelihood of DVT. One must avoid the overstretching (hyperabduction) of the arms to prevent stretching the brachial plexus. Padded foot and shoulder supports may be used to prevent the patient from slipping when the operating table is moved into the Trendelenburg or reverse Trendelenburg position. To reduce the occurrence of DVT, many protocols call for prophylaxis by low-molecular-weight heparin in addition to pneumoboots. This is usually started immediately before surgery and continued for 12 hours into the postoperative period. The stomach is emptied by an orogastric tube prior to emergence from anesthesia, or a nasogastric tube is left in place to reduce gastric contents. Prokinetics such as metoclopramide have been shown to facilitate emptying the stomach, and routine administration of antiemetics decrease postoperative nausea and vomiting.

▶ CONCLUSION

Caring for obese patients remains a challenge for anesthesia care providers despite the availability of newer and better induction drugs, inhalation agents, and neuromuscular relaxants. To perform a safe anesthetic procedure, it is important that anesthesia providers carefully assess the patient preoperatively so as to facilitate proper planning and minimize intra- and postoperative morbidity.

▶ REFERENCES

1. Mokdad AH, Bowman BA, Ford ES, et al: The continuing epidemics of obesity and diabetes in the United States. JAMA 2001;286:1195-2000.
2. Chopra M, Galbraith S, Darnton-Hill I: A global response to a global problem: the epidemic of overnutrition. Bull World Health Organ 2002;802:952-958.
3. Adams JP, Murphy PG: Obesity in anaesthesia and intensive care. Br J Anaesth 2000;85:91-108.
4. Wilson PW, D'Agostino RB, Sullivan L, et al: Overweight and obesity as determinants of cardiovascular risk: the Framingham experience. Arch Intern Med 2002;162:1867-1872.
5. Morricone L, Malavazos AE, Coman C, et al: Echocardiographic abnormalities in normotensive obese patients: relationship with visceral fat. Obes Res 2002;10:489-498.
6. Koch R, Sharma AM: Obesity and cardiovascular hemodynamic function. Curr Hypertens Rep 1999;1:127-130.
7. Bjerkedal T: Overweight and hypertension. Acta Med Scan 1957; 159:13-26.
8. Kolanowski J: Obesity and hypertension: from pathophysiology to treatment. Int J Obes Rel Metabol Dis 1999;23(suppl 1):42-46.
9. Grassi G, Cattaneo BM, Seravalle G, et al: Obesity and the sympathetic nervous system. Blood Press (suppl) 1996;1:43-46.
10. Doll S, Paccaud F, Bovet P, et al: Body mass index, abdominal adiposity and blood pressure: consistency of their association across developing and developed countries. Int J Obes Rel Metabol Dis 2002; 26:48-57.
11. Backman L, Freyshuss V, Halberg D, et al: Cardiovascular function in extreme obesity. Acta Med Scan 1973;193:437-446.
12. Alpert MA: Obesity cardiomyopathy: pathophysiology and evolution of the clinical syndrome. Am J Med Sci 2001;321:225-236.
13. Pickering TG: Principles and techniques of blood pressure measurement. Cardiol Clin 2002;20:207-223.
14. Pickering TG: Effect of standard cuff on blood pressure readings in patients with obese arms: how frequent is arms of a 'large circumference'? Blood Press Monit 2003;8:101-106.
15. Benumof JL: Obstructive sleep apnea in the adult obese patient: implications for airway management. Anesth Clin North Am 2002; 20:789-811.
16. DP White, Sleep related breathing disorders: pathophysiology of obstructive sleep apnea. Thorax 1995;50:797-804.
17. Koenig JS, Thach BT: Effects of mass loading on the upper airway. J App Physiol 1988;64:2294-2299.
18. Boushra NN: Anesthetic management of patients with sleep apnea syndrome. Can J Anaesth 1996;43:599-616.
19. Nandi PR, Charlesworth CH, Taylor SJ, et al: Effect of general anaesthesia on the pharynx.comment. Br J Anaesth 1991;66:157-162.
20. Catley DM, Thornton C, Jordan C, et al: Pronounced, episodic oxygen desaturation in the postoperative period: its association with ventilatory pattern and analgesic regimen. Anesthesiology 1985;63:20-28.
21. Mathru M, Esch O, Lang J, et al: Magnetic resonance imaging of the upper airway: effects of propofol anesthesia and nasal continuous positive airway pressure in humans. Anesthesiology 1996; 84:273-279.
22. Drummond GB: Influence of thiopentone on upper airway muscles. Br J Anaesth 1989;63:12-21.
23. Robinson RW, Zwillich CW, Bixler EO, et al: Effects of oral narcotics on sleep-disordered breathing in healthy adults. Chest 1987;91:197-203.
24. Sharp JT, Henry JP, Sweany SK et al: Total work of breathing in normal and obese men. J Clin Invest 1964;43:728-739.
25. Koenig SM: Pulmonary complications of obesity. Am J Med Sci 2001;321:249-279.
26. American Thoracic Society: Indications and standards for use of nasal continuous positive airway pressure (CPAP) in sleep apnea syndromes, official statement. Am J Respir Crit Care Med 1994; 150:1738-1785.
27. Strollo PJ, Sanders MH, Atwood CW: Sleep disorders: positive pressure therapy. Clin Chest Med 1998;19:55-68.
28. Krieger J, Meslier N, Lebrun T, et al: Accidents in obstructive sleep apnea patients treated with nasal continuous positive airway pressure: a prospective study. Chest 1997;112:1561-1566.
29. Adams JP, Murphy PG: Obesity in anaesthesia and intensive care. Br J Anaesth 2000;85:91-108.
30. Vaughan RW, Bauer S, Wise L: Volume and pH of gastric juice in obese patients. Anesthesiology 1975;43:686-689.
31. Harter RL, Kelly WB, Kramer MG, et al: A comparison of the volume and pH of gastric contents of obese and lean surgical patients. Anesth Analg 1998;86:147-152.
32. Kranke P, Apefel CC, Papenfuss T, et al: An increased body mass index is no risk factor for postoperative nausea and vomiting; a systematic review and results of original data. Acta Anaesthesiol Scand 2001;45:160-166.
33. Gomez Escudero O, Herrera Hernandez MF, Valdovinos Diaz MA: Obesity and gastroesophageal reflux disease. Rev Invest Clin 2002; 54:320-327.
34. Frezza EE, Ikramuddin S, Gourash W, et al: Symptomatic improvement in gastroesophageal reflux disease (GERD) following laparoscopic Roux-en-Y gastric bypass. Surg Endosc 2002;16:1027-1031.
35. Barak N, Ehrenpreis ED, Harrison JR, et al: Gastroesophageal reflux disease in obesity: pathophysiological and therapeutic considerations. Obes Rev 2002;3:9-15.

36. Halsted CH: Obesity: effects on the liver and gastrointestinal system. Curr Opin Clin Nutr Metab Care 1999;2:425-429.

37. Pivalizza EG, Pivalizza PJ, Weavind LM: Perioperative thromboelastography and sonoclot analysis in morbidly obese patients. Can J Anaesth 1997;44:942-945.

38. Clayton JK, Anderson JA, McNicol GP: Preoperative prediction of postoperative deep vein thrombosis. BMJ 1976;2:910-912.

39. Dominguez-Cherit G, Gonzalez R, Borunda D, et al: Anesthesia for morbidly obese patients. World J Surg 1998;22:969-973.

40. Eriksson S, Backman L, Ljungstrom KG: The incidence of clinical postoperative thrombosis after gastric surgery for obesity during 16 years. Obes Surg1997;7:332-335.

41. Adelman RD: Obesity and renal disease. Curr Op Nephrol Hyperten 2002;11:331-335.

42. Hall JE: The kidney, hypertension, and obesity. Hypertension 2003;41:625-633.

43. Maddox DA, Alavi FK, Santella RN, et al: Prevention of obesity-linked renal disease: age-dependent effects of dietary food restriction. Kidney Int 2002;62:208-219.

44. Keyes LE, Frazee BW, Snoey ER, et al: Ultrasound-guided brachial and basilic vein cannulation in emergency department patients with difficult intravenous access. Ann Emerg Med 1999;34:711-714.

45. Amsterdam JT, Hedges JR, Weinshenker E, et al: Evaluation of venous distension device: phase II: cannulation of nonemergent patients. Am J Emerg Med 1988;6:224-227.

46. Alpert MA, Terry BE, Cohen MV, et al: The electrocardiogram in morbid obesity. Am J Cardiol 2000;85:908-910.

47. Eisele JH Jr, Milstein JM, Goetzman BW: Pulmonary vascular responses to nitrous oxide in newborn lambs. Anesth Analg 1986;65:62-64.

48. Heerdt PM, Caldwell RW: The mechanism of nitrous oxide-induced changes in pulmonary vascular resistance in a dog model of left atrial outflow obstruction. J Cardiothorac Anesth 1989;3:568-573.

49. Strollo PJ, and Rogers RM: Obstructive sleep apnea. N Engl J Med 1996;334:99-104.

50. Kitchen S, Preston FE: Standardization of prothrombin time for laboratory control of oral anticoagulant therapy. Semin Thromb Hemost 1999;25:17-25.

51. Ogunnaike BO, Jones SB, Jones DB, et al: Anesthetic considerations for bariatric surgery. Anesth Analg 2002;95:1793-1805.

52. Bray GA, Greenway FL: Current and potential drugs for treatment of obesity. Endocr Rev 1999;20:805-875.

53. Davidson MH, Hauptman J, DiGirolamo M, et al: Weight control and risk factor reduction in obese subjects treated for 2 years with orlistat: a randomized controlled trial. JAMA 1999;281:235-242.

54. Valescia ME, Malgor LA, Farias EF, et al: Interaction between orlistat and antihypertensive drugs. Ann Pharmacother 2001; 35:1495-1496 (letter).

55. Nguyen NT, Goldman C, Rosenquist CJ, et al: Laparoscopic versus open gastric bypass: a randomized study of outcomes, quality of life, and costs. Ann Surg 2001;234:279-289.

56. Fisher A, Waterhouse TD, Adams AP: Obesity: its relation to anaesthesia. Anaesthesia 1975;30:633-647.

57. Voyagis GS, Kyriakis KP, Dimitriou V, et al: Value of oropharyngeal Mallampati classification in predicting difficult laryngoscopy among obese patients. Eur J Anaesth 1998;15:330-334.

58. Davies RJ, Ali NJ, Stradling JR: Neck circumference and other clinical features in the diagnosis of the obstructive sleep apnoea syndrome. Thorax 1992;47:101-105.

59. Karkouti K, Rose DK, Wigglesworth D, et al. Predicting difficult intubation: a multivariable analysis. Can J Anaesth 2000;47:730-739.

60. Buckley FP, Robinson NB, Simonowitz DA, et al: Anaesthesia in the morbidly obese: a comparison of anaesthetic and analgesic regimens for upper abdominal surgery. Anaesthesia 1983;38:840-850.

61. Brodsky JB, Lemmens HJ, Brock-Utne JG, et al: Morbid obesity and tracheal intubation. Anesth Analg 2002;94:732-736.

62. Juvin P, Blarel A, Bruno F, et al: Is peripheral line placement more difficult in obese than in lean patients? Anesth Analg 2003;96:1218.

63. Beebe DS, Ostanniy I, Komanduri V, et al: Continual non-invasive blood pressure monitoring with the Vasotrac™: experience in the morbidly obese. Anesthesiology 1998;89:A565.

64. Sawyer RJ, Richmond MN, Hickey JD, et al: Peripheral nerve injuries associated with anaesthesia. Anaesthesia 2000;55:980-991 (comment).

65. Oberg B, Poulsen TD: Obesity: an anaesthetic challenge. Acta Anaesthesiol Scand 1996;40:191-200.

66. Tsueda K, Debrand M, Zeok SS, et al: Obesity supine death syndrome: reports of two morbidly obese patients. Anesth Analg 1979;58:345-347.

67. Brodsky JB: Positioning the morbidly obese patient for anesthesia. Obes Surg 2002;12:751-758.

68. Frappier J, Guenoun T, Journois D, et al: Airway management using the intubating laryngeal mask airway for the morbidly obese patient. Anesth Analg 2003;96:1510-1515.

69. American Society of Anesthesiologists Task Force on Management of the Difficult Airway: Practice guidelines for management of the difficult airway: an updated report. Anesthesiology 2003;98:1269-1227.

70. Blouin RA, Warren GW: Pharmacokinetic considerations in obesity. J Pharm Sci 1999;88:1-7.

71. Abernethy DR, Greenblatt DJ: Drug disposition in obese humans: an update. Clin Pharmacokinet 1986;11:199-213.

72. Wada DR, Bjorkman S, Ebling WF, et al: Computer simulation of the effects of alterations in blood flows and body composition on thiopental pharmacokinetics in humans. Anesthesiology 1997;87: 884-899.

73. Greenblatt DJ, Abernethy DR, Locniskar A, et al: Effect of age, gender, and obesity on midazolam kinetics. Anesthesiology 1984;61:27-35.

74. Wasan KM, Lopez-Berestein G: The influence of serum lipoproteins on the pharmacokinetics and pharmacodynamics of lipophilic drugs and drug carriers. Arch Med Res 1993;24:395-401.

75. Kanto J, Gepts E: Pharmacokinetic implications for the clinical use of propofol. Clin Pharmacokinet 1989;17:308-326.

76. Saijo H, Nagata O, Kitamura T, et al: Anesthetic management of a hyper-obese patient by target-controlled infusion (TCI) of propofol and fentanyl. Masui 2001;50:528-531.

77. Song D, Whitten CW, White PF: Remifentanil infusion facilitates early recovery for obese outpatients undergoing laparoscopic cholecystectomy. Anesth Analg 2000;90:1111-1113.

78. Salihoglu Z, Demiroluk S, Demirkiran, et al: Comparison of effects of remifentanil, alfentanil and fentanyl on cardiovascular responses to tracheal intubation in morbidly obese patients. Eur J Anaesthesiol 2002;19:125-128.

79. Juvin P, Vadam C, Malek L, et al: Postoperative recovery after desflurane, propofol, or isoflurane anesthesia among morbidly obese patients: a prospective, randomized study. Anesth Analg 2000;91:714-719.

80. Salihoglu Z, Karaca S, Kose Y, et al: Total intravenous anesthesia versus single breath technique and anesthesia maintenance with sevoflurane for bariatric operations. Obes Surg 2001;11:496-501.

81. Torri G, Casati A, Comotti L, et al: Wash-in and wash-out curves of sevoflurane and isoflurane in morbidly obese patients. Minerva Anestesiol 2002;68:523-527.

82. Torri G, Casati A, Albertin A, et al: Randomized comparison of isoflurane and sevoflurane for laparoscopic gastric banding in morbidly obese patients. J Clin Anesth 2001;13:565-570.

83. Bentley JB, Vaughan RW, Gandolfi AJ, et al: Halothane biotransformation in obese and nonobese patients. Anesthesiology 1982;57: 94-97.

84. Bentley JB, Vaughan RW, Cork RC, et al: Does evidence of reductive halothane biotransformation correlate with hepatic binding of metabolites in obese patients? Anesth Analg 1981;60:548-551.

85. Miller MS, Gandolfi AJ, Vaughan RW, et al: Disposition of enflurane in obese patients. J Pharmacol Exp Ther 1980;215:292-296.

86. Higuchi H, Satoh T, Arimura S, et al: Serum inorganic fluoride levels in mildly obese patients during and after sevoflurane anesthesia. Anesth Analg 1993;77:1018-1021.

87. Rose JB, Theroux MC, Katz MS: The potency of succinylcholine in obese adolescents. Anesth Analg 2000;90:576-578.

88. Bentley JB, Borel JD, Vaughan RW, et al: Weight, pseudocholinesterase activity, and succinylcholine requirement. Anesthesiology 1982;57:48-49.

89. Weinstein JA, Matteo RS, Ornstein E, et al: Pharmacodynamics of vecuronium and atracurium in the obese surgical patient. Anesth Analg 1988;67:1149-1153.

90. Kirkegaard-Nielsen H, Lindholm P, Petersen HS, et al: Antagonism of atracurium-induced block in obese patients. Can J Anaesth 1998; 45:39-41.

91. Puhringer FK, Keller C, Kleinsasser A, et al: Pharmacokinetics of rocuronium bromide in obese female patients. Eur J Anaesthesiol 1999;16:507-510.

92. Buckley FP: Anesthetizing the Obese Patient: ASA Refresher Courses, pp. 1-6. Philadelphia, Lippincott, 1989.

93. Ramez Salem M, Joseph NJ, Crystal GJ, et al: Preoxygenation: comparison of maximal breathing and tidal volume techniques. Anesthesiology 2000;92:1845-1847.

94. Benumof JL: Preoxygenation: best method for both efficacy and efficiency. Anesthesiology 1999;91:603-605.

95. Esclamado RM, Glenn MG, McCulloch TM, al: Perioperative complications and risk factors in the surgical treatment of obstructive sleep apnea syndrome. Laryngoscope 1998;99:1125-1129.

96. Lang SA, Duncan PG, Shephard DA, et al: Pulmonary oedema associated with airway obstruction. Can J Anaesth 1990;37:210-218.

97. Rawal N, Sjostrand U, Christoffersson E, et al: Comparison of intramuscular and epidural morphine for postoperative analgesia in the grossly obese: influence on postoperative ambulation and pulmonary function. Anesth Analg 1984;63:583-592.

98. Gelman S, Laws HL, Potzick J, et al: Thoracic epidural vs balanced anesthesia in morbid obesity: an intraoperative and postoperative hemodynamic study. Anesth Analg 1980;9:902-908.

99. McCulloch WJ, Littlewood DG: Influence of obesity on spinal analgesia with isobaric 0.5% bupivacaine. Br J Anaesth 1986;58:610-614.

100. Taivainen T, Tuominen M, Rosenberg PH: Influence of obesity on the spread of spinal analgesia after injection of plain 0.5% bupivacaine at the L3-4 or L4-5 interspace. Br J Anaesth 1990;64:542-546.

101. DeRigg JR, Jamrozik K, Myles PS, et al, MASTER Anaesthesia Trial Study Group: Epidural anaesthesia and analgesia and outcome of major surgery: a randomised trial. Lancet 2002;359:1276-1282.

102. Scholz SE, Sticher J, Haufler G, et al: Combination of external chest wall oscillation with continuous positive airway pressure. Br J Anaesth 2001;87:441-446.

103. Joris JL, Sottiaux TM, Chiche JD, et al: Effect of bi-level positive airway pressure (BiPAP) nasal ventilation on the postoperative pulmonary restrictive syndrome in obese patients undergoing gastroplasty. Chest 1997;111:665-670.

104. Marik P, Varon J: The obese patient in the ICU. Chest 1998;113:492-498.

105. Ebeo CT, Benotti PN, Byrd RP Jr: The effect of bi-level positive airway pressure on postoperative pulmonary function following gastric surgery for obesity. Respir Med 2002;96:672-676.

106. Hunter JD, Reid C, Noble D: Anaesthetic management of the morbidly obese patient. Hosp Med (London) 1998;59:481-483.

15

Perioperative Management of the Bariatric Surgery Patient

J. Patrick O'Leary, M.D., John T. Paige, M.D., and Louis F. Martin, M.D.

The rise in the prevalence of obesity has resulted in a concomitant dramatic increase in the number of bariatric procedures performed to help people lose weight and improve the associated comorbid conditions. In 2001, according to the American Society for Bariatric Surgery (ASBS), approximately 47,000 bariatric operations were performed[1]; in 2005, the projected number was 180,000. Proper perioperative management of these challenging patients is essential to ensure successful outcomes, and that requires familiarity with the pathophysiologic consequences of the obese state and their influence on surgical management and with the potential problems associated with each bariatric procedure. This chapter focuses on the immediate preoperative, intraoperative, and postoperative management of the bariatric patient using a systems-based approach and drawing on available evidence-based data.

▶ PREOPERATIVE PREPARATION

The bariatric surgeon must be familiar with the unique challenges presented by the severely obese patient. The metabolic and physical consequences of the obese state increase the likelihood of many associated comorbid conditions that can have a profound influence on the operative management of the patient.[2] Some individuals may even require an extensive preparatory period prior to surgery. A multidisciplinary approach to this preoperative assessment and preparation has long been recognized as an effective means of identifying and improving risk factors and was included as part of the 1991 National Institutes of Health Consensus Development Conference and the 2005 ASBS Consensus Statement recommendations for the operative treatment of obesity.[3,4] In addition to the bariatric surgeon and internist, such a team includes members from many specialties in the allied health professions, including a dedicated nutritionist, clinic nurse specialist, exercise physiologist, psychologist, and social worker.

Preoperative Review

Before proceeding with operative intervention, the bariatric surgeon should undertake a comprehensive review of the patient's preoperative workup using an organ-based approach to ensure that any comorbidities or other risk factors involving surgery have been properly diagnosed and addressed (Table 15-1). Based on findings from this review, the following recommendations may be helpful. From a pulmonary perspective, obstructive sleep apnea (OSA) and obesity hypoventilation syndrome (OHS) are identified via polysomnography and arterial blood gas (ABG) analysis. If present, OSA may be treated with preoperative continuous positive airway pressure (CPAP). OHS is often treated with CPAP, because the daytime awake hypercarbia may be a physiologic consequence of the nighttime-associated OSA. Patients with OHS, however, sometimes require additional noninvasive positive pressure ventilation and, in extreme cases, a tracheostomy may be needed prior to bariatric intervention. All preoperative patients should undergo training in incentive spirometer use, especially those with any pulmonary-function abnormalities. Finally, all patients should have stopped smoking at least 2 weeks prior to surgery.

The cardiovascular workup should be thorough, given the fact that a large proportion of severely obese patients have major risk factors for coronary artery disease due to their increased adiposity and associated comorbid conditions (Table 15-2).[5] All patients should undergo risk stratification using established criteria, with further cardiac stress testing pursued as indicated. Significant coronary artery disease may require revascularization prior to surgery. Hypertension should be adequately controlled with medications, and any heart failure or pulmonary hypertension identified and medically addressed. Finally, treatment of any venous stasis disease should be initiated using elastic compression stockings or wound care as needed.

The increased intraabdominal pressure (IAP) present in severely obese patients is thought to be responsible for

Table 15-1	PREOPERATIVE CHECKLIST	

ORGAN SYSTEM	DIAGNOSTIC TESTING	PREOPERATIVE INTERVENTION
Pulmonary		
Obstructive sleep apnea	Positive polysomnography	Continuous positive airway pressure
Obesity hypoventilation syndrome	ABG with hypercapnia	Noninvasive positive pressure ventilation vs. CPAP vs. tracheostomy with ventilation
Decreased pulmonary function	Positive pulmonary function tests	Incentive spirometry training, conditioning
Tobacco use	Patient history of smoking	Cessation of smoking
Cardiovascular		
Hypertension	SBP >140, DBP >90	Antihypertensives
Heart failure	Physical signs, positive echocardiography	Preload, afterload reduction, diuresis
Pulmonary hypertension	Positive echocardiography	Reversal of hypoxemia
Venous stasis disease, leg ulcers	Physical signs, positive duplex imaging	Elastic compression stockings, wound care
Coronary artery disease	Positive stress test, positive cardiac catheterization	Angioplasty vs. coronary bypass grafting
Gastrointestinal		
Gastrointestinal reflux disease	History, positive 24-hr pH, EGD	Proton pump inhibitors, H2 blocker therapy
Hepatic steatosis	Abnormal liver function tests, ultrasound	Rule out viral hepatitides, cirrhosis
Cholelithiasis/biliary colic	Positive ultrasound, history	Counseling regarding concomitant procedure
Colorectal polyps, cancer	Positive colonoscopy, barium enema	Polypectomy, treatment of cancer (delay procedure)
Renal		
Chronic renal insufficiency	Elevated creatinine , decreased creatinine clearance	Dietary restrictions, management of associated illnesses
Kidney cancer	Hematuria on urinary analysis, positive computed tomography	Treatment of cancer, delay procedure
Endocrine		
Diabetes mellitus	Elevated Hgb A_1c, positive oral glucose tolerance test	Oral antidiabetic medications, insulin
Hypothyroidism	Elevated TSH	Thyroid replacement therapy
Polycystic ovarian disorder	History of amenorrhea, positive ultrasound	Counseling
Cushing syndrome/disease	Dexamethasone testing, ACTH levels	Treatment of underlying cause, delay procedure
Hematologic		
Anemia	Decreased hemoglobin	Oral iron supplements vs. erythropoietin vs. transfusion
Coagulopathy	Elevated prothrombin, partial thromboplastin, bleeding times	Identification and correction of underlying coagulopathy
Deep vein thrombosis	History, positive duplex ultrasound	Anticoagulation (if present), consideration of vena cava filter
Musculoskeletal		
Degenerative joint disease	Positive radiographs, other imaging	Supportive therapy, increase mobility
Spinal vertebral disease	Positive radiographs, other imaging	Supportive therapy, increase mobility, documentation of neurologic impairment
Genitourinary		
Cervix, uterine, ovarian cancer	Positive Pap smear, biopsy, computed tomography	Treatment of cancer, delay procedure
Breast cancer	Physical exam, mammography, positive FNA or biopsy	Treatment of cancer, delay procedure
Prostate cancer	Physical exam, positive PSA, ultrasound biopsy	Treatment of cancer, delay procedure
Psychiatric		
Depression	Positive Beck Depression Inventory, psychiatric evaluation	Antidepressive therapy, counseling
History of abuse	Positive history	Psychological counseling
Personality disorder	Psychiatric evaluation	Psychiatric/psychological counseling
Other psychiatric illness	Psychiatric evaluation	Pharmacotherapy, counseling

ABG, arterial blood gases; ACTH, adrenocortical hormone; CPAP, continuous positive airway pressure; CRI, chronic renal insufficiency; DBP, diastolic blood pressure; EGD, esophagogastroduodenostomy; FNA, fine needle aspiration; GERD, gastroesophageal reflux disease; Hgb A_1c, hemoglobin A_1c; PSA, prostate-specific antigen; SBP, systolic blood pressure; TSH, thyroid stimulating hormone.

numerous comorbid conditions, including gastrointestinal reflux disease (GERD).[6] If symptoms of GERD are severe, further workup with upper endoscopy and 24-hour pH testing should be pursued. Preoperative treatment with proton pump inhibitors or type 2 histamine receptor (H2R) blockers is indicated. Cholelithiasis is commonly encountered in obese patients and should be screened preoperatively via ultrasonography. Steatosis of the liver does not require any preoperative intervention, but care must be taken to rule out

other causes of hepatic disease and to ensure that severe cirrhosis with alterations in liver function is not present. Routine preoperative upper gastrointestinal tract visualization via radiographs or endoscopy is often performed. Advocates argue that it permits identification of abnormalities that would otherwise be missed and helps with preoperative planning.[7] Its necessity, however, has been questioned.[8]

Severely obese patients with longstanding hypertension and diabetes mellitus are at increased risk for

Table 15-2	**MAJOR CORONARY ARTERY DISEASE RISK FACTORS**		

MAJOR RISK FACTOR	MODIFIABLE	ASSOCIATION WITH OBESITY
Increasing age	No	No
Male gender	No	No
Heredity	No	No
Increased cholesterol	Yes	Yes
Hypertension	Yes	Yes
Physical inactivity	Yes	Yes
Diabetes	Yes	Yes
Obesity/overweight	Yes	Yes
Tobacco use	Yes	No

(Adapted from American Heart Association: Risk Factors and Coronary Heart Disease. www.americanheart.org. Accessed, May 20, 2003.)

microvascular injury to the kidneys. As a result, bariatric patients should be screened for chronic renal insufficiency using blood chemistries, and any abnormalities should be pursued with further workup. Patients with renal insufficiency require optimization of kidney function prior to surgery. Candidates with end-stage renal disease require coordination of dialysis perioperatively.

Insulin resistance secondary to the obese state makes diabetes a common comorbid disorder among the severely obese. These patients require preoperative control of their blood glucose levels using oral antidiabetic medications or insulin therapy. When appropriate, biochemical screening for other endocrine abnormalities should be undertaken, especially conditions prone to cause obesity. In particular, Cushing disease and syndrome should be ruled out. If it is present, surgery should be cancelled, and the illness treated appropriately. Also, hypothyroidism should be identified and treated to attain a euthyroid state before surgery. Finally, polycystic ovarian disease may be encountered in the severely obese female patient, but it does not require specific preoperative therapy.

Hematologic disorders, such as anemia or coagulopathies, should be sought through laboratory investigation when indicated by history and physical examination. If present, the cause must be identified and the abnormality corrected. A history of deep vein thrombosis (DVT) or pulmonary embolus (PE) may require preoperative placement of a vena caval filter. Hamad has even advocated such prophylaxis for patients with pulmonary hypertension greater than 40 mmHg or OHS.[9] No consensus, however, exists on whether such aggressive prophylaxis is necessary.

Severely obese patients often have debilitating joint or spinal disk degenerative disease, further impeding their already compromised mobility. Any patient with spinal disease should have documentation of existing neurologic impairments or radiculopathies. These individuals should have adequate supportive therapy for their often painful conditions, and they should try to increase their mobility and activity. All candidates for bariatric surgery should preoperatively start a modest exercise program tailored to their medical limitations. Oftentimes, this entails increasing activity via a pedometer and performing limited aerobic exercises. Such preoperative optimization of conditioning assists in postoperative recovery.

Obesity and overweight are estimated to account for up to a fifth of deaths from cancer in the United States.[10]

Because bariatric surgery is an elective intervention undertaken to improve comorbidities and potentially prolong survival, it is essential that candidates for the procedure be properly screened for the presence of malignancies associated with obesity. Such screening should be based on established recommendations for the particular cancer or pursued with further workup based on abnormal findings in the history and physical examination. Any patient who has been treated for malignancy should undergo further study to ensure that a recurrence is not present. In general, a patient should be disease free for at least 2 years before undergoing bariatric surgery.

Patients with psychiatric disorders must be properly treated before undergoing an operation. Depression is common and can often be identified using a standardized screening instrument like the Beck Depression Inventory, second edition. Preoperative treatment consists of antidepressant therapy and counseling by a mental health professional. Patient with histories of sexual or physical abuse may require counseling, especially if unresolved issues are identified. Finally, patients with severe personality disorders or other psychiatric illnesses should be on appropriate medications, mentally stable, and followed by a mental health professional willing to assist in the patient's postoperative care. Sociopathic or unstable psychiatric behavior may be considered a contraindication to proceeding with operative intervention.

Laparoscopic Versus Open Bariatric Procedures

Bariatric surgery entered the minimally invasive era in 1993 with the first successful adaptation of adjustable gastric banding to laparoscopy.[11] Minimally invasive versions of Roux en Y gastric bypass (RNYGB)[12] and vertical banded gastroplasty (VBG)[13] soon followed. Today, even the biliopancreatic diversion with duodenal switch (BPD/DS) has a laparoscopic equivalent.[14] Such innovations in the bariatric field have contributed to increased demand for operative therapy among the severely obese. Several randomized studies have revealed important differences between the laparoscopic and open bariatric procedures (Table 15-3).[15-18] In general, even though the minimally invasive approach requires a longer operative time, it results in less postoperative pain, a shorter hospital stay, and a quicker return to work. Furthermore, most studies reveal no difference in overall morbidity, and weight loss is equivalent. Every severely obese patient is, therefore, a potential candidate for minimally invasive surgery. Laparoscopic bariatric procedures, however, can be some of the most technically difficult operations in minimally invasive surgery. As a result, such operations should be performed only by surgeons with advanced laparoscopic expertise.

Absolute contraindications to the laparoscopic approach include severe cardiopulmonary disease, including the possibility of creating pneumoperitoneum, that precludes general anesthesia; severe cirrhosis with portal hypertension; and uncorrectable coagulopathy. Relative contraindications include a hostile abdomen secondary to multiple operations; inadequate working space secondary to hepatomegaly or intraabdominal adiposity; and the presence of a massive paraesophageal hernia. Patients who are candidates for minimally invasive surgery must be willing to undergo open conversion if required. Under no

Table 15-3	RANDOMIZED TRIALS COMPARING LAPAROSCOPIC AND OPEN BARIATRIC PROCEDURES				
AUTHORS	TYPE OF PROCEDURE	NUMBER OPEN/NUMBER LAPAROSCOPIC (CONVERSIONS)	ADVANTAGE OF OPEN APPROACH	ADVANTAGE OF LAPAROSCOPIC APPROACH	NO DIFFERENCE BETWEEN APPROACHES
de Wit et al[15]	Adjustable gastric banding	25/25 (2)	1. Decreased operative time 2. Lower degree of difficulty	1. Decreased mean hospital stay 2. Fewer total readmissions 3. Decreased overall hospital stay	1. Weight loss 2. Overall morbidity
Azagra et al[16]	Vertical banded gastroplasty	34/34 (4)	1. Decreased operative time	1. Decreased incisional hernia 2. Decreased wound infections	1. Weight loss 2. Major morbidity 3. Mean hospital stay
Nguyen et al[17]	Gastric bypass	76/79 (2)	1. Decreased operative time 2. Decreased OR costs 3. Decreased late strictures	1. Decreased hospital stay 2. Decreased intraoperative bleeding 3. Decreased hospital costs 4. Sooner return to work 5. Decreased incisional hernia 6. Decreased wound infections	1. Weight loss 2. Overall morbidity 3. Total costs 4. Quality of life at 1 year
Westling, Gustavsson[18]	Gastric bypass	21/30 (7)	1. Decreased Roux limb obstruction	1. Decreased analgesia 2. Decreased hospital stay 3. Decreased sick leave	1. Weight loss 2. Perioperative bleeding

circumstances should a patient be guaranteed that only the laparoscopic approach will be employed.

Informed Consent

Once the patient is deemed fit for operative intervention, the bariatric surgeon should set up an office visit with the candidate near the date of the elective surgery to obtain informed consent for the proposed procedure. During this meeting, the surgeon should give an overview of the procedure, review the mechanisms of weight loss, discuss general outcomes, and describe expected morbidity and mortality rates. Major complications should be discussed in detail, and a risk-benefit analysis should be presented. Liberal use of diagrams and visual aids should be employed, and no assurances as to outcome should be given. At the end of the discussion, the patient should be given an opportunity to ask questions, which should be answered completely. Finally, preoperative instructions should be given. Thorough documentation of the visit should be made, including the topics covered, the approximate time spent with the patient, the individuals present, and the specific medical issues discussed.

Preoperative Diet

Although not essential, all candidates should be encouraged to follow a preoperative diet. Such a diet helps to decrease the degree of difficulty of any operation in two important ways. First, the weight loss associated with the diet decreases abdominal girth and omental size, improving access to the abdomen. Second, the diet helps to reduce hepatic stores of both glycogen and fat. As a result, the left lateral sector of the liver decreases in size, facilitating exposure of the proximal stomach. Such exposure is especially important in laparoscopic bariatric procedures and can mean the difference between successful completion and open conversion. Another advantage of a preoperative diet is that it introduces the patient to the postoperative dietary discipline necessary for successful recovery. Finally, a preoperative diet helps to identify individuals who may have difficulties with compliance and allows for preoperative discussion and intervention.

▶ INTRAOPERATIVE MANAGEMENT

After ensuring that a patient has been adequately evaluated and prepared for surgery, the bariatric surgeon can proceed with operative therapy. The intraoperative management of severely obese patients can be extremely demanding and, as with preoperative preparation, a systematic approach is essential. The surgeon, in close cooperation with an anesthesiologist experienced in bariatric care, must lead a cohesive team of allied health professionals in ensuring that the bariatric patient undergoes the scheduled procedure successfully. This bariatric operative team should include a dedicated surgical technologist, operating room

| Table 15-4 | ACS EQUIPMENT RECOMMENDATIONS FOR OPERATING ROOM |

ACS RECOMMENDATION	AVAILABLE DEVICES	COMPANY	IMPORTANT CHARACTERISTICS	APPROXIMATE LIST COST
Specialized operating room tables and equipment to accommodate morbidly obese patients	Hercules 6500HD table	Skytron	1000 lb limit; 850 lb articulating limit	$40,000 to $45,000
	Maquet Alphamaxx table	Getinge	800 lb limit; 800 lb articulating limit; dual articulating split leg plates	$55,000 to $60,000
Retractors suitable for bariatric surgical procedures	Omnitract BF200 Upper Abdominal Retractor	Minnesota Scientific, Inc.	Three-step setup; unlimited options for blade positioning	$10,000 to $15,000
	Elite II	Thompson Surgical Instruments	Unlimited height adjustment; interchangeable handles for quick changes	$3,000 to $20,000
Specially designed stapling instruments	Endopath ETS Flex45 Articulating Endoscopic Linear Cutter	Ethicon Endo-surgery	Ability to articulate; use in laparoscopy	$2000 (set of 3 with 3 staple loads)
	Endo GIA Universal with 45 roticulator loads	US Surgical	Ability to articulate; use in laparoscopy	$2200 (set of 3 with 6 staple loads)
Appropriately long surgical instruments	Mayo needle holder (14″)	V. Mueller	Extra long length	$200 to $250
	Metzenbaum scissors (14″)			$450 to $500
	Mayo-Hegar needle holder (14″)	Jarit	Extra long length	$200 to $250
	Metzenbaum scissors (14″)			$200 to $250
Other special supplies unique to the procedure	AirPal Lateral Transfer System	AirPal Patient Transfer Systems	Low-pressure air transfer device	$2500 to $3500
	HM43HS Transfer Mattress	HoverTech International	Low pressure air transfer device	$2500 to $3500

nurse circulator, nurse anesthetist, equipment support technologist, and surgical assistant or cosurgeon. All team members should have a thorough understanding of their particular role in the procedure, and a routine system of care should be instituted to support patient safety and team efficiency in the intraoperative environment. Having such a system in place can be very useful when performing complex, technically challenging bariatric procedures. Finally, the bariatric surgeon must have a good working relationship with the hospital administration. Open, interactive communication between the surgeon and administrators allows for identification and correction of any deficiencies that could potentially affect patient care.

Operating Room Environment

Severely obese patients present unique challenges to operative therapy. These patients often exceed the weight limits of typical operating room tables and are frequently too thick for conventional surgical instruments. Their large mass makes even mundane tasks like patient transfer difficult and complicated. The American College of Surgeons recognized the need for specialized facilities in caring for bariatric patients and has developed recommendations toward this end.[19] The operating room environment alone

requires a plethora of specially designed pieces of equipment for surgery in the severely obese patient and, fortunately, a wide variety are currently available (Table 15-4). The cost of these devices, however, can be high. By some estimates, properly fitting an operating room to accommodate bariatric surgery may require $70,000 to $80,000, not to mention the $3500 per case for disposable laparoscopic instruments.[20] The hospital administration, therefore, must be willing to make a concerted effort to provide appropriate amenities for the bariatric surgeon interested in using its facility. Performing bariatric procedures at a hospital that is not properly equipped for such patients is fraught with potentially devastating problems and should be avoided.

Perioperative Prophylaxis

Antibiotics and DVT prophylaxis are two important considerations in the bariatric patient. Like many aspects in the care of these individuals, management is influenced by the physiologic consequences of increased adiposity. Retrospective data have identified obesity as an independent risk factor for infectious complications in both elective and emergent obstetric surgery.[21] A recent multivariate analysis of data collected from three randomized, prospective, multicenter trials on antibiotic prophylaxis in noncolorectal abdominal surgery reached similar conclusions, finding obesity a risk factor for both superficial wounds and global infections.[22] Perioperative antibiotic prophylaxis, therefore, is essential to help reduce an inherent risk in these patients. The increased body mass of a severely obese patient can potentially result in an increased volume of distribution of certain categories of antibiotics, requiring dose adjustment to higher values. Forse and colleagues revealed that β lactams reached inadequate minimal inhibitory concentrations at common dosages in severely obese patients. By doubling the prophylactic dose of cefazolin from 1 to 2 g, they showed that surgical wound infection rates dropped from 16.5% to 5.6%.[23] An earlier study by Mann and Buchwald suggested that cefamandole be administered at 2 g in the severely obese patient and redosed every 3 hours.[24] Such data emphasize the importance of taking into account the increased size of severely obese patients when determining antibiotic dosing.

In a thorough review of the subject, Wurtz and colleagues suggested using the following formula for determining the dosing weight (DW) of antimicrobials: DW = DWCF (ABW–IBW) + IBW, where DWCF is the dosing weight correction factor, ABW is the actual body weight, and IBW is the ideal body weight (based on the Devine formula).[25,26] The DWCF is different for each antimicrobial category, depending on its hydrophilicity and volume of distribution in adipose tissue. β lactams have a DWCF of 0.3 (the water content of adipose tissue), whereas quinolones have a DWCF of 0.45.[26] The bariatric surgeon, therefore, must adjust the dose of a given antibiotic prophylaxis to accommodate for the patient's excess mass, and redosing should occur during prolonged procedures.

In addition to being an independent risk factor for infectious complications following abdominal surgery, obesity is one of the major risk factors for the development of DVT following surgical intervention (Table 15-5).[27] Elevated levels of fibrinogen and plasminogen activator inhibitor as well as antithrombin III deficiency and decreased fibrinolysis are all thought to be possible contributing factors to increased thrombogenesis in the

obese patient.[9] In addition, Nguyen and colleagues demonstrated that the reverse Trendelenburg position increases venous stasis in the femoral veins of patients undergoing gastric bypass.[28] Combined, these facts suggest that the risk for DVT in bariatric patients is rather high, although a recent prospective analysis of 116 patients undergoing gastric bypass using preoperative and postoperative ultrasonography revealed DVT and PE rates of 1.7% and 0.8%, respectively.[29] Nonetheless, adequate prophylaxis is essential in order to minimize the potentially catastrophic complication of PE. No consensus exists, however, on what the proper prophylaxis should be, as demonstrated by a survey of ASBS members. Although over 95% of respondents used some form of DVT prophylaxis, the type employed varied considerably. Unfractionated heparin (UFH) was the most popular preferred prophylaxis, followed by intermittent pneumatic compression (IPC) devices, low-molecular-weight heparin (LMWH), and alternative methods. Furthermore, only 38% of respondents used a combination of prophylactic measures in their practices, the most common being UFH and IPCs.[30]

Most bariatric surgeons, however, do agree that the dosing of LMWH or UFH requires adjustment secondary to increased adiposity and body mass. In a recent prospective analysis of 700 patients undergoing laparoscopic gastric bypass, Shepherd and colleagues used an adjusted-dose UFH protocol based on antifactor Xa levels in volunteers.[31] No DVTs occurred and the PE rate was 0.4%. Therapy was discontinued in 2.3% of patients secondary to bleeding; 1% required transfusions; and minor hematomas were recognized in only 0.6%. IPC devices were used concomitantly. Scholten and colleagues retrospectively looked at 487 bariatric patients receiving either 40 mg or 30 mg of enoxaparin (LMWH) twice a day in conjunction with IPCs, early ambulation, and compression stockings.[32] They found that the thromboembolism rate was lower (0.6% compared to 5.4%) in the group with the higher dosage. Finally, Kalfarentzos and colleagues conducted a randomized trial to show that a daily dose of 5700 IU of nadroparin (LMWH) alone was adequate for prophylaxis.[33] At this dosage, neither adverse bleeding nor a thromboembolic event occurred in the 30 patients undergoing gastric bypass. Nadroparin is not currently available in the United States. Whatever the dosing regimen, given the lack of large-scale trials in the bariatric population, a prudent thromboembolic prophylactic regimen should utilize a combined approach of early ambulation, IPCs, and either UFH or LMWH.

Anesthetic Considerations

Even though an experienced anesthesiologist is an indispensable member of the operative team, the bariatric surgeon should be familiar with aspects of the anesthetic care of the severely obese patient. Patient positioning and monitoring, intubation techniques, anesthetic agents, and comorbidity management all have potentially profound influences on the intraoperative course of the patient. Care must be taken when positioning the patient for operative intervention. The operating room (OR) table should have an adequate weight limit and be able to articulate a severely obese individual without difficulty. A patient is often able

Table 15-5	MAJOR RISK FACTORS FOR THROMBOEMBOLISM AFTER SURGICAL PROCEDURES
RISK FACTOR	**GREATEST RISK**
Increasing age	Greater than 60 years old
Carcinoma	Pancreatic, female reproductive, colorectal, breast, lung, and prostate cancers
Obesity (BMI >30)	Super-severe obesity (BMI >50)
History of DVT or PE	Multiple episodes of DVT or PE
Recent surgical procedures	Hip or knee replacements, pelvic surgery
Hypercoagulable states	Antiphospholipid syndrome, antithrombin III deficiency, protein C and S deficiency, activated protein-C resistance, hyperhomocystinemia

(Adapted from Green RM: The role of prophylactic anticoagulation in the surgical patient. Curr Probl Surg 2003; 40:92-130.)

BMI, body mass index; DVT, deep vein thrombosis; PE, pulmonary embolus.

to transfer voluntarily onto an OR table at the beginning of a case but not at the end. Using a specialized transfer device, such as the air mattresses now available, greatly simplifies this process and decreases the risk of work-associated injury caused by straining during such transfers. Once on an operating table, the patient must be properly secured to ensure that no slippage occurs during the surgery. In addition to an extra-large table strap at the hips, a footrest is used and the feet are placed in the dorsiflexed position to keep the patient in place when in the reverse Trendelenburg position. Some authors advocate the use of a vacuum beanbag to hold the patient in position.[34] Side extensions may be needed for the table, and an extra-thick table pad may be utilized to provide proper cushioning. Adequate padding of all pressure points is essential to prevent compression injuries, and the padding should be used liberally.

The supine position can dramatically alter the mechanical properties of respiration in a sedated, paralyzed, severely obese patient. The weight of the abdominal contents increases IAP, leading to decreased functional residual capacity and pulmonary compliance. In addition, ventilation-perfusion mismatch is increased.[35] The reverse Trendelenburg position can improve respiratory mechanics, increasing both compliance and functional residual capacity.[36] Severely obese patients should, therefore, be placed on the OR table in a slight reverse Trendelenburg or a semirecumbent position. In addition to having an effect on respiratory mechanics, these positions also seem to increase the apneic time to desaturation in severely obese patients after induction of general anesthesia, helping with intubation.[37]

Bariatric patients require the typical anesthetic monitoring necessary for all major abdominal procedures, including continuous pulsoximetry, telemetry, and intermittent blood pressure readings. Given their large limb size, proper blood pressure cuffs must be employed to ensure accurate measurements. In addition to this monitoring, patients with severe cardiopulmonary problems such as pulmonary hypertension or heart failure may require additional invasive monitoring, including pulmonary and peripheral arterial catheters. Finally, proper intravenous access is necessary in order to administer medications and fluids. Frequently, a central venous catheter is required, given the problematic peripheral access that severely obese patients have. Oftentimes, this catheter can be placed after induction of general anesthesia, especially if a temporary peripheral intravenous site can be obtained preoperatively.

The increased adiposity in the upper oropharynx coupled with the altered respiratory mechanics of a severely obese patient make obtaining an airway particularly hazardous. Bariatric patients must be carefully screened to identify individuals who may be at increased risk for difficult intubation. In a prospective study of 100 patients, Brodsky and colleagues developed a useful system of identification based on neck circumference. Larger neck circumference correlated with an increased probability for a problematic intubation. Such a probability was 5% for a neck circumference of 40 cm, but it rose to 35% for a circumference of 60 cm. Furthermore, they showed that no association existed between "problematic" intubation and increasing body mass index.[38] Proper positioning,

adequate mask ventilation, ready access to a fiberbronchoscope, and a low threshold for performing awake intubation all are important components in safely securing an airway in a bariatric patient. A high body mass index, however, does not necessarily preclude intubation via direct laryngoscopy.

General anesthesia can be maintained during bariatric surgery using either intravenous or inhalational agents. In a randomized trial of 36 patients undergoing laparoscopic gastroplasty, desflurane was found to be superior to both propofol and isoflurane in terms of immediate and intermediate postoperative recovery. In particular, patients recovering after desflurane anesthesia had higher oxygen saturations and better mobility.[39] Another randomized trial comparing sevoflurane to intravenous anesthesia in 30 patients demonstrated superior hemodynamic parameters in the sevoflurane group intraoperatively.[40] A comparison of sevoflurane to isoflurane in 90 severely obese patients undergoing BPD showed that the sevoflurane group had faster extubation times and quicker postoperative recovery.[41] Such data suggest that that both desflurane and sevoflurane are acceptable anesthetic agents in the severely obese population because of their quicker postoperative recovery times compared to intravenous anesthetics.

Finally, the bariatric surgeon must work closely with the anesthesiologist or nurse anesthetist to ensure the proper management of a patient's comorbid conditions intraoperatively. Open communication is essential to identify and treat emerging problems. Such work is facilitated by using a systems-based approach focusing on those illnesses identified preoperatively.

Laparoscopic Considerations

Laparoscopic bariatric procedures require a high degree of technical skill for successful completion. In addition to possessing such skill, the bariatric surgeon performing these procedures must be familiar with the physiologic consequences of pneumoperitoneum in the severely obese patient. Carbon dioxide insufflation exacerbates the already elevated IAP. As a result, venous stasis is increased in the femoral veins secondary to vena caval compression, theoretically increasing the risk of DVT.[28] Urine output is decreased due to altered renal blood flow. This decrease, however, is only transient, recovering after release of pneumoperitoneum, and it does not seem to affect renal function.[42]

Respiratory system compliance is decreased due to elevation of the diaphragm, but the clinical significance of this response is minimal.[43] The increase in the IAP, however, does not seem to cause significant hemodynamic alterations.[44] Overall, the creation of pneumoperitoneum can cause subtle changes in the physiologic function of the severely obese patient that might be misinterpreted by an uninformed bariatric surgeon. One must be aware of these changes and understand that their effects are typically transient. At times, patients can develop dramatic vagal responses due to the stretching of the peritoneum as a result of the insufflation of carbon dioxide. In these situations, the pneumoperitoneum should be immediately released as part of the overall therapy.

Recognizing the appropriate time to provide better intraabdominal access during a laparoscopic procedure is as important as possessing the technical skills to perform one. Options include increasing the number of trocar sites, placing a hand port, and converting to a traditional open approach. An extra trocar may be useful to allow retraction of recessed tissues or provide access for difficult suturing. A hand port is useful in situations where tactile feedback is needed and is a helpful adjunct during a surgeon's initial laparoscopic learning curve. The hand-assisted technique, however, has a complication profile similar to that of the open approach and is more expensive in terms of hospital costs.[45] Indications for open conversion include uncontrollable hemorrhage, major intraoperative complication requiring repair, failure to progress, and inadequate working space.

Technical Considerations

Patients who undergo open bariatric procedures are at high risk for wound complications postoperatively. A randomized controlled trial of 331 bariatric patients undergoing such operations demonstrated the superiority of continuous fascial closure compared to interrupted fascial closure. In this study, patients who underwent continuous closure had a deep wound complication rate of only 3%. In contrast, the rate was 15% among patients randomized to interrupted fascial closure.[46] Subcutaneous drainage using a closed suction device also appears to decrease infection rates in severely obese patients. A randomized controlled trial comparing various techniques of wound closure after cesarean section in 76 obese women revealed a substantially increased relative risk of wound infection (10.2%) in patients without subcutaneous drain placement.[47] A continuous fascial closure coupled with subcutaneous closed suction drainage, therefore, would seem prudent to help mitigate the risk of wound infection following open bariatric operations.

▶ POSTOPERATIVE RECOVERY

Upon successful completion of a bariatric procedure, the surgeon must begin the demanding task of overseeing the postoperative recovery of the severely obese patient. Such work, like all other aspects of the care of the bariatric patient, requires the coordination of a team of allied health professionals familiar with the particular requirements of this patient population. In addition to the surgeon and medical specialists (pulmonary, cardiology, critical care, internal medicine, endocrine, and radiology), this team should include dedicated nutritionists, physical therapists, nursing staff (postanesthesia care unit [PACU], intensive care, and ward), pharmacists, and transport personnel. All members must work in close collaboration to help avoid or overcome potentially difficult postoperative problems.

Hospital Environment

Much like the OR, the rest of the hospital must be adequately equipped to handle severely obese patients. Specialized bariatric beds, wheelchairs, transfer equipment, and monitoring devices must be available. In addition, the fluoroscopy units and computed tomography scanners in the radiology department should be able to accommodate bariatric patients. Properly fitting gowns should be plentiful. Enlarged doorways, ward rooms, and bathrooms are essential. Finally, floor-mounted toilet and shower seats help to avoid embarrassing and sometimes injurious falls that can occur if the facility separates from the wall. Without such amenities, the postoperative care of the bariatric patient can be severely impeded, leading to often devastating results. The creation of a dedicated bariatric postoperative ward incorporating many of these recommendations is ideal, but such an endeavor is unlikely without substantial backing from the hospital administration. A close working relationship between administrators and bariatric surgeons is imperative, therefore, in order to create an accommodating and safe postoperative environment for the bariatric patient.

Postoperative Triage

Most bariatric patients proceed directly to the general surgical ward following a brief recovery in the PACU. Some patients, however, require closer monitoring in either a step-down unit (SDU) or an intensive care unit (ICU). The decision to triage a postoperative bariatric patient to any one of these settings depends on many variables, including the number and severity of concomitant comorbidities, the length and difficulty of the operation, and the immediate postoperative respiratory status. Levi and associates have developed a triage system that divides patients into four classes based on age, important comorbidities, and respiratory problems. Class I patients (those under 40 years of age and without major comorbidities or respiratory problems) typically go directly to the general surgical ward after the PACU, whereas class IV patients (those with syndrome X, pulmonary hypertension, DVT/PE, pseudotumor cerebri, or chronic respiratory failure) always proceed to the ICU. The majority of class II (those between 40 and 50 years of age, with diabetes, venous insufficiency, asthma, or snoring) and class III (those older than 50 years, with a history of DVT/PE, immobility, OSA, OHS, or hypoxemia) invariably spend time in the SDU.[48] Another program reserves the SDU and ICU for patients with high-risk comorbidities, intraoperative complications, or failure to extubate.[49] Whatever triage system is employed, severely obese patients with any respiratory or cardiac comorbidities are best served with continuous oxygen saturation monitoring and telemetry in the early postoperative period. Such monitoring will alert the clinician to potential cardiopulmonary problems before they become severe, allowing timely intervention.

Routine Postoperative Care

The routine postoperative care of the bariatric patient has several important features and requires close cooperation between the surgeon and members of the postoperative team. Comorbidities should be managed using a systems-based approach addressing the conditions identified in the preoperative preparation. Patients with OSA or OHS should continue on their nocturnal CPAP therapy. Oftentimes, it is easier to have these individuals bring in their own calibrated machines from home for use in the perioperative period. Hypertension should initially be managed on an as-needed basis using intravenous medications. Once liquid intake is initiated, the patient can be transitioned to oral antihypertensives. Care must be taken to convert extended-release medications to their more frequently dosed short-acting equivalents because most medications must be crushed or mixed with food to prevent gastric outlet obstruction after most procedures. Any heart failure or pulmonary hypertension should be aggressively treated with appropriate therapies. GERD is oftentimes cured following bariatric intervention but, if necessary, intravenous followed by oral therapy using proton pump inhibitors or H2R blockers can be helpful. Diabetics are initially managed with subcutaneous regular insulin injections following a sliding scale based on periodic finger-stick glucose measurements. This therapy can be transitioned to oral antidiabetics, but oftentimes, especially after RNYGB, these individuals will achieve euglycemia almost immediately following their procedure. Pharmacologic control of diabetes, therefore, is frequently not necessary.

Thyroid replacement therapy should be continued without interruption in patients with hypothyroidism. Any coagulopathies should be corrected using appropriate blood products, and DVT prophylaxis should be continued until discharge. Finally, psychiatric medications should be given orally as soon as the patient is able to tolerate such intake. Some concomitant illnesses, such as seizure disorders, require continuous medical therapy in order to prevent unwanted sequelae.

Unrecognized complications occurring in the immediate postoperative period after bariatric procedures can have devastating consequences. Prompt identification and treatment of complications, therefore, require a high index of suspicion. The diagnosis and treatment of specific complications are addressed in the subsequent section, but a few comments regarding routine postoperative studies are appropriate. All postoperative bariatric patients should have a complete blood count on the first post operative day in order to detect anemia secondary to hemorrhage. In addition, a basic blood chemistry analysis, although not required, should be obtained at the same time to detect any electrolyte, glucose, or renal abnormalities. Further blood chemistry analysis should be based on specific associated comorbid conditions in individual patients.

Perhaps the most controversial topic is the routine use of postoperative contrast studies following bariatric procedures. Several recent studies, both prospective and retrospective, have examined their utility and cost-effectiveness, and conclusions have differed. One large review in Italy examined 413 patients who had undergone a variety of bariatric procedures with routine early contrast studies.[50] Complications ranging from stomal stenosis to postoperative leak were identified in 8.2%. Two patients required reoperation. The authors concluded that routine radiologic study was useful and modified clinical care.

A prospective study of 100 consecutive patients undergoing RNYGB with postoperative contrast swallow study reached a similar conclusion.[51] A large prospective review in Austria of 350 patients undergoing laparoscopic adjustable gastric banding with postoperative radiologic study reached a different conclusion.[52] Early pouch dilatations were found in 1.8%, whereas stomach perforation occurred in 1.2%. All complications occurred during the first 100 cases, and no further abnormalities were noted in the last 250 patients. The authors concluded that routine contrast studies were not necessary in centers that had broad experience, thus decreasing both hospital costs and radiation exposure to the patient. Finally, a retrospective review from Las Vegas of 242 randomly selected, open RNYGB patients undergoing routine postoperative contrast studies calculated a positive predictive value of only 27%.[53] The authors recommended that upper gastrointestinal studies be reserved for patients with clinically suspicious signs. Clearly, no consensus exists regarding the routine use of contrast studies following bariatric procedures. A prudent course would suggest performing such tests during a surgeon's initial learning curve and adopting a more selective approach after considerable clinical experience has been gained.

Adequate pain management following a bariatric procedure is essential to allow mobilization of the severely obese patient. Narcotics are most often employed in the immediate postoperative period. Multiple modalities are available for such care, ranging from nurse-administered suspensions to epidural infusions. Perhaps the most useful approach is intravenous patient controlled analgesia followed by conversion to a nurse-administered liquid oral agent when the patient is able to tolerate one. The bariatric surgeon must be cognizant of the potential for a high degree of tolerance in these postoperative patients, because many have been taking chronic narcotics for debilitating joint and back conditions. The increased body mass of these severely obese patients may also alter drug dosage. A continuous-infusion patient-controlled analgesia with bolus-demand dosing, therefore, may be necessary to provide adequate relief. In addition, narcotics may have to be supplemented with other analgesics, such as local anesthetics or nonsteroidal antiinflammatory drugs. Injection of bupivacaine at the incision sites during a laparoscopic procedure is helpful in reducing postoperative pain. The use of a continuous infusion of local anesthetic at incision sites using the newer slow-release bulb devices can also assist in decreasing immediate postoperative pain. Finally, intravenous or intramuscular administration of the nonsteroidal antiinflammatory drug ketorolac is especially useful in supplementing pain control, but its use should be limited to 72 hours in patients without renal problems. Laparoscopic procedures have been shown to result in less postoperative pain than open procedures, in many instances.[54-56]

Early mobilization of the severely obese patient plays an important role in helping to prevent respiratory and thrombogenic complications in the early postoperative period. Ambulation should begin within hours of the procedure in the stable patient. If ambulation is not immediately possible, mobilization to a chair is performed. Such aggressive return to activity requires close coordination between nursing staff members and the physical therapist. In addition to mobilization, the bariatric patient should receive education regarding exercises and activity when discharged to home. Such counseling prepares the patient for a new emphasis on physical well-being following bariatric intervention.

All bariatric patients must immediately cope with their altered relationship to food after surgical treatment. Limited oral intake of low-fat, low-sugar liquids should be started once the surgeon is satisfied that the patient does not have a complication that would preclude enteral feeding (postoperative leak, delayed emptying, or obstruction). This intake is increased at a predetermined rate with concomitant decrease of intravenous fluid administration.

▶ EARLY POSTOPERATIVE COMPLICATIONS

Early postoperative complications can be divided into two broad categories: (1) complications common to operative intervention in the bariatric population in general and (2) complications unique to specific bariatric interventions.

General Complications

Like any abdominal procedure, bariatric interventions carry the risk for certain complications inherent in undergoing operative therapy. These risks are often best classified using a systems-based approach. Respiratory distress can occur at any time following operative intervention. The primary concern for the bariatric surgeon is to provide adequate supportive care using supplemental oxygenation, nebulizer therapy and, if need be, ventilator support while attempting to identify the cause of the problem. Severely obese patients have poorer respiratory mechanics in the supine position, so any postoperative bariatric patient in respiratory distress should be placed in a reverse Trendelenburg position in order to improve airflow and decrease IAP from abdominal girth. Initial workup after a careful physical examination should include a blood gas analysis and chest radiograph. Potential causes of respiratory distress immediately following a bariatric procedure include hypoventilation secondary to oversedation or incomplete emergence from anesthesia; pneumothorax (especially following a laparoscopic procedure); asthmatic episode; pulmonary embolus; and laryngeal edema. Patients who develop distress in the surgical ward may be experiencing oversedation, pulmonary edema, asthmatic episodes, pulmonary embolus, large pleural effusion, acute respiratory distress syndrome, severe atelectasis, lobar collapse, or pneumonia.

Certain pulmonary complications bear further comment. Severely obese patients are likely to have atelectasis following general anesthesia in the supine position. Clinical examination and radiography of the chest are usually sufficient to diagnose this condition, and therapy consists of aggressive mobilization, incentive spirometry use, and nebulizer therapy. If not properly treated, persistent alveolar collapse can lead to pneumonia. Pneumothorax can occur in patients after laparoscopy, especially after perihiatal and diaphragmatic dissection. This condition may manifest itself by increased peak inspiratory pressures and difficulty with patient ventilation during an operation, and it is often improved by decreasing the pneumoperitoneum pressures. Rarely, decompression is necessary. In the postoperative period, patients may present with decreased oxygenation in the PACU with lack of breath sounds on the affected side. Radiography of the chest can confirm the diagnosis. Finally, patients may develop sympathetic effusions which, if large, can affect respiration. Physical examination and radiography of the chest often lead to the diagnosis. Thoracentesis is indicated for clinically significant effusions unresponsive to noninvasive therapy.

Postoperative hypotension can occur following bariatric interventions. Intravascular depletion secondary to third-spacing or hemorrhage is the most common cause. Physical findings of volume depletion include decreased urine output and persistent tachycardia. A complete blood count should be obtained to determine whether the hemoglobin is decreased. Volume resuscitation is the mainstay of therapy, using crystalloid at first, with progression to colloids and transfusions, as dictated by the patient's clinical response. The bariatric surgeon, however, must also entertain the possibility of cardiogenic hypotension. Acute coronary syndrome (ACS) or heart failure is a possible cause. Patients with ACS present with chest pressure or pain. Diagnosis is made by electrocardiogram and serial cardiac enzymes. Initial therapy includes pain control through narcotics, aspirin therapy, and sublingual nitroglycerin. In the immediate postoperative period, patients with ACS require cardiac catheterization for further therapy, because the risk for bleeding as a result of thrombolytic therapy is too high. Heart failure often presents with pulmonary edema, usually resulting from volume overload. Supportive treatment with afterload reduction and diuresis is essential. Postoperative arrhythmias, usually atrial fibrillation or atrial flutter secondary to fluid overload, are diagnosed by electrocardiogram and treated according to advanced cardiac life support protocols. PE can often manifest as cardiovascular collapse. These patients require aggressive hemodynamic support with either anticoagulation or caval filter placement. Diagnosis can be made using Doppler ultrasonography of the lower extremities, ventilation-perfusion scintigraphy, helical computed tomography, or pulmonary angiography. Finally, some patients may develop hypertensive crises. If inadequate pain control is present, analgesia should be adjusted. Severe crises with clinical signs of headache or neurologic disorders require computed tomography of the head and aggressive treatment using intravenous antihypertensive medications.

Prolonged ileus or delayed gastric emptying may occur following operative intervention. Vagal denervation, especially during RNYGB or VBG, can occur. The large-sleeve gastrectomy performed during BPD/DS can potentially cause some delay in gastric emptying. RNYGB and BPD/DS are more likely to cause ileus, given their more extensive character and enteroenterostomies. Patients should be supported with intravenous fluids, and parenteral nutrition should be instituted if the condition continues.

Renal insufficiency in the postoperative period is commonly secondary to intravascular depletion. Volume resuscitation can correct the problem. If creatinine elevation is persistent, further workup through 24-hour urine collection and determination of fractional excretion of sodium and creatinine clearance should be undertaken. Therapy should be geared toward the cause of the insufficiency (whether prerenal, renal, or postrenal). Patients in acute renal failure should undergo dialysis for metabolic acidosis, hyperkalemia, or volume overload. Electrolyte and acid-base abnormalities can occur following bariatric procedures. For example, metabolic acidosis can result from the administration of normal saline intraoperatively. Serum chemistry analysis permits identification of the specific electrolyte abnormality. Therapy consists of repletion or adjustment of the specific component.

Postoperative hemorrhage is always a concern in the bariatric patient. The stomach has a rich blood supply, and many procedures involve dissection close to the spleen, increasing the potential for intraabdominal bleeding. Additionally, gastrointestinal bleeding can occur at the sites of anastomoses. Such bleeding usually occurs toward the end of the first postoperative week, but it should remain part of the differential diagnosis of perioperative hemorrhage. As discussed earlier, decreased urine output, persistent tachycardia, hypotension, and decreased hemoglobin levels suggest the diagnosis. Oftentimes, nonoperative therapy is possible using volume resuscitation and transfusion support. Patients who are hemodynamically unstable or require multiple transfusions, however, need reexploration, hematoma evacuation, and creation of hemostasis.

Rhabdomyolysis can occur in the severely obese patient undergoing operative therapy.[57] A high index of suspicion is needed to assist in diagnosis. Parathesias and pain are presenting signs. Diagnosis is made by checking serum creatine phosphokinase, serum creatinine, and urine myoglobin. Therapy centers on alkalinization of the urine and fluid support to prevent renal failure. Neuropraxias can also occur in the improperly positioned severely obese patient.[58] Diagnosis is apparent from clinical signs in the postoperative period. Physical therapy and splinting are employed as needed.

Common postoperative infectious complications include pneumonia, urinary tract infection, wound infection, intraabdominal abscess, and central line infection. Cultures should be obtained and appropriate antibiotic therapy initiated. Wound infections and intraabdominal abscesses require drainage. Infected central lines must be removed and alternative access obtained.

Patients may have exacerbation of depression or psychiatric illnesses following bariatric procedures. Diagnosis is usually apparent on clinical evaluation. As mentioned earlier, antidepressant therapy should be continued in the immediate postoperative period. Psychotic episodes should be treated with antipsychotics after ensuring that their cause is not due to a physiologic abnormality.

Complications Unique to Specific Bariatric Procedures

Each bariatric procedure has early postoperative complications unique to it. These considerations are covered in subsequent chapters.

▶ SUMMARY

The perioperative care of the bariatric patient can be challenging, yet rewarding. The bariatric surgeon must lead a team of allied health professionals in the preoperative, intraoperative, and postoperative setting to ensure the effective, safe treatment of the severely obese patient undergoing bariatric interventions. Familiarity with all aspects of the perioperative care of the patient and the use of a systems-based approach to manage comorbidities and complications help the bariatric surgeon to address successfully the multiple issues involved. In this manner, the severely obese patient can undergo a life-changing bariatric procedure in a supportive environment while receiving the best possible care.

▶ REFERENCES

1. Mitka M: Surgery for obesity: demand soars amid scientific, ethical questions. JAMA 2003;289:1761-1762.
2. Kral J: Morbidity of severe obesity. Surg Clin North Am 2001; 81:1039-1061.
3. National Institutes of Health Consensus Development Panel: Gastrointestinal surgery for severe obesity. Ann Intern Med 1991; 115:956-961.
4. Buchwald H, Consensus Conference Panel: Bariatric surgery for morbid obesity: health implications for patients, health professionals, and third-party payers. J Am Coll Surg 2005;200(4):593-604.
5. American Heart Association: Risk factors and coronary heart disease. http://www.americanheart.org/presenter.jhtml?identifier=539. Accessed, May 20, 2003.
6. Sugerman HJ: Effects of increased intra-abdominal pressure in severe obesity. Surg Clin North Am 2001; 81:1063-1075.
7. Frigg A, Peterli R, Zynamon A, et al: Radiologic and endoscopic evaluation for laparoscopic adjustable gastric banding: preoperative and follow-up. Obes Surg 2001; 11:594-599.
8. Ghassemian AJ, MacDonald KG, Cunningham PG, et al: The workup for bariatric surgery does not require a routine upper gastrointestinal series. Obes Surg 1997;7:16-18.
9. Hamad GG: Prophylaxis of venous thromboembolism in morbidly obese patients. In DeMaria EJ, Latifi R, Sugerman HJ (eds). Laparoscopic Bariatric Surgery: Techniques and Outcomes, pp. 38-44. Georgetown, Tex., Landes Bioscience, 2002.
10. Calle EE, Rodriguez C, Walker-Thurmond K, et al: Overweight, obesity, and mortality from cancer in a prospectively studied cohort of U.S. adults. N Engl J Med 2003; 348:1625-1638.
11. Belachew M, Legrand MJ, Defechereux TH, et al: Laparoscopic adjustable silicone gastric banding in the treatment of morbid obesity: a preliminary report. Surg Endosc 1994; 8:1354-1356.
12. Wittgrove AC, Clark GW, Tremblay LJ: Laparoscopic gastric bypass, Roux-en-Y: preliminary report of five cases. Obes Surg 1994; 4:353-357.
13. Cadiere GB, Bruyns J, Himpens J, et al: Laparoscopic gastroplasty for morbid obesity. Br J Surg 1994;81:15–24.
14. Ren CJ, Patterson E, Gagner M: Early results of laparoscopic biliopancreatic diversion with duodenal switch: a case series of 40 consecutive patients. Obes Surg 2000;10:514-523.
15. de Wit LT, Mathus-Vliegen L, Hey C, et al: Open versus laparoscopic adjustable silicone gastric banding: a prospective randomized trial for treatment of morbid obesity. Ann Surg 1999; 230:800-805.
16. Azagra JS, Goergen M, Ansay J, et al: Laparoscopic gastric reduction surgery: preliminary results of a randomized, prospective trial of laparoscopic vs open vertical banded gastroplasty. Surg Endosc 1999; 13:555-558.
17. Nguyen NT, Goldman C, Rosenquist CJ, et al: Laparoscopic versus open gastric bypass: a randomized study of outcomes, quality of life, and costs. Ann Surg 2001;234:279-289.
18. Westling A, Gustavsson S: Laparoscopic vs open Roux-en-Y gastric bypass: a prospective, randomized trial. Obes Surg 2001;11:284-292.
19. Recommendations for facilities performing bariatric surgery. Bull Am Coll Surg 2000;85:20-23.
20. Patterson P: Surgery for the morbidly obese requires a special commitment. OR Manager 2002;18:7-9, 12.
21. Myles TD, Gooch J, Santolaya J: Obesity as an independent risk factor for infectious morbidity in patients who undergo cesarean delivery. Obstet Gynecol 2002;100:959-964.
22. Pessaux P, Msika S, Atalla D, et al: Risk factors for postoperative infectious complications in noncolorectal abdominal surgery: a multivariate analysis based on a prospective multicenter study of 4718 patients. Arch Surg 2003;138:314-324.

23. Forse RA, Karam B, MacLean LD, et al: Antibiotic prophylaxis for surgery in morbidly obese patients. Surgery 1989;106:750-756.

24. Mann HJ, Buchwald H: Cefamandole distribution in serum, adipose tissue, and wound drainage in morbidly obese patients. Drug Intell Clin Pharm 1986;20:869-873.

25. Devine BJ: Gentamicin therapy. Drug Intell Clin Pharm 1974;8:650-655.

26. Wurtz R, Itokazu G, Rodvold K: Antimicrobial dosing in obese patients. Clin Infect Dis 1997;25:112-118.

27. Green RM: The role of prophylactic anticoagulation in the surgical patient. Curr Probl Surg 2003;40:92-130.

28. Nguyen NT, Cronan M, Braley S, et al: Duplex ultrasound assessment of femoral venous flow during laparoscopic and open gastric bypass. Surg Endosc 2003;17:285-290.

29. Westling A, Bergqvist D, Bostrom A, et al: Incidence of deep venous thrombosis in patients undergoing obesity surgery. World J Surg 2002;26:470-473.

30. Wu EC, Barba CA: Current practices in the prophylaxis of venous thromboembolism in bariatric surgery. Obes Surg 2000;10:7-13.

31. Shepherd MF, Rosborough TK, Schwartz ML: Heparin thromboprophylaxis in gastric bypass surgery. Obes Surg 2003;13:249-253.

32. Scholten DJ, Hoedema RM, Scholten SE: A comparison of two different prophylactic dose regimens of low molecular weight heparin in bariatric surgery. Obes Surg 2002;12:19-24.

33. Kalfarentzos F, Stavropoulou F, Yarmenitis S, et al: Prophylaxis of venous thromboembolism using two different doses of low-molecular-weight heparin (nadroparin) in bariatric surgery: a prospective randomized trial. Obes Surg 2001;11:670-676.

34. Ogunnaike BO, Jones SB, Jones DB, et al: Anesthetic considerations for bariatric surgery. Anesth Analg 2002;95:1793-1805.

35. Pelosi P, Croci M, Ravagnan I, et al: Respiratory system mechanics in sedated, paralyzed, morbidly obese patients. J Appl Physiol 1997;82:811-818.

36. Perilli V, Sollazzi L, Bozza P, et al: The effects of the reverse Trendelenburg position on respiratory mechanics and blood gases in morbidly obese patients during bariatric surgery. Anesth Analg 2000;91:1520-1525.

37. Boyce JR, Ness T, Castroman P, et al: A preliminary study of the optimal anesthesia positioning for the morbidly obese patient. Obes Surg 2003;13:4-9.

38. Brodsky JB, Lemmens HJ, Brock-Utne JG, et al: Morbid obesity and tracheal intubation. Anesth Analg 2002;94:732-736.

39. Juvin P, Vadam C, Malek L, et al: Postoperative recovery after desflurane, propofol, or isoflurane anesthesia among morbidly obese patients: a prospective, randomized study. Anesth Analg 2000;91:714-719.

40. Salihoglu Z, Karaca S, Kose Y, et al: Total intravenous anesthesia versus single breath technique and anesthesia maintenance with sevoflurane for bariatric operations. Obes Surg 2001;11:496-501.

41. Sollazzi L, Perilli V, Modesti C, et al: Volatile anesthesia in bariatric surgery. Obes Surg 2001;11:623-626.

42. Nguyen NT, Perez RV, Fleming N, et al: Effect of prolonged pneumoperitoneum on intraoperative urine output during laparoscopic gastric bypass. J Am Coll Surg 2002;195:476-483.

43. Sprung J, Whalley DG, Falcone T, et al: The impact of morbid obesity, pneumoperitoneum, and posture on respiratory system mechanics and oxygenation during laparoscopy. Anesth Analg 2002;94:1345-1350.

44. Casati A, Comotti L, Tommasino C, et al: Effects of pneumoperitoneum and reverse Trendelenburg position on cardiopulmonary function in morbidly obese patients receiving laparoscopic gastric banding. Eur J Anaesthesiol 2000;17:300-305.

45. DeMaria EJ, Schweitzer MA, Kellum JM, et al: Hand-assisted laparoscopic gastric bypass does not improve outcome and increases costs when compared to open gastric bypass for the surgical treatment of obesity. Surg Endosc 2002;16:1452-1455.

46. Derzie AJ, Silvestri F, Liriano E, et al: Wound closure technique and acute wound complications in gastric surgery for morbid obesity: a prospective randomized trial. J Am Coll Surg 2000;191:238-243.

47. Allaire AD, Fisch J, McMahon MJ: Subcutaneous drain vs. suture in obese women undergoing cesarean delivery: a prospective, randomized trial. J Reprod Med 2000;45:327-331.

48. Levi D, Goodman ER, Patel M, et al: Critical care of the obese and bariatric surgical patient. Crit Care Clin 2003;19:11-32.

49. Davidson JE, Callery C: Care of the obesity surgery patient requiring immediate-level care or intensive care. Obes Surg 2001;11:93-97.

50. Toppino M, Cesarani F, Comba A, et al: The role of early radiological studies after gastric bariatric surgery. Obes Surg 2001;11:447-454.

51. Serafini F, Anderson W, Ghassemi P, et al: The utility of contrast studies and drains in the management of patients after Roux-en-Y gastric bypass. Obes Surg 2002;12:34-38.

52. Nehoda H, Hourmont K, Mittermair R, et al: Is a routine liquid contrast swallow following laparoscopic gastric banding mandatory? Obes Surg 2001;11:600-604.

53. Singh R, Fisher BL: Sensitivity and specificity of postoperative upper GI series following gastric bypass. Obes Surg 2003;13:73-75.

54. Trondsen E, Reiertsen O, Andersen OK, et al: Laparoscopic and open cholecystectomy: a prospective, randomized study. Eur J Surg 1993;159:217-221.

55. Weeks JC, Nelson H, Gelber S, et al: Short-term quality-of-life outcomes following laparoscopic-assisted colectomy vs open colectomy for colon cancer: a randomized trial. JAMA 2002;287:321-328.

56. Nilsson G, Larsson S, Johnsson F: Randomized clinical trial of laparoscopic versus open fundoplication: blind evaluation of recovery and discharge period. Br J Surg 2000;87:873-878.

57. Bostanjian D, Anthone GJ, Hamoui N, et al: Rhabdomyolysis of gluteal muscles leading to renal failure: a potentially fatal complication of surgery in the morbidly obese. Obes Surg 2003;13:302-305.

58. Warner MA, Warner ME, Martin JT: Ulnar neuropathy: incidence, outcome, and risk factors in sedated or anesthetized patients. Anesthesiology 1994;81:1332-1340.

16

Postoperative Care of the Bariatric Surgery Patient

Joseph D. DiRocco, M.D., John D. Halverson, M.D., Jessica Planer, R.D., C.D.N.,
Marguerite Walser, F.N.P., and Paul R. G. Cunningham, M.D.

The adequacy of routine postoperative patient care following a bariatric procedure depends upon whether patient selection has been appropriate (relative to overall health and likelihood of compliance with diet and with postoperative instructions); whether preoperative behavioral training in proper dietary regimen has occurred; whether the appropriate operation has been chosen for the patient; whether the patient and procedure have successfully survived the perioperative period; and whether the patient maintains long-term follow-up.

Postoperative care of the morbidly obese patient is an ongoing process that is carried on indefinitely and that is conducted in the context of continued support by the patient's primary caregivers. Follow-up must involve the long-term commitment of surgeons, nutritionists, nurse practitioners, radiologists, gastroenterologists, exercise physiologists, and other health care providers with special training and experience. It is particularly important that the surgeon, as leader of the team, be highly motivated and fastidious in demonstrating to patients and staff alike the importance of long-term follow-up in achieving both good weight-loss results and avoidance of metabolic complications.

The ability of the bariatric surgeon to care effectively for a postoperative patient can be greatly enhanced by proper preoperative preparation of the patient. This includes both dietary training and optimal procedure selection, each of which is integral to the effort to lose weight. For example, all bariatric operations place certain requirements for eating behavior upon the patient and, for follow-up, upon the bariatric team. In the case of an operation with a significant restrictive component, modification of the speed and quantity of oral intake is critical to a good weight result, and failure to make necessary behavior changes will result not only in inappropriate weight loss but also in a sick, often vomiting patient. If a malabsorptive operation is done, it is essential that a patient participate in long-term follow-up, including blood testing, in order to avoid the nutritional complications that may ensue. In either case, compliance is critical, and patients failing to exhibit preoperative understanding and compliance should probably be rejected for surgery.

▶ GUIDELINES FOR FOLLOW-UP OF POSTOPERATIVE PATIENTS

The goal of postoperative follow-up is to evaluate outcomes and to assess the patient for postoperative complications, as well as to provide patient education and support. Immediately postoperatively, patients should be seen as needed (wound checks, suture removal, weigh-in, dietician support, and so forth). It is likely that patients will come from a distance, and the rapport and bonding that take place with the bariatric care team in the preoperative phase will become invaluable in patients' postoperative care. Many times, phone calls to patients who are comfortable with their established relationships with the professional team can eliminate unnecessary concern and, occasionally, significant mishaps.

During the first postoperative year, patients should be seen at least every 3 months. At each visit, a nutrition history should be obtained, and any symptoms or problems the patients have should be evaluated by the appropriate members of the bariatric team. Because improvements in arterial hypertension and glucose handling predictably occur soon after operation, follow-up should include monitoring of these parameters, and regular communication with the patients' primary care physicians should take place. Further, assessing patients for the development of nutrition deficiencies should be carried out. Typically, serum hemoglobin, hematocrit, vitamin B_{12}, folate, thiamine (or erythrocyte transketolase), and iron and total iron-binding capacity should be measured at the 6-month and 1-year intervals and yearly thereafter, unless deficiencies occur.

In the absence of any apparent complication, the frequency of visits may decrease to twice during the second year and annually thereafter. Lifelong follow-up is necessary because this is the only reliable means of ensuring a long-term positive outcome. And only with long-term follow-up can we make valid conclusions regarding outcomes.

Follow-up in the bariatric clinic should be a multidisciplinary effort, and patients should have easy access to the nurse practitioner and surgeon as well as to the dietician and support-group staff. In addition, an exercise physiologist and psychotherapist familiar with the problems experienced by bariatric surgery patients should be available. Most important, nutritional, psychological, and exercise counseling should be coordinated and tailored to suit each individual.

The intensity of this follow-up is greater than that for average surgical patients, but the needs of these patients are subtle, if not unique, and are not well known to most primary care physicians. Further, the increased likelihood of vitamin and mineral deficiencies and actual protein-calorie malnutrition (in the case of the more malabsorptive procedures) make this level of follow-up essential. Although there is no actual proof that closer follow-up leads to better weight loss, the opportunity for the bariatric team to interact with the patient regarding dietary intake probably increases the likelihood of compliance and therefore is more likely to lead to satisfactory weight loss. In addition, the surgical procedures result in profound life changes, some of which continue to require emotional adjustment and professional support.

▶ POSTOPERATIVE DIETARY BEHAVIORAL MODIFICATION

Hereditary factors, endocrine status (metabolic rate), and exercise all influence an individual's weight, but only calories are stored as fat, and only deprivation of calories (relative to the body's daily need) will result in decease of fat and subsequent weight loss. Therefore, preoperative behavioral modification training and close postoperative follow-up to ensure compliance with proper dietary behavior postoperatively are critical.

Most bariatric surgery centers recognize the benefits of having a registered dietitian on the bariatric surgery team. The dietitian can become an essential part of the patient's postoperative course by overseeing diet advancement and by monitoring weight loss. The registered dietitian also assesses adequacy of dietary intake and can help to evaluate dietary problems the patient may be experiencing. Counseling about needed multivitamin and protein supplementation is also an important task. Finally, the registered dietitian can play a role in providing support and encouragement as the patient's lifestyle changes. A support group may serve as the primary setting for this function.

We recommend a mechanistic approach to postoperative dietary intake such that the patient eat a balanced diet and eat this diet very slowly. This is accomplished by teaching the patient to take bites that are teaspoon-sized or smaller, to chew each bite thoroughly (20 times or more), and to wait 5 minutes after swallowing until taking the next bite. In order to avoid overfilling of the pouch (and emesis or stretching of the pouch), we insist that a patient conclude a meal when no longer hungry rather than eating until "full," which may be associated with pain when a small gastric pouch is overfilled.

Common food intolerances may be present, particularly with surgical procedures that combine restrictive and malabsorptive components. With prior coaching, patients will be less likely to select diets that cause distress. Beef, pasta, leavened bread, and alcohol precipitate difficulty in some patients.

▶ DIET AND NUTRITIONAL SUPPORT AFTER A BARIATRIC OPERATION

Bariatric procedures accomplish weight loss either by changing the amount of food eaten or by malabsorption of ingested food or both. Restrictive procedures, such as vertical banded gastroplasty (VBG) and gastric banding, help to limit (by the small proximal gastric pouch) the amount of food that is consumed and, in some cases, the type of food that may be ingested. That is, restrictive procedures may make it difficult to eat foods that must be cut with a knife. These foods (steak and other fibrous meats) may tend to produce a feeling that food is "hanging up" in the esophagus and may occasionally actually block the gastric pouch outlet if inadequately chewed.

Malabsorptive procedures, on the other hand, alter the course of digestion. The jejunoileal bypass of a generation ago bypassed most of the small bowel and produced profound malabsorption (and nutritional deficiencies),[1] but biliopancreatic bypass and duodenal switch operations tend to be safer metabolically.[2] However, both of these malabsorptive operations may, themselves, produce profound deficiencies in some patients, making close follow-up the responsibility of the bariatric surgeon. Roux-en-Y gastric bypass (RYGB), on the other hand, represents an eclectic approach, incorporating real gastric restriction and a modicum of malabsorption.

Opinions vary regarding postoperative feeding of bariatric surgical patients. At one extreme are surgeons who send all patients home on pureed diets, with the rationale that solid food in the postoperative period will be likely to lodge in the small gastric pouch and obstruct. At the other extreme are surgeons who recognize that chewing food (to a pureed consistency) conveys a proprioceptive signal to the brain from muscles of mastication that contribute to a feeling of satiety. Such surgeons will advance their patients to a soft or regular diet sooner postoperatively. Regardless, avoidance of emesis in the immediate postoperative period is important, as increased intragastric pressures during bouts of vomiting may lead to dehiscence of surgical wounds or dislodgement of staples (or, in the case of gastric banding, slippage of the band).

There is no theoretical advantage of pureed food over solid food that has been adequately chewed. In fact, complete mastication may contribute to satiety and lead to fewer long-term complications. Additionally, the consumption of high-calorie liquids (or purees) can circumvent the benefit of bariatric procedures in general and should be avoided except when nutritionally indicated in an individual with limited intake.

Postoperatively, a bariatric surgery patient may find certain food textures unpleasant. Also, some patients (mainly those who have undergone gastric bypass) may experience intolerance to simple sugars, starches, or concentrated beverages. If a patient complains of sweating, dizziness, rapid heart rate and, occasionally, diarrhea after eating such foods, the patient may be experiencing the "dumping syndrome." Preoperative teaching for the RYGB patient should include instruction in the importance of avoiding high-calorie liquid- or sugar-containing foods. A rule of thumb is that if the list of ingredients contains the word sugar within the first three or four ingredients, its consumption should be moderate. Patients who have experienced a dumping state find that it is very unpleasant and in the future will avoid the foods that caused it.

Postoperatively, decreased caloric intake, the avoidance of foods such as meat and dairy products, and malabsorption can lead to various nutritive deficiencies. We start our patients on therapeutic multivitamins and calcium supplementation within 2 to 4 weeks after operation, allowing considerable latitude for the formulations, depending upon the preferences and needs of the patient. Multivitamins reduce the likelihood but do not completely eliminate the possibility of vitamin deficiencies.

▶ MICRONUTRIENT DEFICIENCY

Bariatric surgeons would do well to recall the numerous serious nutritional deficiencies that occurred when jejunoileal bypass was the accepted malabsorptive operation for morbidly obese patients.[1] Not only did patients experience protein-calorie malnutrition, but serious micronutrient deficiencies occurred commonly. Fortunately, the malabsorptive operations done today are less dangerous but, as a rule, the more malabsorption introduced by the operation, the greater the likelihood that a micronutrient deficiency will occur. Further, with the more malabsorptive procedures, unlike with gastroplasty, gastric banding, or gastric bypass, patients may actually develop generalized malnutrition. As a rule, gastroplasty and gastric banding are only rarely associated with micronutrient or nutrition deficiencies.[3] Such deficiencies become progressively more common with gastric bypass, duodenal switch, and biliopancreatic bypass. They are most easily treatable after gastric bypass.

Vitamin B₁₂

Vitamin B_{12} (cobalamin) is a substrate for cofactors of enzymes such as methionine synthase, glutamate mutase, dioldehydratase, and methylmalonyl coenzyme-A mutase and is found in fish, milk and milk products, eggs, meat, and poultry. The recommended daily intake for the general population is 2.4 µg per day. Most multivitamins contain 6 µg B_{12}. In dietary form, it is protein bound. Normally, cleavage occurs in the presence of gastric acid, and the B_{12} then binds with a salivary R-protein, which enhances absorption, possibly by protecting it during its passage to the ileum. In the small intestine, pancreatic proteases release the B_{12} from R-protein. The free B_{12} then binds to intrinsic factor (produced by parietal cells in the stomach) and travels to the ileum, where it is liberated and attaches to special receptor cells on the brush border. The B_{12} is transferred to transport proteins called transcobalamins, which are then taken up by the liver, bone marrow, and blood cells prior to intracellular release and conversion into its bioactive forms.

B_{12} deficiency can lead to neurologic symptoms but more commonly leads to megaloblastic anemia. B_{12} deficiency is found in patients with both restrictive and malabsorptive surgery but is rare after gastroplasty or gastric banding, where the deficiency (when it occurs) is felt to be caused primarily by decreased dietary intake. Gastric bypass procedures appear to have the greatest effect on B_{12} levels, with as many as two thirds of RYGB patients having low levels of B_{12}.[4] The mechanism for this deficiency may be based on the practical absence of significant gastric acid production in the gastric pouch, with subsequent failure to liberate dietary cobalamin.[5] Predigestion with an enzyme mixture improves absorption but simultaneous ingestion of the mixture dies not demonstrate any benefit.[6] A normal Schilling test is typically found in RYGB, suggesting that the remaining gastric antrum produces intrinsic factor that functions in the common channel.

The high incidence of B_{12} deficiency in gastric bypass and biliopancreatic diversion/duodenal switch procedures suggests that routine testing of B_{12} levels should be done. Although only 66% of bariatric surgeons screen for B_{12} deficiencies,[7] all patients should be prospectively studied. Deficiencies in B_{12}, when they occur due to a malabsorptive procedure, usually appear more than a year postoperatively. Therapy is given orally (at least 350 µg daily)[8] or as 1000 µg B_{12} intramuscularly every 2 to 3 months, as indicated by serum B_{12} levels. While the administration of B_{12} in multivitamins preventively does not preclude the possibility of B_{12} deficiency, it does reduce the incidence.[9,10] Many bariatric surgeons treat all of their RYGB patients with B_{12} prophylactically, orally or intramuscularly.

Folic Acid

Folic acid is a pteroylmonoglutamic acid that is found in fortified breakfast cereals, leafy green vegetables, liver, and kidney. Dietary folate is primarily in a polyglutamate form and must be hydrolyzed to monoglutamates before absorption takes place in the jejunum. Folate is a cofactor in reactions that involve transfer of single carbon atoms vital to amino acid metabolism, purine and pyrimidine synthesis, and the formation of S-adenosylmethionine. Its metabolic effect is closely tied with that of vitamin B_{12}, and deficiencies of B_{12} should be ruled out before treatment of a folate deficiency. The symptoms of folate deficiency are generally secondary to anemia.

Deficiencies in patients after weight-loss procedures are believed to be secondary to decreased dietary intake and decreased gastric acid production. Folate deficiencies can lead to higher levels of homocysteine. Hyperhomocysteinemia has been identified as an independent risk factor for atherosclerotic disease. A study of patients 1 year after gastroplasty demonstrated that approximately two thirds of patients showed an increase in homocysteine levels and that this increase was tied directly to reductions in folate levels.[11] Overt folate deficiency does not appear to be necessary to effect these changes. The increased atherosclerosis risk secondary to high homocysteine levels may offset the cardiovascular benefits of the procedure. It is thus recommended that all patients be given a daily folate supplement. Serum levels of folate are generally not useful as they reflect only recent intake. Erythrocyte folate levels are more stable indicators of folate metabolism and correlate more closely with homocysteine levels than serum levels.[12]

Thiamine

Thiamine (vitamin B_1) is found in pork, liver, potatoes, whole-grain cereals, and breads. The daily recommended intake is 1.5 mg per day. Thiamine pyrophosphate is the biologically active derivative of B_1 and is required for the oxidative decarboxylation of pyruvate to form acetyl-coenzyme A, initiating the Krebs cycle. It also functions as a coenzyme for transketolase in the pentose phosphate pathway, an alternative pathway for glucose oxidation. Finally, thiamine pyrophosphate is involved in the oxidative decarboxylation of α-ketoglutarate and branched-chain α-keto acids.

Beriberi (deficiency of thiamine) is seen mostly in alcoholics and in countries where polished rice is the staple food. Its neurologic manifestations fall under the Wernicke-Korsakoff syndrome, which may present as nystagmus, ocular gaze palsies, or sensorimotor polyneuropathy. Late symptoms include ataxia and delirium.

Wernicke-Korsakoff syndrome has been identified in a small number of patients after weight-loss procedures, including gastroplasty, gastric bypass, and biliopancreatic diversion.[13-17] Usually, there was a history of protracted vomiting antecedent to the identification of neurologic changes. For this reason, any patient with significant emesis should receive thiamine supplementation, and all postoperative patients receiving parenteral nutrition should have thiamine added to their formula.

Iron

Iron is a mineral involved in the transport and storage of oxygen. It is found in liver, beef, whole-meal breads, cereals, eggs, and dried fruit and is incorporated into enzymes that mediate energy production and cell diffusion. It also plays a role in the function of the immune and central nervous systems.

Vitamin C consumed in the same meal as inorganic iron improves its absorption by up to 50% and has been used in an attempt to improve the absorption of iron by patients who have undergone gastric bypass.[18] Iron is normally absorbed in the duodenum and proximal jejunum. Iron deficiency leads to a hypochromic, microcytic anemia and is manifested as fatigue and weakness. The best laboratory test of iron deficiency is a serum ferritin. Ferritin levels do not have the same diurnal variation as serum iron levels, and a low result is diagnostic for an iron deficiency.

Iron deficiency is seen in 15% to 50% in patients after gastric bypass, and the incidence after biliopancreatic diversion lies somewhere in this range. It is rare after gastroplasty or gastric banding. Both poor dietary intake and malabsorption of iron seem to play a role in the development of iron deficiency. After a 7-year follow-up of gastric bypass patients, many patients exhibit a mild iron deficiency that seems to correlate with meat intolerance.[19]

Iron-deficiency anemia is the micronutrient complication that seems to give patients the most problems. Whereas B_{12} and folate deficiencies are typically silent in the postoperative patient, iron-deficiency anemia produces a myriad of symptoms adversely affecting quality of life.[20] Prophylaxis with oral iron supplementation is not generally recommended because poor patient compliance makes it ineffective for many. After a bariatric procedure, most iron deficiency occurs in menstruating women. Prophylaxis in these women is recommended.[21] In women with refractory iron-deficiency anemia and menometrorrhagia, consultation with a gynecologist is sometimes warranted, because surgical options may be indicated.

Iron may be given as 200 to 300 mg of iron sulfate daily (although intolerance to this formulation occurs frequently and should be suspected). Pregnancy soon after a bariatric procedure is considered generally contraindicated, but patients who become pregnant should have their iron and hemoglobin closely monitored because they are susceptible to anemia and other deficiencies and may require more aggressive strategies for iron replacement.[22] Communication with the obstetrician is vital because those practicing in this specialty may not be attuned to the special problems of the bariatric patient. The role of intravenous or intramuscular iron replacement has not been well defined but may be necessary in patients intractable to oral supplementation. In some cases, transfusions have been required.

Calcium

Absorption of calcium is dependent on a high calcium gradient and thus requires large quantities of dietary calcium. In a patient who has undergone a malabsorptive procedure, calcium binding to fat in the gut leads to hypocalcemia, which in turn may produce secondary hyperparathyroidism. The outcome may be osteomalacia, because a defect in both calcium absorption and protein synthesis may follow such operations.[23] Routine calcium supplementation should be given to all patients who have undergone malabsorptive procedures. Although gastric restriction is not usually associated with hypocalcemia, dietary intake is probably sufficiently small to warrant prophylaxis in these patients as well. Serum calcium should be monitored periodically in all bariatric surgery patients.

Zinc

A deficiency of zinc may lead to alopecia, diarrhea, emotional disorders, intercurrent infections, dermatitis, and hypogonadism in males. Significant hair loss was noticed in some patients after RYGB. The alopecia was either arrested or reversed after administration of zinc supplements.[24]

Fat-Soluble Vitamins: K, A, D

The malabsorptive procedures function, in part, by decreasing fat absorption. Consumption of fatty foods may lead to malodorous stools or flatus and diarrhea. With decreased intake and processing of dietary fat, deficiencies in fat-soluble vitamins may evolve. These should be provided prophylactically to all patients who have undergone biliopancreatic diversion/duodenal switch procedures. Vitamin D deficiency has been observed as a deficiency of obesity de facto and may not be altered by weight-loss procedures.[25] Vitamin K deficiency, if it occurs, may be identified clinically (bruising, bleeding). Jejunoileal bypass was associated with known occurrences of vitamin D and A deficiency. In the case of vitamin D, the deficiency contributed to the occurrence of osteomalacia. With vitamin A deficiency, night blindness was sometimes identified. It is, therefore, prudent to measure serum vitamin D and vitamin A periodically if a malabsorptive procedure has been carried out.

▶ MACRONUTRIENT (PROTEIN) DEFICIENCY

Protein-calorie malnutrition after bariatric surgery is found almost exclusively in malabsorptive procedures such as distal RYGB and biliopancreatic diversion with or without duodenal switch, but occasionally it may be found after protracted emesis in restrictive procedures.[26] Clinically, protein deficiency results in a reduction of muscle mass and in edema. It may manifest as recurrent or severe infections as a result of subsequent immunodeficiency. Protein-calorie malnutrition is known as marasmus, and protein malnutrition by itself is known as kwashiorkor. Protein malnutrition was seen in 8% of patients with the original biliopancreatic diversion described by Scopinaro.[27] Later modification of this procedure, by lengthening the common channel, increasing gastric volume, or both, decreased the incidence to 3%.[28] Protein malnutrition may be avoided by encouraging high-protein diets and providing protein supplementation and, of course, by avoiding highly malabsorptive procedures in people who might be considered at higher risk. In extreme cases, protein deficiency may be treated with total parenteral nutrition, and occasionally a revision operation is necessary. Routine screening of total protein and albumin levels is recommended in patients who have undergone malabsorptive procedures.

▶ PSYCHOLOGICAL CONSIDERATIONS

A major issue that confronts all bariatric surgery teams is the misperception that morbid obesity is always associated with or is caused by mental illness. As in any population, the morbidly obese can be affected by mental illness, and depression is particularly common. On the other hand, the usual range of human behavior is seen in these patients, from the completely normal to the profoundly psychologically impaired.

For whatever reasons, many patients presenting for bariatric operations are taking psychotropic drugs. Most patients report having had feelings of depression because of their weight, but Gentry and others have shown that depression is lessened after gastric bypass.[29] Conversely, some patients report feeling depressed because their ability to enjoy food has been so radically altered.

A bariatric operation usually produces amelioration of a patient's sense of well-being. Also, improvement in physical appearance, employability, overall health, and even sexual performance produces what many patients describe as a rebirth or a new life, and their functioning becomes increasingly normal.

Phobias may develop postoperatively, including fear of failure, fear of eating, and fear of emesis, and ongoing support by the bariatric team (and perhaps by a clinical psychologist) is important. Reinforcement of an attitude of optimism about postoperative eating may be useful, but adherence to behavioral modification principles learned preoperatively is critical to a good outcome. Although fear of regaining weight is prominent, that fear alone rarely causes patients to become anorexic. The fear of emesis, however, leads many people to curtail not only the speed with which they eat, but also the types of food and the amount eaten. The importance of psychologists, experienced nurse practitioners, and dieticians dedicated to patients with these sorts of problems is obvious, and the overall success of bariatric procedures may well depend upon such support.

▶ SPECIAL POSTOPERATIVE PROBLEMS

Emesis

Postoperative emesis may occur after any bariatric procedure but is most commonly seen after gastric restrictive procedures in patients who do not eat slowly or chew adequately. A combination of small pouch size and narrow outflow tract appears to be the cause. In RYGB, the pouch size is similar to that found in VBG, but the distance of narrowing through which food passes after leaving the pouch is less than the 1-cm-long channel created by a band, which may predispose patients to more frequent lodging of pieces of inadequately chewed food.

Emesis may have a profound influence on a patient's quality of life. Shai and colleagues found that two thirds of patients, after vertical banded gastroplasty, exhibited some vomiting, swallowing difficulties, or reflux symptoms, but that these symptoms did not correlate with patient dissatisfaction.[30] Halverson and Brown, in contrast, found that after either gastric bypass or gastroplasty, two thirds of patients experienced minimal or no emesis if they had been trained carefully preoperatively.[31] Balsiger and colleagues defined significant vomiting as one or more episodes per week and determined the incidence to be 21% according to this definition.[32]

Protracted emesis may lead to malnutrition and should be evaluated urgently. Consistent emesis may indicate an obstructing piece of food or an anatomic abnormality such as an anastomotic stricture. However, emesis after any bariatric procedure with a restrictive component may simply be a marker of patient noncompliance with diet. Extensive preoperative counseling regarding eating habits, with continued postoperative reinforcement, is critical in reducing the incidence and severity of emesis. For patients who experience episodes of vomiting, there are theoretical risks of staple dehiscence, the stretching of the pouch, and the evolution of reflux symptoms. DeMaria and colleagues have expressed concern about the development of achalasia after gastric banding.[33]

Experienced bariatric surgeons ensure careful preoperative training of patients in eating behaviors that promote successful weight loss postoperatively. These behaviors include: (1) eating a well-balanced diet; (2) taking one bite every 5 minutes; (3) chewing each bite at least 20 times; (4) stopping eating when no longer hungry; and (5) consuming no liquids for 45 minutes before and after meals. Postoperative emesis in many instances may be attributed to inappropriate eating habits and may result in food avoidance. Weight loss, however, does not appear to be correlated with the presence or severity of emesis.[31]

Anastomotic Stricture

Narrowing or ulceration of the anastomosis between the stomach and the small bowel after RYGB has been reported to occur in as many as 14% of patients undergoing laparoscopic gastric bypass.[34] The incidence with open RYGB is far less. Such patients experience frequent emesis, usually unremitting, and often require repeated endoscopic dilation. They usually are treated successfully, with only the intractable stricture requiring surgical intervention. A tight outlet following a VBG cannot be dilated and dilation should not be attempted; Silastic rings and Marlex bands do not dilate.

▶ ROLE OF POSTOPERATIVE EXERCISE IN BARIATRIC PATIENTS

Limitation of physical activity is a common complaint of obese patients. The ratio of lean body mass (LBM) to total body mass is lower in the obese patient because most of their excess weight is in the form of fat. Moreover, the obese individual must perform more work than an individual of normal weight to carry out the same activities.

As postoperative weight loss occurs, both fat and LBM are lost, the proportions of which depend upon the type of operation and the length of time since operation. That is, by 1 year postoperatively, restrictive and gastric bypass bariatric procedures are associated with less depletion of LBM than are the more malabsorptive procedures, in which cases protein-calorie malnutrition is more likely to occur.[35] Independent of the type of procedure performed, exercise is an important element in the preservation of muscle mass and in the maintenance of LBM.

The cardiopulmonary reserve of obese patients is also decreased. Cardiac evaluation of morbidly obese patients preoperatively demonstrates that there is a high percentage of left ventricular hypertrophy with high filling pressures, leading to diastolic dysfunction.[36] There is also some degree of systolic dysfunction, with approximately one quarter of patients having a left ventricular ejection fraction of "less than 50%. Furthermore, radionuclide evaluation during exercise demonstrates inducible ventricular wall motion bnormalities, and some patients have histories of anginal symptoms. Coronary angiography failed to reveal any significant atherosclerotic disease in these patients.[37] This suggests that the decreased compliance of the ventricles reduces the vasodilatory capability of coronary vessels. With exercise, there is little change in stroke volume, and cardiac output is determined solely by rate. Echocardiographic evaluation of patients as early as 6 months postoperatively reveals resolution of left ventricular hypertrophy, and radionuclide imaging confirms a decrease in left ventricular mass in nearly all patients.[38,39] Afterload reduction occurs postoperatively, with decreases in systolic blood pressures at rest and during exercise.[40] The observed decrease in left ventricular mass may result from this afterload reduction or may result from a direct effect of weight loss on the myocyte. These changes have been observed in patients who have undergone VBG and RYGB. It remains to be seen whether similar changes occur after other bariatric procedures.

From a respiratory standpoint, the ventilatory requirements of obese patients are notably higher than those of the general population. The ventilatory capacity of obese patients may also be compromised by extrathoracic (i.e., restrictive) pressures. Postoperatively, it can be shown that the peak oxygen consumption (VO_2) and anaerobic thresholds significantly increase, and the resting VO_2 returns to nearly normal values.[41] There is, however, only a moderate improvement in ventilatory capacity.[42]

Weight-loss operations do not, ipso facto, lead to increased activity. Certainly, exercise should become easier as the excess body weight is lost, but encouragement and social support systems are essential for developing positive lifestyle changes. Patients in support groups after VBG engaged in significantly more physical activity than did matched control groups after the same operation. In addition, patients in support groups reported consuming fewer calories and had greater nutritional knowledge. It is surprising that there was no difference in weight loss in the two groups by the time of the study's completion.[43] The inference may be made that the weight loss, at least in the first years, is dependent primarily on the operation, but that long-term maintenance of weight loss (as well as preservation of LBM) may, to a degree, be dependent on continued exercise.

▶ SUPPORT GROUPS

Support groups can become the foundation of a bariatric surgery program. Properly run, they create a setting that provides guidance, education, and enlightenment for both pre- and postoperative patients, and they may lead to higher overall success rates and greater weight loss. Because of the unique nature of these groups of patients, the meetings of support groups for bariatric patients must be held in rooms that are large enough and have chairs that are armless and comfortable. Meetings should be structured and have agendas. Preoperative patients and postoperative patients have different issues, and the needs of both groups should be addressed. Much of the activity of a good support group focuses on education and emotional support, but time should be allowed at the end of each meeting for a social period. This time provides an opportunity for patients to talk among themselves as a group and privately and for certain patients to reach out to others who are less likely to speak up.

Creative use of guest speakers provides an excellent opportunity to provide information about exercise and nutrition. "Support groups are best led by competent, well-trained, educated and positive leaders who understand the surgery, preoperative workup, postoperative management plan and group dynamics."[44] Without these elements, groups may become gossip groups or gripe groups. Patients should be encouraged to become leaders and to develop their own e-mail lists and group bulletins to keep lines of support open among all members.

▶ TAKING CALLS FROM THE POSTOPERATIVE PATIENT

The unique nature of bariatric surgery makes close attention to patients' complaints important in their care. Many routine calls to the bariatric team occur for information about laboratory results, resumption of activities, care of the wound, and other subjects. The majority of contacts, particularly in the first few months after the operation, require special expertise.

Pain

Pain frequently prompts a telephone call to the team, and the usual descriptors (intensity, location, radiation, constancy, factors that affect it) help to determine whether a phone call to the pharmacy, care in a local emergency room, or a trip to the bariatric center is indicated. Incisional pain can be dealt with routinely, but pleuritic pain in these patients bears special scrutiny, given their propensity to develop deep venous thrombosis and pulmonary emboli.

Reports of epigastric or retrosternal pain, when associated with eating, bear special investigation. Satiety or emesis after one or two swallows, or unprovoked emesis, may well indicate stricture of an anastomosis or a foreign body stuck in the outlet channel. Severe or persistent pain, when associated with swallowing or eating, must occasionally be evaluated by upper gastrointestinal series or esophagogastroduodenoscopy. Food lodged in the outlet of the pouch can usually be pushed through with the endoscope, making actual removal unnecessary.

Emesis

Postoperative emesis should be unusual in a patient who has been adequately trained preoperatively and who has been properly selected. Experience indicates that the majority of patients who do vomit are not complying with dietary instructions, rather than manifesting an anatomic problem resulting from the operation. When a patient calls and complains of emesis, one must determine whether the emesis occurs at the onset, during or after intake, and after what quantity of food (or liquid). One must ascertain that the patient is chewing the food adequately (to a pureed state) and that the speed of intake is sufficiently slow to allow passage of the food.

Most patients report vomiting if they chew inadequately or if they eat too fast; hence the importance of teaching behavioral modification preoperatively. Such patients commonly vomit only after consuming solid foods and are able to keep liquids down. If a patient vomits both liquids and solids consistently, the likelihood that a bezoar is blocking the anastomosis (or more commonly, the VBG or gastric band outflow tract) is higher. Intermittency of emesis resulting from a bezoar can occur when there is a "ball-valve" effect, which may persist for weeks or even a few months.

Persistent emesis of both solids and liquids demands quick action to restore the patient to health and also to avoid the dehydration and weakness that will result from the malnutrition that will ensue. Performing an upper gastrointestinal examination may seem reasonable, but it may not detect a foreign body stuck in the pouch outflow tract; esophagogastroduodenoscopy is the most diagnostically effective and the most therapeutically useful investigation to perform in this situation.

Occasionally, patients complain of a mucuslike, frothy, or phlegmonous emesis, denying they see food when they vomit. These people often deny that there is any relationship between the vomiting and their meals. Although this situation is uncommon and almost always resolves by itself, the bariatric team must keep in mind that postnasal drip or chronic sinusitis may be contributing to this kind of complaint and should be appropriately treated.

Last, in some patients who complain of emesis, no cause can be found. Fortunately, this group of patients is small, and the duration of the complaint is usually short. They may be treated with the usual antiemetic regimens.

▶ PSYCHOLOGICAL ISSUES

The usual range of psychological issues occurs in postoperative patients. Postoperative anorexia is rare, if it occurs at all, but bulimia occurs in the occasional patient. When bulimia occurs, it should be recognized not as a rational act designed to make a person lose weight, but rather as a symptom of an underlying psychiatric illness, and help should be sought for the patient.

At the other extreme is severe aversion in which a patient's intake decreases secondary to fear of gaining weight, dislike of the food per se, or even fear of vomiting. Food aversion often starts with a particular type of food (meat, pastry, sauces) but may generalize to many types of foods. Psychiatric consultation should be obtained.

Changes in body image are one of the salutary side effects of bariatric procedures. Stories of patients' self-perception, increased employability, and improved sexual function are legendary and are positive factors for most patients. However, there is a small group of patients in whom an improved appearance or body image has negative connotations because it increases the likelihood of social interaction, raises personal expectations, or even poses a sexual threat. This is particularly true in the cases of patients who have histories of sexual abuse and have not had proper psychological counseling preoperatively. Prior sexual abuse must be dealt with effectively before life-changing events such as a bariatric operation are faced.

An odd but common reaction in postoperative patients is irritability as they lose weight and people start to treat them differently. Although it might be easier to get a job or be promoted, some patients react negatively, recognizing that they are "really the same people they were before," and they do not understand why people are treating them differently.

In general, preoperatively, patients have experienced diminution in sexual function and satisfaction as they have become morbidly obese. Conversely, as they regain their health and achieve more normal weight postoperatively, these factors improve, and marital satisfaction increases.

▶ REFERENCES

1. Halverson JD, Wise L, Wazna MF, et al: Jejunoileal bypass for morbid obesity: a critical appraisal. Am J Med 1978;64:461-475.
2. Marceau P, Hould FS, Lebel S, et al: Malabsorptive obesity surgery. Surg Clin North Am 2001;81:1113-1127.
3. Printen KJ, Halverson JD: Hemic micronutrients following vertical banded gastroplasty. Am Surg 1988;54:267-268.
4. Halverson JD: Micronutrient deficiencies after gastric bypass for morbid obesity. Am Surg 1986;52:594-598.
5. Doscherholmen A, Swaim WR: Impaired assimilation of egg Co 57 vitamin B_{12} in patients with hypochlorhydria achlorhydria and after gastric resection. Gastroenterology 1973;64:913-919.
6. Rhode BM, Arseneau P, Cooper BA, et al: Vitamin B_{12} deficiency after gastric surgery for obesity. Am J Clin Nutr 1996;63:103-109.
7. Brolin RE, Leung M: Survey of vitamin and mineral supplementation after gastric bypass and biliopancreatic diversion for morbid obesity. Obes Surg 1999;9:150-154.
8. Rhode BM, Tamin H, Gilfix BM, et al: Treatment of vitamin B_{12} deficiency after gastric surgery for severe obesity. Obes Surg 1995;5:154-158.
9. Brolin RE, Gorman RC, Milgrim LM, et al: Multivitamin prophylaxis in prevention of post-gastric bypass vitamin and mineral deficiencies. Int J Obes 1991;15:661-667.
10. Provenzale D, Reinhold RB, Golner B, et al: Evidence for diminished B_{12} absorption after gastric bypass: oral supplementation does not prevent low plasma B_{12} levels in bypass patients. J Am Coll Nutr 1992;11:29-35.
11. Borson-Chazot F, Harthe C, Teboul F, et al: Occurrence of hyperhomocysteinemia 1 year after gastroplasty for severe obesity. J Clin Endocrin Metab 1999;84:541-545.
12. Chadefaux B, Cooper BA, Gilfix BM, et al; Homocysteine: relationship to serum cobalamin, serum folate, erythrocyte folate, and lobation of neutrophils. Clin Invest Med 1994;17:540-550.
13. Haid RW, Gutman L, Crosby TW: Wernicke-Korsakoff encephalopathy after gastric plication. JAMA 1982;247:2566-2567.
14. Maryniak O: Severe peripheral neuropathy following gastric bypass surgery for morbid obesity. Can Med Assoc J 1984;131:119-120.
15. Primavera A, Brusa G, Novello P, et al: Wernicke-Korsakoff encephalopathy following biliopancreatic diversion. Obes Surg 1993;3:175-177.
16. Chaves LC, Faintuch J, Kahwage S, et al: A cluster of polyneuropathy and Wernicke-Korsakoff syndrome in a bariatric unit. Obes Surg 2002;12:328-334.
17. Munoz-Farjas E, Jerico I, Pascual-Millan LF, et al: Neuropathic beriberi as a complication of surgery of morbid obesity. Rev Neurol 1996;24:456-458.
18. Rhode BM, Shustik C, Christou NV, et al: Iron absorption and therapy after gastric bypass. Obes Surg 1999;9:17-21.
19. Avinoah E, Ovnat A, Charuzi I: Nutritional status seven years after Roux-en-Y gastric bypass surgery. Surgery 1992;111:137-142.
20. Brolin RE, Gorman JH, Gorman RC, et al: Are vitamin B_{12} and folate deficiency clinically important after Roux-en-Y gastric bypass? J Gastrointest Surg 1998;2:436-442.
21. Brolin RE, Gorman JH, Gorman RC, et al: Prophylactic iron supplementation after Roux-en-Y gastric bypass: a prospective, double-blind, randomized study. Arch Surg 1998;133:740-744.
22. Gurewitsch ED, Smith-Levitin M, Mack J: Pregnancy following gastric bypass surgery for morbid obesity. Obstet Gynecol 1996;88:658-661.
23. Halverson JD, Teitelbaum SL, Haddad JG, et al: Skeletal abnormalities after jejunoileal bypass. Ann Surg 1979;189:785-790.
24. Neve HJ, Bhatti WA, Soulsby C, et al: Reversal of hair loss following vertical gastroplasty when treated with zinc sulphate. Obes Surg 1996;6:63-65.
25. Buffington C, Walker B, Cowan GS Jr, et al: Vitamin D deficiency in the morbidly obese. Obes Surg 1993;3:421-424.
26. Schneider SB, Erikson N, Gebel HM, et al: Cutaneous anergy and marrow suppression as complications of gastroplasty for morbid obesity. Surgery 1983;94:109-111.
27. Scopinaro N, Gianetta E, Adami GF, et al: Biliopancreatic diversion for obesity at eighteen years. Surgery 1996;119:261-268.
28. Scopinaro N, Adami GF, Marinari GM, et al: Biliopancreatic diversion. World J Surg 1998;2:936-946.
29. Gentry K, Halverson JD, Heisler S: Psychological assessment of morbidly obese patients undergoing bypass. a comparison of preoperative and postoperative adjustment. Surgery 1984;95:215-220.
30. Shai I, Henkin Y, Weitzman S, et al: Determinants of long-term satisfaction after vertical banded gastroplasty. Obes Surg 2003;13:269-274.
31. Halverson JD, Brown CA: An analysis of vomiting behavior after gastric stapling for morbid obesity. Obes Surg 2000;10:133.
32. Balsiger BM, Kennedy FP, Abu-Lebdeh HS, et al: Prospective evaluation of Roux-en-Y gastric bypass as primary operation for medically complicated obesity. Mayo Clin Proc 2000;75:673-680.
33. DeMaria EJ, Sugerman HJ, Meador JG, et al: High failure rate after laparoscopic adjustable silicone gastric banding for treatment of morbid obesity. Ann Surg 2001;233:809-818.
34. Perugini RA, Mason R, Czerniach DR, et al: Predictors of complication and suboptimal weight loss after laparoscopic Roux-en-Y gastric bypass: a series of 188 patients. Arch Surg 2003;138:541-546.
35. Palombo JD, Maletskos CJ. Reinhold RV, et al: Composition of weight loss in morbidly obese patients after gastric bypass. J Surg Res 1981;30:435-442.
36. Alaud-din A, Meterissian S, Lisbona R, et al: Assessment of cardiac function in patients who were morbidly obese. Surgery 1990;108:809-820.
37. Murray GL, Cowan GS Jr, Vander-Zwagg R: Exercise-induced wall motion abnormalities and resting left ventricular dysfunction in the morbidly obese as assessed by radionuclide ventriculography. Obes Surg 1991;1:37-45.
38. Boone KB, Kreuger M, Ho T, et al: Obesity and the effects of weight loss on cardiac structure and function. Obes Surg 2003;13:197 (abstract).
39. Kanoupakis E, Michaloudis D, Fraidakis O, et al: Left ventricular function and cardiopulmonary performance following surgical treatment of morbid obesity. Obes Surg 2001;11:552-558.
40. Ben-Dov I, Grossman E, Stein A, et al: Marked weight reduction lowers resting and exercise blood pressure in morbidly obese subjects. Am J Hypertens 2000;13:251-255.
41. Zavala DC, Printen KJ: Basal and exercise tests on morbidly obese patients before and after gastric bypass. Surgery 1984;95:221-229.
42. Refsum HE, Holter PH, Lovig PH, et al: Pulmonary function and energy expenditure after marked weight loss in obese women: observations before and one year after gastric banding. Int J Obes 1990;14:175-183.
43. Rabner JG, Greenstein RJ: Antiobesity surgery: is a structured support group desirable? Obes Surg 1993;3:381-390.
44. Zanders B, Fox K, Fox SR, et al: Choosing and creating bariatric surgery support group lessons that are relevant, informative and fun. Obes Surg 2003;13:196 (abstract).

17

Surgery in the Morbidly Obese Patient

Robert J. Greenstein, M.D., F.A.C.S., F.R.C.S.

As bariatric surgery becomes increasingly accepted as therapy for those suffering from morbid obesity, the challenge to provide this patient population with optimal care arises. The purpose of this chapter is to identify how to provide an appropriate operating room environment for the morbidly obese population. This chapter does not address the preoperative counseling of the patient other than those issues specifically germane to surgery.

▶ PREOPERATIVE EDUCATION AND PREPARATION

Patient preparation is of paramount importance in the performance of bariatric surgery.[1]

Skin Hygiene

Prior to elective surgery, diabetic patients with massively redundant panniculi should ensure that all skin excoriations are healed. Motivating patients to wash under overhanging skin flaps, to maintain skin dryness by wearing cotton underwear, and to correct undertreated diabetes is a simple yet effective preventive measure that decreases wound infections. At an office visit before day-of-admission surgery, patients may be given a betadine- or chlorhexidine-infused surgical scrub brush with which to wash on the morning of their surgery, prior to coming to the hospital.

Venous Thromboembolic Prophylaxis

It is important to explain to patients the absolute necessity of repetitive postoperative mobilization as an important adjunct in preventing blood clots in the legs and the possibility of pulmonary emboli. Patients are willing to perform against pain if their actions will improve their chances of doing well following a potentially life-threatening elective operation. Describing the unique spongelike nature of the calf muscles as they pump blood through veins to minimize blood clot development encourages patients to walk as soon and as often as possible following surgery.

Recovery Room

Patients should be prepared for the atmosphere they will encounter in the recovery room following their surgery. They should be made aware of the possibility of waking up with the endotracheal tube still in place.

Early Mobilization

Patients should be prepared for early mobilization before entering the hospital. Securing a single intravenous line to support patient mobility is preferable prior to transporting patients from the recovery room to the station following operation. If possible, the use of nasogastric tubes and arterial lines should be avoided. It may be preferable for patients to sit in chairs rather than be nursed in bed in the 24 hours following surgery, as patients stand more readily from a sitting than from a recumbent position.

Pulmonary Prophylaxis

Respiratory complications are the most common problems following bariatric surgery.[2] The most propitious time to educate patients about the use of incentive spirometers is before the operative procedure. Depending on the administrative structure at a given institution, the respiratory component of patient preparation can take place during the office visit, during the anesthesiology interview, or during a preoperative visit to the station. If possible, patients should be given incentive spirometers and be instructed in their use, allowing time for practice with the device at home.

▶ POSTOPERATIVE MANAGEMENT

My philosophy of how to manage postoperative bariatric patients was articulated succinctly by Professor E. E. Mason when I visited him in Iowa in 1982, at the beginning of my bariatric surgical career. He mused, "If you treat them as though they are sick, they will get sick."

Recovery Room

It is recommended that patients be progressed expeditiously through the recovery room. As a rule, patients can go to the nursing station from the recovery room; however, certain patients should be considered for admission to the intensive care unit. This is particularly true for patients with respiratory problems and those who have had difficult intubation.

Early Mobilization

The nursing staff is pivotally important in instituting early mobilization, preferably with patients who have been inculcated in the importance of early and repetitive ambulation. In a center where a bariatric program is being initiated, this may require a change in the concepts and behavior patterns of the nursing team.

▶ ANTIBIOTIC PROPHYLAXIS

Preoperative Antibiotics

The American Heart Association has published guidelines for the use and duration of prophylactic antibiotics to prevent endocarditis.[3] These were updated from earlier guidelines from the American Society of Colorectal Surgeons that addressed primarily the impact of intestinal flora.[4] No similar set of guidelines for antibiotic prophylaxis has been instituted by the bariatric surgeon community.

A first-generation cephalosporin is usually acceptable. When there is a preexisting cephalosporin allergy, an aminoglycoside is an appropriate alternative. From the perspective of the bariatric surgeon, documentation of the need to adjust the required dosage of prophylactic antibiotic according to the weight of the patient is vital.[5] As a rule, for a body mass index (BMI) of 40 to 50 kg per m², twice the normally recommended dosage is advisable; for a BMI of 51 to 65 kg per m², two and a half times the normal dosage; and for a BMI greater than 65 kg per m², three times the normal dosage. Preoperative antibiotics should be given intravenously in the operating room prior to induction.

Intraoperative Antibiotics

In the event that the surgery takes more than 2 hours, a repeat dose of antibiotics may be required intraoperatively, depending on the half-life of the antibiotic used.

Postoperative Antibiotics

There are no compelling data that justify the use of postoperative prophylactic antibiotics; however, surgeons employ a wide range of postoperative regimens.

▶ VENOUS THROMBOEMBOLIC PROPHYLAXIS

An estimated 60% to 70% of deaths in bariatric surgery are attributable to pulmonary emboli.[6] Accordingly, the vast majority of bariatric surgeons employ multimodal forms of venous thromboembolic prophylaxis to minimize the appreciable mortality and morbidity resulting from venous thromboembolism.[7-9]

Preoperative

The National Institutes of Health Consensus Development Conference on Venous Thromboembolic Prophylaxis recommends the use of anticoagulation, venous compression stockings, or both.[10] At the time of publication of the Consensus Statement (1986), the recommended dosage of heparin was not prorated for weight; however, studies comparing various doses of enoxaparin, combined with other multimodal venous thromboembolic prophylactics, suggest that higher anticoagulation doses may be more efficacious in the morbidly obese.[11] A weight-based algorithm to determine the appropriate anticoagulation dose may be developed in the future.[12]

Intraoperative

Compression stockings are available commercially, and the manufacturer's instructions list contraindications to their use.[12,13] The bariatric surgeon has to take into account that some morbidly obese patients may have thighs and calves so large that no commercially available thigh or calf compression appliances will fit them. In these instances, the use of calf-only or foot-compression devices should be considered.

Postoperative

Compression boots or stockings as well as heparin or its derivatives are often used postoperatively until the patient is fully mobile. Depending on the nature of the operation and the protocols employed, prophylactic antithrombotic therapy may be continued until discharge from the hospital. In the event that the patient is bed-bound (e.g., in an intensive care unit), both heparin-based anticoagulation and compression stockings are generally continued until the patient is fully mobile.

▶ ANESTHESIA

Anesthesia for the morbidly obese is a subspecialty in its own right. From the perspective of the surgeon, appropriate communication with anesthesia colleagues is particularly important in bariatric surgery. Various means of maintaining gas exchange may be considered, and commonly available volatile agents may be used.[14,15] Although theoretically there may be no need to prorate by the weight of the patient all of the pharmacologic agents that are used, most agents have variable degrees of fat solubility; thus, increasing the dose of some agents will be necessary.

The response of the patient to painful stimuli along with surgeon-anesthesiologist communication are the paramount elements of establishing and maintaining satisfactory anesthesia and patient neuromuscular relaxation. Some anesthesiologists may be reluctant to provide satisfactory relaxation, especially at the time of closure; they are concerned with their ability to perform a rapid extubation at the conclusion of the procedure. At the same time, incisional hernia rates of 8% to 18 % following open bariatric surgery have been reported[16-18] and, anecdotally, many surgeons acknowledge a higher incidence. In part, this high incidence of postoperative ventral hernias may be attributable to inadequate patient relaxation at the time of wound closure.

SPECIALIZED SURGICAL EQUIPMENT

The performance of any operation requires appropriate instrumentation. Operating tables that are capable of holding the weight of the morbidly obese are mandatory. The positioning of the patient in both open and laparoscopic cases often entails having the patient in a reverse Trendelenburg position, which helps to obtain exposure at the esophagogastric junction and improves gas exchange in the morbidly obese.[19]

Open Surgery

Critical to all open procedures is the ability to maintain stable mechanical exposure.[20,21] Several manufacturers make retractor assemblies that are designed specifically for bariatric surgery. Every institution that performs open or laparoscopic bariatric operations must have mechanical retractors capable of achieving and maintaining adequate exposure in a morbidly obese patient. In the event that a laparoscopic procedure has to be converted into an open case, these retractors must be immediately available.

In all bariatric operations, exposure at the esophageal hiatus is necessary. Several retractor blades and tools have been designed to achieve this objective.[22] At the time of closure, particular attention should be paid by both the scrub nurse and the surgeon to achieving an accurate sponge and instrument count, which sometimes proves to be difficult in the morbidly obese patient.[23]

Laparoscopic Surgery

A major difference between general and bariatric laparoscopic surgery is the length of the instruments that may be required. Surgeons should have extra-length trocars available (15 cm rather than 10 cm). If they are actually required, usually it will be only the use of one or two extra-length trocars on the lateral aspect of the abdominal wall. Use of extra-length trocars when not necessary compromises the movement of the blades and is not recommended. In a subset of patients, extra-length (45-cm) laparoscopic instruments are necessary. This is particularly true in men with high BMIs. The surgeon usually does not require extra-length instruments, but their absence in the operating room may preclude the safe conduct of the operation.

Both open and laparoscopic surgery require stable, prolonged mechanical exposure. A few master technicians are able to achieve satisfactory exposure using simple instruments. In my experience, however, these surgeons have the same surgical assistants available to them on a regular basis. These assistants are able to compensate for deficiencies in exposure that would make the operation treacherous for the average surgeon. The laparoscopic surgeon also needs to have the capability of achieving and maintaining stable

mechanical retraction at the esophageal hiatus. Several manufacturers offer instrument assemblies that provide such optimal exposure The most versatile retractor blade for the laparoscopic retraction of the left lobe of the liver appears to be the curiously shaped rods designed by Nathanson of Australia, which possess the dual advantages of being reusable and introducible through a 5-mm port. As in open surgery, when performing laparoscopic surgery, it is wise to use a mechanical device to aid in maintaining exposure; several such devices are commercially available.[24]

BARIATRIC SURGEON

Operating on morbidly obese patients is one of the most technically difficult challenges that a surgeon can encounter. In elective cases, a potential major problem is an increase in wound infections.[25] Altogether, complications may be more common in academic centers, although this is probably a reflection of the patient population undergoing surgery rather than of the bariatric surgeon.[26] The International Federation for the Surgery of Obesity,[27] the American Society of Bariatric Surgeons,[28] and the Society of American Gastrointestinal and Endoscopic Surgeons[28] have issued guidelines concerning the education and proctoring requirements to credential surgeons who wish to perform bariatric surgery. Of particular importance in formulating these principles is the difficulty encountered in revisional bariatric surgery[29,30]; preferably, such cases are performed by experienced bariatric surgeons rather than by neophytes in this field.

ENTEROTOMY: A PRIMARY COMPLICATION

As with all surgery, when an intraoperative complication occurs, it is best dealt with by immediate detection and correction. The most dangerous problem is an undetected enterotomy.[31] Unlike bleeding, which is usually easy to identify, an undetected enterotomy may not manifest itself until several days after surgery. The most treacherous perforation, that of the esophagus, which is commonly caused by passage of oro- or nasoenteric instruments, is particularly difficult to detect. Unfortunately, such perforation often manifests only in the postoperative period. Requesting a postoperative gastrointestinal series with water-soluble contrast is the most reliable course of detection.[14] Unexplained tachycardia in the postoperative period may be the earliest harbinger of a missed perforation. It behooves the surgeon to evaluate a fast pulse rate aggressively.

Detection

There are two techniques to detect an intraoperative perforation. One involves insufflation of air into the gastrointestinal tract via a nasogastric or orogastric tube after the area under suspicion has been covered with normal saline. The surgeon looks for bubbles of air escaping from the viscus. In my experience, this is an unreliable test with an unacceptably high rate of false-positives and false-negatives.

The second technique involves instillation of methylene blue into the lumen of the gastrointestinal tract. When a perforation is suspected, this is my preferred test. It involves requesting that the anesthesiologist dilute 10 ml of methylene blue in 200 ml of normal saline, which is then instilled via an orogastric or nasogastric tube. Segments of the gastrointestinal tract that are inaccessible to the anesthesiologist, such as the excluded stomach in a gastric bypass, may require direct instillation of the dye solution by the surgeon, using a syringe and a small-caliber needle. Following the use of methylene blue, the patient will pass green urine for several days and will have to be assured that there is nothing amiss.

Repair

When an enterotomy is identified, it should be repaired, if possible, at the primary operation. If this is not technically possible, or if a salvage reexploration is being performed, the probability of a breakdown of the repair must be considered. The establishment of adequate drainage is vital and may be life saving. The means of establishing such drainage is left to the discretion of the surgeon. My preference is a sump tube that can be irrigated. In the event that an attempted repair breaks down, and satisfactory drainage has been established, permitting the patient's body to repair the defect while nutrition by parenteral alimentation is maintained is the therapy of choice.

▶ GENERAL CONSIDERATIONS

Secondary (Revision) Cases

Revisional bariatric cases are associated with a higher complication rate than that observed in primary cases.[29-31] In addition to raising a higher index of suspicion, all of the strategies enunciated above apply. Although there are more operative complications during revisional surgery, the long-term consequences are similar to those seen following primary procedures.[30]

Nursing Team

As with any surgical procedure, experienced nursing teams that understand the steps of the procedures and the use of the required equipment make bariatric procedures safer and more expeditious. Nurses should be aware of the increased incidence of retained instruments and laparotomy pads in the obese patient.[23]

Postoperative Emergencies

The most dreaded complication following a bariatric surgical operation is a leak from the gastrointestinal tract. As explained earlier, optimal management entails detection, possible repair, and establishment of drainage. In the event that the leak manifests in the days following surgery, aggressive, rapid management may be the difference between patient salvage and death.

Each case is unique and must be individualized; however, several general principles apply: In secondary procedures there are greater probabilities of complications.[30,32] The earliest indicator of an undetected gastrointestinal leak is tachycardia, which may be associated with a postoperative respiratory problem.[2] The most common bariatric surgery complication is respiratory in nature. In the event that the postoperative tachycardia does not abate with the implementation of forced coughing and the use of an incentive spirometer, pulmonary percussion, and nebulizers, in addition to ambulation, the evaluation should become more aggressive. The most effective investigation for detecting a leak is an upper gastrointestinal series using water-soluble contrast material. The identification of a leak that is not satisfactorily drained mandates reexploration.[14] It is important to remember that a positive test is useful. A test that does not demonstrate a leak may be misleading (e.g., the leak may be in an excluded portion of the gastrointestinal tract). If concern persists, the surgeon should be prepared to reexplore on clinical suspicion alone.

▶ SUMMARY

Bariatric surgery is evolving. Meticulous attention to perioperative management has decreased morbidity and mortality to the point where the risk-benefit ratio of bariatric surgery now favors surgical intervention.

▶ REFERENCES

1. Byrne TK: Complications of surgery for obesity. Surg Clin North Am 2001;81:1181-1193.
2. Mason EE, Renquist KE, Jiang D: Perioperative risks and safety of surgery for severe obesity. Am J Clin Nutr 1992;55:573S-576S.
3. Dajani AS, Taubert KA, Wilson W, et al: Prevention of bacterial endocarditis: recommendations by the American Heart Association. JAMA 1997;277:1794-1801.
4. The Standards Task Force, American Society of Colon and Rectal Surgeons: Practice parameters for antibiotic prophylaxis-supporting documentation. Dis Colon Rect 1992;35:278-285.
5. Forse RA, Karam B, MacLean LD, et al: Antibiotic prophylaxis for surgery in morbidly obese patients. Surgery 1989;106:750-757.
6. Msika S: Surgery for morbid obesity: 2: Complications: results of a technologic evaluation by the ANAES. J Chir (Paris) 2003;140:4-21.
7. Wu EC, Barba CA: Current practices in the prophylaxis of venous thromboembolism in bariatric surgery. Obes Surg 2000;10:7-14.
8. Clagett GP, Reisch JS: Prevention of venous thromboembolism in general surgical patients: results of meta-analysis. Ann Surg 1988;208:227-240.
9. Kumar R, McKinney WP, Raj G: Perioperative prophylaxis of venous thromboembolism. Am J Med Sci 1993;306:336-344.
10. National Institutes of Health, NIH Consensus Development: Prevention of venous thrombosis and pulmonary embolism. JAMA 1986;256:744-749.
11. Scholten DJ, Hoedema RM, Scholten SE: A comparison of two different prophylactic dose regimens of low molecular weight heparin in bariatric surgery. Obes Surg 2002;12:19-24.
12. Smith RC: Risk factors and prophylaxis for the development of venous thromboembolic disease. Consult Pharm 1996;11:565-580.
13. Perkins J, Beech A, Hands L: Vascular surgical society of Great Britain and Ireland: randomized controlled trial of heparin plus graduated compression stocking for the prophylaxis of deep venous thrombosis in general surgical patients. Br J Surg 1999;86:701.
14. Toppino M, Cesarani F, Comba A, et al: The role of early radiological studies after gastric bariatric surgery. Obes Surg 2001;11:447-454.

15. Sollazzi L, Perilli V, Modesti C, et al: Volatile anesthesia in bariatric surgery. Obes Surg 2001;11:623-626.
16. Nguyen NT, Goldman C, Rosenquist CJ, et al: Laparoscopic versus open gastric bypass: a randomized study of outcomes, quality of life, and costs. Ann Surg 2001;234:279-291.
17. De Luca M, de Werra C, Formato A, et al: Laparotomic vs laparoscopic lap-band: 4-year results with early and intermediate complications. Obes Surg 2000;10:266-268.
18. Israelsson LA, Jonsson T: Overweight and healing of midline incisions: the importance of suture technique. Eur J Surg 1997;163:175-180.
19. Perilli V, Sollazzi L, Bozza P, et al: The effects of the reverse Trendelenburg position on respiratory mechanics and blood gases in morbidly obese patients during bariatric surgery. Anesth Analg 2000;91:1520-1525.
20. Tera H: How to use abdominal wall retractors at laparotomy in grossly obese patients. World J Surg 1983;7:555-556.
21. Fisher BL: The Elite II Bariatric Surgery Retractor system: a recent addition to the bariatric surgeon's tool chest. Obes Surg 2001;11:225-228.
22. Greenstein RJ: Mechanical retraction in obesity and esophagogastric surgery. Obes Surg 1991;1:431-433.
23. Gawande AA, Studdert DM, Orav EJ, et al: Risk factors for retained instruments and sponges after surgery. N Engl J Med 2003;348:229-235.
24. Greenstein RJ: Mechanical retraction in laparoscopic surgery: intra-operative cholangiography. J Laparoendoscop Surg 1993;3:233-238.
25. Dindo D, Muller MK, Weber M, et al: Obesity in general elective surgery. Lancet 2003;361:2032-2035.
26. Lopez J, Sung J, Anderson W, et al: Is bariatric surgery safe in academic centers? Am Surg 2002;68:820-823.
27. Cowan GS Jr: The Cancun IFSO Statement on bariatric surgeon qualifications, International Federation for the Surgery of Obesity. Obes Surg 1998;8:86.
28. Society of American Gastrointestinal Endoscopic Surgeons, SAGES Bariatric Task Force: Guidelines for institutions granting bariatric privileges utilizing laparoscopic techniques. Surg Endosc 2003;17:2037-2040.
29. Greenstein RJ: Reexploration following vertical banded gastroplasty: technical observations and comorbidities from smoking, dentition and esophageal dysmotility. Obes Surg 1993;3:265-270.
30. Owens BM, Owens ML, Hill CW: Effect of revisional bariatric surgery on weight loss and frequency of complications. Obes Surg 1996;6:479-484.
31. Buckwalter JA, Herbst CA Jr: Leaks occurring after gastric bariatric operations. Surgery 1988;103:156-160.
32. Kothari SN, DeMaria EJ, Sugerman HJ, et al: Lap-band failures: conversion to gastric bypass and their preliminary outcomes. Surgery 2002;131:625-629.

section V

OPERATIVE PROCEDURES

18

Evolution of Bariatric Procedures and Selection Algorithm

Henry Buchwald, M.D., Ph.D.

By the early 1950s, years of clinical observation had taught physicians that the shortened gut led to massive weight loss. Could the "short-gut," as well as other manipulations of the gut, be harnessed as treatment for the morbidly obese? Bariatric surgery ideally should provide for massive weight loss, eventual weight maintenance, minimal short- and long-term side effects and complications, and reversibility. The complications associated with bariatric surgery procedures determine the cost-benefit ratios of these procedures. Reversibility is an essential prerequisite in order to provide a safe retreat from a potential iatrogenic catastrophe.

Bariatric surgery evolved in the 1950s from the jejunoileal (JI) bypass. This operation was the prototype of the malabsorptive genealogic branch of obesity operations.[1] Malabsorptive procedures are also maldigestive. They limit the small intestine's length and surface area to create decreased digestion of normal foods and decreased absorption of digested food elements. Thus, malabsorptive procedures result in the burning of body mass (preferably fat, not lean body mass). Weight loss ceases when a balance is reached between caloric absorption and expenditure, which is a function of intestinal adaptation and decreased caloric needs for a reduced body mass.

In the 1960s, a separate genus of bariatric operations evolved that combined intestinal malabsorption with gastric restriction (gastric bypass) but relied primarily on gastric restriction for weight loss. A minimum of long-term complications associated with the malabsorptive/restrictive gastric procedures made them preferable to the first generation of malabsorptive operations. The JI bypass is a highly effective weight-reduction operation, but it is associated with gas-bloat syndrome, steatorrhea, electrolyte imbalance, nephrolithiasis, hepatic fibrosis, cutaneous eruptions, and impaired mentation.[1] On the other hand, the gastric bypass causes dumping, iron-deficiency anemia, vitamin B_{12} malabsorption, and loss of the possibility of visualizing the distal stomach and duodenum. Nevertheless, the malabsorptive/restrictive genus of bariatric surgery became the most popular bariatric operation in the 1970s

and early 1980s and has remained so to the present in the United States.[1]

Malabsorptive operations, however, became dormant, rather than extinct. Indeed, JI bypass resurfaced in the 1970s to 1990s when many of its complications were eliminated or minimized in a species of malabsorptive operations—primarily the biliopancreatic diversion and its duodenal-switch modification. These newer malabsorptive procedures provided for two functional limbs of small intestine joined in a common terminal channel, avoiding intestinal stasis, bacterial overgrowth, and toxicemia.[1]

In the 1970s and 1980s, bariatric surgery was simplified by the introduction of purely restrictive gastric operations—gastroplasties, gastric partitioning, banded or vertical gastroplasties, and gastric banding. These operations have the fewest long-term complications, with outlet problems being the main concern. In the late 1990s, a new innovation, neither malabsorptive nor restrictive, was introduced into the armamentarium of bariatric surgery—namely, gastric pacing.

Over the years, certain bariatric operations have failed to be effective in the long term but have provided the germinal idea for future innovations. Others are currently in clinical use, and still others may revolutionize the field of bariatric surgery, creating dramatic offshoots from the genealogical tree of bariatric procedures. The introduction of laparoscopic skills has certainly expanded the field of bariatric surgery not only in the number of operations performed annually but also in the variety of procedures and their potentials. Table 18-1 provides a chronologic overview of the surgical operations for morbid obesity.

With this plethora of options for bariatric operations, can a specific operation be selected for a specific patient? To test this hypothesis, thoughts on the construction of an algorithm are presented. The basic formulation of an algorithm for bariatric surgery presumes that there is no gold-standard bariatric surgery procedure and that the skilled bariatric surgeon should be able to perform more than one kind of bariatric operation.

Table 18-1	CHRONOLOGIC OVERVIEW OF OPERATIONS			
	MALABSORPTIVE	MALABSORPTIVE/RESTRICTIVE	RESTRICTIVE	PACING
1950s	1953 Varco			
	1953 Kremen, Linner, Nelson			
1960s	1963 Payne & DeWind			
	1965 Sherman			
	1966 Lewis, Turnbill, Page	1967 Mason & Ito		
	1969 Payne & DeWind			
1970s	1971 Scott		1971 Mason & Printen	
	1971 Salmon			
	1971 Buchwald & Varco		1976 Tretbar	
	1977 Forestieri	1977 Alden		
	1978 Starkloff	1977 Griffen	1978 Wilkinson	
	1978 Lavorato			
	1979 Scopinaro		1979 Gomez	
			1979 Pace & Carey	
			1979 LaFave & Alden	
1980s	1980 Palmer & Marliss		1980 Wilkinson	
	1981 Eriksson		1981 Fabito	
			1981 Laws	
			1982 Kolle	
			1982 Mason	
		1983 Torres, Oca, Garrison	1983 Molina	
			1985 Bashour	
		1986 Linner & Drew	1986 Eckhout, Willbanks, & Moore	
		1987 Torres & Oca	1986 Kuzmak	
	1988 Cleator & Gourley	1988 Salmon		
	1989 Kral & Dorton	1989 Fobi		
1990s		1991 Fobi		
	1993 Marceau		1993 Catona	
			1993 Forsell	
		1994 Wittgrove & Clark	1994 Hess & Hess	
			1995 Chua & Mendiola	
		1997 Vassallo		
	1998 Hess & Hess		1998 Niville	
		1999 de la Torre & Scott	1999 Cadiere	1999 Cigaina
		1999 Higa		

▶ MALABSORPTIVE PROCEDURES

First Generation

In 1953, Dr. Richard L. Varco of the Department of Surgery at the University of Minnesota performed what was probably the first JI bypass, the original malabsorptive procedure performed specifically to induce weight loss.[1] This operation consisted of an end-to-end jejunoileostomy with a separate ileocecostomy for drainage of the bypassed segment (Fig. 18-1). Varco's contribution was preceded by an intestinal resection specifically for the management of obesity by Victor Henriksson of Gothenberg, Sweden.[2] Neither Varco nor Henriksson published their contributions.

In 1954, Kremen, Linner, and Nelson published a research article on nutritional aspects of the small intestine in dogs.[3] In their discussion section, they described a patient upon whom they had performed an end-to-end jejunoileal bypass for reduction of body weight. These authors, also from the University of Minnesota, can be credited with the first case report publication in bariatric surgery.

After a hiatus of some years, in 1963, Payne, DeWind, and Commons published the results of the first clinical program of massive intestinal bypass for the management of morbidly obese patients.[4] In a series they initiated in 1956, they described bypassing nearly the entire small intestine, the right colon, and half of the transverse colon in 10 morbidly obese female patients. Intestinal continuity was restored by an end-to-side anastomosis of the proximal 37.5 cm of jejunum to the mid-transverse colon. Although weight loss was dramatic, electrolyte imbalance, uncontrolled diarrhea, and liver failure proved prohibitive and required eventual reversal of the bypasses.[5] In actuality, this procedure was originally designed by Payne and DeWind to lead to unlimited weight loss, thereby requiring a second operation to restore additional intestinal length and weight equilibrium when ideal body weight was attained. All patients in this series, following their takedown operations, regained the weight previously lost.[6]

There were several other steps in the development of the JI bypass. In the mid-1960s, Sherman and colleagues,[7] as well as Payne and DeWind,[6] proposed the restoration of intestinal continuity proximal to the ileocecal valve by an end-to-side jejunoileostomy. The aim of these less radical

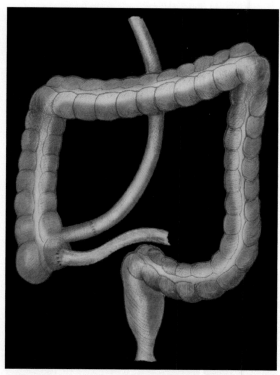

Figure 18-1. Jejunoileal bypass: end-to-end jejunoileostomy with ileocecostomy. 1953, Varco; 1954, Kremen, Linner, Nelson. (From Buchwald and Buchwald: Evolution of operative procedures for the management of morbid obesity, 1950-2000. Obes Surg 2002;12:705-717. By permission.)

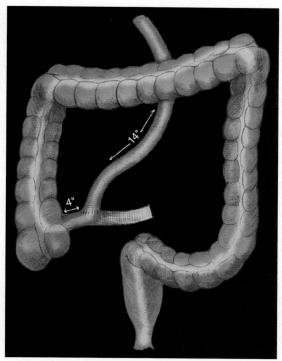

Figure 18-2. Jejunoileal bypass: classic 14″ + 4″ end-to-side jejunoileostomy. 1969, Payne, DeWind. (From Buchwald and Buchwald: Evolution of operative procedures for the management of morbid obesity, 1950-2000. Obes Surg 2002;12:705-717. By permission.)

bypasses was to achieve an eventual balance between caloric intake and the body's caloric needs, eliminating the necessity for a second operation and minimizing postoperative side effects. During this transitional phase, in 1962, Lewis, Turnbull, and Page reported a series of JI bypass procedures in which an end-to-side jejunotransverse colon anastomosis (similar to that originally reported by Payne and DeWind) was performed.[8] Again, significant complications ensued, requiring reversal of these procedures.[5]

In 1966, Lewis, Turnbull, and Page described 11 patients in whom they performed an end-to-side jejunocecostomy, a procedure that foreshadowed the general implementation of a less radical approach to the JI bypass.[9] Completing this evolution, Payne and DeWind entirely abandoned bypass to the colon.[6] In 1969, in a series of 80 morbidly obese patients, Payne and DeWind established what was to become the standard for the end-to-side jejunoileostomy procedure: anastomosis of the proximal 35 cm (14 inches) of jejunum to the terminal ileum, 10 cm (4 inches) from the ileocecal valve. This operation (the so-called 14 + 4 procedure) became the most commonly used bariatric operation in the United States at that time (Fig. 18-2). This procedure allowed for significant weight loss with moderate long-term side-effects and complications and did not require a second, restorative operation.

Although Payne and DeWind's classic JI bypass was widely adopted, nearly 10% of patients did not achieve significant weight loss, possibly due to reflux of nutrients into the bypassed ileum.[5] Thus, Scott and colleagues,[10] Salmon,[11] and Buchwald and Varco[12] independently

returned to the original procedure of Varco and of Kremen and colleagues: an end-to-end anastomosis to prevent reflux into the terminal ileum. In all these end-to-end operations, the ileocecal valve was preserved in order to decrease postoperative diarrhea and electrolyte loss, the appendix was removed, and the jejunal stump was attached to the transverse mesocolon or the cecum to avoid intussusception.[5]

Scott and colleagues' variation consisted of the anastomosis of 30 cm of jejunum to 30 cm of ileum, with the bypassed bowel draining into the transverse or sigmoid colon.[10] Also in 1971, Salmon reported his variation of the end-to-end jejunoileostomy: 25 cm of jejunum anastomosed to 50 cm of ileum, with the bypassed bowel draining into the mid-transverse colon.[11] In the same year, 1971, we reported our series in which 40 cm of jejunum were anastomosed to 4 cm of ileum, with the bypassed bowel draining into the cecum near the ileocecal valve.[12] In addition to producing significant weight loss, this JI bypass caused a marked and lasting reduction in the serum lipids in obese hyperlipidemic patients. Three months postoperatively, hyperlipidemic patients showed an average decrease in cholesterol of 90% (from 898 mg/dl to 90 mg/dl) and a reduction in average triglycerides of 95% (from 7255 mg/dl to 230 mg/dl).

Next there followed a series of modifications rarely performed by physicians other than the primary authors of the reports. Forestieri and colleagues,[13] Starkloff and colleagues,[14] and Palmer and Marliss[15] created various modifications at the jejunoileal anastomosis to prevent reflux into the bypassed segment without the necessity of dividing and separately draining the bypassed segment. Cleator and Gourlay[16] described an ileogastrostomy for drainage of the bypassed small intestine. Kral and Dorton[17] shortened the proximal intestinal segment back to the ligament of Treitz in a duodenoileal bypass modification.

Second Generation

As stated, the JI bypass was gradually abandoned for the gastric bypass because of its side effects and complications. Descendants, however, of the JI bypass flourish today. These modern operations share a key trait: no limb of the small intestine is left without flow through it. The enteric limb contains the flow of food, and the biliopancreatic limb contains the flow of bile and pancreatic juice.

Transition procedures were performed in 1978 by Lavorato and colleagues[18] and in 1981 by Eriksson.[19] Both groups performed an end-to-side JI bypass, with the proximal end of the bypassed segment of the small intestine anastomosed to the gallbladder, thereby diverting bile into the bypassed limb. These biliointestinal bypasses were not widely performed, and the modern malabsorptive operative era began with Scopinaro and colleagues' biliopancreatic diversion (BPD).[20] Nicola Scopinaro, of Genoa, Italy, reported his initial series of 18 patients in 1979,[20] and he subsequently performed thousands of these procedures. The current BPD consists of a horizontal partial gastrectomy (leaving 200 to 500 ml of proximal stomach) with closure of the duodenal stump, a gastrojejunostomy with a 250-cm Roux limb, and anastomosis of the biliopancreatic limb to the Roux limb 50 cm proximal to the ileocecal valve, creating an extremely short common channel (Fig. 18-3).[21]

More than a decade later, the BPD was modified in the United States and Canada by the addition of a duodenal switch. Hess and Hess deviated from the Scopinaro procedure by (1) making a lesser-curvature gastric tube and a greater-curvature gastric resection, rather than performing a horizontal gastrectomy; (2) preserving the pylorus; (3) dividing the duodenum and closing the distal duodenal stump; and (4) anastomosing the enteric limb to the proximal duodenum.[22] Marceau and colleagues performed a similar procedure but cross-stapled the duodenum without dividing it.[23] The Marceau procedure did not prove to be reliable because the cross-stapled duodenum routinely underwent disruption of the staple line and the subsequent loss of operative efficacy. The Hess and Hess procedure is outlined in Figure 18-4.

Even though the biliopancreatic diversion/duodenal switch (BPD/DS) is gaining greater acceptance in the United States and elsewhere and is now also being performed laparoscopically, the specific dimensions for this procedure have not become standard. It is generally agreed that the gastric volume should be approximately 100 ml. There are various measuring formulas, each with its advocates, for the relative lengths of the enteric (Roux) and biliopancreatic limbs. Though the common channel is usually 75 to 100 cm, in clinical practice today the common channel can be as short as 50 cm or as long as 150 cm.

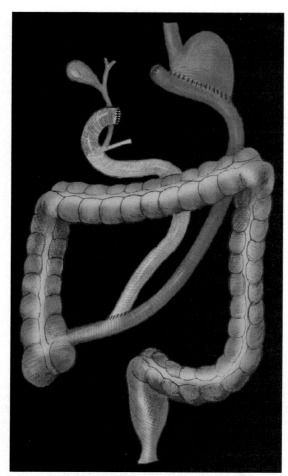

Figure 18-3. Biliopancreatic diversion. 1979, Scopinaro. (From Buchwald and Buchwald: Evolution of operative procedures for the management of morbid obesity, 1950-2000. Obes Surg 2002;12:705-71. By permission.)

▶ MALABSORPTIVE/RESTRICTIVE PROCEDURES

The malabsorptive/restrictive procedures involve a restrictive element consisting of the creation of a small gastric pouch with a small outlet that, on distention by food, causes the sensation of satiety; it is combined with a gastrointestinal bypass as the malabsorptive element. The extent of the bypass of the intestinal tract determines the degree of malabsorption. The minimal amount of intestinal tract bypassed consists of the distal stomach, the entire duodenum, and the first segment of the proximal jejunum. More extensive malabsorptive variations consist of gastric bypasses with a long Roux limb.

Origins

The first gastric bypass was developed by Mason and Ito in 1966, and it represented the origin of a new paradigm in weight-loss induction.[24] In the original Mason and Ito gastric bypass, the stomach was divided horizontally and a loop (not Roux limb) gastrojejunostomy was created between the proximal gastric pouch and the proximal jejunum (Fig. 18-5). The original upper gastric pouch of Mason was 100 to 150 ml in volume, with a stoma 12 mm

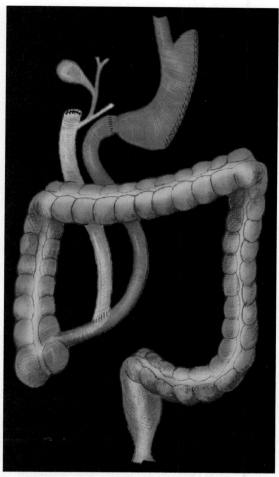

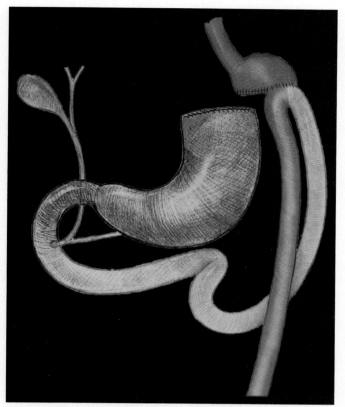

Figure 18-5. Gastric bypass: gastric transection with loop gastrojejunostomy. 1967, Mason, Ito. (From Buchwald and Buchwald: Evolution of operative procedures for the management of morbid obesity, 1950-2000. Obes Surg 2002;12:705-717. By permission.)

Figure 18-4. Duodenal switch with division of the duodenum. 1998, Hess, Hess. (From Buchwald and Buchwald: Evolution of operative procedures for the management of morbid obesity, 1950-2000. Obes Surg 2002;12:705-717. By permission.)

in diameter. Later, Mason and Printen reduced the pouch size to 50 ml to increase weight loss and, by including the acid-secreting mucosa in the distal stomach, reduce ulcer formation.[25]

In 1977, John Alden simplified this procedure by using a horizontal staple-line without gastric division.[26] This modification in a series of 100 patients, without mortality and with minimal morbidity, established the gastric bypass as the dominant procedure in this field.

Roux-en-Y Gastric Bypass

In 1977, Griffen and colleagues added a further modification to the gastric bypass, namely, the construction of a Roux-en-Y gastrojejunostomy, rather than a loop gastrojejunostomy (Fig. 18-6).[27] This gastric bypass, the Roux-en-Y gastric bypass (RYGB) had the advantages of avoiding tension on the loop and of preventing bile reflux into the upper gastric pouch.[28] Both Griffen and colleagues[27] and Buchwalter[29] reported randomized studies demonstrating that RYGB patients were achieving weight loss equivalent to that previously seen after the JI bypass.

Over the next several years, variations of the RYGB were introduced. Torres, Oca, and Garrison stapled the stomach vertically rather than horizontally.[30] Linner and Drew reinforced the gastrojejunal outlet with a fascial band.[31] Torres and Oca reported a modification of the vertical RYGB with the creation of a long Roux limb for individuals who had failed their original procedure.[32] The so-called long-limb RYGB was later popularized as a primary operation for the superobese by Brolin and colleagues.[33] There have been several modifications of the long-limb RYGB that vary with the length of the common channel proposed.

Subsequently, Salmon combined two procedures—a vertical banded gastroplasty (to be discussed) and a long-limb RYGB.[34] In 1989, Fobi introduced the Silastic ring vertical RYGB, creating a small vertical pouch drained by a gastrojejunostomy and containing a restrictive Silastic ring proximal to the gastrojejunostomy.[35] Fobi later modified this RYGB by dividing the stomach and interposing the jejunal Roux limb between the gastric pouch and the bypassed stomach to ensure maintenance of the gastric division (Fig. 18-7).[36] In a further variation, which has not gained popularity, Vassallo and colleagues performed a distal BPD with no gastric resection and with a transient vertical banded gastroplasty constructed using a polydioxanone band that is absorbed within 6 months.[37]

In 1994, Wittgrove, Clark, and Tremblay reported their results with laparoscopic RYGB, introducing the

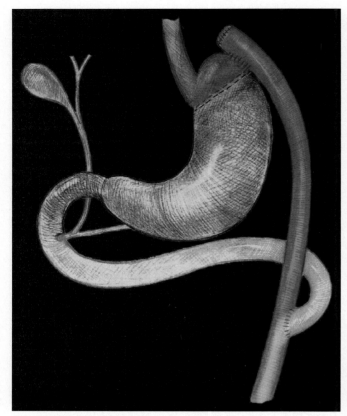

Figure 18-6. Gastric bypass: horizontal gastric stapling with Roux gastrojejunostomy. 1977, Griffen. (From Buchwald and Buchwald: Evolution of operative procedures for the management of morbid obesity, 1950-2000. Obes Surg 2002;12:705-717. By permission.)

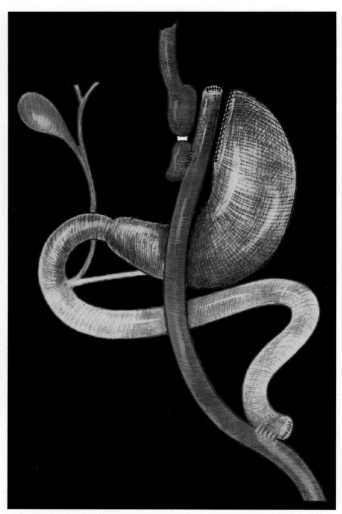

Figure 18-7. Gastric bypass: vertical gastric division with interposed Roux gastrojejunostomy and proximal Silastic ring. 1991, Fobi. (From Buchwald and Buchwald: Evolution of operative procedures for the management of morbid obesity, 1950-2000. Obes Surg 2002;12:705-717. By permission.)

anvil of their end-to-end stapler endoscopically.[38] This procedure was modified by de la Torre and Scott with their introduction of the anvil of the stapler intraabdominally to allow greater precision in anvil placement and avoid esophageal complications.[39] Subsequently, several laparoscopic bariatric surgeons avoided the end-to-end stapler altogether and began to utilize a linear stapler to form the gastrojejunostomy. Finally, in 1999, Higa and colleagues, to avoid the relatively high incidence of gastrointestinal anastomotic leaks in laparoscopic procedures, described a technique for hand-sewing the gastrojejunostomy laparoscopically.[40] Within half a decade, the most common bariatric procedure in the United States, the RYGB, was being performed predominantly by using a laparoscopic technique.

▶ RESTRICTIVE PROCEDURES

Gastroplasties

The primary name in gastric restrictive surgery is again Mason, who, in association with Printen, performed the first known restrictive procedure in 1971. The solely restrictive operations can be performed more rapidly than

a RYGB and are more physiologic because no part of the gastrointestinal tract is bypassed or rerouted. In their 1971 gastroplasty procedure, Printen and Mason divided the stomach horizontally from the lesser curvature to the greater curvature, leaving a gastric conduit at the greater curvature (Fig. 18-8).[41] This procedure was unsuccessful in maintaining weight loss.[41,42] In 1979, Gomez introduced the horizontal gastric stapling modification of the divided gastroplasty and, in addition, reinforced the greater-curvature outlet with a running suture.[42] This, too, did not result in lasting success. Similarly, the gastric-partitioning operation of Pace and colleagues (1979) was unsuccessful because the partitioning created by the removal of several staples from the middle of the stapling instrument was followed by the widening of the gastrogastrostomy outlet.[43] To overcome this problem, in 1979, LaFave and Alden performed a total gastric cross-stapling and a sewed anterior gastrogastrostomy; this operation also was not successful in the long term.[44]

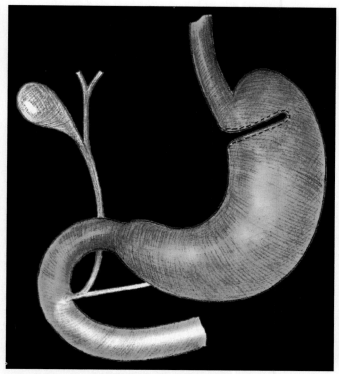

Figure 18-8. Gastroplasty: partial gastric transition with greater-curvature conduit. 1971, Mason, Printen. (From Buchwald and Buchwald: Evolution of operative procedures for the management of morbid obesity, 1950-2000. Obes Surg 2002;12:705-717. By permission.)

Figure 18-9. Gastroplasty: Silastic ring vertical banded gastroplasty. 1981, Laws. (From Buchwald and Buchwald: Evolution of operative procedures for the management of morbid obesity, 1950-2000. Obes Surg 2002;12:705-717. By permission.)

In 1981, Fabito was the first to perform a vertical gastroplasty by employing a modified TA-90 stapler and reinforcing the outlet with seromuscular sutures.[45] That same year, Laws was probably the first to use a Silastic ring as a permanent, nonexpandable support for the vertical gastroplasty outlet (Fig. 18-9).[46]

In 1980, Mason performed his last gastroplasty variation—the vertical banded gastroplasty (VBG).[47] This VBG involved a novel concept: making a window, a through-and-through perforation in both walls of the stomach, with the end-to-end stapling instrument just above the crow's foot on the lesser curvature. This window was used for the insertion of a standard TA-90 stapler to the angle of His to create a small, stapled vertical pouch. The lesser-curvature outlet was banded with a polypropylene mesh collar (1.5 cm wide and 5.5 cm long) through the gastric window and around the lesser-curvature conduit (Fig. 18-10).

The most recent and popular innovation of gastroplasty is the 1986 Eckhout, Willbanks, and Moore Silastic ring gastroplasty (also referred to as a VBG).[48] This method uses a specially constructed notched stapler to avoid the window of the Mason VBG and produce a final result comparable to that of the Laws procedure (see Fig. 18-9). Also, the nonreactive, far narrower (.25 cm wide, 4.4 cm long) Silastic ring prevents the formation of granulation tissue that is at times induced by the polypropylene (Marlex) mesh, causing subsequent outlet obstruction.

In 1994 Hess and Hess,[49] and in 1995 Chua and Mendiola[50] performed the VBG laparoscopically.

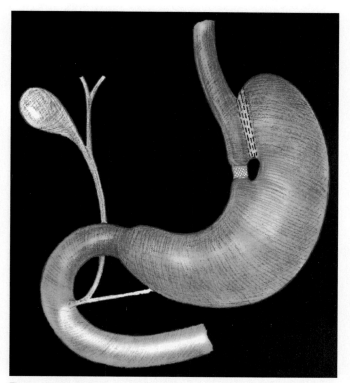

Figure 18-10. Gastroplasty: vertical banded gastroplasty. 1982, Mason. (From Buchwald and Buchwald: Evolution of operative procedures for the management of morbid obesity, 1950-2000. Obes Surg 2002;12:705-717. By permission.)

They utilized the standard Mason technique, adapting available laparoscopic instruments. A different approach was introduced by Champion and colleagues, who resected a triangular wedge of the fundus of the stomach laparoscopically, using the cutting stapler, and banding the elongated lesser curvature of the stomach outlet with polypropylene mesh.[51]

Gastric Banding

Gastric banding (GB) is the least invasive of the gastric restrictive procedures. A small pouch and a small stoma are created by a band around the upper stomach. The stomach is not cut or crushed by staplers and no anastomoses are made. The precursors of GB are found in the fundoplication procedure of Tretbar and colleagues (1976)[52] and in the mesh wrapping of the entire stomach by Wilkinson (1980).[53] Independently, Wilkinson and Peloso (1978),[54] Kolle (1982),[55] and Molina and Oria (1983)[56] initiated actual GB. Their bands were not adjustable, similar to the "gastro-clip" of Bashour and Hill (1985).[57]

In 1986, Kuzmak introduced the inflatable Silastic band connected to a subcutaneous port, which is used for the percutaneous introduction or removal of fluid to adjust the caliber of the gastric band (Fig. 18-11).[58] In 1992-1993, Broadbent and colleagues[59] and Catona and colleagues[60] were probably the first to perform GB laparoscopically, and in 1993 Belachew[61] and Forsell[62] and their colleagues were the first to perform adjustable GB laparoscopically. Niville and colleagues reported placing the posterior aspect of the band at the distal esophagus and constructing a tiny anterior gastric pouch, the so-called virtual gastric pouch.[63] Optimal laparoscopic, adjustable-GB results have been reported with the pars flaccida approach, namely, the construction of a high retrogastric tunnel above the lesser sac with a 15-ml upper gastric pouch,

total band imbrication anteriorly by using at least four gastrogastric sutures, and the delaying of band inflation until 4 weeks postoperatively.[64]

The world of surgical robotics entered the field of bariatric surgery in 1999 with the report by Cadiere and colleagues of the world's first placement of an adjustable GB under robotic control.[65]

▶ GASTRIC PACING PROCEDURES

Another innovation in bariatric surgery has been gastric pacing, first introduced by Cigaina and colleagues in 1996.[66] They were able, in an animal model, to create gastric paresis and weight loss by antral electric stimulation. In this process, an electrode placed into the wall of the stomach between the incisura and the esophagogastric junction along the lesser curvature is connected by a wire lead to a pacer in a subcutaneous pocket that is programmed to deliver a bipolar pulse to the stomach (Fig. 18-12). An alternative hypothesis to the effect of gastric pacing is afferent vagal stimulation of the hypothalamus to produce satiety. Studies of gastric pacing in humans are currently underway in both Europe and the United States.

▶ PATIENT-PROCEDURE ALGORITHM

With the wide current selection of bariatric procedures, some in the field have proposed the construction of algorithms to match a given patient to a given operation. Obviously, these algorithms cannot be absolute, but they may serve as guidelines to help the surgeon and the patient in the decision-making process. The proposed algorithm is the invention of Buchwald; it has not yet been tested in a clinical setting.[73]

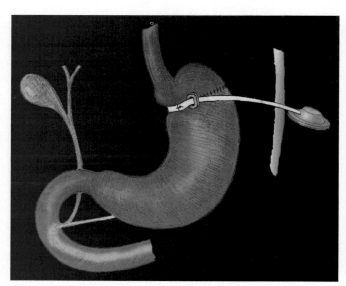

Figure 18-11. Gastric band: adjustable Silastic band was subsequently inserted at a much higher location. 1986, Kuzmak. (From Buchwald: Overview of bariatric surgery. J Am Coll Surg 2002;194:367-375. By permission.)

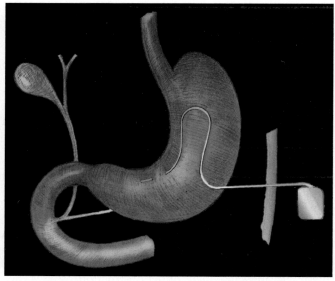

Figure 18-12. Gastric electrode bipolar pulsation. 1999, Cigaina. (From Buchwald and Buchwald: Evolution of operative procedures for the management of morbid obesity, 1950-2000. Obes Surg 2002;12:705-717. By permission.)

Variables

PATIENT VARIABLES

1. Weight. Body mass index (BMI) has six categories: 30 to 34.9; 35 to 39.9; 40 to 44.9; 45 to 49.9; 50 to 54.9; and above 55. A BMI of 30 to 34.9 falls below the current definition of morbid obesity, even in the presence of significant comorbidities. There is, however, impetus today to liberalize the lower limit of morbid obesity.[67] Superobesity is usually been defined as a BMI above 50; however, for this classification system, a BMI above 55 is used.

2. Age. A distinction is made between those less than or more than 40 years of age. For this algorithm, the dividing age has been chosen as 40 because it is customary to consider age above 40 to be a risk factor for elective surgery.

3. Gender/race/body habitus. Gender may be an independent or a dependent (e.g., related to race) variable.[68] Responses to bariatric surgery among racial and ethnic groups may vary. There is evidence that African-Americans do not have a weight response to bariatric surgery comparable to that of Caucasians.[68,69] The same may be true of individuals of Hispanic descent.[70] There is also evidence associating cardiovascular and other risks in the morbidly obese with body habitus, in particular, central obesity in males and android obesity in females.[71,72]

4. Presence of major comorbidities. Type 2 diabetes, hyperlipidemia, hypertension, obstructive sleep apnea, and other disorders are among the major comorbidities that afflict the morbidly obese.

EFFICACY OF WEIGHT LOSS

Few papers in the literature document long-term patient follow-up of more than 5 years or, indeed, longer than 2 years with an adequate percentage of patients followed.[73] Thus, I chose the bias introduced by 1-year follow-up results in order to base the algorithm on a large patient sample with accurate follow-up data. A literature search revealed 16 reports of GB suitable for review, with a total of 4429 patients; the mean and case-weighted mean for percent excess weight loss (%EWL) were 48.6% and 49.5%. Fifteen VBG reports were reviewed, for a total of 3382 patients; the mean and case-weighted mean for the %EWL were 58.3% and 60.2%. Eleven RYGB papers were suitable for review, with a total of 2949 patients; the mean and case-weighted mean for %EWL were 68.6% and 70.1%. Nine BPD/DS reports were suitable for review, with a total of 3903 patients; the mean and case-weighted mean for the %EWL were 68.8% and 71.7%. Finally, the literature for the long-limb RYGB was isolated and consisted of only three suitable reports, with a total of 301 patients; the mean and case-weighted mean for the %EWL were 71.6% and 74.6%.

Algorithm Construction

The first approximation of the construction of the algorithm was for the selection of an operation based solely on the preoperative BMI.[73] The second approximation, or second line in a flow diagram, was based on age, with the assumption that in patients less than 40 years old, the algorithmic decisions lines can be modified to include relatively less definitive procedures, and for patients more than 40 years old, relatively more definitive procedures. By selecting more definitive procedures for the older patients, reoperations on older patients would be minimized. The third approximation in the construction of the algorithm was based on a consideration of gender/race/body habitus. If these combined criteria predict a greater likelihood of refractory %EWL, a more definitive procedure should be selected. If, on the other hand, these factors in a particular body habitus predict a markedly increased operative risk, a simpler, faster operation should be selected. The final formulation is based on the presence of existing preoperative comorbidities. It is to be expected that the fewer

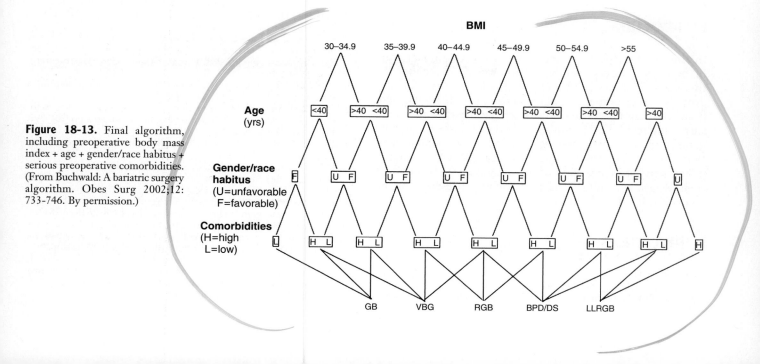

Figure 18-13. Final algorithm, including preoperative body mass index + age + gender/race habitus + serious preoperative comorbidities. (From Buchwald: A bariatric surgery algorithm. Obes Surg 2002;12:733-746. By permission.)

OC = 1.0 + BMI Number (1 to 6) ± 0.5 (age <40>) ± 0.5 (GRH, Favorable or
Unfavorable) ±1 (CoM, Low or High).

Operative category (OC): GB = 0–3; VBG = 2–5; RGB = 3–6; BPD/DS = 4–7; LLRGB = 6–9

BMI: 30–34.9 = 1, 35–39.9 = 2, 40–44.9 = 3, 45–49.9 = 4, 50–54.9 = 5, >55 = 6

Age: <40 = −0.5, >40 = +0.5

Gender, race, body habitus (GRH): Favorable = −0.5, Unfavorable = +0.5

Significant preoperative comorbidities (CoM): Low = −1, High = +1

Figure 18-14. Bariatric algorithm equation. (From Buchwald: A bariatric surgery algorithm. Obes Surg 2002; 12:733-746. By permission.)

serious preoperative comorbidities that exist, the better the patient's long-term prognosis. Such patients can be guided toward the procedures with the lowest operative risk and the fewest long-term operation-engendered morbidities. Conversely, the greater the number of serious existing preoperative comorbidities (and even though it is more likely that the patient's long-term prognosis will be poorer), the better it is to guide a patient toward the more definitive procedures, even though the operative risks and long-term operation-engendered morbidities may be higher.

The fourth and final approximation for a flow-diagram of this algorithm is given in Figure18-13. Except for the lower and upper extremes, each terminal operative designation allows for final selection based on surgeon and patient preference. The flow diagram formulation can be converted into an equation (Fig. 18-14). Counting 0 as an integer, every operative category has 4 degrees of freedom, or relative certainty of selection within an operative category. There is also an overlap among integers to offer further freedom for surgeon and patient preference.

▶ SUMMARY

In this chapter, we have delineated the evolutionary tree of bariatric surgery. In the future, certain branches of this tree will become obsolete and will show no further growth. Other branches will engender new offshoots. And branches may be grafted onto this tree, bearing new and surprising fruit. The evolution of bariatric surgery mirrors general medical progress—innovation, trial, standardization, and obsolescence. Bariatric surgeons and bariatric patients living in this state of flux may be greatly aided in their decision-making reasoning by the presence of an algorithm for the selection of operation.

▶ REFERENCES

1. Buchwald H, Rucker RD: The rise and fall of jejunoileal bypass. In Nelson RL, Nyhus LM (eds): Surgery of the Small Intestine, pp. 529-541. Norwalk, CT, Appleton Century Crofts, 1987.
2. Henriksson V: Kan tunnfarmsresektion forsvaras som terapi mot fettsot? Nordisk Medicin 1952;47:744. (Can small bowel resection be defended as therapy for obesity? Obes Surg 1994;4:54.)
3. Kremen AJ, Linner LH, Nelson CH: An experimental evaluation of the nutritional importance of proximal and distal small intestine. Ann Surg 1954;140:439-444.
4. Payne JH, DeWind LT, Commons RR: Metabolic observations in patients with jejunocolic shunts. Am J Surg 1963;106:272-289.
5. Deitel M: Jejunocolic and jejunoileal bypass: an historical perspective. In Deitel M (ed): Surgery for the Morbidly Obese Patient, pp. 81-89. Philadelphia, Lea & Febiger, 1998.
6. Payne JH, DeWind LT: Surgical treatment of obesity. Am J Surg 1969;118:141-147.
7. Sherman CD, May AG, Nye W: Clinical and metabolic studies following bowel bypassing for obesity. Ann N Y Acad Sci 1965;131:614-622.
8. Lewis LA, Turnbull RB, Page LH: "Short-circuiting" of the small intestine. JAMA 1962;182:77-79.
9. Lewis LA, Turnbull RB, Page LH: Effects of jejunocolic shunt on obesity, serum lipoproteins, lipids, and electrolytes. Arch Intern Med 1966;117:4-16.
10. Scott HW, Sandstead HH, Brill AB: Experience with a new technique of intestinal bypass in the treatment of morbid obesity. Ann Surg 1971;174:560-572.
11. Salmon PA: The results of small intestine bypass operations for the treatment of obesity. Surg Gynecol Obstet 1971;132:965-979.
12. Buchwald H, Varco RL: A bypass operation for obese hyperlipidemic patients. Surgery 1971;70:62-70.
13. Forestieri P, DeLuca L, Bucci L: Surgical treatment of high degree obesity: our own criteria to choose the appropriate type of jejuno-ileal bypass: a modified Payne technique. Chir Gastroenterol 1977;11:401-408.
14. Starkloff GB, Stothert JC, Sundaram M: Intestinal bypass: a modification. Ann Surg 1978;188:697-700.
15. Palmer JA, Marliss EB: The present status of surgical procedures for obesity. In Deitel M (ed): Nutrition in Clinical Surgery, pp. 281-292. Baltimore, Williams & Wilkins, 1980.
16. Cleator IGM, Gourlay RH: Ileogastrostomy for morbid obesity. Can J Surg 1988;31:114-116.
17. Kral JG: Duodenoileal bypass. In Deitel M (ed): Surgery for the Morbidly Obese Patient, pp. 99-103. Philadelphia, Lea & Febiger, 1998.
18. Lavorato F, Doldi SB, Scaramella R: Evoluzione storica della terapia chirurgica della grande obesita. Minerva Med 1978;69:3847-3857.
19. Eriksson F: Biliointestinal bypass. Int J Obes 1981;5:437-447.
20. Scopinaro N, Gianetta E, Civalleri D: Biliopancreatic bypass for obesity. II. Initial experiences in man. Br J Surg 1979;66:618-620.
21. Scopinaro N, Adami GF, Marinari GM, et al: Biliopancreatic diversion: two decades of experience. In Deitel M, Cowan SM Jr (eds): Update: Surgery for the Morbidly Obese Patient, pp. 227-258. Toronto, FD-Communications, 2000.

22. Hess DW, Hess DS: Biliopancreatic diversion with a duodenal switch. Obes Surg 1998;8:267-282.
23. Marceau P, Biron S, Bourque R-A, et al: Biliopancreatic diversion with a new type of gastrectomy. Obes Surg 1993;3:29-35.
24. Mason EE, Ito C: Gastric bypass in obesity. Surg Clin North Am 1967;47:1345-1352.
25. Mason EE, Printen KJ: Optimizing results of gastric bypass. Ann Surg 1975;182:405-413.
26. Alden JF: Gastric and jejuno-ileal bypass: a comparison in the treatment of morbid obesity. Arch Surg 1977;112:799-806.
27. Griffen WO, Young VL, Stevenson CC: A prospective comparison of gastric and jejunoileal bypass procedures for morbid obesity. Ann Surg 1977;186:500-507.
28. McCarthy HB, Rucker RD, Chan EK, et al: Gastritis after gastric bypass surgery. Surgery 1985;98:68-71.
29. Buckwalter JA: Clinical trial of jejunoileal and gastric bypass for the treatment of obesity: four-year progress report. Am Surg 1980;46:377-381.
30. Torres JC, Oca CF, Garrison RN: Gastric bypass: Roux-en-Y gastrojejunostomy from the lesser curvature. South Med J 1983;76:1217-1221.
31. Linner JR, Drew RL: New modification of Roux-en-Y gastric bypass procedure. Clin Nutr 1986;5:33-34.
32. Torres J, Oca C: Gastric bypass lesser curvature with distal Roux-en-Y. Bariatr Surg 1987;5:10-15.
33. Brolin RE, Kenler HA, Gorman JH, et al: Long-limb gastric bypass in the superobese: a prospective randomized study. Ann Surg 1992;21:387-395.
34. Salmon PA: Gastroplasty with distal gastric bypass: a new and more successful weight-loss operation for the morbidly obese. Can J Surg 1988;31:111-113.
35. Fobi MA: The surgical technique of the banded Roux-en-Y gastric bypass. J Obes Weight Reg 1989;8:99-102.
36. Fobi MA: Why the operation I prefer is Silastic ring vertical banded gastric bypass. Obes Surg 1991;1:423-426.
37. Vassallo C, Negri L, Della Valle A, et al: Biliopancreatic diversion with transitory gastroplasty preserving duodenal bulb: 3 years experience. Obes Surg 1997;7:30-33.
38. Wittgrove AC, Clark GW, Tremblay, LJ: Laparoscopic gastric bypass, Roux-en-Y: preliminary report of five cases. Obes Surg 1994;4:353-357.
39. de la Torre RA, Scott JS: Laparoscopic Roux-en-Y gastric bypass: a totally intra-abdominal approach—technique and preliminary report. Obes Surg 1999;9:492-497.
40. Higa KD, Boone KB, Ho T: Laparoscopic Roux-en-Y gastric bypass for morbid obesity in 850 patients: technique and follow-up. Obes Surg 2000;10:146 (abstract, p. 34).
41. Printen KJ, Mason EE: Gastric surgery for relief of morbid obesity. Arch Surg 1973;106:428-431.
42. Gomez CA: Gastroplasty in morbid obesity. Surg Clin North Am 1979;59:1113-1120.
43. Pace WG, Martin EW, Tetirick CE, et al: Gastric partitioning for morbid obesity. Ann Surg 1979;190:392-400.
44. LaFave JW, Alden JF: Gastric bypass in the operative revision of the failed jejuno-ileal bypass. Arch Surg 1979;114:438-444.
45. Fabito DC: Gastric vertical stapling. Read before the Bariatric Surgery colloquium, Iowa City, Iowa, June 1, 1981.
46. Laws HL, Piatadosi S: Superior gastric reduction procedure for morbid obesity: a prospective, randomized trial. Am J Surg 1981;193:334-336.
47. Mason EE: Vertical banded gastroplasty. Arch Surg 1982;117:701-706.
48. Eckhout GV, Willbanks OL, Moore JT: Vertical ring gastroplasty for obesity: five-year experience with 1463 patients. Am J Surg 1986;152:713-716.
49. Hess DW, Hess DS: Laparoscopic vertical banded gastroplasty with complete transection of the staple-line. Obes Surg 1994;4:44-46.
50. Chua TY, Mendiola RM: Laparoscopic vertical banded gastroplasty: the Milwaukee experience. Obes Surg 1995;5:77-80.
51. Champion JK, Hunt T, Delisle N: Laparoscopic vertical banded gastroplasty and Roux-en-Y gastric bypass in morbid obesity. Obes Surg 1999;9:123(abstract).
52. Tretbar LL, Taylor TL, Sifers EC: Weight reduction: gastric plication for morbid obesity. J Kans Med Soc 1976;77:488-490.
53. Wilkinson LH: Reduction of gastric reservoir capacity. J Clin Nutr 1980;33:515-517.
54. Wilkinson LH, Peloso OA: Gastric (reservoir) reduction for morbid obesity. Arch Surg 1981;116:602-605.
55. Kolle K: Gastric banding. OMGI 7th Congress, Stockholm,1982; 145;37(abstract).
56. Molina M, Oria HE: Gastric segmentation: a new, safe, effective, simple, readily revised and fully reversible surgical procedure for the correction of morbid obesity. 6th Bariatric Surgery Colloquium, Iowa City. 2-3 June 1983;15(abstract).
57. Bashour SB, Hill RW: The gastro-clip gastroplasty: an alternative surgical procedure for the treatment of morbid obesity. Tex Med 1985;81:36-38.
58. Kuzmak LI: Silicone gastric banding: a simple and effective operation for morbid obesity. Contemp Surg 1986;28:13-18.
59. Broadbent R, Tracy M, Harrington P: Laparoscopic gastric banding: a preliminary report. Obes Surg 1993;3:63-67.
60. Catona A, Gossenberg M, La Manna A, et al: Laparoscopic gastric banding: preliminary series. Obes Surg 1993;3:207-209.
61. Belachew M, Legrand M, Jacquet N: Laparoscopic placement of adjustable silicone gastric banding in the treatment of morbid obesity: an animal model experimental study; a video film; a preliminary report. Obes Surg 1993;3:140(abstract).
62. Forsell P, Hallberg D, Hellers G: Gastric banding for morbid obesity: initial experience with a new adjustable band. Obes Surg 1993;3:369-374.
63. Niville E, Vankeirsblick J, Dams A, et al: Laparoscopic adjustable esophagogastric banding: a preliminary experience. Obes Surg 1998;8:39-42.
64. Belachew M, Legrand MJ, Vincent V: History of Lap-Band®: from dream to reality. Obes Surg 2001;11:297-302.
65. Cadiere GB, Himpens J, Vertruyen M: The world's first obesity surgery performed by a surgeon at a distance. Obes Surg (England) 1999;9:206-209.
66. Cigaina V, Pinato G, Rigo V: Gastric peristalsis control by mono situ electrical stimulation: a preliminary study. Obes Surg 1996;6:247-249.
67. Buchwald H, for the Consensus Conference Panel: Bariatric surgery for morbid obesity: health implications for patients, health professionals, and third-party payers. J Am Coll Surg 2005;200:593-604.
68. DeMaria EJ, Sugerman HJ, Meador JG, et al: High failure rate after laparoscopic adjustable silicone gastric banding for treatment of morbid obesity. Ann Surg 2001;233:809-818.
69. Sugarman HS, Londrey GL, Kellum JM, et al: Weight loss with vertical banded gastroplasty and Roux-en-Y gastric bypass for morbid obesity with selective vs random assignment. Am J Surg 1989; 157:93-102.
70. Capella RF, Capella JF: Ethnicity, type of obesity surgery and weight loss. Obes Surg 1993;3:375-380.
71. Khaodhiar L, Blackburn GL: Obesity assessment. Am Heart J 2001;142:1095-1101.
72. Schapira DV, Kumar NG, Lyman GH, et al: Upper-body fat distribution and endometrial cancer risk. JAMA 1991;266:1808-1811.
73. Buchwald H: A bariatric surgery algorithm. Obes Surg 2002;12:733-746.

19

Laparoscopic Adjustable Gastric Banding

Mitiku Belachew, M.D.

Attempts to restrict intake surgically by means of a gastric band for the treatment of morbid obesity can be traced back to the early 1980s. Wilkinson and Peloso (1981),[1] Kolle (1982),[2] and Molina and Oria (1983)[3] have been credited with initiating the nonadjustable gastric banding approach to restrictive bariatric surgery.[4] Yet one group discontinued use of the Molina nonadjustable gastric band early on because it seemed to require a high percentage of reoperations.[5] Then, an *adjustable* gastric banding technique was introduced; it was based on a liquid-filled Silastic cuff. This approach was tested for the first time in mini pigs by Szinicz and colleagues.[6,7]

The first adjustable gastric banding systems successfully developed for use in humans were the adjustable silicone gastric band (ASGB)[8,9] and the Swedish adjustable gastric band (Swedish band),[10,11] both initially placed by open surgery. A preliminary report comparing the Kuzmak ASGB with the already established vertical banded gastroplasty (VBG) indicated that complications were minor and rare in both groups and that weight-loss outcomes were similar in the two types of procedures.[12]

It was inevitable that the next phase in bariatric surgery would be the development of laparoscopic adjustable gastric banding. In our bariatric surgical experience we had performed hundreds of VBG procedures. The choice then was whether the VBG or the ASGB would be the more appropriate operation to develop for laparoscopic application. We chose to work with the adjustable gastric band because, in addition to being as effective in producing weight loss as the VBG, gastric band surgery was also less invasive of the stomach, totally reversible, and offered a stoma adjustable to the patient's ongoing needs. In addition, we presumed that the gastric banding procedure would be easier to perform and standardize laparoscopically than the stapling procedure.

First, we developed an animal model for the laparoscopic technique using a series of band prototypes specifically designed for insertion through laparoscopic trocars and passage behind the stomach.[13] We then proceeded to the development and application of the laparoscopic

ASGB (which became the LAP-BAND) for use in obese patients.[14-16] Meanwhile, Cadiere and colleagues went ahead with laparoscopic placement of the Kuzmak ASGB in an obese female patient.[17] Laparoscopic gastric banding for the treatment of obesity was also reported by Catona and collaborators, first using variations of nonadjustable bands and then using the open ASGB[18] and the Swedish band.[19]

These activities have led to the commercial development and current marketing of the following laparoscopic adjustable gastric bands:

- LAP-BAND, Inamed Health (formerly BioEnterics), United States
- Swedish Adjustable Gastric Band, Obtech Medical (acquired by Ethicon Endo-Surgery [Johnson & Johnson]), Switzerland
- MIDBAND, Médical Innovation Développement, France
- Heliogast Adjustable Gastric Ring, Hélioscopie, France
- AMI Band, Agency for Medical Interventions, Austria
- Pier Band, Minimizer, Germany

▶ DESCRIPTION OF THE LAPAROSCOPIC ADJUSTABLE GASTRIC BAND

My practical experience with laparoscopic adjustable gastric banding has involved the development and implementation of a single device, the LAP-BAND System[20]; thus, the main focus of the chapter is on this system. Published information is sparse for banding systems other than the LAP-BAND and the Swedish band.

Design

The main components of the LAP-BAND are the silicone elastomer band, access port, and kink-resistant

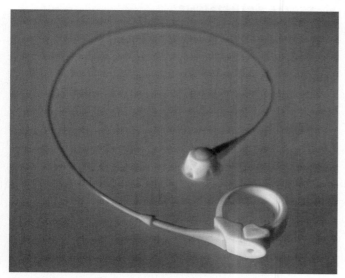

Figure 19-1. The main components of the LAP-BAND are the silicone elastomer band, access port, and kink-resistant tubing.

tubing (Fig. 19-1). The LAP-BAND design has changed little over the years other than in some subtle, yet meaningful, enhancements of the design. For example, to allow for variations in port placement techniques and to increase the port's durability, continuous improvements have been made to the access port tubing transition.

Principle and Mode of Action

Adjustable gastric banding devices are implanted laparoscopically to create an adjustable restricted opening (stoma) and a small gastric pouch to limit food consumption and induce early satiety (Fig. 19-2).[21] There may be another mechanism, in addition to mechanical restriction, that explains satiety. The presence of a foreign body in contact

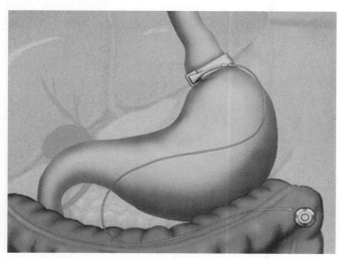

Figure 19-2. Adjustable gastric banding devices are implanted laparoscopically to create an adjustable restricted opening (stoma) and a small gastric pouch to limit food consumption and induce early satiety.

with the gastric wall, which has afferent as well as efferent vagus nerve fibers, may explain the postoperative reduction of hunger. This assumption has to be confirmed by electrophysiologic research on the banded stomach.

Features

The advantages of laparoscopic abdominal surgery are well known and have been widely proclaimed for cholecystectomy,[22] adjustable gastric banding,[16,23] vertical banded gastroplasty,[24] and Roux-en-Y gastric bypass.[25]

Advantages

The specific advantages of adjustable gastric banding in bariatric surgery include:

- Being the least invasive type of bariatric surgery
- Lack of stomach stapling, cutting, and intestinal rerouting
- Absence of permanent changes to the gastrointestinal tract
- Complete reversibility
- Adjustable stoma constriction
- Short operating time and hospital stay
- Few hospital readmissions during follow-up
- Good weight loss
- Low rates of early and late complications
- Rarity of life-threatening complications
- Low risk for nutritional deficiencies and malnutrition

Disadvantages

The specific disadvantages of adjustable gastric banding in bariatric surgery include:

- Necessity for some modification in eating and drinking habits
- Slower initial weight loss than with gastric bypass
- Critical need for regular follow-up (band adjustments in order to utilize the adjustability) to produce optimal results

▶ PLACEMENT TECHNIQUES

As previously mentioned, the design of the LAP-BAND has changed little since its introduction in 1993. By contrast, the technique for its placement has undergone numerous changes. These changes resulted from the initially high rate of late complications, which were related primarily to enlargement of the gastric pouch and to gastric prolapse (also called gastric herniation and band slippage).

PERIGASTRIC TECHNIQUE

The perigastric dissection technique employed in the early years was found to be technically difficult and often resulted in a higher rate of pouch dilatation or prolapse.[26-29] Dissection begins directly on the lesser curve at the midpoint (equator) of the calibration balloon. Dissection is completed behind the stomach toward the angle of His under direct visualization. Avoidance of the lesser sac is important. Retrogastric suturing is an option.

PARS FLACCIDA TECHNIQUE

The pars flaccida technique is now the most commonly utilized technique and is the procedure generally recommended. It is easier to teach and to perform than the perigastric technique, and it is associated with a much lower risk for gastric prolapse and erosion.[30-32] Details of the pars flaccida procedure, including photographs of the various stages, have been published by Fielding and Allen.[32]

Dissection begins directly lateral to the equator of the calibration balloon in the avascular space of the pars flaccida. After seeing the caudate lobe of the liver, blunt dissection is continued under direct visualization until the right crus is seen, followed immediately by the left crus over to the angle of His.

PARS FLACCIDA TO PERIGASTRIC TECHNIQUE (WEINER TWO-STEP)

Some surgeons prefer to use a combination technique in which an initial pars flaccida dissection is performed but is ultimately modified so that the band is brought closer to the gastric wall next to the lesser curve.[33-35] This is done to prevent postoperative dysphagia and outlet obstruction caused by an excess of adipose tissue inside the band.

Dissection begins with the pars flaccida technique. A second dissection is made at the midpoint (equator) of the balloon near the stomach until the perigastric dissection, limited to a simple opening next to the lesser curve, intercepts the pars flaccida dissection. The band is then placed from the angle of His through to the perigastric opening.

VARIATIONS

The number, size, and placement of trocars used for laparoscopic adjustable gastric banding vary according to individual surgeon preference. The laparoscopic Nissen fundoplication procedure can be used as a model.[32]

Various technical modifications have been introduced over the years, including the following:

- A very small initial pouch, less than 15 ml (the "virtual pouch") was created.
- Posterior dissection is performed above the peritoneal reflection of the bursa omentalis; at this level, the stomach wall is naturally fixed to the crura and there is no need for posterior-wall suturing.
- Suture-fixation of the anterior wall is performed to completely embed the silicone band; at least four gastrogastric sutures are needed.
- There is partial or complete deflation of the band at operation to prevent excessive constriction of the stoma due to postoperative edema.

To ensure that surgeons new to laparoscopic adjustable gastric banding take advantage of the most current surgical procedures and technical refinements, training at an approved center is recommended. Surgeon training includes mentoring by experienced bariatric surgeons with advanced laparoscopic skills and places particular emphasis on the placement of the band and its subsequent adjustment. Training also involves guidance in postoperative long-term patient management.[36]

▶ STOMA ADJUSTMENT

One of the most important advantages of laparoscopic adjustable gastric banding over other gastric restrictive procedures is the ability to adjust the size of the stoma without reoperation. The size of the stoma can be readily adjusted by injecting or withdrawing saline via the percutaneous access port, thereby inflating or deflating the inflatable portion of the silicone band (Fig. 19-3).[37] This process requires no anesthesia and normally takes 5 to 10 minutes in the office. Periodic adjustment permits optimization of the stoma size to provide sustained weight loss, reasonable food tolerance, and minimization of complications for the individual patient.

Nevertheless, the timing of inflation or deflation, as well as the quantity of saline injected or withdrawn for an optimal stoma size, may be difficult to determine. An optimally sized stoma guarantees sustained weight loss and reasonably good food tolerance. A stoma diameter that is too small results in severe food intolerance and may be responsible for pouch dilatation or gastric slippage; however, a stoma diameter that is too large is associated with insufficient weight loss. Adjustment of stoma size should not be decided on the basis of subjective criteria. A patient's history of increased food tolerance is not enough to warrant adjustment. Patients often request to be "tightened up" because of subjective perception of increased food tolerance, feelings of hunger, or comparison with other patients or simply to quicken weight loss. The decision to adjust stoma size should be based on objective criteria, including documented dietary inquiry, postoperative weight-loss curves, and radiologic studies.

The guidelines for stoma-size adjustment after LAP-BAND placement areas are as follows:

1. Completely or partially deflate the balloon at operation in order to avoid early food intolerance related to postoperative edema.

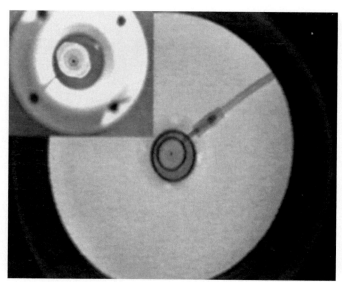

Figure 19-3. The size of the stoma can be readily adjusted by injecting or withdrawing saline via the percutaneous access port, thereby inflating or deflating the inflatable portion of the silicone band (*inset*).

Table 19-1	**PERCENTAGE OF EXCESS WEIGHT LOSS**								
					MONTHS AFTER SURGERY				
STUDY	N	12	18	24	36	48	60	72	84
Belachew et al 2002[64]	763						50-60*		
O'Brien et al 2002[78]	706	47	51	52	53	52	54	57	
Cadiere et al 2002[79]	652	38		62					
Vertruyen et al 2002[80]	543	38		61	62	58	53		52†
Dargent 1999[81]	500	56		65	64				
Toppino et al 1999[82]	361	42							
Fielding et al 1999[57]	335	52	62						
Paganelli et al 2000[83]	156	43							
Niville/Dams 1999[84]	126	48	58						
Berrevoet et al 1999[85]	120	46	53						

*Percentage of reduction of excess weight in patients with more than 5-year follow-up.
†Percentage at 86 months.

2. After operation, wait at least 2 months for capsule formation around the band before reinflating it.
3. Never overinject saline at a refilling session.

Adjustment is performed either in the operating room (my preference) or in the radiology department. The injection port is located using radioscopy, and a coin or a metal ring is placed on the skin above the radiologic image of the port. A circle is drawn on the skin in front of the injection port around the coin and the coin or the metal ring is taken away. No local anesthesia is needed. Under sterile conditions, the non-coring needle is introduced into the injection port. The content of the balloon is aspirated and the initial volume and final volume of fluid are measured and recorded. The placement of the access port (reservoir) depends, to some extent, on the individual surgeon's preference. Suitable placement sites include the left upper quadrant and subxiphoid region.[38]

▶ **WEIGHT LOSS**

A comprehensive, systematic review comparing outcomes of laparoscopic adjustable gastric banding (LAP-BAND and Swedish band), VBG, and Roux-en-Y gastric bypass was conducted by an expert panel under the auspices of the Royal Australasian College of Surgeons (ASERNIP-S Report).[39] Based on a search of electronic databases for references to these types of bariatric surgery, the panel found the overall quality of the evidence to be "average" (up to 4 years of follow-up). The panel found that laparoscopic adjustable gastric banding, like the other two procedures, was considered to be effective for up to 4 years. At 2 years, though, the laparoscopic adjustable gastric band had not produced the weight loss of Roux-en-Y gastric bypass. Between 2 and 4 years, the panel determined there was insufficient evidence to conclude that the Roux-en-Y procedure remained more effective than laparoscopic adjustable gastric banding. In terms of short-term mortality, the panel concluded that laparoscopic adjustable gastric banding was safer than VBG and Roux-en-Y gastric bypass.

Three international trials have accumulated 5-year postsurgery data that show an average 56% excess weight loss (%EWL) with the LAP-BAND (Table 19-1). These results are comparable to Roux-en-Y gastric bypass outcomes that average 59% at 5 years (four reports).[40] Table 19-2 shows weight loss after LAP-BAND placement expressed as reduction in body mass index (BMI). A medium-term prospective study (ongoing) showed mean %EWL values of 52% at 24 months, 53% at 36 months, 52% at

Table 19-2	**REDUCTION IN BODY MASS INDEX**									
						MONTHS AFTER SURGERY				
STUDY	N	BASE BMI	12	18	24	36	48	60	72	84
Angrisani et al 2001[86]	1265	44	35	33	30	32	32			
Favretti et al 2002[87]	830	46	37		36	37	37	36	40	29
Belachew et al 2002[64]	763	42	32		30		30	<30		
Vertruyen 2002[80]	543	44	33.2		31.3	30.1	31.4	31.2		32.1*
Abu-Abeid/Szold 1999[88]	391	43	32	30						
Belachew et al 1998[16]	350	43	30							
Hauri et al 2000[89]	207	43	35							
Furbetta et al 1999[90]	201	43	35	33	33					
Weiner et al 2003[33]	184	48	32	30	28					
Gambinotti et al 1998[91]	162	43	32							
Nowara 2001[92]	108	49			35					

*Percentage at 86 months.

Table 19-3	REDUCTION IN BODY MASS INDEX	
YEAR	GASTRIC BYPASS	GASTRIC BANDING
Baseline BMI	45	45
1	29	36
2	29	32
3	29	31
4	29	32
5	29	30

(From National Institute of Clinical Excellence: Assessment Report on the Clinical and Cost-Effectiveness of Surgery for People With Morbid Obesity. www.nice.org.uk. Accessed July 19, 2002.)

48 months, 54% at 60 months, and 57% at 72 months.[41] With increased and accumulated experience, data from U.S. studies show a similar pattern of improved outcomes, demonstrating mean weight-loss values of approximately 40%EWL at 12 months[42,43] and over 50%EWL at 36 months.[42] In addition, a study published by the National Institute for Clinical Excellence in England[44] showed that adjustable gastric banding weight loss is comparable to Roux-en-Y gastric bypass at 5 years (Table 19-3). Nevertheless, it is generally accepted that Roux-en-Y gastric bypass affords better weight loss than the LAP-BAND, excluding all other inconveniences and risks.

COMORBIDITIES

It has been well established that weight reduction after bariatric procedures such as gastric bypass is able to ameliorate or, in some cases, completely reverse comorbid conditions.[45,46] This ability has also been demonstrated with gastric restrictive procedures.[47] The use of the LAP-BAND System has been shown to reverse several major comorbidities,[48] including diabetes,[49,50] hypertension and hypercholesterolemia,[50] clinical depression,[51] sleep apnea, and gastroesophageal reflux.

QUALITY OF LIFE

Following LAP-BAND surgery, clear improvements in various quality-of-life indexes have been demonstrated (e.g., by the Rand SF-36,[52] by the BAROS score,[53] and by

body image[54]). Equivocal results concerning quality of life have also been reported (at 2 years).[55]

COMPLICATIONS

Reported complications specific to the adjustable gastric band can be divided between early and late complications. Early complications include:

- Gastrointestinal perforation
- Hepatic or splenic injury (now very rare)

Late complications include:

- Pouch dilatation due to overinflation of band or excessive food intake
- Band slippage (gastric prolapse, herniation) due to improper band positioning
- A combination of pouch dilatation and band slippage
- Band erosion
- Port leakage or migration

As with any surgical procedure, the incidence of complications decreases with the experience of the individual surgeon (the learning curve).[56] In addition, complication rates have generally decreased over the years with improvements in surgical technique.[57,38] Thus, initial rates of band slippage (gastric prolapse) have decreased from the early reported rates of around 22% to less than 5%.[15,26,32,58] For example, Dargent reported that changing from the perigastric to the pars flaccida procedure produced a decrease in band slippage from 5.2% to 0.6%.[59] Dargent stated that he had benefited from previous surgeons' experiences and was able to achieve lower rates of band slippage by placing the band higher than at the beginning of his series. Similarly, by changing to the pars flaccida technique, another bariatric surgery group reduced the incidence of gastric prolapse from 15% to 1.8%.[32] The most frequently reported complications associated with the LAP-BAND are summarized in Table 19-4.

Improper placement of the access port can lead to a port rotation of up to 180 degrees or to fractures at the tube junction. Satisfactory placement, with suturing to the fascia, ensures access for adjustments, patient comfort and convenience, and stabilization.[38,60] Complications with the access port affect the integrity of the LAP-BAND System

Table 19-4	COMPLICATIONS OF LAPAROSCOPIC ADJUSTABLE GASTRIC BANDING (LAP-BAND) IN VARIOUS STUDIES				
STUDY	N	GASTRIC PROLAPSE/POUCH DILATATION (%)	ESOPHAGEAL DILATATION OR DYSMOTILITY (%)	EROSION (%)	ACCESS PORT PROBLEMS (%)
FDA Trial[93]	299	24.0	10	1.0	6.0
Belachew et al 2002[64]	763	8.0	NR	0.9	2.6
Cadiere et al 2002[79]	652	3.8	NR	0.3	2.7
Dargent 1999[81]	500	5.0	NR	1.6	1.0
Favretti et al 2002[87]	830	10.0	NR	0.5	11.0
Fielding et al 1999[57]	335	3.6	NR	0	1.5
O'Brien et al 1999[56]	302	9.0	NR	NR	3.6
Vertruyen 2002[80]	543	4.6	NR	1.0	3.0
Weiner et al 2003[33]	184	2.2	NR	1.1	3.2

and compromise effective weight loss. Many of these problems are preventable.[61]

LAP-BAND erosion is rare and may occur months after placement. One possible cause is minute injury to the gastric wall during the initial procedure.[62] Mortality following LAP-BAND placement is virtually nonexistent and is zero in many series, both large and small.

More recent experience in the United States shows complication rates closer to those in large international series than to the rates reported in the initial U.S. clinical trial, which was conducted to obtain the approval of the Food and Drug Administration. For example, the gastric prolapse rate was 14.2% (9 of 63 over 3 years) in one early, single-surgeon study[42] and was 2% (2 of 115 over 12 months) in a collaborative study involving four surgeons and a total of 500 consecutive patients.[43] This improvement can be attributed to the impact of the learning curve because most of the surgeons participating in the FDA trial had less experience with the procedure and with laparoscopic surgery than those reporting the later studies.

Esophageal dilatation related to the LAP-BAND has been reported in recent years, especially by authors in the United States.[63] These reports came from small series within the Food and Drug Administration's clinical trial of the LAP-BAND, from investigators with limited experience, and during a period of an inadequate policy concerning band adjustment.

It is also noteworthy that reoperation in laparoscopic banding does not have the same significance as in other bariatric surgery procedures. Actually, in more than 80% of patients, the complications can be corrected by minimally invasive (laparoscopic) surgery.[64] Operations such as band removal, band repositioning, and conversion to Roux-en-Y gastric bypass may be performed laparoscopically after LAP-BAND complications.

▶ OTHER ADJUSTABLE GASTRIC BANDS

Surgeons choosing to perform laparoscopic adjustable gastric banding have to choose a band, so it is appropriate to review the literature concerning bands other than the LAP-BAND. Although there are more than 1100 publications, including presentation abstracts, relating to experience with the LAP-BAND, there exist few reports on other gastric banding systems. Most of those that do exist describe experience with the Swedish band.

The group that developed the Swedish adjustable gastric band reported their 4-year follow-up results in 46 out of 50 patients initially operated upon by laparotomy. The mean weight loss was 54 kg, equivalent to a decrease in BMI of 18.5 kg per m².[65] This paper provided limited discussion of complications, which included incisional hernia, abdominal reoperation, accidental perforation of the connecting tube, and vomiting due to overconstricted stoma.

In the long-term follow-up report of this same series, of 326 Swedish-band patients, 296 patients had no significant complications. For this subset, mean excess weight loss was 68%.[66] Complications requiring reoperation included band dislocations (0.6%), band leakages (1.8%), and band migrations or erosions (4.6%). Band slippage was attributed mainly to the overfilling of the band system. The most common complication not requiring reoperation was reflux (4.7%). In cases in which there was a small gastric pouch, this did not appear to be a serious problem. The authors concluded that the complication rate could be reduced further by making improvements in operating technique and by practicing closer follow-up. In particular, reoperation for band migration should be avoidable by not overfilling the band.

In a 5-year prospective study, 824 patients had the Swedish band placed laparoscopically, with 97% available for follow-up.[67] Mean excess weight loss was 30%, 41%, 49%, 55%, and 57% after 1, 2, 3, 4, and 5 years, respectively. The perioperative complication rate was 1.2%. The long-term complication rate was 23.3%, with 16.4% band-related and 6.8% access-port-related. There were no intraoperative or postoperative deaths (up to 30 days) in this series. Mittermair and colleagues[68] achieved a mean excess weight loss of 72% (a decrease in BMI of 16.6 kg/m²) after 3 years in a 6-year follow-up of 451 patients undergoing laparoscopic Swedish band surgery. Complications requiring reoperation occurred in 7.9% of patients.

Two studies compared the Swedish band with the LAP-BAND. In one study using comparable surgical techniques, the LAP-BAND (29 patients) appeared to show better weight-loss characteristics over 12 to 18 months, but the authors found the Swedish band (41 patients) easier to handle and less prone to causing dysphagia or slippage.[69] Another prospective study compared 49 patients receiving the Swedish band with 52 patients receiving the LAP-BAND, most of them placed laparoscopically.[70] Excluding patients with leakage of the Swedish band due to technical failure, mean weight loss was similar at 6 months, 1 year, and 2 years for the two groups. The complication rates and profiles were similar.

There are two published reports of experience with the Heliogast adjustable gastric band. A prospective, randomized study compared outcomes for the LAP-BAND (n = 30) and the Heliogast band (n = 30).[71] The devices were implanted using the two-step technique (pars flaccida to perigastric). There were no differences in operating times, intraoperative complications, or weight loss during the initial 4 weeks after surgery. However, with increasing time, there were more complications with the Heliogast band, and differences in weight loss favoring the LAP-BAND (n = 30) became increasingly significant. At 12 months, the mean excess weight loss was 41.7% for the LAP-BAND group and 28.3% for the Heliogast group (P < 0.0001). The baseline patient demographics were similar in the two groups. Even after a change in Heliogast design early in the study, the authors were still unable to achieve a functional stoma size in 26 of the 30 patients, despite increasing the fill volume over the standard amount stated in the manufacturer's recommendation. Wasserberg and colleagues[72] found similar rates of anterior slippage, requiring band repositioning for the LAP-BAND and the Heliogast adjustable gastric band, of 2.1% and 2.7%, respectively. However, the authors thought that the design of the Heliogast locking mechanism allowed for more straightforward reopening and repositioning (salvage) than the LAP-BAND, which requires considerable operative skill and is not always successful.

DISCUSSION

The overall complication rate is lower in laparoscopic adjustable gastric banding than in VBG, and much lower than that in gastric bypass or other highly invasive bariatric procedures. Also, the types of complications associated with gastric banding are, on the whole, less severe than those following gastric bypass and are rarely life threatening. The short-term weight loss (up to 2 years) in laparoscopic adjustable gastric banding appears to fall between that in VBG and gastric bypass. Medium-term weight-loss outcomes (2 to 4 years) have yet to be fully established for laparoscopic adjustable gastric banding, but as more and more longer term studies are published, the data are beginning to show weight loss with adjustable gastric banding and Roux-en-Y gastric bypass to be comparable at 5 years.

As with gastric bypass and VBG procedures, laparoscopic adjustable gastric banding has demonstrated significant reversal of comorbidities and improvements in quality of life. These may prove to be the critical factors in long-term patient benefit, rather than the rate or extent of weight loss.

Determining the suitability of patients for one type of bariatric surgery procedure or another has been somewhat controversial. There is no doubt that laparoscopic adjustable gastric banding requires commitment by the patient and family to adhere to a suitable diet and to attend regular follow-up visits for evaluation and for band adjustment, as needed. In nonsocialized medical systems this can impose an additional financial burden. However, inappropriate eating habits can also reduce the effectiveness of VBG and gastric bypass surgery.[73] Further, gastric bypass and other malabsorptive procedures also necessitate lifelong nutritional augmentation with supplements such as iron and vitamin B_{12}.

Major complications, such as staple-line leaks (in VBG) and anastomotic leaks and intraabdominal sepsis (in gastric bypass), are not seen following laparoscopic adjustable gastric banding. Also, the early mortality rate in gastric bypass is much higher than in the LAP-BAND procedure. Early on, many surgeons were reluctant to perform laparoscopic adjustable gastric banding on superobese patients because of the risk for increased perioperative complications and presumed insufficient weight loss. However, recently many surgeons have successfully performed laparoscopic banding procedures in these patients.[74,75]

There has been debate about the psychological profile of candidate patients. For example, obese patients prepared to accept the risks associated with a surgical procedure requiring general anesthesia have biopsychosocial profiles statistically different from the profiles of those who are not willing to accept these risks.[76] Some clinically obese patients will not accept major and permanent revisions in internal anatomy. Others, for professional or social reasons, prefer minimal procedures that allow them to return quickly and discreetly to normal activities.

Dixon and O'Brien have reviewed the criteria for selecting the optimum patient for LAP-BAND placement.[77] The issues described in this chapter apply equally to the other laparoscopic adjustable gastric banding systems. It is not possible to compare, in any systematic manner, the safety and efficacy of the various gastric banding systems available because there have been very few head-to-head studies and even fewer prospective, randomized trials comparing one band with another.

Furthermore, the preponderance of LAP-BAND reports and the paucity of studies of other bands prohibit meaningful metaanalyses to compare outcomes. Until comparative data from rigorously conducted clinical studies are available, individual surgeon preference and the marketplace will determine the status of each of the laparoscopic adjustable gastric banding systems.

The introduction of laparoscopic adjustable gastric banding into bariatric surgery on September 1, 1993, was a considerable breakthrough. Along with the innovations of total reversibility and adjustability, it introduced the notion of minimal invasiveness. It is not by mere chance that the laparoscopic band gave a new impetus to bariatric surgery in general and to laparoscopic surgery in particular. Today, 13 years later, more than 250,000 LAP-BANDs have been placed worldwide.

The introduction of laparoscopic adjustable gastric banding into the therapeutic arsenal of surgical techniques that can be used in morbid obesity has enhanced the interest of endocrinologists, other internists, and general practitioners, as well as the public, in surgery for morbid obesity. Obviously, it is not a panacea in the field of obesity surgery. Weight loss after a restrictive procedure such as banding is initially less than it is in the malabsorptive procedures. Nevertheless, as confirmed by its outstanding international appeal and its extensive use since its emergence, laparoscopic adjustable gastric banding deserves a prominent place in the surgical treatment of morbid obesity.

REFERENCES

1. Wilkinson LH, Peloso OA: Gastric (reservoir) reduction for morbid obesity. Arch Surg 1981;116:602-605.
2. Kolle K: Gastric banding, OMGI 7th Congress, Stockholm. 1982;37:145 (abstract).
3. Molina M, Oria HE: Gastric segmentation: a new, safe, effective, simple, readily revised and fully reversible surgical procedure for the correction of morbid obesity. 6th Bariatric Surgery Colloquium Iowa City, June 2-3, 1983;(abstract).
4. Buchwald H: Overview of bariatric surgery. J Am Coll Surg 2002;194:367-375.
5. Vassallo C, Andreoli M, La Manna A, et al: 60 reoperations on 890 patients after gastric restrictive surgery. Obes Surg 2002;11:752-756.
6. Szinicz G, Muller L: A new method in the surgical treatment of pathologic obesity: results of animal experiments. Proceedings of the XI Annual Meeting of the European Society for Artificial Organs, Sept. 9-12, 1984, Alpbach-Innsbruck, Austria, p. 322. London, W.B. Saunders, 1984.
7. Szinicz G, Muller L, Erhart W, et al: "Reversible gastric banding" in surgical treatment of morbid obesity: results of animal experiments. Res Exp Med (Berl) 1989;189:55-60.
8. Kuzmak LI: Silicone gastric banding: a simple and effective operation for morbid obesity. Contemp Surg 1986;28:13-18.
9. Kuzmak LI: A review of seven years' experience with silicone gastric banding. Obes Surg 1991;1:403-408.
10. Forsell P, Hallberg D, Hellers G: A gastric band with adjustable inner diameter for obesity surgery: preliminary studies. Obes Surg 1993;3:303-306.
11. Forsell P, Hallberg D, Hellers G: Gastric banding for morbid obesity: initial experience with a new adjustable gastric band. Obes Surg 1993;3:369-374.

12. Belachew M, Jaquet P, Lardinois F, et al: Vertical banded gastroplasty vs adjustable gastric banding in the treatment of morbid obesity: a preliminary report. Obes Surg 1993;3:275-278.

13. Belachew M, Legrand, Jacquet N: Laparoscopic placement of adjustable silicone gastric banding in the treatment of morbid obesity: an animal model experimental study, a video film, a preliminary report. Obes Surg 1993;3:140 (abstract).

14. Belachew M, Legrand MJ, Deffechereux TH, et al: Laparoscopic adjustable silicone gastric banding in the treatment of morbid obesity. Surg Endosc 1994;8;1354-1356.

15. Belachew M, Legrand M, Vincent V: Laparoscopic placement of adjustable silicone gastric band in the treatment of morbid obesity: how to do it. Obes Surg 1995;5:66-70.

16. Belachew M, Legrand M, Vincent V, et al: Laparoscopic adjustable gastric banding. World J Surg 1998;22:955-963.

17. Cadiére GB, Bruyns J, Himpens J, et al: Laparoscopic gastroplasty for morbid obesity. Br J Surg 1994;81:1524.

18. Catona A, Gossenberg M, La Manna A, Mussini G: Laparoscopic adjustable gastric banding: preliminary series. Obes Surg 1993;3:207-209.

19. Catona A, La Manna L, Forsell P: The Swedish adjustable gastric band: laparoscopic technique and preliminary results. Obes Surg 200;10:15-21.

20. Belachew M, Legrand MJ, Vincent V: History of Lap-Band®: from dream to reality. Obes Surg 2001;11:297-302.

21. BioEnterics (INAMED): LAP-BAND® Adjustable Gastric Banding System, U.S. approved labeling, June 13, 2001.

22. Soper NJ, Stockmann PT, Dunnegan DL, et al: Laparoscopic cholecystectomy: the new "gold standard"? Arch Surg 1992;127:917-921.

23. Suter M, Giusti V, Heraief E, et al: Laparoscopic gastric banding. Surg Endosc 2003;17:1418-1425.

24. Morino M, Toppino M, Bonnet G, et al: Laparoscopic adjustable silicone gastric banding versus vertical banded gastroplasty in morbidly obese patients: a prospective randomized controlled clinical trial. Ann Surg 2003;238:835-841.

25. Wittgrove AC, Clark GW: Laparoscopic gastric bypass, Roux-en-Y: 500 patients: technique and results, with 3-60-month follow-up. Obes Surg 2002;10:233-239.

26. Favretti F, Cadiere G, Segato G, et al: Laparoscopic adjustable silicone gastric banding (LAP-BAND®): how to avoid complications. Obes Surg 1997;7:352-358.

27. Wiesner W, Schlumpf R, Schob O, et al: Gastric pouch dilatation: complications after laparoscopic implantation of a silicon gastric band in pathologic obesity. Rofo Forschr Geb Rontgenstr Neuen Bildgeb Vefahr 1998;169:479-483.

28. Niville E, Dams A: Late pouch dilation after laparoscopic adjustable silicone gastric banding: incidence, treatment, and outcome. Obes Surg 1999;9:381-384.

29. DeMaria EJ, Sugerman HJ, Meador JG, et al: High failure rate after laparoscopic adjustable silicone gastric banding for treatment of morbid obesity. Ann Surg 2001;233:809-818.

30. Zimmermann JM, Michel G, Grimaldi JM, et al: Complications of laparoscopic gastric banding and how to manage them. Obes Surg 1998;8:164 (abstract).

31. Belachew M, Zimmermann J-M: Evolution of a paradigm for laparoscopic adjustable gastric banding. Am J Surg 2002;184:21S-25S.

32. Fielding GA, Allen JW: A step-by-step guide to placement of the LAP-BAND adjustable gastric banding system. Am J Surg 2002;184:26S-30S.

33. Weiner S, Engert R, Weiner S, et al: Outcome after laparoscopic adjustable gastric banding: 8 years experience. Obes Surg 2003;13:427-434.

34. Rubin M, Benchetrit S, Lustigman H, et al: Laparoscopic gastric banding with Lap-Band for morbid obesity: two-step technique may improve outcome. Obes Surg 2001;11:315-317.

35. Spivak H, Rubin M: Laparoscopic management of Lap-Band slippage. Obes Surg 2003;13:116-120.

36. Belachew M: Les dix commandements pour éviter les complications de la chirurgie bariatrique sous laparoscopie. J Coelio-Chirugie 1999;29:58-60.

37. Belachew M, Ernould D: Directives pour l'ajustement de l'anneau modulable laparoscopique. J Coelio-Chirurgie 2002;42:5-11.

38. Spivak H, Favretti F: Avoiding postoperative complications with the LAP-BAND system. Am J Surg 2002;184:31S-37S.

39. Chapman A, Kiroff G, Game P, et al: Laparoscopic adjustable gastric banding in the treatment of obesity: a systematic review. Surg 2004;135:326-351.

40. O'Brien PE, Dixon JB: Lap-Band: outcomes and results. J Laparoendosc Adv Surg Tech A 2003;13:265-270.

41. O'Brien PE, Dixon JB: Weight loss and early and late complications: the international experience. Am J Surg 2002;184:42S-45S.

42. Rubenstein RB: Laparoscopic adjustable gastric banding at a US center with up to 3-year follow-up. Obes Surg 2002;12:380-384.

43. Ren CJ, Horgan S, Ponce J: US experience with the LAP-BAND system. Am J Surg 2002;184:46S-50S.

44. National Institute of Clinical Excellence: Assessment report on the clinical and cost-effectiveness of surgery for people with morbid obesity. www.nice.org.uk. Accessed July 19, 2002.

45. Pories WJ, Swanson MS, MacDonald KG, et al: Who would have thought it? An operation proves to be the most effective therapy for adult-onset diabetes mellitus. Ann Surg 1995;222:339-350.

46. Buchwald H, Avidor Y, Braunwald E, et al: Bariatric surgery: a systematic review and meta-analysis. JAMA 2004;292:1724-1737.

47. Wolf AM, Beisiegel U, Kortner B, et al: Does gastric restriction surgery reduce the risks of metabolic diseases? Obes Surg 1998;8:9-13.

48. Dixon JB, O'Brien PE: Changes in comorbidities and improvements in quality of life after LAP-BAND placement. Am J Surg 2002;184:51S-54S.

49. Dixon JB, O'Brien PE: Health outcomes of severely obese type 2 diabetic subjects 1 year after laparoscopic adjustable gastric banding. Diabetes Care 2002;25:358-363.

50. Bacci V, Basso MS, Greco F, et al: Modifications of metabolic and cardiovascular risk factors after weight loss induced by laparoscopic gastric banding. Obes Surg 2002;12:77-82.

51. Dixon JB, Dixon ME, O'Brien PE: Depression in association with severe obesity. Arch Intern Med 2003;163:2058-2065.

52. Dixon JB, Dixon ME. O'Brien PE: Quality of life after Lap-Band placement: influence of time, weight loss, and comorbidities. Obes Res 2001;9:713-721.

53. Nini E, Slim K, Scesa JL, et al: Evaluation of laparoscopic bariatric surgery using the BAROS score. Ann Chir 2002;127:107-114 (in French).

54. Dixon JB, Dixon ME, O'Brien PE: Body image: appearance, orientation, and evaluation in the severely obese: changes with weight loss. Obes Surg 2002;12:65-71.

55. Horchner R, Tuinebreijer MW, Kelder PH: Quality-of-life assessment of morbid obese patients who have undergone a Lap-Band operation: 2-year follow-up study: is the MOS SF-36 a useful instrument to measure quality of life in morbidly obese patients? Obes Surg 2001;11:212-218.

56. O'Brien PE, Brown WA, Smith PJ, et al: Prospective study of a laparoscopically placed, adjustable gastric band in the treatment of morbid obesity. Br J Surg 1999;85:113-118.

57. Fielding GA, Rhodes M, Nathanson LK: Laparoscopic gastric banding for morbid obesity: surgical outcome in 335 cases. Surg Endosc 1999;13:550-554.

58. O'Brien PE, Brown WA, Smith PJ, et al: Prospective study of a laparoscopically placed, adjustable gastric band in the treatment of morbid obesity. Br J Surg 1999;85:113-118.

59. Dargent J: Pouch dilatation and slippage after adjustable gastric banding: is it still an issue? Obes Surg 2003;13:111-115.

60. Furbetta F, Gambinotti G: New positioning of the port system. Obes Surg 2001;11:430.

61. Susmallian S, Ezri T, Elis M, et al: Access-port complications after laparoscopic adjustable gastric banding. Obes Surg 2003;13:128-131.

62. Abu-Abeid A, Szold A: Laparoscopic management of Lap-Band erosion. Obes Surg 2001;11:87-89.

63. DeMaria EJ, Sugerman HJ: A critical look at laparoscopic adjustable silicone gastric banding for surgical treatment of morbid obesity: Surg Endosc 2000;14:697-699.

64. Belachew M, Belva PH, Desaive C: Long-term results of laparoscopic adjustable gastric banding for the treatment of morbid obesity. Obes Surg 2002;12:564-568.

65. Forsell P, Hellers G: The Swedish adjustable gastric banding (SAGB) for morbid obesity: 9-year experience and a 4-year follow up of patients operated with a new adjustable band. Obes Surg 1997;7:345-351.

66. Forsell P, Hallerback B, Glise H, et al: Complications following Swedish adjustable gastric banding: a long-term follow-up. Obes Surg 1999;9:11-16.

67. Steffen R, Biertho L, Ricklin T, et al: Laparoscopic Swedish adjustable gastric banding: a five-year prospective study. Obes Surg 2003;13:404-411.

68. Mittermair RP, Weiss H, Nehoda H, et al: Laparoscopic Swedish adjustable gastric banding: 6-year follow-up and comparison to other laparoscopic bariatric procedures. Obes Surg 2003;13: 412-417.

69. Hesse UJ, Berrevoet F, Ceelen W, et al: Adjustable silicone gastric banding (ASGB, Bioenterics) and Swedish adjustable gastric banding (SAGB, Obtech) in the treatment of morbid obesity. Chirurg 2001;72:14-18 (in German).

70. Ponson AE, Janssen IM, Klinkenbijl JH: Laparoscopic adjustable gastric banding: a prospective comparison of two commonly used bands. Obes Surg 2002;12:579-582.

71. Blanco-Engert R, Weiner S, Pomhoff I, et al: Outcome after laparoscopic adjustable gastric banding, using the Lap-Band® and the Heliogast® band: a prospective, randomized study. Obes Surg 2003;13:776-779.

72. Wasserberg N, Nudelman I, Fuko Z, et al: Laparoscopic repositioning of Heliogast® gastric band after anterior slippage. Obes Surg 2003;13:780-783.

73. Sugerman HJ, Starkey JV, Birkenhauer R: A randomized prospective trial of gastric bypass versus vertical banded gastroplasty for morbid obesity and their effects on sweets- versus non-sweets-eaters. Ann Surg 1987;205;613-624.

74. Fielding G: Laparoscopic adjustable gastric banding for massive super obesity. ANZ J Surg 2003;73(suppl):A61.

75. Moose D, Lourie D, Powell W, et al: Am Surg 2003;69:930-932.

76. Martin LF: The biopsychosocial characteristics of people seeking treatment for obesity. Obes Surg 1999;9:235-243.

77. Dixon JB, O'Brien PE: Selecting the optimum patient for LAP-BAND placement. Am J Surg 2002;184:17S-20S.

78. O'Brien P, Dixon J, Brown W, et al: The laparoscopic adjustable gastric band (LAP-BAND): a prospective study of medium-term effects on weight, health and quality of life. Obes Surg 2002;12: 652-660.

79. Cadiere GB, Himpens J, Vertruyen M, et al: Laparoscopic gastroplasty (adjustable silicone gastric banding). Semin Laparosc Surg 2002;7:55-65.

80. Vertruyen M: Experience with LAP-BAND system up to 7 years. Obes Surg 2002;12:569-572.

81. Dargent J: Laparoscopic adjustable gastric banding: lessons from the first 500 patients in a single institution. Obes Surg 1999;9:446-452.

82. Toppino M, Morino M, Bonnet G, et al: Laparoscopic surgery for morbid obesity: preliminary results from SICE registry (Italian Society of Endoscopic and Minimally Invasive Surgery). Obes Surg 1999;9:62-65.

83. Paganelli M, Giacomelli M, Librenti MC, et al: Thirty months' experience with laparoscopic adjustable gastric banding. Obes Surg 2000;10:269-271.

84. Niville E, Dams A: Late pouch dilation after laparoscopic adjustable gastric and esophagogastric banding: incidence, treatment, and outcome. Obes Surg 1999;9:381-384.

85. Berrevoet F, Pattyn P, Cardon A, et al: Retrospective analysis of laparoscopic gastric banding technique: short-term and mid-term follow-up. Obes Surg 1999;9:272-275.

86. Angrisani L, Alkilani M, Basso N, et al: Laparoscopic Italian experience with the LAP-BAND. Obes Surg 2001;11:307-310.

87. Favretti F, Cadiere GB, Segato G, et al: Laparoscopic banding selection and technique in 830 patients. Obes Surg 2002;12:385-390.

88. Abu-Abeid S, Szold A: Results and complications of laparoscopic adjustable gastric banding: an early and intermediate experience. Obes Surg 1999;9:188-190.

89. Hauri P, Steffen R, Ricklin T, et al: Treatment of morbid obesity with the Swedish adjustable gastric band (SAGB): complication rate during a 12-month follow-up period. Surgery, 2000;127:484-488.

90. Furbetta F, Gambinotti G, Robortella EM: 28-month experience with the lap-band technique: results and critical points of the method. Obes Surg 1999;9:56-58.

91. Gambinotti G, Robortella ME, Furbetta F: Personal experience with laparoscopic adjustable silicone gastric banding in the treatment of morbid obesity. Eat Weight Disord 1998;3:43-45.

92. Nowara HA: Egyptian experience in laparoscopic adjustable gastric banding (technique, complications and intermediate results). Obes Surg 2001;11:70-75.

93. FDA Approval Letter: Trial of LAP-BAND, 2001. Department of Health and Human Services. http://www.fda.gov/cdrh/pdf/p000008a.pdf. Accessed June 14, 2005.

20

Vertical Banded Gastroplasty

Andrew C. Jamieson, M.D.

It is curious that the procedure from which the vertical banded gastroplasty (VBG) evolved was neither vertical nor banded. Mason had a limited experience with jejunoileal bypass from 1954 on and then developed gastric bypass in 1966. In 1971 he reasoned that if the mechanism of weight loss in gastric bypass was food intake reduction, then a small-sized gastric pouch emptying directly into the distal stomach should be equally effective in promoting weight loss. The complications of bypass, such as micronutrient deficiency and peptic ulceration, would be avoided and the surgery would be simpler and safer. Gastroplasty (Fig. 20-1), as it was called, divided the stomach into a small upper section and a large distal part connected by a channel on the greater curve. Because of inadequate weight loss, only 59 operations were performed before the procedure was abandoned and Mason returned to the gastric bypass. Gomez resurrected gastroplasty in 1977, initially using a Dacron mesh collar around the stomal channel, but when stomal stricturing was abandoned, he changed to a running polypropylene suture.[1] This had the disadvantage sometimes of eroding into the stomach. Pace tried a different approach by removing a few staples from the center of a cartridge and stapling across the upper stomach.[2] Stomal widening through the unzipping of the staple line from the

stoma was invariable, despite attempts at staple-line reinforcement, and this operation was also abandoned.

In 1976, Tretbar and colleagues (Fig. 20-2) reported an extended Nissen-type fundoplication in which the greater curve was progressively wrapped around the lesser curve from the cardia to the incisura.[3] Despite reportedly good early results, he was soon performing what was probably the first vertical, stapled gastroplasty with a lesser-curve stoma, placing staples parallel to the lesser curve and creating an esophageal extension 180 cm in length with an unsupported stoma. The results of this procedure were never published. Johnston reproduced Tretbar's operation independently, with significant modifications, from 1987 on as the Magenstrasse and Mill procedure (Fig. 20-3), which showed impressive medium-term results but no long-term results.[4]

Long, in 1978 (see Fig. 20-2), placed an oblique staple line from the fundus to the lesser curve, initially unsupported but soon with Prolene stomal-supporting sutures and a progressively more vertical staple line.[5] Fabito, in 1979, began using a staple line with a lesser-curve stoma reinforced by a Prolene suture, and Laws used the Silastic ring in an attempt to reduce the risk of suture erosion.[6] Around 1980, Wynne-Jones was performing hand-sewn,

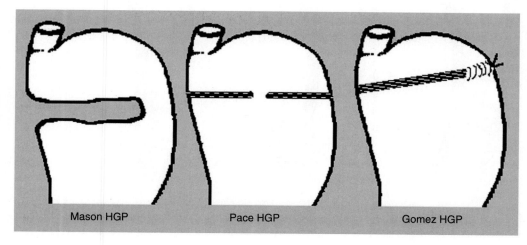

Figure 20-1. The horizontal gastroplasties: Mason, 1971; Pace, 1979; Gomez, 1977.

Mason HGP   Pace HGP   Gomez HGP

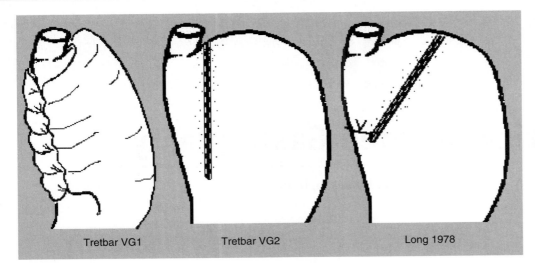

Tretbar VG1 Tretbar VG2 Long 1978

Figure 20-2. Early open vertical gastroplasties: Tretbar's extended plication, 1976; Tretbar's gastroplasty, 19; Long's gastroplasty, 1978.

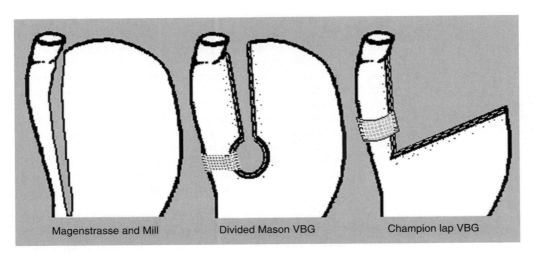

Magenstrasse and Mill Divided Mason VBG Champion lap VBG

Figure 20-3. Divided gastroplasties: Johnston's Magenstrasse and Mill (open); Mason's VBG (open or laparoscopic); Champion's wedge excision (laparoscopic).

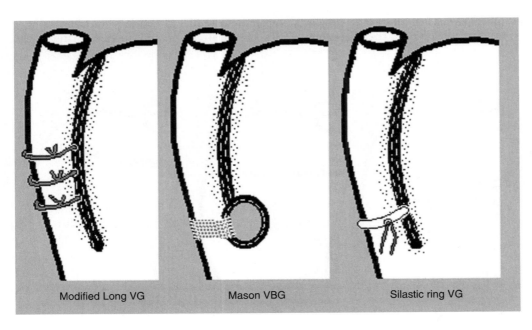

Modified Long VG Mason VBG Silastic ring VG

Figure 20-4. The current standard open gastroplasties: modified Long VBG; Mason VBG; Silastic ring VBG.

divided vertical gastroplasty 10 to 12 cm long alongside a 32F bougie, with a nylon or Teflon-coated, stainless-steel wire stomal suture 10 cm from the angle of His.[7] Apart from the original Mason 1971 gastroplasty, this seems to have been the first divided gastroplasty.

Mason began using the VBG (Fig. 20-4) in 1980, employing a lesser-curve stoma supported by a Marlex band passed through a window created by a circular stapler with the partition extended upwards.[8] This soon became the gold-standard operation for morbid obesity, although other surgeons attempted various modifications with sometimes less than satisfactory results. Mason justifiably complains that the results of these series are unfairly used to argue that VBG should no longer be performed. In the 1990s, VBG was adapted to laparoscopic technique by Chua and Mendiola (see Fig. 20-3), who performed their first in February 1993.[9] A different laparoscopic approach was described by Melissas[10]; a linear cutter is used to excise a wedge of stomach from the greater curve and fundus, leaving a vertical pouch along the lesser curve (see Fig. 20-3). This operation was first performed by Champion in Atlanta in 1996 and has the advantage of being easier and quicker to perform than the standard laparoscopic VBG.

▶ SURGICAL PRINCIPLES OF GASTROPLASTY

It became clear early on in the evolution of gastroplasty that certain technical principles were of vital importance for the success of the operation. Mason stated four basic principles in his monumental book, *Surgical Treatment of Obesity*, published in 1981.[11] They were (1) a measured volume of 50 ml or less; (2) a calibrated outlet between 10 and 12 mm in diameter; (3) a secure partition; and

(4) reinforcement to prevent dilatation of the stoma. These principles remain valid today, although pouch volumes of less than 20 ml are now used. The gastroplasties most commonly performed now (see Fig. 20-4) all involve vertical partitions and lesser-curve stomata. They are the modified Long vertical gastroplasty (MLVG), the Mason VBG, and the Silastic ring VBG (SRVG). In the Mason VBG a doughnut of stomach is cut out using a circular stapling device to allow a linear stapler to be slid upward, parallel to the lesser curve, to the angle of His, creating the pouch. Initially two-row stapling devices were used, but a significant incidence of staple-line failures resulted in the development of a four-row device. With the development of linear cutting staplers, division of the stomach became more feasible and safer, almost eliminating partition failure but perhaps increasing the risk for early leak.

Long, in 1977, found that a linear stapler could be rotated into position from the angle of His downward through a window in the gastrosplenic ligament and placed parallel to a bougie lying along the lesser curve (Fig. 20-5). The small puncture wound caused by the locking pin of the stapling gun can easily be oversewn anteriorly, although Long and I have not usually practiced this unless there was obvious leakage. The posterior pinhole is a little more difficult to oversew and is ignored. With more than 4000 cases in our combined experience, the posterior pinhole has never been shown to be the cause of a leak. This is probably because of the thickness of the gastric wall close to the lesser curve, where the three layers of smooth muscle prevent leakage.

The pinhole was avoided totally in the SRVG, in which the staple gun was placed inferiorly on the lesser curve up to the angle of His. To avoid complete partitioning of the stomach, some staples were removed or part of

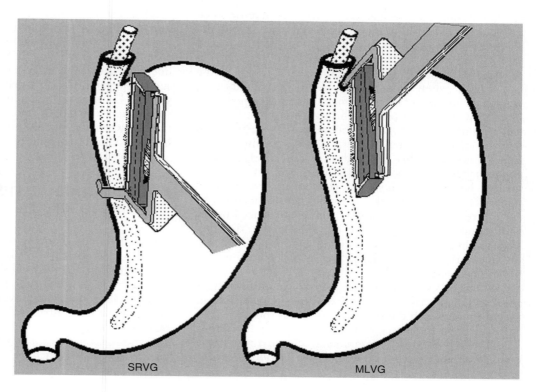

Figure 20-5. Staple gun application: SRVG from below up with (notched) TA-90-BN stapler; MLVG from angle of His downward.

SRVG

MLVG

the cartridge was cut away, allowing for a stoma. Later, notched linear staplers (see Fig. 20-5) were developed to overcome this problem.

Measured Volume of 20 ml or Less

Mason learned with gastric bypass and again with his 1971 gastroplasty that small pouch size was vitally important for success. Mason has strongly advocated the measurement of pouches, and he developed a straightforward method of doing this.[12] As a result of these measurements, there was a steady decrease in pouch volume in his series to an average of 14 ml at a pressure of 70 cm of water. It is more difficult to measure pouch volume in the MLVG and SRVG. However, if the partition is constructed close to a bougie lying along the lesser curve, consistently small pouches will be obtained.

Pouch size inevitably increases with time, and this is fortunate because otherwise, excess weight loss and malnutrition would occur in the long term. What is unpredictable is the distensibility of the pouch, and after many years some patients develop very large pouches or occasionally what almost appear to be wide-necked diverticuli of the pouches. Whether this is a function of the elasticity of the stomach or of the pouch's having been constructed too large initially or is an indication of chronic overeating has not been determined.

Calibrated Outlet With Reinforcement

Calibration of the stomal outlet is necessary to determine the rate of drainage of masticated food out of the pouch. That is partly a function of the distance of the partition from the lesser curve, but because the stomach wall is elastic, the tightness of the stomal-reinforcing support is the ultimate determining factor in the ease of passage of food through the stoma. Generally, a bougie between 34F and 38F (11 to 12 mm in diameter) is placed along the lesser curve, and the staple line or the division is placed parallel and close to it. It was learned in 1971 that the unsupported stoma would inevitably dilatate, and in the late 1970s, when gastroplasty began its renaissance, various techniques of reinforcement were developed. The simplest was a suture passing through the staple line and tied around the stoma, with a bougie inside the stoma so that the effective stomal diameter was that of the bougie. Long employed this method in 1978, initially with polypropylene sutures and later with braided polyester sutures. Jamieson extended the concept in 1983 to form a stomal channel rather than a two-dimensional stoma by using three Ethibond sutures 12 mm apart, placed nearly halfway up the staple line (see Fig. 20-4)—the MLVG.[13] This modification improved weight loss, but whether it was due to the channel effect or the smaller pouch or both has not been established.

In the SRVG, Fabito used a Prolene suture initially and Laws instituted the use of a 2.2-mm-diameter Silastic tube through which the Prolene suture was threaded. The length of the Silastic tube varies, but it is generally 45 mm. The Proring band is a premolded Silastic ring that is radiopaque and more flexible and has fixation points to prevent slippage.[14]

The classic Mason VBG stoma is reinforced by a Marlex mesh band encircling the stoma through the window and sutured to itself. Three band lengths (4.5, 5.0, and 5.5 cm) have been used, and 5 cm is generally agreed to be the most satisfactory, the larger length resulting in poorer weight loss and the shorter in excess regurgitation. SRVG and MLVG have the advantage over the Mason VBG of easier technique, less cost and, if necessary, easier revisional surgery.

Band or suture erosion can occur with any type of band or suture and is probably a consequence of infection, abscess formation, and rejection of foreign material. Although the stomach is generally sterile, the placement of the stomal sutures in MLVG and SRVG so that they pass through the staple line and not through the lumen of the stomach would be, logically, very important. Erosion per se is rare if meticulous technique is followed.

Secure Partition

The security of the partition is essential for the success of gastroplasty, and this became evident when linear staplers were used to partition the stomach. The cause of staple-line failure remains unproved, and various techniques have been tried to prevent it. Early unpublished work by the author who studied dogs' stomachs showed that the early Auto-Suture TA-90 staple gun, which had a screw-down anvil, did not cause splitting of the gastric mucosa alongside the staple line unless it was tightened beyond the recommended setting. This left mucosa in apposition, with mucosa between the staples. It was postulated that splitting the mucosa on both layers of the stomach was necessary to allow apposition of the submucosal layers and scar formation to strengthen the integrity of the staple line. The Auto-Suture Premium staple gun resulted in better mucosal splitting, and experience showed a reduced incidence of staple-line failure with this instrument. The introduction of the four-row staple line reduced the incidence of staple-line failure further, though it has not eliminated it. Techniques such as reinforcing the staple line with sutures were generally not successful, although superimposing two or three staple lines has had some success. Division of the stomach has become the ultimate technique for avoiding staple-line failure, though fistulation between the pouch and the remainder of stomach has been known to occur, presumably due to infection and abscess formation.

▶ MECHANISM OF GASTROPLASTY AND EATING TECHNIQUES

Gastroplasty and its many variants depend for success on the physical restriction of food intake, initially severe, to achieve weight loss by radical reduction of energy intake over the first year and then moderate restriction to allow weight stabilization and prevent future weight regain. The attraction of this restrictive approach, when compared to pure malabsorption or mixed malabsorption/restrictive operations, is that in the short and the long terms, micronutrient deficiencies (such as iron, potassium, vitamin B_{12}, calcium, protein) are less likely to occur and, if they do occur, are easy to correct. In addition, fully malabsorptive procedures in the short and medium term often result in diarrhea, which may cause significant morbidity.

It has long been established that a pouch volume of about 20 ml or less is important for good weight loss; however, the calorie restriction can be overcome by several factors. The first of these is dilatation of the pouch with time, and this will occur normally because of the stretching of the smooth muscle of the gastric wall. It is likely that chronic overfilling of the pouch may lead to more dilatation, although this has never been proved. The other cause of excess pouch dilatation is that the pouch was too large to start with. It must be recognized that the gastric pouch is a dynamic structure that has an inlet and a stomal outlet as well as its own inherent motility and peristalsis. Liquids pass easily and rapidly through the empty pouch according to their viscosity and the rate at which they enter the pouch. Solids pass through much more slowly, according to the particle size of the swallowed food and on its consistency and the degree of holdup at the stoma. After eating solid food, patients describe a feeling of fullness and satiety or an epigastric or low-retrosternal discomfort, which indicates pouch fullness. At this point, the patient must observe the first rule of eating (Table 20-1). If eating continues, discomfort increases until voluntary or spontaneous regurgitation of the excess food occurs. There is no nausea, but there is a feeling of relief after the regurgitation, and patients should be advised to eat no more until the next meal.

The effect on satiety of filling the gastric pouch is a very important factor in weight loss. The obese almost invariably admit to excessive hunger, a powerful sensation that has evolved to ensure that animals have the desire to eat and thus survive. The lack of success in dieting without surgery is hardly surprising in this setting, and if hunger were not reduced by surgery, the hungry patient would soon out-eat the operation and gain weight. Satiety is dependent on the thickness and consistency of the food eaten; hence, patients who take mainly liquid diets usually have poor weight loss, whereas those who can cope with solid food do much better. The rate of drainage of the gastric pouch is also influential, and if the gastric stoma is made too large, weight loss is poor. Similarly, if there is breakdown of the partition or of the stoma, patients report an increase in hunger and an earlier loss of postprandial satiety as well as an increased volume of intake accompanying their weight regain. Functional reversal of gastroplasty can be achieved by removing the stomal support; an increase in hunger and a regain of weight are almost invariably the consequences.

Patients must be advised to avoid eating and drinking at the same time; if a small amount of solid food is followed by a mouthful of liquid, the food will be washed through into the distal stomach. Satiety will not be achieved, and the sequence can be repeated over and over, resulting in excessive intake of food. Some patients use this strategy so as to appear to be eating more normally when coping with socially difficult situations, but if used at all meals, weight loss will be inadequate. If patients fill the pouch with solid food and then drink liquids, discomfort, regurgitation, and sometimes heartburn may occur. They must, therefore, be advised to drink before a solid meal and then wait at least 90 minutes before attempting to drink again, by which time the pouch will be empty enough to tolerate the liquid.

The most important rule of eating is that all solid food must be reduced into particles smaller than the size of the gastric stoma; otherwise obstruction will occur. If obstruction occurs, patients complain of spasmodic and unpleasant epigastric discomfort or pain, often accompanied by hypersalivation and even watering of the eyes. It is presumed that this response reflects spasm of the gastric smooth muscle. Sometimes there will be a sudden relief of the symptoms accompanied by audible borborygmi, reflecting the passage of the obstructing bolus through the stoma. If there is no relief, spontaneous or self-induced retching will occur until the obstruction is relieved. A large proportion of the vomitus is swallowed saliva. Generally, resolution occurs in minutes, but occasionally the obstruction may last for days, result in dehydration, and require endoscopy. The offending bolus can be retrieved by a basket snare or polyp forceps. Alternatively, it may be broken up if soft and pushed through the stoma with the endoscope. A J-maneuver of the gastroscope in the pouch should always be attempted because lumps may hide high in the cardia. Large enteric-coated tablets may occasionally cause obstruction and be impossible to snare endoscopically. Having the patient steadily drink up to a liter of 10% sodium bicarbonate solution to alkalinize the environment usually results in the dissolution of the tablets.[15]

Patients vary widely in their abilities to cope with solid food; the variations depend on type of food available, dentition, preoperative eating habits, and psychosocial factors. Bohn and colleagues found that there is a consistent hierarchy in ease of food consumption, with unminced red meat being the most difficult and liquids the easiest.[16] Hard or crunchy foods such as nuts or biscuits are easy to manage, but soft solids such as fresh bread or scrambled eggs frequently result in regurgitation. They also found that careful counseling and dietitian-supervised meals improved the ability of patients to tolerate the more difficult foods. Poor teeth make mastication difficult, and strategies such as cutting up food finely or mincing it can help; however, patients in this category may resort to softer foods and soups, with a corresponding reduction in weight loss. Inattention to chewing along with stress, depression, and the need to eat quickly are also associated with difficulty in the tolerance of some solids.

Gastric motility may play a part in the rate of drainage of the gastric pouch, and excessive motility may be responsible for poor weight loss in some cases. The anticholinergic propantheline was associated with excellent weight loss in two patients with anatomically normal gastroplasties but very poor weight loss.[17] The variability in weight loss after gastroplasty and, indeed, after all restrictive operations

Table 20-1	THE RULES OF EATING AFTER GASTROPLASTY

1. Stop eating when feeling full or uncomfortable.
2. Do not drink and eat at the same time.
3. Do not drink for at least an hour and a half after eating.
4. Chew thoroughly and check oral contents before swallowing.

brings home the fact that the final amount of weight loss depends on patient-controlled factors as much as it does on the operation. The lack of instructions to patients in the correct use of the operation may result in poor weight loss. Surgery does not control

- the type or calorie content of food eaten; fats, oils, and sugary foods are easy to chew.
- the frequency of eating; small amounts taken frequently add up to a large amount.
- the amount or quality of liquids; liquids can be drunk almost without limit.
- the amount of exercise done by patients; patients with severe disabilities that prevent physical exercise often lose a disappointingly small amount of weight.
- the unrelenting pressure in Western society and increasingly in the rest of the world to consume food and drink beyond what is needed for adequate nutrition.

With these factors able to act against gastroplasty or any other form of surgery for obesity, it is perhaps surprising that patients do as well as they do.

▶ PATIENT ASSESSMENT AND PREPARATION

Preoperative assessment is discussed in other chapters of this book; however, three specific factors are particularly important in relation to restrictive operations. The first of these is motivation which, of course, has to be assessed subjectively. Surgeons must remember that they can only facilitate the weight-loss process by their operations; gastroplasty can easily be defeated, and poor weight loss is the result. Fortunately, this situation is unusual, but it may occur in patients who are severely depressed and bent on self-harm or occasionally in patients with personality disorders. The ability to regurgitate easily by failing to masticate or by eating excessively can be used in a manipulative way by some patients to gain the attention and sympathy of family members or medical attendants. Organic obstruction must, of course, be excluded by endoscopy or contrast radiology, but if these investigations are normal psychological help may be needed.

Patients must also have the ability and willingness to be able to adapt their eating to the gastroplasty. This may bear little relationship to intelligence. Some patients with low intelligence comply with dietary instructions, and the converse certainly occurs too. Good teeth are vital if solid foods are to be consumed, and patients must be encouraged to care for their teeth, which will deteriorate if regurgitation is frequent or tooth brushing is neglected. The possession of dentures or even the absence of teeth does not contraindicate gastroplasty surgery but does necessitate more careful instruction and dietary advice for those patients. Such patients often suffer more frequent regurgitation and a consequent avoidance of solids, with reliance on liquids and soft foods and predictably less weight loss.

There are no absolute contraindications for gastroplasty (except for Prader-Willy syndrome), as long as the patient will survive the anesthetic. The simpler open gastroplasties such as SRVG and MLVG, which can be performed rapidly through a small incision and with very little postoperative morbidity, can be excellent solutions for the morbidly obese who have severe respiratory disorders, ischemic heart disease, or poorly controlled diabetes.

Preoperative education is most important for success. The effects of the surgery on eating techniques must be explained to patients, bearing in mind that eating is often a social activity. Explanatory brochures and well-organized, supervised support groups are important aids in preparation for surgery.

▶ POSTOPERATIVE MANAGEMENT AND FOLLOW-UP

After the experience of more than 3200 patients, I have found that if there are no complications, recovery is rapid and need not be traumatic to patient or surgeon. Proper respiratory management is vital, particularly in a patient who is of android body shape, where pressure from intraabdominal fat and often hepatic steatosis is transmitted through the diaphragm and significantly reduces respiratory reserve, increasing the work of breathing when the patient is recumbent. It is essential that a patient have full reversal of relaxant anesthesia at the completion of the operation and be placed in the sitting position in the hospital bed. The temptation to leave the patient intubated and transfer him or her to the intensive care unit should be strongly resisted. Oxygen must be given judiciously, particularly when the pCO_2 is elevated, as in pickwickian syndrome; otherwise respiratory drive may be reduced, leading to hypoxia and hypercarbia. Narcotic analgesia must not be excessive so as to avoid reducing consciousness. Local anesthetic infiltration by intercostal or rectus sheath blocks or by continuous infusion into the wound is very useful. Continuous narcotic infusions may lead to oversedation, nausea, and hallucinations, but patient-controlled analgesia may be worthwhile. Nonsteroidal antiinflammatory drugs (paracetamol or aspirin, rectally or orally) effectively and cheaply contribute to pain relief and allow early mobilization. Large recliner chairs are often more comfortable than most hospital beds and they make nursing care easier.

Patients should be encouraged to mobilize early and take themselves to the toilet; routine urinary catheters are unnecessary and may lead to bladder infection. Patients should be carefully monitored for the first few days, with particular attention being paid to heart rate, temperature, and oxygen saturation, all of these being indicators of intraabdominal or respiratory mischief. Low-dose heparin or low-molecular-weight heparin for the duration of hospital stay and early mobilization reduces thromboembolic complications to a minimum, though some surgeons add compression stockings or intraoperative electric calf stimulation.

Various dietary regimens are recommended, but oral fluids can be commenced on the day of operation and pureed foods on the day after. A study showed solid foods could be administered under the direct supervision of a dietitian on the day after surgery; however, the more usual practice is to commence solids, after suitable instruction, 1 to 2 weeks after surgery. If patients accidentally ingest a large bolus in the first week and regurgitate, it will cause excessive pain in the healing abdominal wound. Rarely will patients repeatedly regurgitate as soon as fluid or food is commenced, and this may be due to a perigastric hematoma or stomal edema. This will resolve after 6 to 7 days but intravenous fluids will be necessary until then.

Gastroplasty is an excellent antireflux operation, provided the pouch is small and the stoma not too tight, but some patients complain of heartburn or epigastric pain after swallowing in the first week or two. This can be controlled by preprandial antacid, H_2 antagonists, or proton pump inhibitors.

After open operation, patients can be discharged as early as 2 days after surgery, and with laparoscopic surgery, even earlier. However, patients should be established on a pureed diet and be confident with their eating before going home.

Patients must be followed until weight stabilization is achieved, normally by 1 year. The change from uncontrolled eating to severe restriction in type and volume of food is dramatic, and most patients require regular counseling to be able to adapt without undue problems of regurgitation. As well as advice on the required technique of eating, patients must be encouraged to exercise regularly and to avoid bad eating habits. They may also need support and advice on the social and psychological consequences of massive weight loss.

▶ POSTOPERATIVE COMPLICATIONS

Four major postoperative complications may be seen after gastroplasty.

Bleeding, which generally emanates from the pinhole or from the staple line, usually presents as melena. As a rule, it is self-limited with the aid of antacids and fluid replacement, although rarely bleeding may require intervention, initially in the form of endoscopy. Injection of the bleeding area with adrenalin solution is usually effective but if not, laparotomy and oversewing of the bleeding area, possibly with endoscopic guidance to the bleeding point, may become necessary.

Leakage from the stomach can be a catastrophic complication unless it is immediately diagnosed and treated. The first and most important sign of a leak is a tachycardia of about 120, usually accompanied by severe abdominal pain and preceding an elevation in body temperature. Breathing is painful and there may be pain at the left shoulder tip due to diaphragmatic irritation. Oxygen saturation soon drops and generalized abdominal tenderness and distension follow. Tachycardia alone is a sufficient indication to perform a Gastrografin swallow or a computed tomography scan. Contrast radiology is most useful in the diagnosis of leaks using water-soluble contrast (barium is contraindicated), preferably under fluoroscopy. Computed tomography has the advantage of localizing fluid collections as well as demonstrating leaks, and in some situations it can be used to guide drainage. If a leak is detected, immediate laparotomy or laparoscopy is necessary. At operation, a leak may be very difficult to detect, and methylene blue instilled into the stomach through a nasogastric tube is useful. If the leak is found, it should be

carefully oversewn, and omentum may be placed over this for reinforcement.

Thorough lavage of the peritoneal cavity, including the pelvis, reduces the chances of abscess formation. One or more large suction or sump drainage tubes are placed close to the site of the leak. If a leak cannot be found, the abdomen should be lavaged and drained by multiple drains, including drainage of the subphrenic spaces and the pelvis. A percutaneous gastrostomy tube is useful for decompression of the stomach and possibly later for feeding, and it eliminates the need for a nasogastric tube. The cause of a leak is often unclear. A tear of the stomach may be caused by the pin of the TA-90 Premium staple gun; it is evidenced by a 2-cm linear defect in the middle part of the pouch anteriorly. More often, leaks are only a few millimeters in size and generally close to the staple line. The development of acute dilatation of the stomach may be the cause of some leaks.

Subphrenic abscess may be part of the aftermath of a gastric leak, usually on the left side and usually accompanied by atelectasis and pleural effusion, which may later become infected to form an empyema. Subphrenic abscess is amenable to drainage by the interventional radiologist; however, open drainage is the time-tested option. The larger and the more chronic the abscess, the longer the cavity will take to resolve, and sinograms are useful for following progress. A gastric fistula may sometimes develop through an abscess cavity and out a drain tube, but once the cavity has collapsed, the drain tube can be gradually withdrawn and the fistula usually resolves. If the fistula arises from the gastric pouch, it may persist if the patient is fed. In this situation, a tube gastrostomy into the distal stomach allows for enteral feeding, encouraging the fistula's closure.

Thromboembolic disease is uncommon but potentially lethal and many regimens of prophylaxis are recommended. The least expensive is probably the most effective: early mobilization by insisting that the patient get out of bed and walk to the toilet (this means no urinary catheter), walk around the ward every day, and move the calves frequently. This is well accepted by patients who are educated preoperatively. Low-dose heparin (5000 U two or three times daily) for the duration of the hospital stay, intraoperative electrical calf stimulation, and the use of soluble aspirin as an analgesic are other simple preventive measures. Elastic and sequential compression stockings may be used and some surgeons have advocated vena caval filters in high-risk cases.

▶ GASTROPLASTY FAILURE AND REVISIONAL SURGERY

Anatomic failure of gastroplasty inevitably has its impact on weight loss or on the patient's quality of life and may require corrective surgery. The aim of revisional surgery is to restore the anatomic integrity of the gastroplasty and, in the case of MLVG and SRVG, is generally not difficult. The surgery is commonly more problematic in the Mason VBG, where mesh stomal support is used, and in cases in which there has been more than one previous operation on the stomach. Adhesions tend to form between the greater omentum, the falciform ligament, and the inferior surfaces of the liver and the stomach, particularly in the region of the stoma. The interposition of omentum between the stoma and the liver makes separation of these structures much easier if revision is later necessary. Dissection of these structures should be aimed at dissecting just outside the capsule of the liver, taking care to avoid damage to the pancreas and also the vessels supplying the lesser curve.

Adhesions may virtually obliterate the lesser sac, making the mobilization of the stomach and the positioning of a new staple line difficult and also putting the pancreas at risk. It may sometimes be useful to divide the greater omentum inferior to the antrum so as to allow better access to the lesser sac. Passage of an orogastric bougie into the stomach is essential to aid in the identification of the gastric anatomy and the position of the stoma. Finally, adhesion of omentum or of the greater curve of the stomach to the spleen poses the risk for hemorrhage of that organ, usually as a result of a traction injury.[18]

Staple-line dehiscence has been a problem ever since the introduction of stapling instruments, but there has been a progressive reduction in its incidence with improvements in instrument design, and there has been virtual elimination of this complication with the performing of divided gastroplasties. In the beginning, staple-line failure was an early occurrence; since the development of better instruments, the symptoms of failure and weight regain develop after 3 to 6 years or even longer. Surgical correction usually involves the further application of staples to create a new small pouch. If the pouch is large, a new gastroplasty may be created inside the old, together with a new stoma (Fig. 20-6). If the pouch is still small and the dehiscence high, a new staple line may be used to isolate the failed area while preserving the old stoma. The Mason VBG may be more simply and safely converted to MLVG or SRVG[19] rather than windowing the stomach again and applying a new mesh in the presence of dense adhesions around the stomal area. Care must be taken to ensure there is no intersection of the new and the old staple line, which would result in excluding a section of stomach. A gastrogastrostomy relieves this situation if it occurs.

If the stoma created is too wide, weight loss is slow from the start and there is early regain. If the stoma loses its support and dilatates, it is usually caused by erosion, and weight gain is the almost invariable result. If the pouch is not too dilatated, a new stomal support is usually the solution, but it should be placed higher up on the staple line so as to reduce pouch volume.

If the patient complains of increased appetite and capacity for food, early loss of satiety after meals, and easier tolerance of solid food, together with weight regain, the cause is usually partition failure or stomal dilatation. Pouch dilatation with a normal stoma often results in slow weight regain and increasing capacity for food, but any existing food intolerance is maintained. Excessive pouch dilatation may lead to the anomalous situation of poor weight loss accompanied by excessive regurgitation. This situation may be due to a sump effect (Fig. 20-7), in which the filling of the large pouch has the effect of closing the stoma. This is characteristically associated with nocturnal reflux and may even lead to aspiration symptoms of cough, choking, or pneumonia in a situation analogous to pyloric stenosis. In certain patients there may be a progressive and, in some, excessive weight loss. Stomal stenosis usually manifests itself in a progressive deterioration in the ability to cope with solid foods and an increase in the frequency of regurgitation. Heartburn and esophagitis are common consequences, and the patient tends to retreat to a liquid diet. Its onset after weeks of solid-food intolerance accompanied by heartburn or indigestion is indicative of stomal-support erosion; however, if it occurs over hours and is accompanied by hypersalivation, a bolus obstruction is likely.

Stenosis may be due to infection of the stoma-supporting material and the reaction of the scar tissue around it. It may eventually lead to the erosion of the stoma-supporting material, which is usually accompanied by indigestion and the worsening of the regurgitation. Some patients cannot tolerate a normal stoma; this situation is commonly found in association with poor teeth or poor concentration on the task of mastication. Endoscopy is generally diagnostic and can be therapeutic if an eroded suture or ring can be cut by endoscopic scissors and removed. Eroding mesh, however, usually requires laparotomy for removal. Removal of only the stomal support

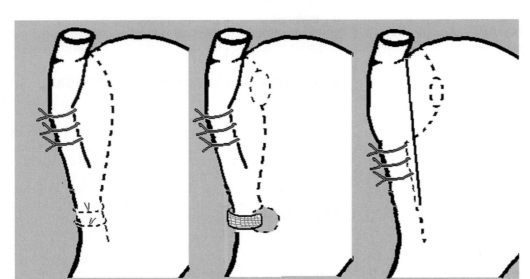

Figure 20-6. Repeat gastroplasty, within dilated pouch, for staple line dehiscence in large and small pouches.

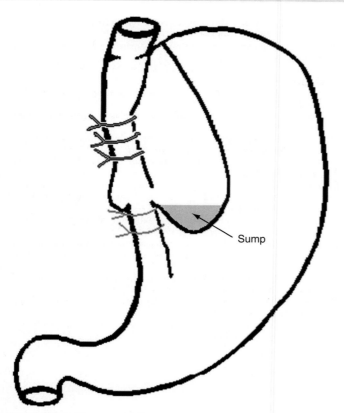

Figure 20-7. The sump effect in gastroplasty that results in stomal obstruction through pressure on the stoma by sump contents.

the view is only two-dimensional. The most useful means of investigating a gastroplasty is endoscopy. It allows the length of the pouch to be measured and an estimate of its width made; this can lead to the diagnosis of pouch dilatation and sump effect. The presence of staple-line failure is usually easily seen either from within the pouch or from the body of the stomach by means of a J-maneuver. If the gastroscope just traverses the stoma, the stomal diameter can be assumed to be adequate; however, very easy passage of the stoma suggests that the stoma is too large. It is strongly recommended that obesity surgeons perform the endoscopies on their own patients because the reports of physicians naïve about gastroplasty are often confusing or misleading.

CONVERSION OPERATIONS

Reversal of gastroplasty is requested by about 4% of patients, usually as a result of food intolerance. Others are under the misapprehension that having lost their excess weight, they will be able to control their weight without the help of the gastroplasty. Functional reversal of gastroplasty is usually achieved easily and can be performed laparoscopically by removing or even just dividing the stomal support.[20] This allows for easy passage of food into the distal stomach and the ability to tolerate all foods in increasing quantities as the unsupported stoma dilates. Even in the best-motivated patient, weight regain invariably occurs, and some patients request further surgical help. An alternative method of reversal is to make an antral gastrotomy and pass a cutting linear stapler on either side of the stoma, thus dividing the partition. Removal of the whole staple line is unnecessary to reverse a gastroplasty.

In the event of failure due to a clearly identifiable and clearly correctable cause in a patient who has had good weight control and good tolerance of the gastroplasty, there is no indication to convert to another procedure. If the patient has had a significant problem with food intolerance, conversion to gastric bypass or to a malabsorptive procedure may be advisable. If the pouch is small and intact, a Roux-en-Y limb can be attached to it and the distal stomach excluded by division with a cutting linear stapler. If the pouch is dilatated or disrupted, a Fobi pouch or similar operation may be feasible. This particular conversion is indicated in the setting of esophagitis associated with bile reflux.

In the event of multiple revisional surgeries, the stomach may be so encased by adhesions that further surgery is dangerous. An effective and surgically simple solution is to convert it into an ileogastrostomy.[21] The only required access to the stomach is the antrum, which is generally minimally affected by encasing adhesions. If necessary, the stomal support can be removed. In this operation all but 70 cm of small bowel is excluded from the food stream and the excluded segment empties isoperistaltically into the antrum, avoiding bacterial overgrowth and blind loop syndrome. The conversion of gastroplasty into gastric banding, both open and laparoscopic, has been described but long-term results have not been published.

Gastric banding can be converted into gastroplasty after removal of the band; however, the thick, fibrous

essentially reverses the gastroplasty, and weight regain is inevitable.

Endoscopic dilation of the stoma is often attempted but usually has no long-term benefit and may worsen the situation by causing damage to and further scarring of the stoma. Most endoscopes are 1 cm in diameter, and the comfortable passage of the endoscope through the stoma denies the diagnosis of stenosis. For some patients, however, a 1-cm stoma is still too tight, and revision may be necessary.

Revision normally involves locating the stomal support, removing it, and refashioning the stoma so it is larger. This is easier in the SRVG and MLVG; a bougie in the stoma is used to gauge the new size of the stoma. In the Mason VBG the old mesh has to be removed and a longer one inserted, a more difficult procedure.

Acute regurgitation may occur without warning in a patient otherwise doing well. It is usually caused by obstruction resulting from a bolus of food. Endoscopy diagnoses and usually relieves the situation. Total extraction of teeth may create the same situation until dentures or dental implants are fitted. New medication, particularly if the tablets are large and enteric-coated, may also cause acute vomiting.

A barium swallow may reveal staple-line failure, but the early films should be taken with the patient in the lateral decubitus position so as to demonstrate the passage of contrast though the staple line before too much contrast has filled the stomach, obscuring the staple line. A barium swallow is of very little value in assessing the stoma because capsule of the band must be disrupted to allow the stomach to expand and facilitate placement of the staple line. Gastric bypass can be converted into gastroplasty, particularly in the situation of gross pouch dilatation, but only with difficulty because gastric continuity must be reinstated and a new pouch and stoma constructed.

▶ REFERENCES

1. Gomez CA: Gastroplasty in the surgical treatment of morbid obesity. Am J Clin Nutr 1980;33:406-415.
2. Pace WG, Martin EW, Tetirick T, et al: Gastric partitioning for morbid obesity. Ann Surg 1979;190:392-400.
3. Tretbar LL, Taylor TL, Sifers EC: Gastric plication for morbid obesity. J Kans Med Soc 1976;77:488-490.
4. Johnston D, Dachtler J, Sue-Ling H, et al: . Obes Surg 2003;13:10-16.
5. Long M, Collins JP: The technique and early results of high gastric reduction for obesity. Aust N Z J Surg 1980;50:146-148.
6. Laws HL: Standardized gastroplasty orifice. Am J Surg 1981;141:393-394.
7. Wynne-Jones G: Vertical ligated gastroplasty by clamp, cut and suture: a series of 504 cases dating back to 1977. Obes Surg 1994;4:344-348.
8. Mason EE: Development and future of gastroplasties for morbid obesity. Arch Surg 2003;138:361-366.
9. Chua TY, Mendiola RM: Laparoscopic vertical banded gastroplasty. Obes Surg 1995;5:77-80.
10. Melissas J: Technical modification of laparoscopic vertical banded gastroplasty. Obes Surg 2003;13:132-135.
11. Mason EE: Surgical treatment of obesity. Major Probl Clin Surg 1981;26:480.
12. Mason EE, Doherty C: Vertical banded gastroplasty for morbid obesity. Dig Surg 1997;14:355-360.
13. Jamieson AC: Weight loss after gastroplasty. Probl Gen Surg 1992;9:290-297.
14. Urbain P: The Proring band, a new device in the field of restrictive surgery: preliminary experience. Obes Surg 2002,12:588-591.
15. Jamieson AC: Unusual clinical problem associated with obesity surgery. Med J Aust 1993;159:632.
16. Bohn M, Way M, Jamieson AC: The effect of practical dietary counseling on food variety and regurgitation frequency after gastroplasty for obesity. Obes Surg 1993;3:23-29.
17. Jamieson AC: Propantheline as an adjuvant to weight loss after vertical gastroplasty. Obes Surg 1997;7:359-362.
18. Lord MD, Gourevitch A: The peritoneal anatomy of the spleen, with special reference to the operation of partial gastrectomy. Br J Surg 1965;52:202-204.
19. Mason EE, Cullen JJ: Management of complications in vertical banded gastroplasty. Curr Probl Surg 2003;60:33-37.
20. Bird PA, Jamieson AC: Functional laparoscopic reversal of a Long gastroplasty. Aust N Z J Surg 1997;67:734-735.
21. Cleator IGM, Gourlay RH: Ileogastrostomy for morbid obesity. Can J Surg 1988;31:114-116.

21

Laparoscopic Vertical Banded Gastroplasty

J. K. Champion, M.D., F.A.C.S. and Michael Williams, M.D.

Gastric restrictive surgery for weight loss has undergone continuous evolution since its introduction in the form of a horizontal gastroplasty in 1971 by Mason and associates at the University of Iowa.[1] Ten years passed before the vertical orientation of the gastric pouch emerged in 1981, and another 6 years were required to further refine the configuration to the form recommended by Mason in 1986—that of a vertically oriented, calibrated and measured, undivided pouch of less than 30 ml with an outlet stabilized by a polypropylene mesh band of 1.5 cm × 5.0 cm, as seen in Figure 21-1.[2]

Mason emphasized the technical aspects of the operation and made a point of recommending the use of a 32F bougie to form the pouch, utilizing a four-row, noncutting, 90-mm stapler, measuring the exact length of the 1.5-cm-wide band for external calibration of the outlet (not around a bougie), and employing a band of a single layer of polypropylene mesh that would become incorporated in the wall of the outlet to minimize the risk of erosion. In comparing the reports of various surgeons, these specific points are important to keep in mind because the technique varies widely and is not standardized. Evolution and experimentation arose because of overall poor weight loss coupled with high morbidity and revision rates that have been inherent in purely gastric restrictive bariatric surgery since its inception. Wound complications, including infection, seroma, dehiscence, and incisional hernia, were significant sources of associated morbidity, when using the open approach, in up to 30% of patients, so it was not surprising that ultimately, a minimally invasive technique would be advocated so as to allow the procedure to further evolve and to reduce complications.

Chua and Mendiola were the first surgeons to perform a laparoscopic vertical banded gastroplasty (VBG), in February 1993, but they did not publish their results until 1995.[3] The first two cases were performed using a laparoscopy-assisted technique that utilized a small midline incision for application of the circular stapler and placement of the band, but in April 1993 they performed the first totally laparoscopic procedure. They attempted to replicate the Mason technique by measuring 9 cm from the angle of His along the lesser curve and creating a window with a circular stapler fired alongside a 32F dilator; they

stabilized the outlet with a prosthetic band, though the pouch was not measured and the band was polytetrafluoroethylene (PTFE) that was measured by internal calibration around the 32F bougie. In addition, the staple line was divided using a cutting linear endoscopic stapler. They reported difficulties because of limited instrumentation and technical issues surrounding the creation of the circular window. The circular stapler required a 33-mm port, and the limitation of movement imposed by the ports, along with the decrease in tactile sensation associated with laparoscopy, made manipulation of the anvil and formation of the window challenging, which resulted in poor pouch and outlet construction, both critical for success with VBG.

Lonroth and colleagues also reported performing a laparoscopic VBG in October 1993 but did not publish their results until 1996.[4] They described their technique as "the traditional according to Mason"; however, significant technical differences were described. The site chosen for the creation of the circular window was reported to be 4 to 5 cm below the angle of His and 3 cm from the lesser curve, with the circular stapler being fired after insertion of a 27F dilator along the lesser curve of the stomach. The band

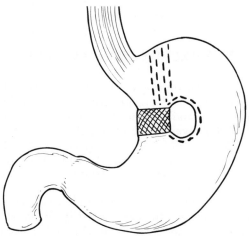

Figure 21-1. Laparoscopic Mason VBG.

utilized was PTFE, and the diameter was determined by internal calibration around a 32F bougie, not by measurement of overall length. The pouch was not measured or calibrated but was undivided with a four-row, noncutting, 60-mm, linear endoscopic stapler. Although the laparoscopic VBG was described as "technically feasible," significant technical issues in attempting to adapt an open technique to a minimally invasive approach remained. Lonroth and colleagues reported an 8% conversion to open surgery and an 8% early reoperation rate due to staple-line and infection issues.

We began performing laparoscopic VBG in 1995, after having refined the technique in the animal laboratory and in fresh cadavers.[5] We observed that the creation of a window near the lesser curve and division of the proximal stomach to form a short tubular structure was the same in the VBG and the Collis gastroplasty (utilized for esophageal-lengthening procedures in management of complex gastroesophageal reflux disease). We employed the circular stapler technique for both procedures because at that time, the primary focus of our practice was reflux surgery. We quickly discovered the same technical issues reported by Chua and Mendiola, namely, difficulty in manipulating the anvil and in accurately placing it alongside the bougie to create a consistent, reproducible outlet and pouch size. In our experience, the circular staple line commonly disrupted at the site where the linear staple line crossed it, and suturing was required to reinforce and repair it, which did not inspire confidence in the product. In addition, the large incision required for laparoscopic introduction of the circular handle required closing with suture, which was difficult in a morbidly obese patient and remained a potential ventral hernia site in the future.

We returned to the laboratory and devised a laparoscopic technique that eliminated the circular stapler and employed only a linear stapler inserted through 12-mm ports to allow "wedging" of a 5 × 5-cm segment of the upper fundus. This technique created a reproducible, small gastric tube, calibrated to 20 ml, that could be utilized for an esophageal-lengthening procedure or a VBG. This modification is technically simpler, avoids the problems with the circular stapler and incision, and recreates a sharp angle of His that may aid in preventing reflux. This chapter reviews the laparoscopic technique and the outcomes of both the Mason-like circular window VBG and the wedge VBG utilizing only a linear stapler.

▶ PATIENT SELECTION AND EVALUATION

Candidates for laparoscopic VBG first must conform to National Institutes of Health criteria for consideration for surgery to handle clinically severe obesity. Patients should be 100 lb over ideal body weight or have body mass indexes (BMIs) of 40 kg per m^2 or greater if they have no associated comorbid conditions. Patients with BMIs of 35 to 39 kg per m^2 may be considered if they have associated clinically significant comorbidities. Examples of significant comorbidities include but are not limited to hypertension, sleep apnea, diabetes mellitus, hyperlipidemia, or severe osteoarthritis (i.e., the need for total joint replacement or vertebrae fusion).

Additional consideration should include whether the patient is a "sweet-eater" or has a BMI of 50 kg per m^2 or greater. Sugerman and colleagues demonstrated in a randomized trial that sweet-eaters and patients with BMIs over 50 kg per m^2 have significantly less weight loss than do non-sweet-eaters and those in lower BMI cohorts.[6] We strongly discourage individuals in these two subgroups from considering gastric restriction surgery but will comply with their decisions if they persist after an intensive informed consent process that outlines alternatives and outcomes. Patients who are less than ideal candidates for VBG may oppose having any procedure that incorporates a malabsorptive component, such as the Roux-en-Y gastric bypass, and their wishes should be respected. We also discourage patients with diabetes mellitus, hyperlipidemia, and severe reflux disease from having VBGs because the gastric bypass provides better long-term control of these conditions.

There are additional restrictions to consider when choosing candidates for a minimally invasive technique. In general, patients with BMIs of less than 50 kg per m^2 or weights of less than 350 lb, with a gynecoid body habitus, and with no previous open abdominal surgery yield the best chances of success in laparoscopic VBGs performed by less experienced surgeons. As experience is gained in minimally invasive bariatric techniques, heavier patients who have an android body habitus or who have had previous open abdominal surgery can be considered as candidates. Massive hepatomegaly is a significant risk for conversion to an open procedure. In our experience, liver size can be reduced preoperatively by encouraging patients to lose weight and reduce their carbohydrate intake by avoiding starches, pasta, and sweets for 10 days prior to surgery. In addition, surgeons must be proficient in laparoscopic suturing and advanced two-handed dissection techniques to complete the procedure with safety. Surgeons should become proficient in performing an open VBG, then complete a laparoscopic bariatric preceptorship and be proctored on their initial laparoscopic cases in order to reduce patient morbidity during the early learning curve. Probably 100 or more cases are required to obtain proficiency. Laparoscopic revisional surgery should not be considered until the surgeon has successfully completed at least 100 primary laparoscopic bariatric operations involving suturing and stapling. No additional evaluation is required for a laparoscopic approach other than the surgeon's standard preoperative bariatric regimen.

▶ SURGICAL TECHNIQUE

Technique for Laparoscopic Wedge VBG

The patient is admitted the morning of surgery and receives a prophylactic antibiotic and low-molecular-weight heparin (enoxaparin 40 mg). The patient is placed under general endotracheal anesthesia and a Foley catheter is inserted. The patient is positioned supine on the table with a footboard, to allow maximal reverse Trendelenburg tilt. The surgeon and camera operator stand on the patient's right side, with the assistant surgeon and scrub nurse positioned on the left.

The initial trocar site is for the camera. It is a 12-mm incision made 15 cm below the xiphoid process, just to the left of the midline and within the left rectus sheath. An Optiview trocar (Ethicon Endosurgery, Cincinnati, Ohio) is utilized to enter the abdomen under direct visualization utilizing a 10-mm zero-degree scope without insufflation. Insufflation to 15 mm is begun and the abdomen is carefully inspected. The remaining 5 trocars are inserted under direct visualization in the positions indicated in Figure 21-2. There are a total of four 5-mm ports and two 12-mm ports, with the second 12-mm port positioned in the left upper quadrant below the costal margin, to be used as the stapling port.

The patient is positioned in the reverse Trendelenburg position and a 5-mm ratcheted Allis clamp is passed through the xiphoid trocar under the left lobe of the liver and attached to the diaphragm just above the esophageal hiatus for retraction. The assistant retracts the fundus of the stomach laterally, and the surgeon takes down the peritoneal attachments along the left crus and angle of His with monopolar electrocautery. This defines the angle of His and assists in the application of the stapler for the final firing and transection of the upper pouch. A measurement is then made 5 cm inferiorly from the angle of His along the lesser curve, and a window is created into the lesser sac directly alongside the gastric wall, utilizing gentle blunt dissection and bipolar electrocautery for hemostasis. This window will be used to position the band around the pouch at the end of the case and is used as a landmark while stapling the pouch.

The dissection now proceeds horizontally from the lesser-curve window to the greater curve of the stomach. The short gastric vessels are taken down along the upper fundus all the way to the left crus and angle of His. We utilize bipolar cautery to obtain hemostasis, but any energy source is appropriate. A 50F bougie is then positioned along the lesser curve of the stomach to form and calibrate the pouch during stapling. The 12-mm linear stapler (Endo GIA-2, USSC, Norwalk, Conn.), with a 45-mm 3.5 load, is inserted via the 12-mm port in the left subcostal position and is applied transversely to the stomach from the greater curve directly horizontal with the window on the lesser curve. The stapler is fired horizontally for two or three firings until the end of the stapler rolls off the bougie at the lesser curvature. The stapler is now repositioned vertically alongside the bougie and fired repeatedly up through the angle of His, transecting and removing a 5 × 5-cm wedge of stomach. With a little manipulation, the transected segment can be withdrawn through the 12-mm port in the left upper abdomen without enlarging the port orifice. If any enlargement is required, the site should be closed with suture at the end of the case. The staple line along the pouch is oversewn with a running 2-0 silk because the patient is begun on liquids immediately postoperatively. The 50F bougie is removed and replaced with a 30F bougie for placement of the band around the pouch.

A band is constructed of polypropylene mesh that is 1.5 cm × 7.0 cm. The band will be overlapped 1 cm on the ends to create a 5-cm band circumference; therefore, the band is marked with a stay suture 1 cm from each end to aid in placement. The band is inserted via a 12-mm port and positioned around the distal pouch through the window 5 cm below the esophagogastric junction. The band is overlapped 1 cm and sutured with two horizontal mattress sutures of 0 Ethibond (Ethicon, Sommerville, N.J.) tied extracorporeally. The completed procedure is illustrated in Figure 21-3. The bougie is removed and an intraoperative esophagogastroscopy is performed to ensure that pouch and stoma size are proper and that there are no leaks from the staple lines. The band is then covered anteriorly with an omental patch, which is sutured in place with a medial suture. The abdomen is irrigated with saline and all trocars are removed under direct visualization to rule out bleeding. Trocars sites are not closed at the fascia level. Skin incisions are closed with 3-0 plain subcuticular sutures and Steri-Strips.

Technique for Laparoscopic Mason VBG

To perform the traditional technique using a circular stapler, the trocar placement, the dissection with creation of a lesser-curve window 5 cm below the angle of His, and

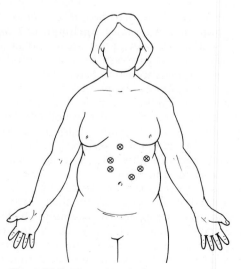

Figure 21-2. Trocar sites for laparoscopic VBG.

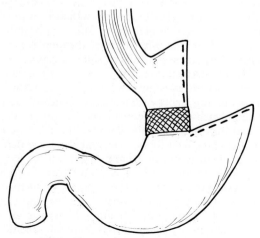

Figure 21-3. Laparoscopic wedge VBG.

the mobilization of the short gastric vessels are the same as described earlier. The window serves as a landmark for pouch creation and is the ultimate site of band placement. A 50F bougie is positioned along the lesser curve, and a horizontal mattress suture is placed alongside the bougie at the level of the window to tightly reapproximate the anterior and posterior walls of the stomach and to allow for easy insertion of the circular stapler anvil. A 2-cm incision is made in the midclavicular line of the left upper abdomen, just below the costal margin. The anvil of a 21-mm circular stapler with a sharp spike attached is lowered into the abdomen via the incision, and air leakage is controlled by clamping the site temporarily with two towel clips. The anvil is positioned posterior to the stomach in the lesser sac, and the sharp spike and anvil shaft are driven through the stomach alongside the bougie at the level of the gastric window. The spike is removed and the anvil mated to the stapler shaft by inserting it through the abdominal wall via the 2-cm anterior incision after removing the towel clips. The stapler is closed, fired, and removed. The incision is again approximated with towel clips for continued insufflation. A 45-mm 3.5 linear stapler (Endo GIA-2, USSC, Norwalk, Conn.) is inserted via the 12-mm port in the left upper abdomen, is positioned through the circular window alongside the bougie vertically, and is fired. Multiple firings are continued until the pouch is completely transected except for the distal outlet along the lesser curve. The staple line is oversewn with 2-0 silk sutures, and the distal pouch is banded as described earlier. The 2-cm anterior abdominal wall incision is closed with a peritoneal needle and permanent suture, and the remaining port sites are managed as previously described.

EQUIPMENT

Laparoscopic bariatric surgery necessitates longer instrumentation than standard 32-cm laparoscopic instruments because of the patients' increased girth and the elevated position of the gastroesophageal junction in morbid obesity. Graspers, needle drivers, and scissors should be 45 cm in length. Trocars should also be longer, with 15-cm lengths now available in both 5-mm and 12-mm diameters. The issue of how best to retract the liver is controversial. We utilize a ratcheted Allis clamp, which is applied via a subxiphoid port and attached to the diaphragm above the esophageal hiatus. This simple, inexpensive, reusable device has worked every time in our experience of more than 1300 laparoscopic bariatric cases over the past 8 years, and it requires no assistant to hold the retractor and no special stabilizing arms or clamps. A method of laparoscopic hemostasis must be considered by the surgeon, who has electrocautery, harmonic scalpels, and metallic clips as options. All work well in experienced hands; which to use is a matter of surgeon preference and training.

A 45-degree angled lens is mandatory for adequate visualization, particularly at the top of the stomach, and the new 60-cm-long lens is very useful for patients with BMIs above 60 kg per m2. The angled lens also allows the scope to remain near the anterior abdominal wall and allows

the surgeon's instruments to work beneath it for suturing. Extra-long 45-cm linear staplers are now available, and appropriate laparoscopic staplers, which articulate and can be loaded with a variety of staple sizes and lengths, are required. Two insufflators and the capability to have dual suction setups are necessary if brisk bleeding is encountered during the procedure, but we normally only employ one of each during a routine case. An open instrument setup should be available, if needed, for emergency conversion to open surgery. Laparoscopic bariatric surgery requires appropriate operating room tables for extra weight, and oversized beds, chairs, scales, and so forth.

POSTOPERATIVE CARE AND CLINICAL PATHWAY

The implementation of a clinical pathway for care of the bariatric surgery patient can provide benefits to the patient, hospital, and physician.[7] A clinical pathway is an anticipated patient-management plan that includes all medical personnel involved in the care of the patient. The pathway serves as a guide, or preplanned course of action, that can reduce medication and treatment errors by the use of clearly printed instructions; can reduce costs by omitting unnecessary tests and procedures; and can reduce the physicians' workload if standardized orders are utilized. An example of our clinical pathway for laparoscopic VBG is demonstrated in Table 21-1.

Postoperatively, patients receive intravenous fluids and pain medication overnight and are begun on a clear liquid diet immediately, as tolerated. Sequential compression devices are employed to reduce the risk for pulmonary embolus. The following morning, patients are discharged if they can tolerate liquids and pain medications by mouth and are clinically stable. If there is any clinical sign of a leak (e.g., fever over 101°F, persistent tachycardia of 120 for more than 4 hours, or persistent nausea), we perform a Gastrografin swallow study.

Patients are discharged on oral pain medication and a proton-pump inhibitor for 30 days. The postoperative diet consists of 2 weeks of liquids and 3 weeks of a soft diet before advancing to regular food. They are instructed to contact the office in the presence of a fever over 101°F, persistent vomiting for more than 6 hours, or a significant change in abdominal pain. They are to avoid all nonsteroidal antiinflammatory drugs and aspirin products so as to prevent pouch ulceration and band erosion.

Patients are contacted by phone at 5 days for postdischarge evaluation, and they return for follow-up at 3 weeks, 3 months, 6 months, and 1 year. Blood tests (including complete blood count, routine serum chemistries, iron, and B_{12} levels) are monitored at 6 months and 1 year and then yearly thereafter for life. Dietary counseling is performed at each office visit.

Patients are instructed not to lift heavy objects for 3 weeks, after which they may resume their normal physical activities. An exercise program, beginning with walking 20 minutes per day, 5 days per week, is initiated upon discharge and is increased to 45 minutes of aerobic exercise, as tolerated. Patients may return to work within 1 week.

| Table 21-1 | CLINICAL PATHWAY MODEL FOR LAPAROSCOPIC GASTRIC BYPASS |

INDICATOR	PREOP DAY 1	PREOP, DAY OF SURGERY	POSTOP, DAY OF SURGERY	POSTOP DAY 1	POSTOP DAY 2
Consults, evaluations	Anesthesia Medical clearance, if indicated				
Tests	H & P Chest radiograph, CBC, ECG, complete chemistry, iron, B_{12} ABG if sleep apnea				
Treatments	Stop NSAIDs, ASA, 7 days prior to surgery Preop teaching Aftercare contract Informed consent Bari Bed if >350 lb	SCD hose to or per bed	Insert Foley if patient has not voided in 6 hr; SCD hose; IV F at 100 ml/hr; IS q 4 hr; VS q 4 hr; O_2 to keep SAT 90% (continuous-pulse O_2 if BMI >60 or sleep apnea); CPAP if sleep apnea at preop; Accucheck q 6 hr if diabetic	D/C O_2 CBC Gastrografin swallow if pulse >120, temperature >100.5°F or intractable vomiting or nausea *Otherwise:* D/C IV D/C meds D/C SCDs if ambulating Inspect wounds Empty, record JP q shift	Remove JP if no leak Inspect incisions for redness, bleeding, or drainage
Medication	Fleets if BMI >60 or weight over 400 lb	Prevacid 30 mg PO; IV F at 100 ml per hr; Lovenox 40 mg SQ; Levoquin 500 mg IV; Flagyl 500 mg IV	IV F at 100 ml per hr; Flagyl 500 mg IV q 6 hr × 3 Reglan 10 mg IV q 8 hr × 3; Phenergan 25 mg IM/IV q 3 hr prn for nausea; Analgesia: PCA per anesthesia, or IM q 3 hr prn pain; Zofran 4 mg IV q 6 hr × 3 doses; Apresoline 10 mg IM q 4 hr prn; Systolic BP >190: sliding-scale insulin (Humilin R) 0-150, none; 151-200, 6 units; 201-250, 10 units; 251-300, 14 units; >301, 18 units; Benadryl: 25 mg IV q 4 hr prn for itching/rash	Tylenol 10 g liquid PO q 4 hr prn for pain, Fever>101°F; Percocet-5 1 PO q 4 hr prn for pain; Prevacid 30 mg PO hs q d; Reglan 10 mg PO, tid if nauseated; Mylanta II 30 ml PO q 4 hr prn for gas; Lovenox 40 mg SQ q am	Percocet -5 1 PO q 4 hr prn for pain; Lovenox 40 mg SQ q d
Diet	Liquid supper NPO at midnight	NPO	NPO except ice chips	Clear liquids if indicated	Clear liquids
Activity	ad lib	ad lib	Ambulate to restroom	Ambulate in hall Shower	Ambulate in hall Shower
Teaching	Postop diet Behavior modification Review vitamins, Ca^+, protein supplement	IS preop teaching	Instruct in IS Instruct in how to use SCDs	Postop diet instructions reinforced	Reinforce diet, vitamins, protein No lifting for 3 weeks
Discharge summary	Transportation needs assessed			Discuss home transport Case manager's assessment	Discharge if tolerates diet and oral meds Rx for pain meds PPIs, Ab if indicated Phone check in 5-7days Return in 3-4 weeks Call if temp >101°F, vomiting or abdominal pain longer than 4 hours

Ab, antibiotics; ABG, arterial blood gases; ASA, aspirin; BP, blood pressure; BMI, body mass index; CBC, complete blood ount; CPAP, continuous positive airway pressure; ECG, electrocardiogram; D/C, discontinue; IVF, intravenous fluid; IS, incentive spirometry; JP, Jackson-Prath; H&P, history and physical; hs, hour of sleep; IV, intravenous; NSAID, nonsteroidal antiinflammatory drug; PCA, patient-controlled analgesics; PPIs, proton pump inhibitors; Rx, prescription; SCD, sequential compression device; VS, vital sings.

▶ OUTCOMES

Assessments of outcomes in laparoscopic VBG are hampered by the small number of procedures performed, the wide variations in technique, and the short follow-up to date.

A randomized prospective trial of Mason open versus laparoscopic VBG with short-term follow-up was reported by Azagra and colleagues; it demonstrated a significant reduction in postoperative wound infections (10.8% vs. 3.3%, $P = 0.04$) and in incisional hernias (15.8% vs. 0%, $P = 0.04$) with the laparoscopic approach.[8] However, the laparoscopic technique did require significantly longer operating-room times (150 min vs. 60 min, $P = 0.001$). The paper reported no significant difference in percent excess weight loss or reduction in mean BMI between the two groups, but absolute values and length of follow-up were not disclosed.

Table 21-2 illustrates 5-year outcomes for laparoscopic VBG from Olbers and colleagues, utilizing the Mason technique (109 patients with undivided pouches and 30 with divided pouches), and my results, using the wedge divided approach.[9,10] We experienced no wound infections and no incisional hernias in our group. Olbers' report does not mention the incidence of wound morbidity in his series. Mean percent excess weight loss was nearly identical in the two series. The incidence of late reoperations in Olbers' group was due to staple-line disruptions in 3 of 11 and poor weight loss in the other 8. Our reoperations were due to outlet stenosis and reflux in 2 of 4 and poor weight loss in the other 2, although we had 3 awaiting insurance approval for revisions for poor weight loss. Evaluation of our symptomatic patients and weight-loss failures by means of barium upper gastrointestinal series and flexible endoscopy revealed no gastric erosions or gastric fistulas.

Olbers reported a mean pouch volume of 80 cc on radiologic exam at 6 months postoperatively and 45% (5 of 11) of revisions for poor weight loss were due to dilatated pouches. Staple-line disruptions were responsible for another 27% of revisions. Thus, overall, 73% of revisions were secondary to technical pouch-construction issues. They subsequently abandoned the undivided staple line for their last 30 cases in this series.

We had a similar early experience with technical problems in getting the circular stapler positioned properly for the laparoscopic Mason procedure, and we were concerned that we had inadequate control over pouch volume. We quickly abandoned this approach for the laparoscopic wedge VBG so we could construct an accurate pouch volume and eliminate staple-line disruptions. Despite the improved technical construction, our mean percentage of excess weight loss and incidence of late reoperations are similar to those in Olbers' group, which again highlights the fact that gastric restrictive surgery is associated with poorer weight loss and a higher incidence of revision. Naslund and colleagues reported, in a series of revisions of failed open VBGs, that repair or revision back to a VBG resulted in no improvement in weight loss,[11] so we have either reversed the failed VBG or converted it into a gastric bypass. The introduction of the laparoscopic technique in either the Mason circular stapler technique or the wedge approach reduces wound morbidity but has failed to improve the efficacy of the procedure.

Complications in Laparoscopic VBG

The laparoscopic VBG has unique complications that are associated with a minimally invasive technique and also has the traditional morbidity of open gastroplasty.[12,13] The traditional complications of the open VBG are covered elsewhere.

Conversion to open surgery in experienced hands occurs principally because a large liver is obscuring visualization of the gastroesophageal junction or because instruments, including staplers, are too short to reach the angle to His and transect the pouch in patients with high BMIs or android body habitus. Of 55 patients, we have experienced one conversion to open surgery (1.8%) because of an enlarged liver in a patient weighing 423 lb. Others have reported conversions in 6 of 139 patients (4%) undergoing laparoscopic VBG, also due to enlarged left lobe of the liver.[9,10]

Trocar localization is important in the laparoscopic approach to ensure adequate camera, instrument, and stapler length to expose the upper stomach for the stapling, as the gastroesophageal junction is often positioned high under the diaphragm at the level of the fourth intercostal space in morbidly obese patients. The camera port needs to be located no more than 15 cm from the xiphoid process for the standard 33-cm laparoscope to reach the upper fundus, but can be 2 to 3 cm lower if a 60-cm lens is available. The umbilicus should not be utilized as a landmark for camera placement because in morbidly obese patients the umbilicus may be quite some distance from the xiphoid process. If the new extra-long staplers are too short to completely transect the stomach at the angle of His, an additional 2 to 3 cm can be obtained by removing the trocar and inserting the stapler directly through the abdominal wall. It may also

Table 21-2	**FIVE-YEAR OUTCOMES IN LAPAROSCOPIC VBG**				
AUTHOR	%EWL,* 2 YEARS	REDUCTION OF BMI	LATE REOPS*	OPEN CONVERSIONS	LEAKS + SD*
Olbers et al[9] n = 139	50%	41 to 32	8.0%	4.0%	2.7% SD = 2% Leaks, 0.7%
Champion n = 58	49%	46 to 34	7.3%	1.8%	1.8%

* %EWL, percent excess weight loss; reops, reoperations; SD, staple line disruption.

help to reduce the intraabdominal insufflation pressure to 8 to 10 mm to allow additional length, or to have the camera operator press inward against the camera port to compress the abdominal wall for several extra centimeters.

Intraoperative complications unique to the laparoscopic approach include staple-line bleeding, staple misfiring, uncontrolled intraabdominal bleeding, trocar injury, and abdominal wall bleeding as well as pouch misconstruction. Endoscopic staplers are mechanical devices with a definite incidence of malformed staples, misfirings, and malfunctions.[14] Laparoscopic surgeons must be prepared to deal with suture repair of stapler misfirings by performing intracorporeal oversewing of staple lines. Surgeons who are not proficient in laparoscopic suturing should not attempt this advanced procedure. A rare complication may involve the locking of a stapler in place, which requires an open conversion to dislodge the device.

Staple-line bleeding is a commonly observed intraoperative event and is controlled by hemaclips or individual sutures. To avoid delayed postoperative bleeding, the staple line must be meticulously dry at the end of the case if preoperative anticoagulants were administered for prophylaxis of deep-vein thrombosis. Electrocautery or use of ultrasonic energy sources on staple lines is discouraged, as the contribution to leaks is unknown, particularly if a two-row stapler is employed. Postoperative bleeding can occur due to intraperitoneal bleeding presenting as hypotension, or due to internal staple-line bleeding, with intraintestinal bleeding also presenting as hypotension, possibly with hematemesis or melena. Differentiation between the two causes can be difficult, and blood may not be evident in drains, even with significant hemorrhage. Persistent bleeding warrants an exploration, particularly if hypotension is present. Bleeding usually stops with induction of anesthesia, so definitive identification of the bleeding site is difficult. All the staple lines should be oversewn to ensure that there is no recurrence of bleeding, and drains should be placed. Anticoagulants should be discontinued.

Uncontrolled intraabdominal bleeding can occur secondary to (1) the perigastric dissection for the band placement; (2) the division of the short gastric vessels; (3) splenic injury; or (4) the dissection of the lesser sac from branches of the splenic vessels, which may perforate the posterior gastric wall. Control of massive unexpected bleeding can be achieved by laparoscopic compression, good suction, and waiting for 4 to 5 minutes if temporary control is achieved. Invariably, the bleeding point will slow at that point and permanent ligation can be achieved. Persistent bleeding of more than 500 ml and intraoperative hypotension are managed by conversion to open surgery. *Conversion to an open procedure is not a complication but, rather, exhibits good surgical judgment in the face of a problem.*

Trocar injuries have not occurred in our series with the utilization of an optical trocar and a 10-mm 0-degree scope inserted under direct visualization via the left rectus sheath without insufflation. This is so in spite of the fact that more than 50% of our cases had had prior open abdominal surgery. A direct open cut-down technique is difficult in the morbidly obese and is to be avoided, in my opinion. An alternative is to use a Veres technique, with insertion of the insufflation needle and initial trocar in the left upper abdomen where the abdominal wall is thinner. Trocar site

bleeding is not uncommon and must be evaluated prior to cessation of the case. We routinely inspect each trocar site for bleeding and remove each trocar under direct visualization before allowing the abdomen to deflate. Bipolar cautery is commonly required to control an abdominal wall vessel. Occasionally, a suture ligation will be necessary; a transabdominal needle passer is used.

Improper pouch construction results in failure to lose weight. Pouch misconstruction can occur with the laparoscopic technique if pouch and stoma calibration is not employed. The pure gastric-restrictive bariatric operations rely on the accurate construction of a vertically oriented pouch of less than 30 ml with a controlled outlet that is calibrated and measured. A mistake made by many surgeons is to "eyeball," or free-hand, the pouch without using a calibration technique. Laparoscopic surgery is hindered by impaired depth perception and decreased tactile sensation, which can result in inaccurate visual estimates. We calibrate the pouch by measuring with a laparoscopic ruler and calibrating with a bougie. Calibrating balloons are also useful but are more expensive than the reusable bougies. The band is externally calibrated by cutting a band 1.5×7.0 cm and overlapping 1 cm on either end to create a 5-cm diameter band to stabilize the outlet at 12 mm. A 30F bougie is placed across the outlet to prevent suturing the posterior wall with band closure. This again calibrates the stoma outlet to prevent technical errors and ensure a high-quality procedure. The final quality control of pouch construction is verification on endoscopy during surgery that the pouch is the appropriate volume, that there is no staple-line bleeding or leak, and that the stoma is patent and allows a 10-mm gastroscope to pass into the distal stomach.

We also feel it is extremely difficult to achieve accurate pouch construction by using a circular stapler. The end-to-end anastomosis anvil and "spike" are difficult to insert close to the bougie, as is required for calibration of pouch diameter. We abandoned the circular technique in 1996 for both laparoscopic VBG and Collis gastroplasty in favor of a linear stapler technique due to our concerns about pouch calibration and the additional 2-cm abdominal wall incision required to insert the circular stapler with its inherent risk of ventral herniation.[5]

A postoperative leak is the most dreaded complication in bariatric surgery, and it has been reported to occur more frequently in certain laparoscopic series.[15] A laparoscopic VBG can now be accomplished by creating an undivided or a divided pouch.[8-10] We employ a divided VBG to avoid late staple-line disruptions and weight regain, just as we do for laparoscopic gastric bypass, and we feel strongly that healing is better and there is less risk for leak if a six-row stapler is employed. We do oversew the staple line with a running 2-0 silk suture because we create a pseudoobstruction with the constricting band on the pouch. We also recommend that surgeons drain the area with a Jackson-Pratt drain until experience has been gained.

Routine intraoperative esophagogastroscopy assessment for leaks can also reduce postoperative leak rates. We identified intraoperative leaks in 4.1% of our laparoscopic bariatric procedures but have seen only three postoperative leaks (0.36%) in 985 laparoscopic bariatric surgical cases to date.[16] A routine postoperative Gastrografin series on day 1 may help to identify leaks early, but a negative result does not rule out a leak. Early recognition, repair, and drainage are key to reducing morbidity. Postoperatively, if a patient exhibits persistent tachycardia (>120) or fever or appears ill, we explore immediately to rule out a leak because the Gastrografin series has a high false-negative rate. Avoidance of pouch division does not eliminate the possibility of leaks.[9]

Other than leaks, the early complications, which may vary with the laparoscopic approach, are early non-leak-related infections, either intraabdominal or incisional. In our opinion, the incidence of intraabdominal infections can be decreased by the routine utilization of preoperative prophylactic antibiotics. We use one preoperative dose of Levaquin (500 mg) and Flagyl (500 mg) to cover gram-negative and anaerobic bacteria associated with oral flora. In addition, we add neomycin (1 g) and kanamycin (500 mg) to our irrigation fluid to reduce the risk of inadvertent bacterial infection, which can occur when using the laparoscopic approach. In a series of 63 laparoscopic gastric bypasses, we established that 23% of the patients had positive intraabdominal peritoneal cultures at the termination of the case. We have, therefore, adopted routine antibiotic lavage for all our laparoscopic bariatric procedures that involve gastric stapling.[17] We have experienced no postoperative intraabdominal or wound infections in our laparoscopic VBG cohort.

Late complications after laparoscopic VBGs are the same as those associated with the open approach, with the exception of trocar hernias.[3-5] We do not suture our 5-mm trocar sites and rarely close our 12-mm sites unless they require enlargement for specimen removal. We have seen no trocar hernias in our laparoscopic VBG group (348 trocar sites) and have had only one hernia in more than 5400 trocar sites in the laparoscopic gastric bypass. Suture closure of trocar sites adds needless expense, time, and patient discomfort to the procedure.

▶ REFLECTION

Laparoscopic VBG can be accomplished by various techniques, and it reduces the incidence of wound morbidity compared to open surgery, but it does not improve efficacy. Just as with gastric bypass or adjustable gastric banding procedures, there is no standardized technique, and significant variations exist among surgeons, making comparisons difficult. Further evidence-based studies are needed in bariatric surgery, and randomized prospective clinical trials are required to determine whether the wedge VBG technique or the Mason procedure offers a clinical advantage and whether the latest restrictive bariatric procedure, the adjustable gastric band, offers an advantage over either of the static-banded VBGs.[18]

Restrictive gastric surgery for weight loss is characterized by poorer weight loss when compared to malabsorptive procedures, and it is associated with a significant revision rate for side effects such as reflux, chronic vomiting, or technical errors.[12,13] For that reason, we feel that the VBG should have a limited role in bariatric surgery, and should not be the only technique in the surgeon's repertoire. The laparoscopic VBG does offer advantages over an open VBG and may replace it over time as surgeons gain experience with the minimally invasive technique.

▶ REFERENCES

1. Mason EE, Doherty C, Cullen JJ, et al: Vertical gastroplasty: evolution of vertical banded gastroplasty. World J Surg 1998;22:919-924.
2. Buchwald H, Buchwald JN: Evolution of operative procedures for the management of morbid obesity 1950-2000. Obes Surg 2002;12:705-717.
3. Chua TY, Mendiola RM: Laparoscopic vertical banded gastroplasty: the Milwaukee experience. Obes Surg 1995;5:77-80.
4. Lonroth H, Dalenback J, Haglind E, et al: Vertical banded gastroplasty by laparoscopic technique in the treatment of morbid obesity. Surg Laparosc Endosc 1996;6:102-107.
5. Champion JK, Hunt T, Delisle N: Laparoscopic vertical banded gastroplasty and Roux-en-Y gastric bypass in morbid obesity. Obes Surg 1999;9:123 (abstract)
6. Sugerman HJ, Starkey JV, Birkenhauer R: A randomized prospective trial of gastric bypass versus vertical banded gastroplasty for morbid obesity and their effects on sweet- versus non-sweet-eaters. Ann Surg 1987;205:613-624.
7. Huerta S, Heber D, Sawiki M, et al: Reduced length of stay by implementation of a clinical pathway for bariatric surgery in an academic health care center. Am Surg 2001;12:1128-1135.
8. Azagra JS, Goergen M, Ansay J, et al: Laparoscopic gastric reduction surgery. Surg Endosc 1999;13:555-558.
9. Olbers T, Lonroth H, Dalenback J, et al: Laparoscopic vertical banded gastroplasty: an effective long-term therapy for morbid obesity patients? Obes Surg 2001;11:726-730.
10. Champion JK: Laparoscopic vertical banded gastroplasty. In Cohen RV, Schiavon A, Schauer P (eds): Videolaparoscopic Approach to Morbid Obesity. Sao Paulo, Via Letera Medica, 2002.
11. Naslund E, Backman L, Granstrom L, et al: Seven-year results of vertical banded gastroplasty for morbid obesity. Eur J Surg 1997;163:281-286.
12. Sugerman HJ, Londrey GL, Kellum JM, et al: Weight loss with vertical banded gastroplasty and Roux-en-Y gastric bypass for morbid obesity with selective versus random assignment. Am J Surg 1989;157:93-102.
13. Balsinger BM, Poggio JL, Mai J, et al: Ten and more years after vertical banded gastroplasty as primary operation for morbid obesity. J Gastrointest Surg 2000;4:595-605.
14. Champion JK: Incidence of endostapler misfires during laparoscopic bariatric surgery. Obes Surg 2000;10:143.
15. Chae FH, McIntyre RC: Laparoscopic bariatric surgery. Surg Endosc 1999;13:547-549.
16. Champion JK, Hunt T, Delisle N: Role of routine intraoperative endoscopy in laparoscopic bariatric surgery. Surg Endosc 2000;16:1663-1665.
17. Williams M, Champion JK: Experience with routine intra-abdominal cultures during laparoscopic gastric bypass with implications for antibiotic prophylaxis. Surg Endosc 2003;17:S229.
18. Gentileschi P, Kini S, Catarci M, et al: Evidence based medicine: open and laparoscopic bariatric surgery. Surg Endosc 2002;16:736-744.

22

Open Roux-en-Y Gastric Bypass

Ward O. Griffen, Jr., M.D., Ph.D.

In 1972, I was asked by a medical colleague to interview his brother as a patient, with the possible intent of providing a surgical solution to his brother's continuing medical problem. He was 27 years old and morbidly obese. Although gainfully employed, he had suffered from hypertension for several years and recently had been found to have an elevated blood glucose level but no glycosuria. His story was typical of so many patients with morbid obesity—many diets, temporary success, but a continuing increase in weight over many years.

At that time, the jejunoileal bypass (JIB) was in its ascendancy; a gastric bypass procedure (GBP) had been described by Mason and Ito[1] in 1969 but was performed in only a few patients. I elected to do the less technically demanding JIB on my colleague's brother. He actually did very well, so I performed several more small-bowel bypasses. However, in follow-up, the patients seemed to lack energy and began to show substantial postoperative consequences, which we all have come to recognize as significant abnormalities peculiar to the JIB.

Having further studied the GBP and talked to Dr. Mason extensively about the gastric bypass, as well as to Dr. H. William Scott, an ardent proponent of the JIB,[2] I decided that a randomized trial comparing JIB to GBP was warranted. I enlisted the assistance of a psychiatrist and a registered dietitian and had many discussions with anesthesiologists and other physicians interested in obesity. Together, we developed a clinical protocol to be presented to the Institutional Review Board at the University of Kentucky Medical Center.

The protocol called for a brochure that included an artist's depiction of the two procedures and text describing them in understandable language. Two important features of the surgical approach to morbid obesity were emphasized in the brochure. First, although the JIB would not modify patients' eating behavior, it would have a profound effect on their bowel movement pattern, whereas the GBP would alter their eating habits, a form of behavior modification, if you will. And second, patients could not reach their ideal body weight without initiating and continuing an exercise program once it was possible to do so. In the brochure was also a listing of the complications of the two operations, beginning with the possibility of dying

postoperatively but also including anastomotic leak and its consequences; various infections; and problems such as diarrhea, strictures at the gastrojejunostomy, and so forth. There was also a schedule of predicted weight loss after each procedure and a list of some of the medications that were usually required postoperatively. The unexpected amelioration or resolution of certain of the more common comorbidities was described. Candidates were also told that they would be interviewed not only by the surgeon but also by a dietitian and a psychiatrist.

Once the Institution Review Board approved the protocol, we began to interview patients in groups of six to eight, and they were randomized by hospital number to either GBP or JIB. All operations were performed as open procedures. In the first seven patients undergoing gastric bypass, the operation was performed according to the method of Mason and colleagues—transecting the stomach at a high level and then anastomosing the stomach pouch to a loop of jejunum brought up behind the colon. For several reasons, this technique seemed awkward, and I reasoned that a Roux-en-Y configuration could be done safely and with more technically satisfying results. First, there are fewer parietal cells in the cardia of the stomach (the part of the stomach used for the gastric pouch), so that marginal ulceration should not pose a great threat. Second, only a single limb of jejunum would be brought up through the mesocolon, making for a more secure closure of the mesenteric defect and preventing internal hernia. Thus the retrocolic Roux-en-Y gastric bypass operation was born. It was first reported as part of the comparative study at the American Surgical Association meeting in May 1977 and published in October of that year.[3] I believe that report was instrumental in ending the use of the JIB and establishing the prominence of the GBP.

In the early days of serious bariatric surgery, the criteria for selecting candidates for a weight-reduction operation were neither entirely precise nor comparable from one study to another. All bariatric surgeons, indeed all physicians, knew how to identify a patient who was morbidly obese, but no well-defined measurement system for morbid obesity existed. Thus, my early writings indicated that being 100 lb, or 45 kg, over ideal body weight was the sufficiently elevated level at which patient and doctor were willing to accept the significant risk of a surgical operation to achieve permanent weight reduction. Today, the concept of body mass index (BMI), correlating height and weight, allows for bariatric surgery reports to be compared on a more scientifically sound basis. In retrospect, it is clear that candidates undergoing the Roux-en-Y GBP in earlier days met the BMI criteria established by the 1991 National Institutes of Health consensus conference on severe obesity.[4] All of the patients operated upon had to bring documentation of serious attempts to lose weight on one or more diet regimens. Moreover, patients with comorbidities such as hypertension, diabetes, or arthritis were strongly encouraged to have the operation.

▶ TECHNIQUE

All bariatric surgeons who perform the GBP have stressed the importance of gastric pouch size; it should be no more than 30 ml, or "as small as possible." The size of the stoma for the gastrojejunostomy has also been emphasized. It should be no greater than 1 cm. I agree with both of these features of the properly performed GBP. I often stressed what I think is the key to the continuing success of the GBP over other operations on the stomach for morbid obesity. The divergence of the food stream from the gastric pouch directly into the jejunum promotes the dumping syndrome, which often occurs when other than isotonic material is presented to the jejunum. For example, when foods with high sugar content are ingested, the unpleasant symptoms of tachycardia, sweating, feeling faint, and other symptoms occur, and the patients quickly learn to avoid such foods. Recent evidence shows that a hormone, ghrelin, which is a stimulus for eating and is elaborated by the stomach, is high before eating and decreases postprandially. Perhaps the stomach bypass eliminates this stimulant for eating, which may not occur after purely restrictive gastric operations, and that may be an additional explanation for the differences in permanent weight loss seen after different bariatric procedures.

Before the days of same-day surgery, we admitted the patient the night before the operation for preoperative blood tests and radiographs. Overnight patients received intravenous fluids containing an antibiotic, usually a cephalosporin, and 5000 U of subcutaneous heparin upon call to the operating room. If the patient had not had a previous cholecystectomy but now had any demonstrable abnormality of the gallbladder, the operative permit included cholecystectomy. Other procedures, such as ventral hernia repair, might be included in the operative permit. If the patient had symptoms of a sliding hiatal hernia, no repair of the hernia would be attempted.

I stood on the patient's right and preferred a bilateral transverse or "rooftop" incision because it seemed to give better exposure to the upper part of the abdominal cavity. Most surgeons today employ a midline incision for the open GBP. After the incision is made, the patient is placed in a reverse Trendelenburg position to permit the fatty abdominal viscera to "drag" the stomach away from the diaphragm. The short gastric vessels are identified and ligated for about 7 cm along the upper greater curvature. This serves to eliminate the angle of His and straighten out the greater curvature of the stomach so that a very small gastric pouch can be fashioned. Invariably, two or three vessels on the posterior aspect of the stomach also need to be ligated. Using the index and second fingers of the right hand, the surgeon then bluntly dissects directly on the posterior surface of the stomach and the lesser curvature, close to the esophagogastric junction, in order to make an opening between the lesser curvature and the superior branch of the left gastric vessels as well as the left vagus nerve. A Penrose drain is used to encircle the upper portion of the stomach through the opening in the lesser-curvature mesentery.

After reflecting the transverse colon superiorly, the ligament of Treitz is identified and, 15 cm distal to the ligament, the vessels in the mesentery of the jejunum are cleared and the jejunum is transected with a stapler. Oversewing the distal cut edge of the jejunum can be done at the preference of the surgeon. The right hand is then placed on the superior aspect of the transverse mesocolon and an opening is made by blunt dissection in the mesocolon, just to the left of the ligament of Treitz. The distal limb of the jejunum is then fed through that opening and brought up posterior to the stomach. Using the Penrose drain, the stomach is pulled downward while the jejunal limb is brought upward and into approximation with the uppermost portion of the previously cleared greater curvature of the stomach. A side-to-side anastomosis between the jejunum and stomach is then made to create an opening no larger than 1 cm.

I usually made the anastomosis in three layers. Four or five interrupted seromuscular sutures of 3-0 nonabsorbable material were placed as a posterior row. Then, beginning in the middle of this posterior row, a double-armed 3-0 nonabsorbable suture was placed as a continuous Lembert suture out to each corner of the posterior row. Openings were then made in the approximated stomach and jejunum and, using absorbable suture, the cut mucosal edges of the stomach and jejunum were approximated with a running suture on the posterior row. Then, the previously inserted nasogastric tube was fed into the jejunum for about 10 cm, after which an inverting Connell suture of the anterior wall of the stomach and jejunum was used to complete the inner row of the anastomosis. The middle continuous row of nonabsorbable suture was then completed, followed by several interrupted nonabsorbable Lembert sutures to finish the anastomosis. The nasogastric tube was then moved up and down to make sure that no sutures had been placed into the tube and to ensure that the stoma was no larger than 1 cm.

The Penrose drain was then removed, and a stapler was placed through the opening in the lesser-curvature mesentery to the greater-curvature side of the upper stomach, distal to the gastrojejunostomy, or from the greater-curvature side of the stomach to the opening in the lesser-curvature mesentery. The stapler was pushed as far cephalad on the stomach as feasible so as to create as small a gastric pouch as possible. I did not perform any maneuvers to measure the pouch size, as advocated by Alder and Terry,[5] for two reasons: (1) it seemed cumbersome and time-consuming; and (2) the accuracy of the measurements always seemed questionable, given the receptive relaxation capability of the stomach and the difficulty of

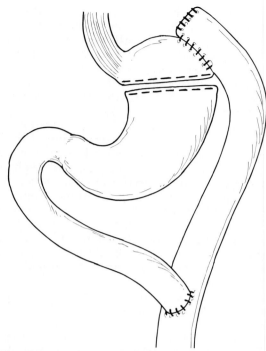

Figure 22-1. During the randomized trial, a second double row of staples was placed on the stomach parallel and distal to the previously placed row of staples. After the stapler was fired, the stomach was transected between the two staple lines.

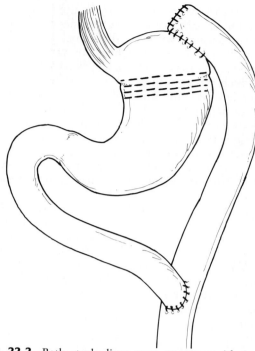

Figure 22-2. Both staple lines were oversewn with interrupted 3-0 nonabsorbable Lembert sutures. As experience with the operation and staplers grew, two double rows of staples were placed adjacent to each other, and the stomach was not transected. This became the standard for the procedure on the stomach for our version of the Roux-en-Y gastric bypass.

closing off all the fluid-escape channels. The pouch is constructed to be as small as possible. After satisfactory placement of the stapler, the stapler was fired, providing for a double row of staples (currently, four rows of staples).

During the randomized trial, a second double row of staples was placed on the stomach parallel and distal to the previously placed row of staples. After the stapler was fired, the stomach was transected between the two staple lines (Fig. 22-1). Both staple lines were then oversewn with interrupted 3-0 nonabsorbable Lembert sutures. As experience with the operation and staplers improved, two double rows of staples were placed adjacent to each other, and the stomach was not transected (Fig. 22-2). This became the standard for the procedure on the stomach in our version of the Roux-en-Y GBP.

After these surgical maneuvers on the stomach were completed, the transverse colon was reflected upward. The jejunal limb was pulled inferiorly until fairly straight. A point on that limb 45 cm from the gastrojejunostomy was identified, and an end-to-side anastomosis between the cut end of the proximal jejunum and the side of the jejunal Roux limb was accomplished. I always preferred to perform the anastomosis by hand in a typical two-layer manner, placing a posterior, seromuscular, Lembert interrupted row first and then cutting the staple line of the proximal jejunum off, making an appropriate opening in the side of the jejunal limb; thus, a running Connell absorbable suture could be used to approximate the mucosal edges circumferentially. The anastomosis was then completed with an anterior row of interrupted,

nonabsorbable Lembert sutures. Today, the standard Roux limb is made about 75 cm in length and is commonly performed before the construction of the gastrojejunostomy. The jejunojejunostomy is currently performed with a linear stapler in a side-to-side manner, with or without oversewing the staple line.

The opening in the transverse mesocolon was then closed circumferentially around the jejunal limb using interrupted nonabsorbable sutures and taking care not to injure any blood vessels in the transverse mesocolon. All portions of the bowel were inspected to make sure that they were of good color, and the incision was closed. No drains were used.

▶ COMPLICATIONS

Early Postoperative Complications

The usual complications following any abdominal surgical operation sometimes occurred, such as atelectasis, urinary tract infections, deep venous thrombosis, and others. Early in our experience, the patients were placed in the intensive care unit and remained intubated for at least 48 hours. This was done primarily at the insistence of the anesthesiologists, but as they became more familiar with taking care of these obese patients, they usually extubated the patients at the end of the procedure or in the recovery room. Soon the patients were no longer sent to the intensive care unit, but to a surgical floor for close monitoring.

Vigorous measures were taken to make the patient cough frequently and breathe deeply. The patients got out of bed the night of surgery with an abdominal binder if the panniculus was particularly weighty. The urinary catheter was removed as soon as feasible. In addition to the low-dose heparin, which was continued in the postoperative period until the patient was fully ambulating, pneumatic stockings were used during and after the operation. The latter measures were done routinely on all patients but were particularly important in patients who had a history of lower-extremity venous problems because they were considered to be at a high risk for pulmonary emboli. All of these maneuvers managed to bring the incidence of these complications to less than 3%.

On the other hand, wound infection in these patients, although occurring in only about 5% of them, was a major problem. The size of the incision and the extensive amount of subcutaneous fat made the open wound a major problem. We used absorbable sutures to close the subcutaneous space at first. After the initial wound infection and because of the supposed dead space in the wound, we started using subcutaneous suction catheters placed in the wound during the closure. The wound infection rate rose to more than 10%. Therefore, we abandoned the catheters and the subcutaneous sutures and simply let the fat fall together as it would. Thereafter, the infection rate plummeted and never rose above 5%. Often, we accomplished the operation in 50 to 100 consecutive patients without a wound problem. At the first sign of infection, the wound was opened widely and packed open. Wet-to-dry dressings were then used to avoid fascial breakdown, which led invariably to a ventral hernia. Other techniques of closure have been employed by others with equal success.

The most dreaded complication of the gastric bypass was an anastomotic leak. The leak could occur at any anastomosis or at a staple line. However, the most common site for a leak to occur was at the gastrojejunostomy. During our initial experience, we tended to wait for fairly clear evidence of a problem such as fever, pain in the abdomen or the left shoulder, and elevated white blood cell count before taking action. Upon further analysis it became obvious that the first sign of an anastomotic leak was tachycardia, particularly out of keeping with the general clinical picture. Standard procedure then became a Gastrografin swallow in any postoperative patient who exhibited a heart rate above 110 beats per minute. In the more than 1000 patients who underwent the Roux-en-Y GBP between 1974 and 1990, there were 11 anastomotic leaks, 2 of which proved fatal because of overwhelming sepsis. Most, but not all, leaks required reoperation; a small, well-contained leak demonstrated radiographically usually responded to watchful waiting. Reoperation was directed toward cleansing as thoroughly as possible any contaminated areas and providing adequate drainage without actually attempting to repair the anastomotic defect.

Late Postoperative Complications

The usual weight-loss pattern is described in the next section. However, if a patient seemed to be doing well during the first several postoperative months and then showed a marked weight gain in a short period of time, a disruption of the staple line was the most likely cause. This did not happen in our early experience, when the stomach was transected, but it did occur nine times when we used a double row of staples below the gastric pouch. When we went to two double rows of staples (four staple lines across the stomach below the gastric pouch), this particular complication virtually disappeared.

The first 3 or 4 weeks after the operation were often characterized by vomiting, usually due to the fact that the patients had not yet modified their habit of eating large quantities of food in large bites. If enough solid food is ingested quickly, the very tiny gastroenteric anastomosis becomes obstructed and the patient vomits the recently ingested material. However, if the vomiting persists, it may be due to stricture of the gastrojejunostomy anastomosis. Endoscopy should be performed, and if the anastomosis is tight, it can be dilated. A protruding stitch or other foreign body may be found and can be removed at that time.

The opposite of gastrojejunostomy stricture is enlargement which, like staple-line disruption, can lead to inadequate weight loss. In this instance the weight gain is gradual, almost insidious, but should be suspected if the patient stops losing weight after 3 or 4 months. Again, endoscopy can be performed. If a dilated anastomosis was found, we usually reoperated upon the patient to place more secure constricting sutures around the anastomosis. Our experience with reoperative gastric operations, however, even in the face of demonstrated surgically correctible situations in these patients, has not been rewarding.[6] Conversion to a distal Roux GBP may be indicated as an alternative. In the future, it is likely that a dilated anastomosis may be treated with restricting sutures placed endoscopically. I did not see pouch enlargement as a common complication of the Roux-en-Y GBP as I have described doing it. At this point, I have seen disappearance of the symptoms of gastroesophageal reflux in the patients who had it preoperatively, which is why no repair of a sliding hiatal hernia was undertaken at the initial procedure.[7]

Vitamin and mineral deficiencies are an expected consequence of any bypass procedure that removes the distal stomach and duodenum from the food stream. The distal stomach, with its rich abundance of oxyntic cells, the source of intrinsic factor, is essential for proper absorption of vitamin B_{12}. The duodenum contains the mucosa specifically designed for maximum efficiency in absorbing both calcium and iron. Therefore, GBP patients should be started on replacement therapy as soon as feasible. Adequate calcium and iron replacement can usually be accomplished by oral ingestion of those minerals, although it may take some individual adjustments to find the right combination of pills to take. Megadoses of oral vitamin B_{12} may remedy a deficiency in that vitamin, but a monthly injection of vitamin B_{12} is an alternative means of avoiding megaloblastic anemia. Folate also needs to be orally supplemented. It is best to start these medications as soon as possible, rather than wait for the deficiencies to cause symptoms. Once adequate oral intake is established, the other vitamins and minerals are ingested in food in sufficient amounts to avoid any deficiencies.

▶ RESULTS

Weight Loss

The majority of GBP patients showed a similar pattern of weight loss. During the first 3 to 6 months, the loss of excess weight ranged between 25% and 40%. Weight loss then slowed so that at 12 months, the loss of excess weight was 50% to 60%. Between 12 and 18 months, the maximum weight loss is seen in these patients, and most of them achieve BMIs of 40 kg per m² or less. Only rarely do they reach BMIs of 25 kg per m² or less. Nevertheless, the percentage of excess weight loss seen in these patients was often accompanied by amelioration of comorbidities, especially diabetes and hypertension. This improvement in diabetes and hypertension was particularly pronounced if the condition had been fairly recent in onset.

When a patient fails to exhibit this pattern or one similar to it, an explanation for the failure should be sought. As noted in the previous section, the cessation of weight loss or the gain of weight 4 to 8 months after the operation may be due to staple-line disruption or dilatation of the gastrojejunostomy stoma. These can be corrected surgically but, in our hands, doing so did not always ensure that continued weight loss would be achieved.[6] However, more puzzling and frustrating to patients and surgeons alike are the patients whose anatomic operative result seems to be satisfactory but who fail to lose weight appropriately. At first, this seemed a dilemma to me, but as others have shown, patient selection for this operation may play an enormous role in its success. For example, patients who preoperatively consume a large amount of carbohydrates, so-called sugar-eaters, may not lose weight satisfactorily after a gastric bypass.[8] Finally, any patient is capable of out-eating any bariatric operation.

Exercise Programs

As mentioned earlier, the initiation and continuance of exercise programs are important for these people who commonly have led very sedentary lives for many years. Convincing them to start exercise programs is another matter. These patients need guidance by professionals who are knowledgeable in physical exercise and motivation. Patients often cannot be depended upon to continue to exercise without monitoring and, perhaps, without some sort of reward plan. This issue introduces two important aspects of being a complete bariatric surgeon that need to be considered seriously by any surgeon contemplating entering the field.

Total Patient Care

An essential feature of being a successful bariatric surgeon is that the surgeon may become the obese patient's physician for the foreseeable future. The surgeon sometimes becomes the patient's hero and is asked questions that have little to do with obesity, comorbidities associated with obesity, the physiologic changes that have occurred as a consequence of the operation, or anything characteristically associated with postoperative surgical care. Another important aspect of bariatric surgery, and one that should be spearheaded by the bariatric surgeon, is the establishment of an obesity support group. At the beginning, the surgeon should be a very visible member of the group. There is nothing more effective than having someone who has had an operation some time ago talk to someone who has just had the same operation or to someone who is thinking about having the operation.

Long-Term Follow-Up

This chapter would be incomplete without some comments about following patients after obesity surgery. Even today, papers are being published describing patients who have had only a median or mean follow-up of 12 months. Those short-term follow-up reports are not terribly enlightening to those in the field. Further, articles that report a 70% to 75% follow-up may be helpful; however, such a 25% to 30% lost-to-follow-up rate may not make the data overly meaningful. Patients do not return for a variety of reasons, but even if only half of those who are lost to follow-up have an unsatisfactory result, that figure must be added to the reported failures. Eventually it will become imperative that articles reporting 25- to 30-year follow-up, with at least 90% patient contact, be reported in the literature.

Roux-en-Y Gastric Bypass Procedure as the Optimal Procedure

Until a nonsurgical solution to the problem of morbid obesity is found, we are still faced with having to offer morbidly obese patients a surgical option. It is clear that pure small-bowel bypassing is no longer a feasible choice. Gastric restrictive operations, while attractive because of their simplicity and their minimal physiologic change, may not induce permanent weight reduction over many years. The fact that the food stream continues in a normal fashion (e.g., esophagus to stomach to duodenum to small and large bowel) may be the very reason for the ultimate failure of these procedures. The GBP operation—channeling ingested food directly into the jejunum and thereby creating the dumping syndrome potential—may provide the optimal balance between purely restrictive and purely malabsorptive procedures.

▶ CONCERNS

At least two major concerns about the long-term effects of the Roux-en-Y GBP exist. The first and most prominent is what happens to these patients who have such an altered gastrointestinal physiologic arrangement. We already know that they show some vitamin and mineral deficiencies, which are generally correctable. Are there other adverse consequences? Will all these patients develop cholelithiasis because the normal gallbladder contractile stimulus has been bypassed? Will they eventually develop some form of liver disease similar to that seen after the JIB? What is the effect of long-term exposure of the jejunum to nonisosmotic substances? All of these questions and others can be answered only by complete follow-up over the long term.

The other major concern is whether these patients will develop some form of cancer as a consequence of the operation. In our series, we are aware of five patients who have developed malignancies—two pancreatic and three colonic—at ages earlier than would be expected. Is this just a coincidence or is it a result of the procedure? Does abnormal postprandial pancreatic stimulation lead to changes in the pancreatic parenchyma that may result in a malignancy? With this new postoperative anatomic configuration, does an excess of bile salts (a known carcinogen) enter the colon? Again, the answers will come only from long-term follow-up.

▶ REFERENCES

1. Mason EE, Ito C.: Gastric bypass in obesity. Ann Surg 1969;170: 329-339.

2. Scott HW Jr, Sandstead HH, Brill AB, et al: Experience with a new technique of intestinal bypass in the treatment of morbid obesity. Ann Surg 1971;174:560-572.

3. Griffen WO Jr, Young VL, Stevenson CG: A prospective comparison of gastric and jejunoileal bypass procedures for morbid obesity. Ann Surg 1977;186:500-509.

4. National Institutes of Health Conference, Consensus Development Conference Panel: Gastrointestinal surgery for severe obesity. Ann Intern Med 1991;115:556-561.

5. Alder RL, Terry BE: Measurement and standardization of the gastric pouch in gastric bypass. Surg Gynecol Obst 1977;144:762-768.

6. Schwartz RW, Strodel WE, Simpson WS, et al: Gastric bypass revision: lessons learned from 920 cases. Surgery 1988;104:806-812.

7. Procter CD, Bell RM, Bivins BA, et al: Gastroesophageal reflux in the morbidly obese. J Ky Med Assoc 1981;79:146-148.

8. Sugerman HJ, Starkey JV, Birkenhauer R: A randomized prospective trial of gastric bypass versus vertical banded gastroplasty for morbid obesity and their effects on sweets eaters versus non-sweets eaters. Ann Surg 1987;205:613-624.

23

Current Status of Laparoscopic Gastric Bypass

Tomasz Rogula, M.D., Stacy A. Brethauer, M.D., Paul A. Thodiyil, M.D., Samer G. Mattar, M.D., and Philip Schauer, M.D.

The laparoscopic approach to bariatric surgery emerged in the late 1990s following Wittgrove's initial description of five Roux-en-Y gastric bypasses (RYGBs) performed laparoscopically in 1994.[1] Initially, the complexity of laparoscopic RYGB (LRYBG) resulted in slow acceptance of this technique into the mainstream of bariatric surgery. In recent years, though, the number of LRYGB procedures performed has increased dramatically. The laparoscopic approach requires dedicated and intensive training to develop the necessary advanced skills, and this is achieved primarily through formal fellowship training. Extensive experience with this technique in the United States over the past 5 years has allowed us to review the safety and efficacy of the LRYGB and discuss the risks and benefits of the procedure.

▶ RATIONALE FOR SURGICAL MANAGEMENT OF OBESITY

Most surgeons and health insurance providers today perform or pay for bariatric surgery based on the report of the 1991 National Institutes of Health (NIH) Consensus Conference on Gastrointestinal Surgery for Severe Obesity.[2] That panel reviewed the long-term safety and efficacy data of medical and surgical weight loss and concluded that surgical therapy should be offered on the basis of specific criteria. This recommendation was based largely on the realization that nonsurgical weight loss, with or without behavioral modification or drug therapy, has an unacceptably high recidivism rate within 2 years. Despite the introduction of newer medical therapies for weight loss since that time, medical weight loss for the morbidly obese patient has disappointing results. According to the NIH guidelines, patients are eligible for surgery if they have failed attempts at nonsurgical weight loss and have body mass indexes (BMIs) above 35, with obesity-related comorbidities, or BMIs above 40, with or without comorbidities. Based on data available at the time, gastric

bypass and vertical banded gastroplasty were the recommended procedures.

It has been 15 years since the NIH Consensus Conference. At that time, few surgeons could conceive of performing RYGB laparoscopically. Since then, though, advances in instrumentation, techniques, and experience have allowed surgeons to perform this procedure safely, with the appropriate training. Most important, the increasing numbers of patients undergoing RYGB in the past 5 years has allowed us to carefully examine the remarkable improvements in comorbidities and quality of life that result from this operation. The 2004 American Society for Bariatric Surgery Consensus Conference report rectified the omissions and brought up to date the 1991 NIH recommendations.[3]

▶ HISTORICAL REVIEW OF BARIATRIC SURGERY

Surgery for morbid obesity was developed in the late 1950s. Initially, long segments of intestine were bypassed to produce malabsorption. The initial jejunocolic bypass caused electrolyte imbalances, intractable diarrhea, and liver failure in a large number of patients and frequently required reversal. This led to the development of the jejunoileal bypass, in which the proximal jejunum was anastomosed to the ileum, leaving a long proximal static loop. Liver failure occurred after this procedure too, particularly in patients who developed protein-calorie malnutrition, as did other problems, such as oxalate renal stones and gas-bloat syndrome.[4]

Gastric bypass was first performed by Mason in 1967 using a loop gastrojejunostomy to the gastric pouch.[5] Over the past 4 decades, this procedure has undergone many modifications to eliminate bile gastritis and reduce the rates of marginal ulcers and staple-line disruptions.[6] The Roux-en-Y divided gastric bypass is now the most commonly performed bariatric procedure in the United States, and the laparoscopic approach to this operation has rapidly gained popularity over the past 5 years.

Horizontal gastroplasty was developed to restrict food intake but frequently failed due to proximal fundal pouch dilatation, outlet dilatation, or staple-line failure.[7] In the early 1980s, Laws performed a vertical ringed gastroplasty,[8] and Mason began performing the vertical banded gastroplasty.[9] This restrictive procedure consists of a stapled proximal pouch with a small banded outlet. Although early complication rates are low and early weight loss is good, late complications of vertical banded gastroplasty have resulted in a 17% to 30% reoperation rate. These complications include gastroesophageal reflux, stomal stenosis, staple-line disruption, band migration, and intractable vomiting. Because of poor long-term weight loss and the high late-complication rate, vertical banded gastroplasty is performed successfully by only 5% of bariatric surgeons in the United States.

Gastric banding was developed in the late 1970s and initially used fixed banding material to create a proximal gastric pouch. The modern version of this procedure[10] lends itself very well to the laparoscopic approach, and the laparoscopic adjustable gastric band allows titration of gastric restriction and weight loss in balance with symptoms of dysphagia, vomiting, and reflux. The laparoscopic adjustable gastric band has been used successfully in Europe and Australia and was approved for use in the United States by the Food and Drug Administration in 2001.

Scopinaro developed the biliopancreatic diversion procedure in the late 1970s. This malabsorptive procedure involves dividing the small bowel 250 cm proximal to the ileocecal valve and anastomosing the distal limb to a 200- to 400-ml gastric pouch. An enteroenterostomy is created using a Roux-en-Y configuration to create a 50- to 100-cm common channel.[11] The biliopancreatic diversion produces the most effective and sustained weight loss of any bariatric surgery to date, but it occurs at the cost of a higher complication and mortality rate. Duodenal switch was developed to overcome the relatively high rates of marginal ulceration and dumping seen with biliopancreatic diversion.[12] In the duodenal switch, a sleeve gastrectomy is performed leaving the pylorus intact and a duodenoileostomy is constructed. This procedure is malabsorptive as well, and a 50- to 100-cm common channel is typically used.

▶ BENEFITS OF LAPAROSCOPY

The use of laparoscopic techniques for any procedure should be carefully scrutinized to determine the specific advantages (or disadvantages) of that operation. In general, though, there are some well-documented benefits of laparoscopy compared to open surgery. Several fundamental differences between open and laparoscopic surgery seem obvious. Specifically, less tissue trauma occurs in laparoscopy with less handling of and trauma to the viscera. If postoperative intraabdominal pressure is used as an indication of early postoperative tissue injury and edema, laparoscopy produces less trauma than open surgery after gastric bypass.[13] Another measure of tissue trauma is the systemic inflammatory response that follows surgery. Nguyen and colleagues evaluated the systemic stress response and inflammatory markers after open and laparoscopic gastric bypass.[14] Both groups had increased stress responses after surgery (elevated tumor necrosis factor-α, interleukin-8, dopamine, epinephrine, insulin, glucose, cortisol, and norepinephrine). However, the open group had significantly higher levels of adrenocorticotropic hormone, norepinephrine, C-reactive protein, and interleukin-6 in the first 1 to 3 days after surgery. The elevated levels of these acute-phase reactants, cytokines, and metabolic markers of stress suggest that there is less tissue injury after LRYGB than after open surgery. Other studies have demonstrated decreased C-reactive protein and interleukin-6 levels after laparoscopic cholecystectomy,[15,16] laparoscopic colectomy,[17] and laparoscopic gynecologic procedures.[18]

▶ LAPAROSCOPIC VERSUS OPEN GASTRIC BYPASS

More than 50 years of experience with open bariatric surgery has produced effective operations with acceptably low complication rates. Pulmonary compromise and wound problems continue to be important considerations after open bariatric surgery, however.[19]

Postoperative wound infections and incisional hernias occur in up to 20% of patients[18,20] after open bariatric surgery. Given the decreased postoperative pain and decreased wound-related complications in other advanced laparoscopic procedures, it was a logical step to apply this technique to gastric bypass so as to achieve the same advantages in this high-risk population of patients.

Only three randomized, controlled trials have been performed comparing open and laparoscopic gastric bypass.[13,21,22] One of these studies[22] was performed after the group had performed only 10 laparoscopic gastric bypasses (10 cases), and the learning curve was strongly reflected in their high complication rates and 3.3% mortality rate.

Abdominal-wall complications occur less commonly after LRYGB than after open RYGB. Randomized, controlled trials[13,21] comparing open to LRYGB have demonstrated a significant reduction in the number of postoperative incisional hernias with the laparoscopic approach. In a review of 3464 LRYGBs in 10 series, Podnos and colleagues reported a 3% wound infection rate (compared with 6.6% for open RYGB) and also found a significant advantage of LRYGB over the open technique for incisional hernia (0.5% vs. 8.5%).[23]

It has been well established that open abdominal surgery can lead to significant pulmonary impairment as measured by spirometry and blood gas analysis.[24] This physiologic impairment can lead to significant morbidity, particularly in patients with baseline pulmonary compromise such as the morbidly obese. One of the major advantages of laparoscopy is that it produces less postoperative pain. This reduction in pain results in better pulmonary function than is found in open surgery.

Nguyen and colleagues evaluated pulmonary function in a randomized trial of patients who had undergone laparoscopic versus open gastric bypass.[25] Analgesic requirements were also evaluated in this study, and there was significantly less pain in the laparoscopic group on the first 2 postoperative days. The LRYGB group had significantly less postoperative pulmonary impairment, and pulmonary function returned to normal sooner (7 days) in the laparoscopic group (Fig. 23-1). Similar pulmonary benefits produced by the laparoscopic approach have also been demonstrated after laparoscopic cholecystecomy[26] and laparoscopic colectomy.[27]

Other outcomes comparing open and laparoscopic gastric bypass have also been examined. Mean operative time is consistently longer for LRYGB, but length of hospital stay is typically shorter (3 vs. 4 days). LRYGB patients also return to normal daily activities and work sooner than patients undergoing open RYGB. Operative costs are higher for LRYGB, but hospital costs are lower.[13]

Weight loss at 1 year is the same for open and LRYBG. Two studies have demonstrated increased excess weight loss (EWL) at 6 months for LRYGB over open RYGB, but EWL at 1 year was similar (69% EWL for LRYGB and 62 to 65% EWL for open RYGB).[13,28] Similar weight loss for open and LRYGB has also been reported at 3 years.[21]

An anastomotic leak after RYGB can be a highly morbid or lethal complication. The anastomotic leak rate for both

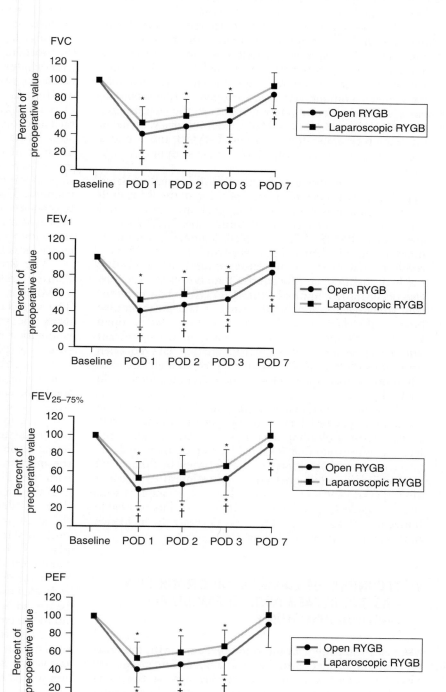

Figure 23-1. Postoperative spirometry (FVC, FEV₁, FEV₂₅₋₇₅%, and PEF) after laparoscopic and after open Roux-en-Y gastric bypass (RYGB). *$P<0.05$ compared with baseline value; + $P<0.05$ compared with laparoscopic RYGB.

FEV₁, forced expiratory volume in 1 sec; FEV₂₅₋₇₅%, forced expiratory volume at midexpiratory phase; FVC, forced vital capacity; PEF, peak expiratory flow; POD, postoperative day.

(From Nguyen NT, Lee SL, Goldman C, et al: Comparison of pulmonary function and postoperative pain after laparoscopic versus open gastric bypass: a randomized trial. J Am Coll Surg 2001;192:469-477. By permission.)

open and LRYGB is currently less than 5%. Initial reports of higher leak rates after LRYGB reflected the difficulty level of the operation, and these early series often included the surgeon's learning curve. In Podnos and colleagues' review, the anastomotic leak rate for open and LRYGB[13] were 1.7% and 2.1%, respectively.[23] In Nguyen's randomized, controlled trial, major complications occurred in 7.6% of LRYGB and 9.2% of open RYGB. There was one anastomotic leak in each group. Leak rates with the laparoscopic technique decrease with surgeons' experience, as demonstrated by Higa and colleagues' report of no leaks in their most recent 1500 LRYGB cases.[29]

The incidence of anastomotic stricture after RYGB depends on the technique used to create the gastrojejunostomy and other variables, including tension and ischemia at the anastomosis. Stricture rates are higher with the laparoscopic approach. In Nguyen's randomized study, the circular stapler technique was used for open and laparoscopic cases, and the stricture rate was higher in the laparoscopic group (11.4% vs. 2.6%, $P = 0.06$).[13] Podnos' review included different techniques for open and LRYGB and found a higher rate of stenosis with LRYGB than with open (4.7% vs. 0.7%).[23]

Early bowel obstruction after RYGB is usually related to technical factors involving the position of the Roux limb or the formation of the jejunojejunostomy. Early bowel obstruction occurs more commonly after LRYGB than after open RYGB.[23] The stapled jejunojejunostomy is more technically demanding laparoscopically, and this may result in a narrowing or angulation of the anastomosis that rarely occurs in open procedures. Late bowel obstructions also occur more commonly after LRYGB.[30] Two randomized trials have found higher rates of late postoperative bowel obstruction with LRYGB than with open RYGB.[13,21] Podnos and colleagues also found a significant differences in late bowel obstruction that favored open surgery (3.1% vs. 2.1%).[23] This may be attributed to less adhesion or inadequate closure of mesenteric defects in LRYGB.

Gastrointestinal hemorrhage from the staple lines can occur after open or LRYGB. In Nguyen's randomized trial, gastrointestinal bleeding occurred more commonly in the laparoscopic group (3.8% vs. 0%),[13] but another randomized trial showed no difference.[21] The review by Podnos did show a significantly higher rate of gastrointestinal bleeding after RYGB (1.9% vs. 0.6%).[23] The use of staplers with shorter staple heights and the addition of bioabsorbable buttress material to staple lines may decrease the incidence of this complication in LRYGB.[23]

▶ TECHNIQUE OF LAPAROSCOPIC ROUX-EN-Y GASTRIC BYPASS WITH LINEAR STAPLED GASTROJEJUNOSTOMY

We place the patient in the supine position with the arms secured on padded arm boards. The patient's legs are placed together, with the feet resting against the footboard. Padding is placed between the legs and knees, and the legs are taped together to maintain the normal anatomic position and to keep the feet placed properly on the footboard. After the patient is secured to the bed, the table is placed in steep Trendelenburg position prior to draping to ensure that the patient is safely restrained on the operating table.

Abdominal access is obtained using a 15-mm trocar or a left upper-quadrant Veress needle, and the remaining ports are placed under direct vision after needle localization and infiltration of local anesthetic. The left lobe of the liver is retracted using a 5-mm Nathanson liver retractor that is then anchored to the bed with a mechanical retractor holding system. The patient is then placed in steep reverse Trendelenburg position to allow visualization of the foregut.

After laparoscopic inspection of the peritoneal cavity, the procedure begins with formation of the Roux limb and jejunojejunostomy. The greater omentum and transverse colon are passed to the upper abdomen and the ligament of Treitz is identified. The proximal small bowel is then placed in a C configuration to aid in identifying the proximal and distal segments. The jejunum is then divided 30 to 50 cm distal to the ligament of Treitz using a 45-mm linear stapler (2.5-mm staples). Two additional firings of the 45-mm linear stapler with vascular loads (2.0-mm staples) are used to further transect the mesentery of the jejunum. This allows a sufficient length of mesentery for tension-free passage of the Roux limb to the gastric pouch. We sew a 6-cm piece of Penrose drain to the corner of the Roux limb to mark it and to facilitate passage up to the gastric pouch.

The Roux limb is then measured distally from the Penrose drain for a distance of 75 cm. In a patient with a BMI over 50 kg per m[2] we create a 150-cm Roux limb. The stretched bowel is measured in 10-cm increments using the tip of an endoscopic grasper with a 10-cm landmark. Once the appropriate length is measured, a stay suture is placed to approximate the biliopancreatic limb and the Roux limb side by side. A small enterotomy is made in both segments of bowel and a 60-mm linear staple (3.5-mm staples) is fired in the lumens to create a side-to-side anastomosis. The remaining common enterotomy is managed by placing stay sutures in the corners and the middle to stabilize the tissue while another firing of the linear stapler is used to close the defect and complete the anastomosis. Care is taken not to narrow either lumen with this final firing of the stapler. This enterotomy can also be hand-sewn or closed using the Endostitch device (Ethicon Endo-Surgery, Cincinnati, Ohio). Once this anastomosis is completed, it is inspected for kinking or obvious staple-line failures, and stabilizing sutures can be placed. If there are no problems with the anastomosis, the mesenteric defect is then closed with a running suture. To minimize tension on the Roux limb, the greater omentum is divided using ultrasound dissection so the Roux limb can be passed between the leaves of the divided omentum and up to the gastric pouch.

The gastric pouch is then created. A window is opened in the clear space of the gastrohepatic ligament with the ultrasonic shears, and a 60-mm linear stapler is fired toward the lesser curvature of the stomach. Once the lesser curvature is reached, a retrogastric space is developed to allow the passage of the jaw of the linear stapler. One horizontal firing of the stapler is started 2 cm below the gastroesophageal junction. Once this is complete, two or three vertical firings of the 60-mm linear stapler (4.8-mm staples) to the angle of His creates a 15 ml to 30 ml vertically oriented gastric pouch. The final vertical staple firing is guided by an angled instrument placed behind the staple line and exiting at the angle of His. The small gastric pouch and the gastric remnant are then gently dissected away from each other. Posterior adhesions are lysed and the pouch is freed from attachments to the left crus to provide sufficient distance between the two staple lines in an effort to minimize the chances of the development of a gastrogastric fistula.

The patient is then placed in the supine position and the Roux limb is brought up through the previously created space above the transverse colon in an antecolic, antegastric fashion. The retrocolic, antegastric or retrocolic, retrogastric placements can be used when tension on the Roux limb dictates. These techniques require more operative time and create the need to close the Petersen space, a potential site for internal hernia between the mesenteries of the Roux limb and transverse colon. Using the Endostitch, the Roux limb is sutured to the posterior wall of the gastric pouch using a running 2-0 absorbable suture. A gastrotomy and enterotomy are then made adjacent to one another to allow passage of the linear stapler and creation of the anastomosis. A 60-mm linear stapler is placed 1.5 cm into each lumen and then closed and fired (Fig. 23-2) The remaining opening is then closed in two continuous layers of absorbable suture over an endoscope. The endoscope sizes the anastomosis to 30F, allows inspection for anastomotic bleeding at the time of the procedure, and provides insufflation for leak testing. A bowel clamp is placed distal to the anastomosis and the anastomosis is submerged in irrigation fluid. The bowel is insufflated and the anastomosis is checked for leaks as evidenced by bubbling. If detected, the defect can be oversewn. A Jackson-Pratt drain is placed posterior to the anastomosis and omentum is placed over the top of the anastomosis. We close all port sites 12 mm or greater with absorbable suture using a suture-passer.

▶ **POSTOPERATIVE MANAGEMENT**

We obtain an upper gastrointestinal study on postoperative day 1 to evaluate the gastrojejunal anastomosis. If it is normal, clear liquids are initiated and advanced to a soft diet as tolerated over the following week. The average length of stay after LRYGB is 3 days. Patients are then seen in the clinic in 1 week, 1 month, 3 months, 6 months, 9 months, and 12 months, and then annually thereafter. Early postoperative visits focus on identifying any complications and addressing the major dietary changes that the patients are required to make. Later visits emphasize nutrition and the importance of compliance with supplementation and physical activity as well as the identification of late complications. Patients are placed on daily supplements of calcium, iron, vitamin B_{12}, and a multivitamin. Nutritional status is evaluated twice a year by laboratory testing. Patients who still have their gall bladders are placed on Actigall for 6 months postoperatively to reduce the incidence of gallstone formation during the rapid-weight-loss period.

▶ **OUTCOMES AFTER LAPAROSCOPIC GASTRIC BYPASS**

Weight Loss

Loss of excess weight after LRYGB is similar to that seen with the open technique and ranges from 68% to 80%.[30] In a study by Schauer and colleagues,[31] the mean EWL in 275 patients who underwent LRYGB was 83% at 1 year and 77% at 30 months. Higa and colleagues reported outcomes of 1500 consecutive LRYGBs that showed an average EWL of 69% at 1 year,[29] and similar results were reported by DeMaria and colleagues in 281 consecutive patients with 70% EWL at 1 year (72% follow-up).[32]

Weight loss after LRYGB in superobese patients (BMI >50) is generally less than in patients with BMIs less than 50 and ranges from 51% to 69% EWL.[33,34] Biertho and colleagues[35] reported 66% EWL in patients with BMIs above 50 compared to 81% EWL in patients with BMIs between 40 and 50 at 18 months. Excess weight loss was 67% at 1 year for 14 patients in this study who had BMIs above 60. Farkas and colleagues[36] reported 53% EWL in patients with BMIs above 60 at 1 year. There was a trend toward higher complication rates in this group of patients, however, compared to those in patients with BMIs above 60.

The long-term durability (>10 years) of the LRYGB has not been established, as it has been for the open technique,[37] but it is reasonable to expect similar results, given the identical anatomic changes involved in both techniques. Pories and colleagues have the longest reported follow-up for open gastric bypass, at 14 years, in which they report 49% EWL.[38]

In a prospective controlled study, the Swedish Obese Subjects study compared surgery (including gastric bypass) to nonsurgical treatment for obesity. The 10-year follow-up of 1268 patients in this study revealed a weight increase of 1.6% in the control group and a weight decrease of 16.1% in the surgery group, when compared to preoperative weight.[39]

Improvement in Comorbidities

Many obesity-related comorbidites improve or resolve after LRYGB. The major benefits of LRYGB are shown in Table 23-1.

Type 2 diabetes and glucose intolerance resolve 82% to 98% of the time after LRYGB.[32,40,41] This operation has a profound effect on glucose metabolism and diabetes control that often precedes weight loss, and the precise mechanisms involved are being investigated actively. Hypertension resolves 52% to 92% of the time[32,40,41] after LRYGB and seems to correlate with the rapid weight loss in the first year after surgery.

Hypercholesterolemia improves in 33% of patients and resolves in 63% of patients[31]; similar results are seen with hypertriglyceridemia. LRYGB is very effective in eliminating gastroesophageal reflux disease. In our study, 24% of patients had improvement in their symptoms and 72% had resolution.[31] Other studies have shown greater than 95% resolution of gastrointestinal reflux disease

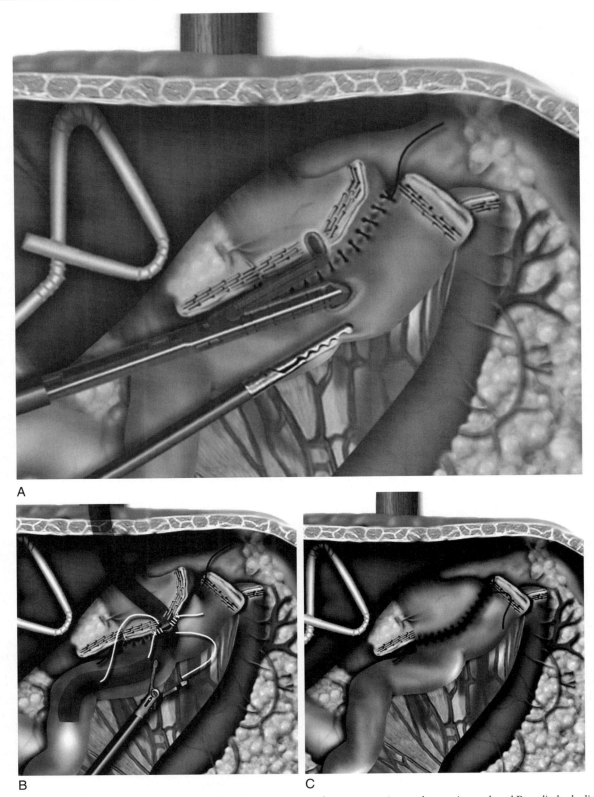

A

B   C

Figure 23-2. A, B, C. Linear stapled gastrojejunostomy. After a posterior row of suture approximates the gastric pouch and Roux limb, the linear stapler is placed into a small gastrotomy and enterotomy for a distance of 1.5 cm. The stapler is closed and fired to create the anastomosis. The anastomosis is closed in two layers over an endoscope.

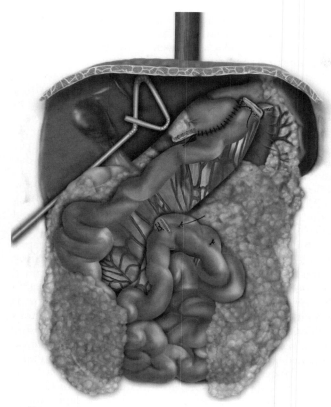

Figure 23-3. Completed laparoscopic Roux-en-Y gastric bypass.

symptoms after LRYGB.[32,40] Patients who are being evaluated for gastrointestinal reflux disease and are morbidly obese should be considered for an LRYGB to treat their reflux and induce weight loss with the same procedure.[42]

Obstructive sleep apnea resolves in 75% to 98% of patients,[40,42] and osteoarthritis improves in 47% and resolves in 41% to 76% of patients after weight loss.[31,32] Stress urinary incontinence resolves in 44% to 88% of patients, and migraine headaches improve in 29% and resolve in 57% of patients after LRYGB.[31]

Table 23-1	BENEFITS OF LAPAROSCOPIC ROUX-EN-Y GASTRIC BYPASS
Excess weight loss, %	68-80 (12-60 month follow-up)
EWL for BMI >50, %	51-66 (12-36 month follow-up)
Hospital stay	2-4 days
Resolution of comorbidities	
Diabetes, %	82-98
Hypertension, %	52-92
Hypercholesterolemia, %	63
Gastroesophageal reflux, %	72-98
Sleep apnea, %	74-100
DJD, %	41-76
Urinary incontinence, %	44-88

BMI, body mass index; DJD, degenerative joint disease; EWL, excess weight loss.

Quality of Life

Most studies evaluating quality of life after LRYGB use the SF-36 assessment, and many reports document significant improvement in quality of life after RYGB.[43] Nguyen compared quality of life after open and LRYGB and found more rapid improvements in quality of life in the laparoscopic group and that it persisted at 1 and 3 months after surgery.[13] At 6 months postoperatively, both groups had scores comparable to U.S. norms. When compared to open RYGB, hospitalization was 1 day less for LRYGB (3 vs. 4 days), and return to daily activities was 8.4 days in Nguyen's study and 9.1 days in our series of 275 patients.[13,31] This was significantly shorter than the return to daily activities after open RYGB (17.7 days in Nguyen's study). Return to work also occurs earlier after LRYGB.[13,31] The earlier improvement in quality of life leads to earlier physical activity and may account for the more rapid early weight loss in LRYGB compared to open surgery.

Mortality

The mortality rate for LRYGB in larger series (n >100) ranges from 0 to 0.9%.[32,40,44,45] This is similar to the mortality rates in the literature for open RYGB (0% to 1.5%). A metaanalysis of all bariatric procedures found an overall mortality rate of 0.5% among 5644 patients undergoing laparoscopic or open gastric bypass.[46]

Fernandez and colleagues reviewed mortality rates in open and LRYGB and found that despite a lower mortality rate in the laparoscopic group (0.7% vs. 1.9%), the access method did not independently predict death in multivariate analysis.[47] They found that preoperative weight and hypertension, postoperative leak, and pulmonary embolism were independently predictors of death for the entire series (which included 884 superobese patients), but only postoperative leak and pulmonary embolus predicted postoperative mortality in the laparoscopic group of 580 patients.

▶ MANAGEMENT OF COMPLICATIONS

Surgeons involved in the management of obese patients after LRYGB should have a very low threshold to investigate for postoperative complications. Clinical manifestations, especially those of intraabdominal septic complications, are more subtle than the signs and symptoms seen in nonobese patients. Bariatric surgeons should have a management strategy for common or serious complications, with the goal of identifying the complication early and treating it aggressively. The risks of LRYGB and the rates of some common complications are shown in Table 23-2.

Venous Thromboembolism

Morbidly obese patients are at higher risk for thromboembolism. Laparoscopic surgery, in spite of its many advantages, typically takes longer to perform than open surgery, especially early in a surgeon's laparoscopic experience. This longer operative time in the reverse Trendelenburg position, with prolonged pneumoperitoneum, increases

Table 23-2	RISKS AND COMPLICATIONS OF LAPAROSCOPIC ROUX-EN-Y GASTRIC BYPASS	
Conversion to open, %		0-8
Early postoperative complication rate (major and minor), %		4.2-30
Bleeding, %		0.4-4
Anastomotic leak, %		0-4.4
Wound infection, %		0-8.7
DVT/PE, %		0-1.3/0-1.1
Late complication rate (major and minor), %		8.1-47
Anastomotic stricture, %		2-16
Marginal ulcer, %		0.7-5.1
Bowel obstruction, %		1.1-10.5
Reoperation rate, %		0-13.8
Iron deficiency, %		6-52
Vitamin B_{12} deficiency, %		3-37
Mortality rate, %		0-2

DVT, deep vein thrombosis; PE, pulmonary embolus.

venous stasis in the lower extremities and may put the patient at higher risk for deep venous thrombosis or pulmonary embolism.[48] Prophylactic methods include low-molecular-weight heparin in combination with mechanical calf compression.[49] The incidence of pulmonary embolism after LRYGB ranges from 0 to 1.1%,[24,30] accounting for between 30% and 50% of all deaths after gastric bypass.[50,51] For patients at particularly high risk for venous thromboembolism (lower limb venous stasis, BMI >55, history of previous venous thromboembolism, and obesity hypoventilation syndrome), prophylactic placement of a vena caval filter should be considered.[52-54]

Confirming the clinical diagnosis may be difficult because most computed tomography (CT) and nuclear medicine scanners are unable to accommodate patients who weigh more than 300 lb. In this situation, it is safer to start full anticoagulation empirically, accepting an 11% risk for major hemorrhage (of which 3% will be fatal) for 5 days of intravenous heparin compared to an overall 6% risk for death and 2% risk for serious permanent disability associated with pulmonary embolism.[55] Unmonitored therapy with low-molecular-weight heparin provides an equivalent practical alternative.[56]

Intestinal Leaks

Anastomotic leaks occur 0% to 5.1% of the time after LRYGB.[13,29,30-32,35,40,44] There are several potential causes for a leak at the gastrojejunostomy, including compromising the vascular supply to the gastric pouch and creating an anastomosis under tension. Careful dissection, placement of the Roux limb in the appropriate position (retrocolic or retrogastric, if necessary) to minimize tension, and checking the anastomosis for leaks intraoperatively are fundamental maneuvers that minimize this complication. Buttressing the staple lines with absorbable material may be beneficial in reducing leak rates.

Not all leaks result in overt peritonitis and sepsis, and the majority have less obvious manifestations. Excessive abdominal pain, shoulder-tip pain, hiccups, and a sense of impending doom are ominous symptoms. Persistent tachycardia, tachypnea, or hypoxia should prompt a search for a leak, even in the absence of these symptoms or of laboratory abnormalities.

An upper gastrointestinal series performed on the first postoperative day can detect up to 33% of all leaks with a specificity of 100%,[57] and this early detection translates to less morbidity[58] and significantly shorter hospital stays.[57] Because the peak incidence of leaks (by clinical or radiologic criteria) is on postoperative day 5,[31] a negative upper gastrointestinal (UGI) study on the first postoperative day should not prevent a thorough reevaluation if the patient's clinical condition changes.[59] When an early contrast study is not performed, the average time to diagnosis for a leak at the gastrojejunostomy is 7 days, and this is associated with a 10% mortality rate.[60]

If radiologic evaluation (UGI and CT) is negative and a leak is suspected clinically, laparoscopic exploration should be performed. In the presence of a contained and adequately drained leak in a hemodynamically unstable patient, supporting nonoperative management is recommended.[31,61] Management consists of intravenous antibiotics, parenteral feeding or feeding via a gastrostomy tube placed under radiologic or laparoscopic guidance. Localized collections can be drained percutaneously under CT guidance.

In our experience with 40 leaks in 2675 consecutive LRYGBs, only 10% of leaks required a laparotomy; 30% required laparoscopic feeding access placement (i.e., a gastrostomy tube), and 60% were managed nonoperatively, with no deaths or long-term morbidity. This approach differs from the more aggressive stance advocated by others[62] who propose early operative intervention in all patients with leaks.

An uncontained leak associated with hemodynamic instability requires urgent operative intervention. It should consist of the repairing of the leak if possible, the placement of drains, and the creation of enteral feeding access. If tissue inflammation prohibits repair of the leak, irrigation and careful placement of close suction drains should be completed. If the patient is hemodynamically stable, this can be performed laparoscopically.

Gastrointestinal Hemorrhage

Upper gastrointestinal bleeding usually results from inadequate hemostasis at the gastric remnant staple line or the gastrojejunostomy. This occurs in 0.4% to 4% of LRYGBs.[13,32,35,40] The use of low-molecular-weight heparin after induction of anesthesia can predispose the staple line to bleeding. Operative intervention may be necessary in about 40% of patients, depending on the rate of blood loss and hemodynamic stability.[63] Endoscopic examination should quickly be performed to evaluate the gastrojejunostomy and pouch for bleeding. Angiographic embolization is usually unsuccessful in the highly vascular stomach, but we have used it to help control bleeding in selected cases.

Intestinal Obstruction and Internal Hernias

The rate of postoperative bowel obstruction following laparoscopic bariatric surgery ranges from 1.1%

to 10.5%.[13,23,31,32,35,40,44,45,64] The mean time to presentation is variable, with some series reporting early obstruction (within 15 weeks) after a retrocolic approach,[65] but others reporting later presentation with the antecolic approach (1 to 3 years).[66]

Unlike open bariatric procedures where adhesive obstruction is most common, intestinal obstruction after laparoscopic gastric bypass is caused primarily by nonadhesive disease. Causes of post-LRYGBP intestinal obstruction include internal hernias, formation of mesocolic constrictions, anastomotic strictures, intussusception and volvulus, or kinking of the bowel distal to the Roux limb at the site of the jejunojejunostomy.

Internal hernias constitute the most common cause of intestinal obstruction after laparoscopic bariatric surgery and may be explained by the relative lack of adhesions which, in the open situation, facilitate fixation of the Roux-limb, thus preventing its displacement and closing mesenteric defects.[67] The high proportion of adhesive obstruction (38%) in the series reported by Champion and colleagues[66] may be a reflection of the fact that 55% of their obstructed patients had previously undergone open abdominal procedures.

The most common site of obstruction in a retrocolic Roux loop is the mesocolic window, especially through the dorsal and lateral aspects of the defect.[65] Internal hernias can occur at any of the defects created during a gastric bypass procedure. These defects include the transverse mesocolic window, the jejunojejunostomy mesenteric defect, and the space between the transverse mesocolon and the mesentery of the Roux limb (the Petersen defect). Some internal hernias occur at more than one site.[67] Furthermore, rapid weight reduction following gastric bypass may result in decreased intraperitoneal fat, which may enlarge the mesenteric defect, facilitating hernia formation.[61]

Intestinal obstruction may be incomplete or intermittent. Internal hernias often present with intermittent postprandial abdominal pain, and contrast radiology may be normal in up to 20% of cases.[67] The initial investigation should be an UGI contrast study. Delay of contrast at the gastrojejunostomy is an indication for endoscopic evaluation, whereas delay of contrast in the Roux limb or dilatation of the Roux limb indicates obstruction at the mesocolic defect where a retrocolic Roux passes through it. A CT scan can assist in making the diagnosis, particularly if the obstruction is distal to the Roux limb.

Access to the gastrointestinal tract and its evaluation may be very challenging after LRYGB, and imaging is a practical starting point to assess most concerns. Helical CT assesses normal postoperative gastrointestinal anatomy and complications such as leaks, staple line dehiscence, bowel obstruction, abscess, hepatic or splenic infarction, and hernia.[68] Anatomic structures, including the gastric pouch, the excluded stomach, the entire course of the Roux limb, and the distal jejunojejunal anastomosis, are easily identified. When the fundus of the excluded stomach is filled with air or fluid, it can be misinterpreted as a loculated fluid collection.

Patients who present with intestinal obstruction after RYGB should undergo surgical exploration. Laparoscopic exploration can successfully determine the cause and treat the obstruction in the majority of these cases[45] and is our preferred approach. Operative treatment includes primarily hernia reduction and closure of any mesenteric defects. Early and aggressive management of intestinal obstruction after gastric bypass is essential to prevent closed loop obstructions or acute dilatation of the gastric remnant. Morbidity remains high, with the incidence of perforations at 9.1% and death at 1.6%.[67]

Internal hernias can be prevented by meticulous closure of all potential defects using a continuous running technique.[67] The adoption of nonabsorbable sutures resulted in a decrease of 50% in internal hernia formation.[45] Kinking of the jejunum distal to the jejunojejunostomy may be prevented by placing a single nonabsorbable stitch between the jejunum immediately distal to the anastomosis and the stapled end of the biliary limb (the Brolin stitch).[69] Antecolic placement of the Roux limb is associated with a lower risk of obstruction (0.43%) compared to the retrocolic position (4.5%).[66]

Acute Gastric Dilatation

Acute dilatation of the gastric remnant is an uncommon (0.6%) but potentially catastrophic event resulting from obstruction of the biliopancreatic limb.[70] Severe epigastric pain in conjunction with gastric dilatation on a plain abdominal radiograph or CT scan is diagnostic. Acute gastric dilatation leads to rapid clinical deterioration, with blow-out of the staple line and hemodynamic instability that may rapidly progress to cardiac arrest.[71] The treatment is urgent percutaneous gastrostomy tube decompression and subsequent management of the underlying biliary limb obstruction.[72]

Rhabdomyolysis

This is a rare complication typically affecting the super-obese male patient who lies supine during a long operative procedure. It results from a gluteal compartment syndrome resulting in myonecrosis.[73-75] It carries a 50% mortality that rises to 100% in those progressing to renal failure.[69,73] Preventive measures include adequate buttock padding and reducing the duration of the surgical procedure, especially in the superobese male. Early identification requires a high index of suspicion and serial creatinine phosphokinase (CPK) measurements. The median CPK rise in postoperative patients without this problem is 1200 IU/l (SD 450-9000), but in affected patients CPK ranges from 26,000 to 29,000 IU/l. If CPK rises above 5000, aggressive hydration and forced mannitol diuresis should be started.[73]

Gastrojejunal Anastomotic Strictures

Overall, this complication occurs in 3% to 12% of patients undergoing gastric bypass. In recent laparoscopic series, stricture rates range from 2% to 16%.[13,31,32,40,44-77] Patients can present with gastric pouch obstruction between 3 and 60 weeks after surgery,[78-80] but most strictures occur between 1 and 3 months after surgery. These lesions are believed to result from ischemia at the site of the anastomosis or from subclinical anastomotic leaks. There may be an association between anastomotic technique and stricture rate.[81] The circular stapler, particularly the 21-mm size, has demonstrated higher stricture rates than hand-sewn or linear stapled techniques.[82] Others have reported equal stricture rates with linear and circular staplers.[83] Several series have reported higher stricture rates with LRYGB than with open RYGB.[13,23]

Painless postprandial regurgitation is the principal presenting symptom and should lead to an UGI contrast study. The diagnosis is confirmed by the inability to pass a 9-mm endoscope through the anastomosis.[80]

Treatment consists of endoscopic balloon dilation (13 to 18 mm) of the anastomosis.[80,82,84,85] An average of two separate procedures relieves the obstruction in 95% of cases of strictures presenting early,[78] but restenosis occurs in 3% of these patients.[80] Strictures presenting after 3 months are still amenable to endoscopic dilation, but up to a third of these patients may require operative revision.[85] Fluoroscopy-guided dilation is an alternative treatment, achieving sustained patency in 71% of patients after one dilation.[86]

Marginal Ulcers

Ulcers at the site of the gastrojejunal anastomosis complicate between 1% and 16% of isolated gastric bypasses,[87,88] with the highest risk occurring in the first 2 months after surgery.[79] This complication may develop as late as 10 years after surgery.[79] Its cause is multifactorial, and it has been associated with the use of nonabsorbable suture material,[89] gastric pouch size larger than 50 ml,[90,91] nonsteroidal antiinflammatory drugs, and *Helicobacter pylori*. Patients who were preoperatively screened and treated for *H. pylori* had a significantly lower incidence of marginal ulcers at 3 years (2.4%) compared to those who were not screened for *H. pylori*.[92] Alcohol and smoking have also been causally implicated in patients with marginal ulcers.[93]

Pouch ulceration heals with proton pump inhibitors, sucralfate, or both, along with cessation of nonsteroidal antiinflammatory drug intake and smoking. In a patient with a large pouch, ulcer recurrence with medical therapy alone is common, and in such cases consideration should be given to reduction of the pouch size along with excision of the ulcer.[87,90] Recurrent ulceration associated with foreign bodies (including sutures) requires removal of the foreign bodies.

Incisional Hernias

One of the main advantages of laparoscopic gastric bypass is the decreased incidence of incisional hernias (0.7%).[31] In open gastric bypass, the rate of this complication has ranged from 15% to 20%.[20,40] A 10-mm port site can present with a Richter type of hernia.[94] A port site hernia following the laparoscopic approach has a small defect that renders it prone to intestinal strangulation. Herniations at the trocar sites are best-demonstrated radiologically, using anterior abdominal wall ultrasound or CT scan. Prevention includes closing the fascia of 10-mm and 12-mm port sites using nonabsorbable sutures.[94] Once recognized, this complication should be managed urgently with laparoscopic reduction and suture repair of the hernia defect, using a nonabsorbable material.

Metabolic Bone Disease

Metabolic consequences of LRYGB may include increased bone turnover.[95] Markers of bone turnover were significantly elevated in patients after LRYGB compared with controls. Bone-mineral density also decreased significantly. Within 3 to 9 months after LRYGB, morbidly obese patients have an increase in bone resorption associated with a decrease in bone mass.

This is an insidious long-term complication of gastric bypass that arises from calcium or vitamin D malabsorption or both.[96,97] Loss of bone mass, resulting from osteoporosis or osteomalacia, is preceded by secondary hyperparathyroidism and is asymptomatic until complicated by pathologic fractures. Elevation in serum immunoreactive parathyroid hormone associated with low or normal calcium levels is the earliest indicator of this condition and should prompt dietary supplementation with calcium and vitamin D and close monitoring of lumbar spine and femoral neck bone mineral density.[98]

Nutritional Deficiencies

Deficiency of iron, folate, and vitamin B_{12} are common postoperatively and contribute to the development of anemia found in up to 54% of patients.[99,100] Iron-deficiency anemia occurs in up to 22% of men and 51% of women,[99] with a higher proportion in menstruating women.[52] The routine administration of micronutrient supplementation following gastric bypass is recommended.

Long-limb gastric bypass with a 50-cm common channel results in protein-calorie malnutrition in 28.5% of patients.[101] Low serum levels of albumin and phosphate indicate depletion in total body proteins. Excessive malabsorption may be reversed by conversion to a 150- to 200-cm common channel. It is important to pay attention to thiamine replacement and to avoid the refeeding syndrome.[102-104]

Cholelithiasis

Routine cholecystectomy concomitant with a LRYGB remains controversial.[105,106] Weight loss following LRYGB is accompanied by a rise in the incidence of gallstones, with 38% to 52.8% of patients in certain series developing stones in the 12 months after surgery.[107,108] Between 15% and 27% of all patients, irrespective of gallstone status at LRYGB surgery, require urgent cholecystectomy within 3 years.[107,109]

▶ INADEQUATE WEIGHT LOSS

When considering contraindications to the combined procedure, it should be noted that it nearly doubles length of hospital stay and adds about 50 minutes to the operation.[110,111] The prophylactic use of oral ursodiol at 600 mg daily for the first 6 months after LRYGB significantly reduces the incidence of gallstones (2% vs. 32% in placebo, $P<0.01$).[112]

Failure of weight loss after LRYGB occurs in 5% to 10% of patients. It is thought to arise from a progressive dilatation of the pouch outlet and the pouch itself and is probably related to poor eating habits.[35,88,113] Patients can also defeat the restrictive component of the operation by consuming sweets or other high-calorie foods despite feeling full. This can be a difficult problem with no satisfactory solution. The best results are achieved by frequent patient supervision and close cooperation with the nutritionist, the psychologist, and support groups. The value of reducing the pouch or stoma size, either operatively or endoscopically, remains unproven despite some reports to the contrary.[35,114] Conversion to a long-limb gastric bypass is an option.

▶ CONCLUSION

We have reviewed the current knowledge with respect to LRYGB. We have provided a detailed description of how to perform the procedure utilizing a linear stapled gastrojejunostomy. LRYGB has become the most popular bariatric procedure in the United States, and its influence is spreading in the rest of the world.

▶ REFERENCES

1. Wittgrove AC, Clark GW, Tremblay LJ: Laparoscopic gastric bypass, Roux-en-Y: preliminary report of five cases. Obes Surg 1994;4:353-357.
2. Consensus Development Conference Panel, National Institutes of Health: Gastrointestinal surgery for severe obesity: Ann Intern Med 1991;115:956-961.
3. Buchwald H, for the Consensus Development Conference Panel, National Institutes of Health: Bariatric surgery for morbid obesity: health implications for patients, health professionals, and third-party payers. J Am Coll Surg 2005;200:593-604.
4. Buchwald H, Rucker RD: The rise and fall of jejunoileal bypass. In Nelson RL, Nyhus LM (eds): Surgery of the Small Intestine, pp. 529-541. Norwalk, Conn., Appleton Century Crofts, 1987.
5. Mason EE, Ito C: Gastric bypass. Ann Surg 1969;170:329-339.
6. Griffen WO, Young VL, Stevenson CC: A prospective comparison of gastric and jejunoileal bypass operation for morbid obesity. Ann Surg 1977;186:500-507.
7. Printen KJ, Mason EE: Gastric surgery for relief of morbid obesity. Arch Surg 1973;106:428-431.
8. Laws HL, Piatadosi S: Superior gastric reduction procedure for morbid obesity: a prospective, randomized trial. Am J Surg 1981;193:334-336.
9. Mason EE: Vertical banded gastroplasty. Arch Surg 1982; 117: 701-706.
10. Kuzmak LI: Silicone gastric banding: a simple and effective operation for morbid obesity. Contemp Surg 1986;28:13-18.
11. Scopinaro N, Gianetta E, Civalleri D: Biliopancreatic bypass for obesity: II. Initial experiences in man. Br J Surg 1979;66:618-620.
12. Hess DW, Hess DS: Biliopancreatic diversion with a duodenal switch. Obes Surg 1998;8:267-282.
13. Nguyen NT, Goldman C, Rosenquist CJ, et al: Laparoscopic versus open gastric bypass: a randomized study of outcomes, quality of life, and costs. Ann Surg 2001;234:279-291.
14. Nguyen NT, Goldman CD, Ho HS, et al: Systemic stress response after laparoscopic and open gastric bypass. J Am Coll Surg 2002;194:557-567.
15. Karayiannakis AJ, Makri GG, Mantzioka A, et al: Systemic stress response after laparoscopic or open cholecystectomy: a randomized trial. Br J Surg 1997;84:467-471.
16. Bruce DM, Smith M, Walker CB, et al: Minimal access surgery for cholelithiasis induces an attenuated acute phase response. Am J Surg 1999;178:232-234.
17. Leung KL, Lai PB, Ho RL, et al: Systemic cytokine response after laparoscopic-assisted resection of rectosigmoid carcinoma: a prospective randomized trial. Ann Surg 2000;231:506-511.
18. Malik E, Buchweitz O, Muller-Steinhardt M, et al: Prospective evaluation of the systemic immune response following abdominal, vaginal, and laparoscopically assisted vaginal hysterectomy. Surg Endosc 2001;15:463-466.
19. Christou NV, Jarand J, Sylvestre JL, et al: Analysis of the incidence and risk factors for wound infections in open bariatric surgery. Obes Surg 2004;14:16-22.
20. Sugerman HJ, Kellum JM Jr, Reines HD, et al: Greater risk of incisional hernia with morbidly obese than steroid-dependent patients and low recurrence with prefascial polypropylene mesh. Am J Surg 1996;171:80-84.
21. Lujan JA, Frutos MD, Hernandez Q, et al: Laparoscopic versus open gastric bypass in the treatment of morbid obesity: a randomized prospective study. Ann Surg 2004;239:433-437.
22. Westling A, Gustavsson S: Laparoscopic vs open Roux-en-Y gastric bypass: a prospective, randomized trial. Obes Surg 2001;11:284-292.
23. Podnos YD, Jimenez JC, Wilson SE, et al: Complications after laparoscopic gastric bypass: a review of 3464 cases. Arch Surg 2003;138:957-961.
24. Latimer RG, Dickman M, Day WC, et al: Ventilatory patterns and pulmonary complications after upper abdominal surgery determined by preoperative and postoperative computerized spirometry and blood gas analysis. Am J Surg 1971;122:622-632.
25. Nguyen NT, Lee SL, Goldman C, et al: Comparison of pulmonary function and postoperative pain after laparoscopic versus open gastric bypass: a randomized trial. J Am Coll Surg 2001;192:469-477.
26. Schauer PR, Luna J, Ghiatas AA, et al: Pulmonary function after laparoscopic cholecystectomy. Surgery 1993;114:389-399.
27. Schwenk W, Bohm B, Witt C, et al: Pulmonary function following laparoscopic or conventional colorectal resection: a randomized controlled evaluation. Arch Surg 1999;134:6-13.
28. Courcoulas A, Perry Y, Buenaventura P, et al: Comparing the outcomes after laparoscopic versus open gastric bypass: a matched paired analysis. Obes Surg 2003;13:341-346.
29. Higa KD, T Ho, KB Boone: Laparoscopic Roux-en-Y gastric bypass: technique and 3-year follow-up. J Laparoendosc Adv Surg Tech A 2001;11:377-382.
30. Schneider BE, Villegas L, Blackburn GL, et al: Laparoscopic gastric bypass surgery: outcomes. J Laparoendosc Adv Surg Tech A 2003; 13:247-255.
31. Schauer PR, Ikramuddin S, Gourash W, et al: Outcomes after laparoscopic Roux-en-Y gastric bypass for morbid obesity. Ann Surg 2000;232:515-529.
32. DeMaria EJ, Sugerman HJ, Kellum JM, et al: Results of 281 consecutive total laparoscopic Roux-en-Y gastric bypasses to treat morbid obesity. Ann Surg 2002;235:640-647.
33. Oliak D, Ballantyne GH, Davies RJ, et al: Short-term results of laparoscopic gastric bypass in patients with BMI > or = 60. Obes Surg 2002;12:643-647.
34. Parikh, MS, Shen R, Weiner M, et al: Laparoscopic bariatric surgery in super-obese patients (BMI>50) is safe and effective: a review of 332 patients. Obes Surg 2005;15:858-863.
35. Biertho L, Steffen R, Ricklin T, et al: Laparoscopic gastric bypass versus laparoscopic adjustable gastric banding: a comparative study of 1,200 cases. J Am Coll Surg 2003;197:536-545.
36. Farkas DT, Vemulapalli P, Haider A, et al: Laparoscopic Roux-en-Y gastric bypass is safe and effective in patients with a BMI > or =60. Obes Surg 2005;15:486-493.
37. White S, Brooks E, Jurikova L, et al: Long-term outcomes after gastric bypass. Obes Surg 2005;15:155-163.
38. Pories WJ, Swanson MS, MacDonald KG, et al: Who would have thought it? An operation proves to be the most effective therapy for adult-onset diabetes mellitus. Ann Surg 1995; 222:339-352.
39. Sjostrom L, Lindroos AK, Peltonen M, et al: Lifestyle, diabetes, and cardiovascular risk factors 10 years after bariatric surgery. N Engl J Med 2004;351:2683-2693.
40. Wittgrove AC, Clark GW: Laparoscopic gastric bypass, Roux-en-Y: 500 patients: technique and results, with 3-60 month follow-up. Obes Surg 2000;10:233-239.
41. Schauer PR, Burguera B, Ikramuddin S, et al: Effect of laparoscopic Roux-en Y gastric bypass on type 2 diabetes mellitus. Ann Surg 2003;238:467-485.

42. Schauer PG, Hamad G, Ikramuddin S: Surgical management of gastroesophageal reflux disease in obese patients. Semin Laparosc Surg 2001;8:256-264.

43. Livingston EH, Fink AS: Quality of life: cost and future of bariatric surgery. Arch Surg 2003;138:383-388.

44. Papasavas PK, Hayetian FD, Cuashaj PF, et al: Outcome analysis of laparoscopic Roux-en-Y gastric bypass for morbid obesity: the first 116 cases. Surg Endosc 2002;16:1653-1657.

45. Higa KD, Boone KB, Ho T: Complications of the laparoscopic Roux-en-Y gastric bypass: 1,040 patients—what have we learned? Obes Surg 2000;10:509-513.

46. Buchwald H, Avidor Y, Braunwald E, et al: Bariatric surgery: a systematic review and meta-analysis. JAMA 2004;292:1724-1737.

47. Fernandez AZ Jr, Demaria EJ, Tichansky DS, et al: Multivariate analysis of risk factors for death following gastric bypass for treatment of morbid obesity. Ann Surg 2004;239:698-703.

48. Nguyen NT, Cronan M, Braley S, et al: Duplex ultrasound assessment of femoral venous flow during laparoscopic and open gastric bypass. Surg Endosc 2003;17:285-290.

49. Wu EC, Barba CA: Current practices in the prophylaxis of venous thromboembolism in bariatric surgery. Obes Surg 2000;10:7-14.

50. Melinek J, Livingston E, Cortina G, et al: Autopsy findings following gastric bypass surgery for morbid obesity. Arch Pathol Lab Med 2002;126:1091-1095.

51. Bajardi G, Ricevuto G, Mastrandrea G, et al: Postoperative venous thromboembolism in bariatric surgery. Minerva Chir 1993;48:539-542 (in Italian).

52. Sugerman HJ, Sugerman EL, Wolfe L, et al: Risks and benefits of gastric bypass in morbidly obese patients with severe venous stasis disease. Ann Surg 2001;234:41-46.

53. Sapala JA, Wood MH, Schuhknecht MP, et al: Fatal pulmonary embolism after bariatric procedures for morbid obesity: a 24-year retrospective analysis. Obes Surg 2004;15:819-825.

54. Baumann D: IVC filter placement in bariatric patients. Endovasc Today 2005;54-63.

55. Kearon C, Hirsh J: Management of anticoagulation before and after elective surgery. N Engl J Med 1997;336:1506-1511.

56. The Columbus Investigators: Low-molecular-weight heparin in the treatment of patients with venous thromboembolism. N Engl J Med 1997;337:657-662.

57. Sims TL, Mullican MA, Hamilton EC, et al: Routine upper gastrointestinal Gastrografin swallow after laparoscopic Roux-en-Y gastric bypass. Obes Surg 2003;13:66-72.

58. Ovnat A, Peiser J, Solomon H, et al: Early detection and treatment of a leaking gastrojejunostomy following gastric bypass. Isr J Med Sci 1986;22:556-558.

59. Hamilton EC, Sims TL, Hamilton TT, et al: Clinical predictors of leak after laparoscopic Roux-en-Y gastric bypass for morbid obesity. Surg Endosc 2003;17:679-684.

60. Marshall JS, Srivastava A, Gupta SK, et al: Roux-en-Y gastric bypass leak complications. Arch Surg 2003:138:520-524.

61. Blachar A, Federle MP, Pealer KM, et al: Gastrointestinal complications of laparoscopic Roux-en-Y gastric bypass surgery: clinical and imaging findings. Radiology 2002;223:625-632.

62. Arteaga JR, Huerta S, Livingston EH: Management of gastrojejunal anastomotic leaks after Roux-en-Y gastric bypass. Am Surg 2002;68:1061-1065.

63. Nguyen NT, Rivers R, Wolfe BM: Early gastrointestinal hemorrhage after laparoscopic gastric bypass. Obes Surg 2003;13:62-65.

64. Higa KD, Boone KB, Ho T, et al: Laparoscopic Roux-en-Y gastric bypass for morbid obesity: technique and preliminary results of our first 400 patients. Arch Surg 2000;135:1029-1034.

65. Filip JE, Mattar SC, Bowers SP, Smith CD: Internal hernia formation after laparoscopic Roux-en-Y gastric bypass for morbid obesity. Am Surg 2002;68:640-643.

66. Champion JK, Williams M: Small bowel obstruction and internal hernias after laparoscopic Roux-en-Y gastric bypass. Obes Surg 2003;13:596-600.

67. Higa KD, Ho T, Boone KB: Internal hernias after laparoscopic Roux-en-Y gastric bypass: incidence, treatment and prevention. Obes Surg 2003;13:350-354.

68. Yu J, Turner MA, Cho SR, et al: Normal anatomy and complications after gastric bypass surgery: helical CT findings. Radiology 2004;231:753-760.

69. Brolin RE: The antiobstruction stitch in stapled Roux-en-Y enteroenterostomy. Am J Surg 1995;169:355-357.

70. Jones KB: Biliopancreatic limb obstruction in gastric bypass at or proximal to the jejunojejunostomy: a potentially deadly, catastrophic event. Obes Surg 1996;6:485-493.

71. Olbers T, Lonroth H, Fagevik-Olsen M, et al: Laparoscopic gastric bypass: development of technique, respiratory function, and long-term outcome. Obes Surg 2003;13:364-370.

72. Maingot R, Zinner M: Maingot's Abdominal Operations, ed 10. Stamford, Conn., Appleton & Lange, 1997.

73. Bostanjian D, Anthone GJ, Hamoui N, et al: Rhabdomyolysis of gluteal muscles leading to renal failure: a potentially fatal complication of surgery in the morbidly obese. Obes Surg 2003;13:302-305.

74. Wiltshire JP, Custer T: Lumbar muscle rhabdomyolysis as a cause of acute renal failure after Roux-en-Y gastric bypass. Obes Surg 2003;13:306-313.

75. Torres-Villalobos G, Kimura E, Mosqueda JL, et al: Pressure-induced rhabdomyolysis after bariatric surgery. Obes Surg 2003;13:297-301.

76. Nguyen T, Ho HS, Palmer LS, et al: A comparison study of laparoscopic versus open gastric bypass for morbid obesity. J Am Coll Surg 2000;191:149-157.

77. Nguyen NT, Stevens C, Wolfe BM: Incidence and outcome of anastomotic stricture after laparoscopic gastric bypass. J Gastrointest Surg 2003;7:997-1003.

78. Go MR, Muscaralla P 2nd, Needleman BJ, et al: Endoscopic management of stomal stenosis after Roux-en-Y gastric bypass. Surg Endosc 2003;18:56-59.

79. Sanyal AJ, Sugerman HJ, Kellum JM, et al: Stomal complications of gastric bypass: incidence and outcome of therapy. Am J Gastroenterol 1992;87:1165-1169.

80. Ahmad J, Martin J, Ikramuddin S, et al: Endoscopic balloon dilation of gastroenteric anastomotic stricture after laparoscopic gastric bypass. Endoscopy 2003;35:725-728.

81. Abdel-Galil E, Sabry AA: Laparoscopic Roux-en-Y gastric bypass: evaluation of three different techniques. Obes Surg 2002; 2:639-642.

82. Gonzalez R, Lin E, Venkatesh KR, et al: Gastrojejunostomy during laparoscopic gastric bypass: analysis of 3 techniques. Arch Surg 2003;138:181-184.

83. Shope TR, Cooney RN, McLeod J, et al: Early results after laparoscopic gastric bypass: EEA vs GIA stapled gastrojejunal anastomosis. Obes Surg 2003;13:355-359.

84. Barba CA, Butensky MS, Lorenzo M, et al: Endoscopic dilation of gastroesophageal anastomosis stricture after gastric bypass. Surg Endosc 2003;17:416-420.

85. Sataloff DM, Lieber CP, Seinige UL: Strictures following gastric stapling for morbid obesity: results of endoscopic dilation. Am Surg 1990;56:167-174.

86. Holt PD, de Lange EE, Shaffer Jr HA: Strictures after gastric surgery: treatment with fluoroscopically guided balloon dilation. AJR Am J Roentgenol 1995;164:895-899.

87. Sapala JA, Wood MH, Sapala MA, et al: Marginal ulcer after gastric bypass: a prospective 3-year study of 173 patients. Obes Surg 1998;8:505-516.

88. Christou NV, Sampalis JS, Liberman M, et al: Surgery decreases long-term mortality, morbidity, and health care use in morbidly obese patients. Ann Surg 2004;240:416-424.

89. Capella JF, Capella RF: Gastro-gastric fistulas and marginal ulcers in gastric bypass procedures for weight reduction. Obes Surg 1999;9:22-28.

90. Printen KJ, Scott D, Mason EE: Stomal ulcers after gastric bypass. Arch Surg 1980;115:525-527.

91. Jordan JH, Hocking MP, Rout WR, et al: Marginal ulcer following gastric bypass for morbid obesity. Am Surg 1991;57:286-288.

92. Schirmer B, Erenoglu C, Miller A: Flexible endoscopy in the management of patients undergoing Roux-en-Y gastric bypass. Obes Surg 2002;12:634-638.

93. Scopinaro N, Gianetta E, Adami GF, et al: Biliopancreatic diversion for obesity at eighteen years. Surgery 1996;119:261-268.

94. Matthews BD, Heniford BT, Sing RF: Preperitoneal Richter hernia after a laparoscopic gastric bypass. Surg Laparosc Endosc Percutan Tech 2001;11:47-49.

95. Coates P, Fernstrom JD, Fernstrom MH, et al: Gastric bypass surgery for morbid obesity leads to an increase in bone turnover and a decrease in bone mass. J Clin Endocrinol Metab 2004;89:1061-1065.

96. Goldner WS, O'Dorisio TM, Dillon JS, et al: Severe metabolic bone disease as a long-term complication of obesity surgery. Obes Surg 2002;12:685-692.

97. Ott MT, Fanti P, Malluche HH, et al: Biochemical evidence of metabolic bone disease in women following Roux-en-Y gastric bypass for morbid obesity. Obes Surg 1992;2:341-348.

98. Shaker JL, Norton AJ, Woods MF, et al: Secondary hyperparathyroidism and osteopenia in women following gastric exclusion surgery for obesity. Osteoporos Int 1991;1:177-181.

99. Brolin RE, Gorman JH, Gorman RC, et al: Are vitamin B_{12} and folate deficiency clinically important after Roux-en-Y gastric bypass? J Gastrointest Surg 1998;2:436-442.

100. Bloomberg RD, Fleishman A, Nalle JE, et al: Nutritional deficiencies following bariatric surgery: what have we learned? Obes Surg 2005;15:145-154.

101. Sugerman HJ, Kellum JM, DeMaria EJ: Conversion of proximal to distal gastric bypass for failed gastric bypass for superobesity. J Gastrointest Surg1997;1:517-525.

102. DeMaria EJ, Schauer P, Patterson E, et al: The optimal surgical management of the super-obese patient: the debate. Surg Innov 2005;12:107-121.

103. Mason EE: Starvation injury after gastric reduction for obesity. World J Surg 1998;22:1002-1007.

104. Terlevich A, Hearing SD, Woltersdorf WW, et al: Refeeding syndrome: effective and safe treatment with phosphates polyfusor. Aliment Pharmacol Ther 2003;17:1325-1329.

105. Mason EE, Renquist KE: Gallbladder management in obesity surgery. Obes Surg 2002;12:222-229.

106. Fobi M, Lee H, Igwe D, et al: Prophylactic cholecystectomy with gastric bypass operation: incidence of gallbladder disease. Obes Surg 2002;12:350-353.

107. Shiffman ML, Sugerman HJ, Kellum JM, et al: Changes in gallbladder bile composition following gallstone formation and weight reduction. Gastroenterology 1992:103:214-221.

108. Iglezias Brandao de Oliveira C, Adami Chaim E, Borges da Silva B: Impact of rapid weight reduction on risk of cholelithiasis after bariatric surgery. Obes Surg 2003;13:625-628.

109. Amaral JF, ThompsonWR: Gallbladder disease in the morbidly obese. Am J Surg 1985;149:551-557.

110. Hamad GG, Ikramuddin S, Gourash WF, et al: Elective cholecystectomy during laparoscopic Roux-en-Y gastric bypass: is it worth the wait? Obes Surg 2003;13:76-81.

111. Papavramidis S, Deligianidis N, Papavramidis T, et al: Laparoscopic cholecystectomy after bariatric surgery. Surg Endosc 2003;17:1061-1064.

112. Sugerman HJ, Brewer WH, Shiffman ML, et al: A multicenter, placebo-controlled, randomized, double-blind, prospective trial of prophylactic ursodiol for the prevention of gallstone formation following gastric-bypass-induced rapid weight loss. Am J Surg 1995;169:91-97.

113. Holzwarth R, Huber D, Majkrzak A, et al: Outcome of gastric bypass patients. Obes Surg 2002;12:261-264.

114. Spaulding L: Treatment of dilated gastrojejunostomy with sclerotherapy. Obes Surg 2003;13:254-257.

24

Laparoscopic Roux-en-Y Gastric Bypass: The Linear Technique

Sayeed Ikramuddin, M.D.

Obesity surgery has become widespread over the past decade. The reasons for this probably are related to the increase in public awareness of the disease of morbid obesity and also to the patient-driven demand for minimally invasive approaches to bariatric surgery. According to Steinbrook approximately 140,000 procedures were performed in 2004.[1] Although not suitable for all patients, particularly those with multiple previous abdominal operations, the laparoscopic Roux-en-Y gastric bypass has gained tremendous popularity.

The first recorded case was performed by Wittgrove and colleagues in 1994. They reported a circular-stapled gastrojejunostomy with a retrogastric, retrocolic Roux-en-Y gastric bypass.[2] There are other approaches to this operation, including a linear-stapled technique for the gastrojejunal anastomosis with the Roux limb passed either retrocolically or antecolically.[3] There is also an approach in which the Roux limb can be passed retrocolically and then placed antegastrically over the gastric remnant and then sutured to the gastric pouch. A totally hand-sewn procedure has also been described.[4]

The wide availability of suturing devices, as well as robot technology, makes the linear technique or hand-sewn technique palatable. Regardless of the technique, it is important that surgeons master one approach to the operation and be at least as familiar with other techniques, should technical complications during surgery warrant them. A fundamental knowledge of intracorporeal suturing is necessary in order to perform safe, reliable bariatric surgery.

▶ TECHNIQUE

We perform a laparoscopic Roux-en-Y bypass with an antecolic, antegastric Roux limb with a linear-stapled gastrojejunostomy, the enterotomy of which is oversewn in two layers over a 30F stent, typically a 30F endoscope. We use a stapled jejunojejunostomy that is performed at variable distances for the Roux limb and biliopancreatic limb,

based on the patient's body mass index and comorbid conditions.

Our procedure is as follows. We use a six-port technique. The surgeon stands on the right. We begin with a Veress needle in the left upper quadrant. After instilling a mixture of ½% Marcaine and lidocaine, we place a 150-mm Veress needle (AutoSuture, Norwalk, Conn.) into the left upper quadrant. (We avoid this approach in a patient who has had left upper quadrant surgery or large ventral hernia repair with mesh or a history of a bowel obstruction.) We insufflate the abdomen to a maximum pressure of approximately 5 mmHg. We insert a 5-mm nonbladed trocar (Ethicon Endo-Surgery, Cincinnati, Ohio) into this area 15 to 20 cm below the xiphoid. We then place an 11-mm nonbladed trocar to reduce the rate of herniation.

The patient is then placed into a steep reverse Trendelenburg position. Another left lateral 5-mm port is placed just inferiorly and just subcostal on the left side, more lateral to the first trocar site. Two ports are then placed for the surgeon, one below the right subcostal margin, and another just paramedian, roughly at the same level as that placed for the camera port. The two working ports are 5 mm and 12 mm, respectively. One 5-mm lateral port is placed for the liver retractor. We use an angulating triangular liver retractor (Genzyme, Cambridge, Mass.) held in place with a side clamp to the table. Figure 24-1 shows the port sites.

After retracting the left lateral segment of the liver, we begin the procedure by incising the hepatogastric ligament with the Harmonic Scalpel (Ethicon Endo-Surgery, Cincinnati, Ohio). Adhesions at the angle of His are taken down sharply with scissors. We use a 45-degree endoscope to perform the procedure because it allows great ease in navigating around complex angles. The lesser sac is entered using the Harmonic Scalpel. In most cases, the lesser sac is free of adhesions, but in a patient who has a history of pancreatitis or gall bladder disease, there tend to be some significant adhesions. Sometimes, sharp and blunt dissection is necessary. Care is taken to avoid injury to the splenic artery and to the pancreas.

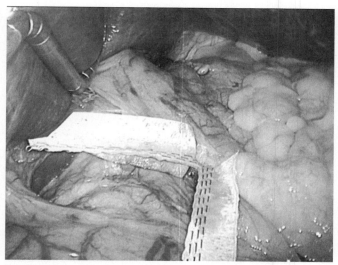

Figure 24-1. Division of lesser curvature, with bovine pericardial reinforcement.

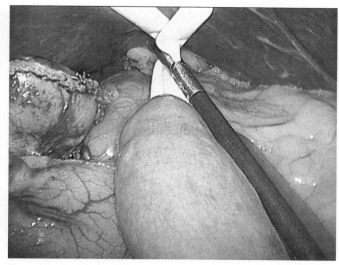

Figure 24-3. Loop of intestine 100 cm distal to ligament of Treitz being brought up to gastric pouch; the loop will be divided after the back wall of the gastrojejunostomy is sewn. The proximal portion will be the biliopancreatic limb.

We begin formation of the gastric pouch immediately below the left gastric artery unless we find it to be aberrant, in which case we start about 3 cm down from the esophagogastric junction on the right side (Fig. 24-2). We use an Endocutter (Ethicon Endo-Surgery) with a wide load with three rows of staples reinforced by a seam guard (W.L. Gore, Flagstaff, Ariz.) to divide the lesser curvature's blood supply. The division and dissection continue just up to the lesser curvature of the stomach.

Dissection is carried up to the angle of His with the aim of constructing a very small, narrow, gastric pouch. The final pouch is approximately 5 to 20 ml in size. The Harmonic Scalpel is used to dissect free the posterior gastric adhesions. Care is taken not to injure the left gastric artery, which may be found quite medially.

With the patient supine, we divide the transverse omentum just to the right of midline with the Harmonic Scalpel. We then identify the ligament of Treitz, elevating the mesentery just above it to confirm clear identification. A Maryland dissector is then passed just below the mesentery of the small bowel. The biliopancreatic limb is to the left, and what is to become the Roux limb will be to the right of this loop. A Penrose drain is then dragged below the bowel, encircling the small bowel and allowing us to place traction on the loop to bring it up to the gastric pouch and begin the suturing of the back row (Fig. 24-3).

The back wall suture is run between the gastric pouch and the loop of small bowel with the Penrose drain still in place to prevent traction. The Endostitch (Autosuture) is used to perform this maneuver. The Penrose drain is then removed from the field, and a reticulating, 60-mm, wide-load Autostapler (Autosuture) is used to divide the small bowel, essentially maintaining what is to the left as the biliopancreatic limb and what is to the right as the Roux limb. The Harmonic Scalpel is used to dissect down along the mesentery, enlarging the mesenteric defect by about 1 cm, with care taken carefully to coagulate the small vessels and care taken not to migrate to the right or to the left into the mesentery.

The bowel that is attached to the gastric remnant is run downstream. In patients with body mass indexes greater than 50 kg per m^2 and in patients with type 2 diabetes, we use a longer Roux limb of 150 cm. The biliopancreatic limb is reconnected to the Roux limb about 150 cm downstream with an Endostitch.

Enterotomies are made using the Harmonic Scalpel, and an endogastrointestinal, wide-load, 60-mm, three-row stapler is inserted into the lumen of each bowel segment and fired. The resultant enterotomy is approximated with the Endostitch, and the entire enterotomy is rotated between 100 and 180 degrees to the left upper quadrant. A wide-load 60-mm stapler is used to close the common enterotomy (Fig. 24-4). An antiobstruction stitch of

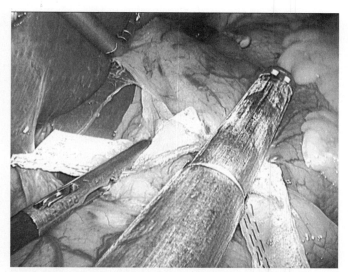

Figure 24-2. Beginning division of stomach to create gastric pouch 1 cm distal to left gastric anastomosis.

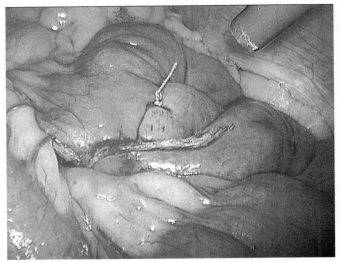

Figure 24-4. Stapled completion of jejunojejunostomy prior to the placement of the antiobstruction stitch.

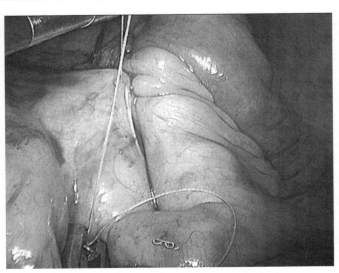

Figure 24-6. Mesenteric closure of jejunojejunostomy.

2-0 Prolene is made, and then a running closure of the jejunojejunostomy mesenteric defect is performed to completely close the jejunojejunostomy mesenteric defect (Figs. 24-5 and 24-6).

At this point, the patient is brought into the steep reverse Trendelenburg position. Enterotomies are made with the Harmonic Scalpel in the gastric pouch as well as in the Roux limb, and an Endocutter (Ethicon Endo-Surgery) blue load is inserted to 1.5 cm and fired (Fig. 24-7). In the process, the upper stitch from the back-wall anastomosis is held and pulled directly to the left upper quadrant toward the left shoulder. This facilitates the proper angle of closure.

The Endostitch is used to begin the anastomosis from the patient's right and the patient's left, beginning at the right corner of the anastomosis and the left corner of the anastomosis. The ends are brought together without tying.

The endoscope is then passed into the Roux limb os. It is 30F in size, and the suture is snugged down. A second layer, using the Endostitch, is used to oversew the anastomosis to complete a two-layer anastomosis.

The anastomosis is tested under saline to inspect for any evidence of bubbling or leakage. Small holes can be oversewn. Figure 24-8 demonstrates the anastomosis being tested under saline, with no evidence of bubbling.

The limitations of the procedure arise when a very thickened small bowel or very short mesentery is found; in these cases it is preferable to use the retrocolic, retrogastric position. An additional advantage of this approach is that when there are multiple adhesions in the lower abdomen, with potential hernias and fat stuck in the hernia defect, it is prudent not to remove those contents unless definitive repair of the hernia can be contemplated at that time.

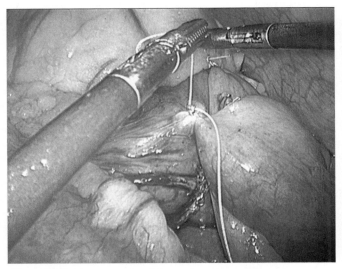

Figure 24-5. Placement of antiobstruction stitch at jejunojejunostomy.

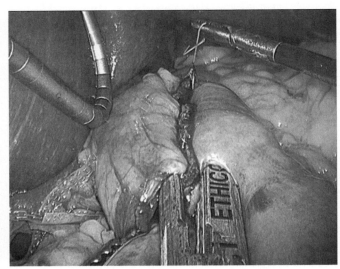

Figure 24-7. The gastrojejunostomy.

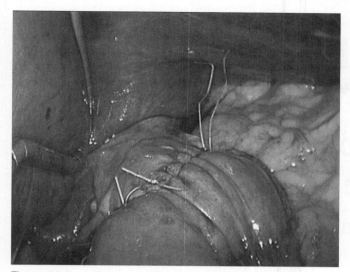

Figure 24-8. Complete gastrojejunostomy anastomosis oversewn in two layers.

▶ CONCLUSION

It is important that surgeons be familiar with multiple techniques in performing the laparoscopic Roux-en-Y gastric bypass. The linear technique is one of the most common techniques being used today.

▶ REFERENCES

1. Steinbrook R: Surgery for severe obesity. N Engl J Med 2004;350: 1075-1079.
2. Wittgrove AC, Clark GW, Tremblay LJ: Laparoscopic gastric bypass, Roux-en-Y: preliminary report of five cases. Obes Surg 1994;4:353-357.
3. Schauer PR, Ikramuddin S, Gourash WF: Laparoscopic Roux-en-Y gastric bypass: a case report at one-year follow-up. J Laparoendoscop Adv Surg Tech A 1999;9:101-106.
4. Higa KD, Boone KB, Ho T: Complications of the laparoscopic Roux-en-Y gastric bypass: 1,040 patients: what have we learned? Obes Surg 2000;10:509-513.

25

Laparoscopic Gastric Bypass Using the Circular Stapler

G. Wesley Clark, M.D.

Gastric bypass, initially using a loop reconstruction, was first proposed by Mason in 1967[1] as a means of treating morbid obesity, and the Roux-en-Y modification was introduced by Griffen in 1977.[2] From those beginnings, the gastric bypass, in particular the Roux-en-Y gastric bypass, has evolved in concept and technique, as thoughtful surgeons have observed and studied the effects of the surgery they performed. Good short-term results have sometimes been followed by longer term disappointments, as patients experienced increasing functional gastric capacity and recurrence of obesity. Gradual anatomic enlargement of the gastric pouch is a common correlative feature of this failure.

Surgeons have responded by reducing initial pouch size and altering the anatomy of pouch construction to eliminate the innate elasticity of the fundus and greater curvature. The modern gastric pouch is based on the lesser curvature, the least distensible part of the stomach. Stability of pouch size and maintenance of a small functional gastric volume, which limits rapid food intake, appear to be important to the maintenance of weight loss. Stomal size appears to be a factor in early weight loss, although its role in long-term weight maintenance is probably less significant.[1]

Fistula formation between the proximal pouch and the distal stomach has been another cause of weight-control failure. Division of the stomach appears to minimize this long-term complication, whereas stapling in continuity has been reported to be associated with fistula formation in up to 48% of patients, over the long term.[3] Because gastric division is not associated with significant increased morbidity and may technically facilitate the formation of the gastroenterostomy, there is little reason to choose not to divide the stomach.

Roux-en-Y reconstruction has been the mainstay of gastric bypass surgery for more than 20 years. Bile and pancreatic secretions are completely diverted away from the sensitive gastric pouch and the gastroenterostomy. Even if the lower esophageal sphincter were to remain incompetent, the tiny gastric pouch empties rapidly of liquids, secretes very little acid, and can suffer no bile reflux because of the length of the Roux limb. Preoperative reflux symptoms are characteristically relieved beginning on the day of surgery.

A major benefit of the proximal Roux-en-Y construction is the profound satiety response that patients experience shortly after ingestion of food, especially proteins. It has long been observed that food, particularly proteins, in the distal duodenum and proximal jejunum produces a satiety response, which is thought to be mediated by gut hormones, probably operating on the regulatory centers of the hypothalamus. Roux-en-Y construction transplants the hypothesized source of hormonal secretion in the proximal jejunum just distal to the rate-limiting gastric pouch. The patient experiences early fullness due to the distention of the pouch, which is followed by rapid satiety resulting from the secondary gut reflex initiated immediately when food leaves the proximal pouch.

Recently, the role of ghrelin, a polypeptide hormone affecting hunger, has been recognized as a factor in the favorable hormonal physiology following gastric bypass. This gastrointestinal hormone has been shown to be associated with hunger, to be chronically elevated after weight-reduction by dieting, and to be markedly reduced after gastric bypass.[4]

These observations lead to a strategy for technical construction of the gastric bypass that produces optimal early weight loss and long-term weight control:

- Minimal calibrated pouch size (15 ml calibrated volume)
- Calibrated stomal size
- Roux limb of sufficient length to prevent reflux
- Proximal Roux-en-Y reconstruction.

These guidelines apply independent of the means of access chosen to accomplish the operation. Fundamental to the concept of laparoscopic surgery from its very inception has been the principle that the performance of an operation by means of this new surgical access technique should not alter or compromise the underlying procedure or its physiology. This principle, applied to laparoscopic gastric bypass, initially led to the use of the circular stapler and placement of the stapler anvil through the mouth in order to satisfy the requirement of minimal pouch size and to provide precise calibration of the gastroenterostomy lumen.[5] Alternative anastomotic techniques inevitably require a larger pouch size simply to provide adequate tissue for closure, and calibration of lumen size may be erratic.

INSTRUMENTATION

Efficient performance of laparoscopic surgery relies heavily on the availability and choice of high-quality instrumentation to a much greater extent than do traditional open techniques. The design of graspers that permit secure manipulation of tissue without slippage or laceration is critical to avoid tissue injury as well as to avoid wasted motion and time.

The design of complex instruments such as linear and circular staplers actually affects the technique of the procedure. In particular, we consider the construction of the anvil of the standard end-to-end anastomosis stapler to be unacceptable and unsafe for use in the oral technique of anvil insertion.

TECHNIQUE

The patient is placed in the position illustrated in Figure 25-1, with both arms out to the sides of the table. Port placement sites are shown in Figure 25-2. The positioning of the camera port must allow the scope to reach the cardia of the stomach and also to view the infracolic region for construction of the enteroenterostomy; the best compromise is approximately one handbreadth below the base of the xiphoid process. The location of the umbilicus, especially in the obese patient, has little relationship to

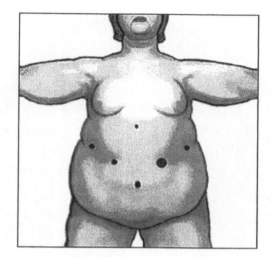

Figure 25-2. Port placement.

the position of fixed retroperitoneal structures, including the cardia and the ligament of Treitz.

The gastric transection is initiated laparoscopically by insertion through the mouth of the calibration tube and inflation of its balloon with 15 to 20 ml of air.[5] The balloon is drawn snugly into the cardia, and dissection of the lesser curvature is initiated at its lower pole, a point that usually coincides with the location of the first gastric vascular arcade and is approximately 2 to 3 cm below the gastro-esophageal-mucosal junction (Fig. 25-3). The lower edge of the fat pad overlying the cardia commonly coincides with the level at which transection is performed. Selection of a level higher than this landmark should alert one to increased risk for esophageal injury.

Dissection may be made cephalad to the upper recess of the lesser peritoneal sac, or entry into the sac may be chosen. In either instance, the initial transection is made in

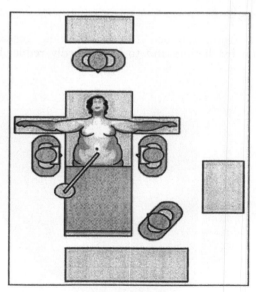

Figure 25-1. Operating room setup.

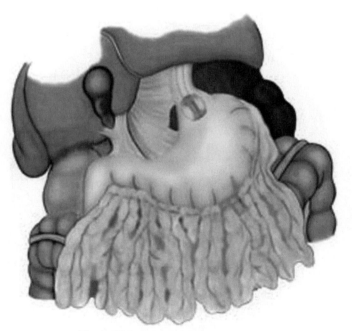

Figure 25-3. Lesser-curvature dissection.

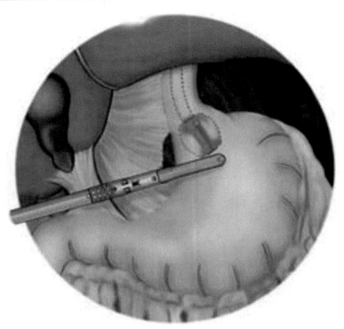

Figure 25-4. Transverse stapler application.

a horizontal direction, the subsequent staple line being turned cephalad to intersect the fundus at the angle of His, leaving only a tiny cuff of stomach lateral to the esophagus (Figs. 25-4 and 25-5).

The Roux limb is constructed by first transecting the jejunum a few centimeters distal to the peritoneal reflection at the ligament of Treitz. The proximal stub of bowel should be kept short so as to preserve the length of functional bowel (Fig. 25-6). The enteroenterostomy is constructed by means of a side-by-side anastomosis (functional end-to-side). The Roux limb is brought through the transverse mesocolon

and across the lesser sac, posterior to the colon and the distal stomach, where it will lie in close relation to the proximal stomach, without tension (Fig. 25-7).

The completed gastric pouch is endoscoped, the bottom of the pouch typically being found to be approximately 2 cm distal to the gastroesophageal-mucosal junction. Using a method originally developed for percutaneous gastrostomy, the gastric pouch is penetrated with a percutaneous needle-catheter assembly. A looped pull-wire is threaded into the lumen and then retrieved, using an endoscopy snare, through the mouth (Fig. 25-8). The pull-wire loop is then inserted into the stem of an ECS-21 stapler; the anvil is placed in the oropharynx and drawn downward into the gastric pouch by gentle traction on the pull-wire. Passage through the upper esophageal sphincter and retrolaryngeal area is facilitated by elevation of the angle of the jaw to open the posterior pharynx.

When the Roux limb has been constructed, the body of the circular stapler is inserted in its lumen, the penetrator exiting through its antimesenteric aspect to mate with the stem of the anvil, extruded through the stomach wall (Fig. 25-9). Closure and discharge of the circular stapler completes a gastroenterostomy that is symmetrically well-formed and that has an initial lumen of 12 mm. The opened end of the Roux limb is closed by transverse application of the linear stapler, a small fragment of bowel being excised (Fig. 25-10). This construction may be further reinforced by external suturing to imbricate the

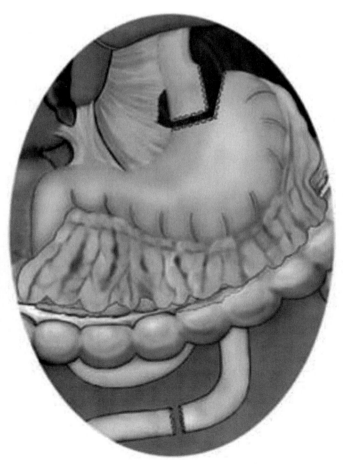

Figure 25-6. Division of small bowel.

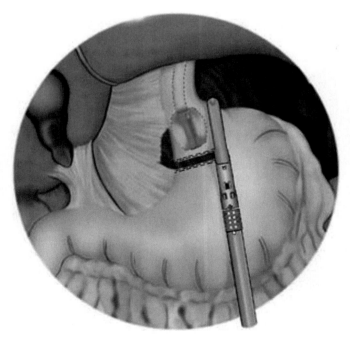

Figure 25-5. Vertical stapler application.

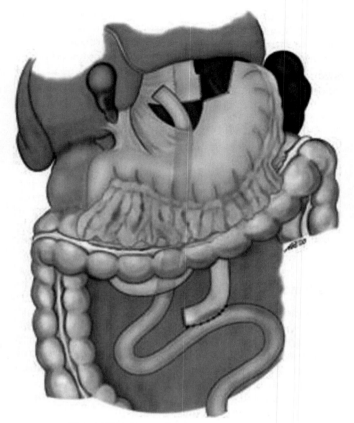

Figure 25-7. Retrocolic passage of Roux limb.

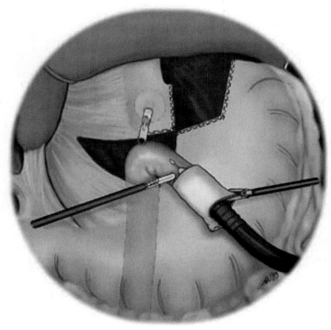

Figure 25-9. Circular stapler inserted, mating with anvil.

staple lines or by forming narrow tissue bridges against adjacent serosa. This suturing further reduces the ultimate size of the pouch as tissue is reefed within suture lines.

The completed gastric bypass construction is illustrated in Figure 25-11. Endoscopic anvil placement makes endoscopic examination and testing of the completed anastomosis readily achievable. With the distal lumen occluded, the endoscope is used to inspect visually the esophagus and gastric pouch. The gastroenterostomy can be submerged in irrigating solution in the abdomen while the endoscope

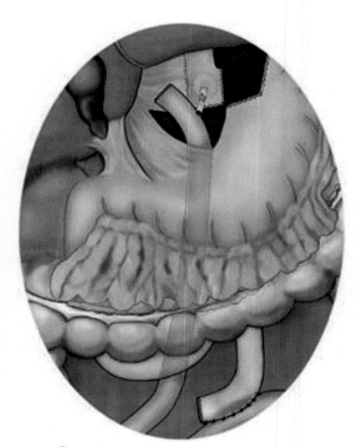

Figure 25-8. Insertion of stapler anvil via the mouth.

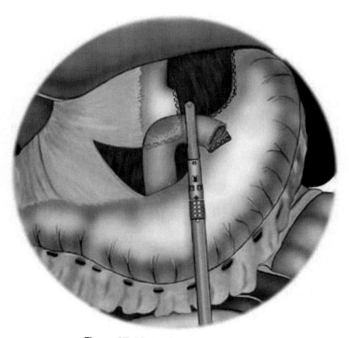

Figure 25-10. Reclosure of Roux limb.

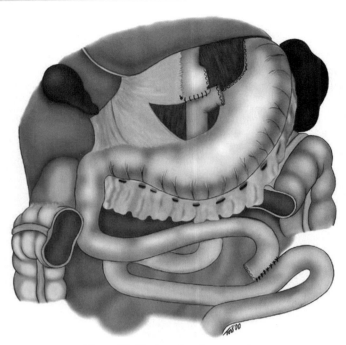

Figure 25-11. Completed construction.

is used to insufflate and pressurize the complex so it can be observed for air leaks. This is a sensitive and easily achieved test of immediate anastomotic integrity.

▶ COMPLICATIONS AND NEGATIVE ASPECTS

Difficulty of Anvil Passage

Passage of the anvil is greatly facilitated by the maneuver of elevating the angles of the jaw anteriorly as the anvil is passed through the posterior pharynx and upper esophageal sphincter. Occasionally, the cuff of the endotracheal tube must also be deflated to allow the anvil to pass the upper esophageal inlet. Despite these actions, impaction of the anvil at the level of the upper esophageal sphincter has occurred in two cases of a series of more than 2400 insertions. In one case, the anvil was retrieved by an endoscopic snare insinuated around it from above. The anvil was reinserted, and passed without difficulty. In the second case, use of the snare was unsuccessful, and retrieval required laparotomy, the anvil being easily dislodged by retrograde passage of an esophageal dilator and retrieved by the anesthesiologist. A sutured gastroenterostomy anastomosis was then performed.

It is likely that the very rare occurrence of anvil impaction can be treated successfully, with avoidance of laparotomy, by inserting the laparoscopic irrigating cannula into the gastric pouch lumen and instilling irrigating solution into the gastric and esophageal lumen to dislodge the anvil by hydrostatic pressure from below.

Gastric Tear

Manipulation of the circular stapler, once mated with the anvil, must be performed with great care to avoid inadvertent

traction on the anvil and the tearing of the gastric wall. Most such injuries can be successfully repaired by laparoscopic suturing. With experience and standardization of the technique, this technical complication has become very rare.

Inadequate Anastomotic "Doughnuts"

The circular stapler should be inspected after firing for confirmation of complete anastomotic "doughnuts." An incomplete doughnut is not necessarily indicative of a defective anastomosis, but it should occasion careful inspection and oversuture of any suspect area.

The relative positions of the linear gastric staple line and the circular gastroenterostomy may lead to narrow points or an isthmus of gastric tissue that is subject to ischemia. Areas such as this should always be protected by imbrication, using adjacent small bowel and gastric wall, to minimize potential sources of leakage.

Anastomotic Leakage

Anastomotic leakage can be expected at a rate of approximately 1% to 2%, as reported in numerous large series.[6] Although technical factors account for some of these occurrences, it is likely that unforeseeable and uncontrollable factors, such as focal ischemic necrosis or leakage around sutures or staples, are often the cause.

Insufflation testing of the gastroenterostomy complex, as described earlier, can minimize technical defects, often surprising the surgeon with a stream of bubbles where a technically sound construction had been confidently assumed.

Port Site Infection

Performance of the circular-stapler technique involves passage of the anvil through the mouth and oropharynx, where contamination of the device inevitably occurs. Cultures of the gastric pouch lumen or of the enteroenterostomy often yield minimal or no flora, whereas cultures of the anvil after extraction typically show that it is teeming with oral flora, which are potentially pathogenic when introduced into the abdomen or subcutaneous tissues. Every effort should be made to minimize contact of the anvil with subcutaneous tissues.

The left lower port site, through which the stapler is inserted and removed, is the port most susceptible to postoperative infection. Wound care should be scrupulous, with avoidance of excessive dissection and dead-space formation and thorough irrigation to remove fibrinous detritus and devitalized fragments of fatty tissue. An intraabdominal drain may be led out through this wound to provide simultaneous wound drainage.

▶ ADDITIONAL MANAGEMENT ISSUES

Intraabdominal Drainage

Placing a drain in proximity to the gastroenterostomy while avoiding actual contact remains a valid management option. The accumulation of any fluid or blood postoperatively, with its inevitable contamination, can result in a localized collection that will seek egress either by penetration of staple and suture lines or via a surgical drain—much the preferable route. Even were a leak to occur, a well-localized and well-drained leak can usually be managed nonoperatively, with minimal septic risk and short hospitalization.

Management of Anastomotic Leak

Conventional surgical wisdom holds that any evidence of an anastomotic leak at the gastroenterostomy demands immediate reoperation, repair of the leak, and establishment of drainage. In practice, attempts at repair often lead to further tissue damage and potentially to further delay in healing. A well-placed drain inserted at the initial procedure obviates the need for a second operation to insert one. Many instances of minimal leakage, with local containment and adequate drainage of the extravasated material, may be successfully managed nonoperatively.

Patients with manifestations of leakage should be evaluated by means of a water-soluble contrast study, which may indicate the site of leakage and aids in estimating the extent of dissemination of the extravasated gastrointestinal contents. Tachycardia, fever, leucocytosis, and increased fluid demand are indicators of disseminated leakage and inadequate drainage. Early operation is demanded. Laparoscopic reexploration can usually be accomplished.

Minimal contained leakage that is well-drained, associated with stable vital signs and the absence of or rapid improvement in leucocytosis, usually argues for nonoperative management by antibiotics, limitation of oral intake, and close observation. A localized area of contamination injudiciously disrupted by reexploration may actually result in dissemination of contaminated material throughout what was previously a sterile general peritoneal cavity.

Acute Gastric Dilatation

Dilatation of the distal gastric remnant due to ileus, obstruction of the enteroenterostomy, or intraluminal bleeding may urgently require either percutaneous gastrostomy or reexploration. Disruption of the gastric remnant is usually a catastrophic event that is associated with sudden and severe peritoneal contamination by stagnant gastric contents overgrown with multiple enteral flora.

Gastrostomy

Gastrostomy into the distal gastric remnant should be performed whenever the security of the gastroenterostomy is not certain and whenever reoperation is necessary. Severe sleep apnea and the need for perioperative continuous positive airway pressure may also be an indication. Gastrostomy is readily accomplished as an adjunct to the laparoscopic procedure.

Embolism Prophylaxis

The risk for pulmonary embolism can be reduced by conscientious attention to patient management. All obese patients are at increased risk consequent to increased abdominal pressure and decreased mobility. Predisposing conditions, such as venous stasis disease or a history of embolism, are more common in the obese.

▶ THE OPERATION AS A TOOL

Bariatric surgery requires that the surgeon transcend the usual concept of healing by surgical technique. Most general surgery procedures are fundamentally extirpative: a malfunctioning or diseased organ, or a portion thereof, is surgically removed to restore health. Follow-up is generally brief, and the goal of treatment is restoration of the patient's accustomed health and lifestyle

Bariatric surgery aims to alter body physiology and the patient's lifestyle permanently. It aims to counteract the inborn genetic and associated behavioral processes that have given rise to the disease of obesity. To achieve effective therapy, the patient must be led to use the benefits of altered physiology to achieve a permanent positive lifestyle change. Habitual negative patterns of food-seeking behavior must be identified and challenged in the therapy process. Simultaneously, the patient must learn to adjust to an altered body image and to the changes and stresses in his or her support system that are the inevitable consequence of dramatic metamorphosis. The successful bariatric surgeon learns to broaden the focus of therapy to incorporate a comprehensive treatment program that features support of patients through revolutionary life changes.

▶ REFERENCES

1. Mason EE, Ito C: Gastric bypass in obesity. 1967. Obesity Research 1996;4:316-319.
2. Buchwald H, Buchwald JN: Evolution of operative procedures for the management of morbid obesity 1950-2000. Obes Surg 2002; 12:705-717.
3. MacLean LD, Rhode BM, Nohr C, et al: Stomal ulcer after gastric bypass. J Am Coll Surg 1997;185:1-7.
4. Cummings DE, Weigle DS, Frayo RS, et al: Plasma ghrelin levels after diet-induced weight loss or gastric by pass surgery. N Engl J Med 2002;346:1623-1630.
5. Wittgrove AC, Clark GW: Combined laparoscopic/endoscopic anvil placement for the performance of the gastroenterostomy. Obes Surg 2001;11:565-569.
6. Schneider BE, Villegas L, Blackburn GL, et al: Laparoscopic gastric bypass surgery: outcomes. J Laparoendo Adv Surg Tech 2003;13: 247-255.

26

Laparoscopic Roux-en-Y Gastric Bypass: Hand-Sewn Gastrojejunostomy Technique

Kelvin Higa, M.D.

The current popularity of bariatric surgery is attributable, in part, to the minimally invasive solutions developed in the 1990s. In previous decades, although surgeons had demonstrated excellent results and low complication rates, medical professionals, third-party payers, and the public demonstrated little acceptance of these procedures. Currently, the limitations of medical management and the exponential rise in obesity rates have contributed to a demand that far outweighs the supply of bariatric surgeons. It was estimated in 2001 that there may be as many as 20,000 prospective patients per bariatric surgeon.[1] Therefore, it is important that surgeons maintain or improve operative efficiency when adopting new techniques while more surgeons are trained in this specialty.

The minimally invasive revolution began in 1993 when Wittgrove, Clark, and Tremblay first performed a proximal gastric bypass laparoscopically.[2] Later, they were able to show that this technique was viable and produced weight loss and reduction in comorbidities equal to or better than many open series.[3] As discussed in Chapter 25, the laparoscopic/endoscopic anvil-placement technique for the creation of the gastrojejunal anastomosis was the foundation for most other procedures that followed. Initial anastomotic leakage rates of up to 5% were observed,[4] but rates improved with experience.[5]

In 1999, de la Torre and Scott published a series of laparoscopic Roux-en-Y gastric bypass procedures utilizing a totally intraabdominal approach for the formation of the gastrojejunal anastomosis with a circular stapler.[6] Champion, and later Schauer, developed the linear-cutter technique that obviates the need for transoral passage of instrumentation, thus avoiding the potential for esophageal injury while creating a stable, calibrated anastomosis.[7]

In 1996, we began development of the hand-sutured technique because of our concerns regarding failure rates of stapled anastomoses. We performed our first procedure in 1998.[8] The design of the procedure paralleled the open Roux-en-Y procedures that we were performing. Based on this experience and the extrapolation of theories of gastric pouch formation,[9] we adopted the basic configuration described by MacLean and colleagues.[10] Knowing that small changes in anatomy or technique might have pronounced effects on short- and long-term results and complications, it was important for us to emulate the open configuration as closely as possible, given the limitations of available laparoscopic instrumentation at that time.

The basis for this technique is the formation of a linear, vertically oriented pouch excluding the distensible fundus of the stomach. This provides a serviceable platform from which a hand-sewn anastomosis to the Roux limb can be performed. This technique has been reproduced and adopted by many centers but is not as popular as are the stapled techniques. The long learning curve and inexperience with advanced laparoscopic suturing are the major drawbacks. However, once mastered, these techniques enable the surgeon to resolve almost all complications related to bariatric surgery (or other complex foregut surgery, for that matter) laparoscopically, and with a greater degree of precision. This technique also allows the surgeon to achieve an operative efficiency that surpasses the open equivalent (Table 26-1).

▶ INDICATIONS AND SELECTION CRITERIA FOR SURGERY

We follow the National Institutes of Health Consensus Development Conference Statement[11] and the 2004 American Society for Bariatric Surgery Consensus Conference[12] guidelines for gastrointestinal surgery for severe obesity in association with the American Society for Bariatric Surgery and the Society of American Gastrointestinal Endoscopic Surgeons recommendations for surgical intervention.

Contraindications to the laparoscopic approach are relatively few in our center (Table 26-2). Larger patients may be more challenging, but the added benefits of avoiding the morbidity of a large incision make this approach worthwhile. Likewise, patients who have had previous open surgery benefit from the mobilizing of adhesions

Table 26-1	**ADVANTAGES AND DISADVANTAGES OF HAND-SEWN TECHNIQUE**

ADVANTAGES	DISADVANTAGES
• Low leak rate in open series; familiarity and comfort with the technique • Complications (stenosis, etc.) already defined • Is less expensive than stapled anastomosis • Does not require endoscopy equipment • Does not require enlargement of port or incur increased infections due to contamination of port site by endomechanical device • Allows for a small, linear gastric pouch • Can be performed by a single surgeon without a skilled surgeon as assistant • Avoids esophageal instrumentation • Enables secondary or revision surgery • Allows surgeon to develop important skills necessary to resolve complications	• Long learning curve

laparoscopically rather than lengthening an already extensive incision. The role of bariatric surgery in the adolescent (younger than 18 years) and the elderly (older than 60 years) age groups has not been well defined, but evolving experience indicates results similar to those in standard age groups.[13] Similarly, ethnic and cultural differences as related to outcomes are currently being evaluated.

▶ PREPARATION FOR SURGERY

The treatment of morbid obesity requires a dedicated multidisciplinary team consisting of the surgeon, psychologist, nutritionist, physical therapist, anesthesiologist, and others. More important, the patient must be an active participant in the bariatric surgical program if optimal outcomes are to be achieved. Optimization of preoperative nutrition and cardiopulmonary performance is advisable and can help to limit one of the major causes of laparoscopic conversions—hepatic enlargement that limits visualization of the proximal stomach. Medical weight reduction, although limited in long-term management alone, may be quite helpful in decreasing the size of the liver and the amount of intraperitoneal fat preoperatively, thus enabling the surgeon to perform the procedure

Table 26-2	**CONTRAINDICATIONS TO LAPAROSCOPIC BARIATRIC SURGERY**

• Unsuitable candidate for bariatric surgery in general; e.g., inadequate cardiopulmonary reserve to tolerate the procedure, uncontrolled drug or alcohol dependency, impaired intellectual capacity, etc.
• Presence of large incisional hernias that would require repair at the time of bariatric procedure
• Presence of intraabdominal adhesions preventing laparoscopic visualization and dissection in general
• Abdominal compartment syndrome or potential for inadequate pneumoperitoneum

laparoscopically with safety while establishing sound nutritional and exercise habits that are beneficial after surgery.

Bowel preparation is unnecessary. A liquid diet 24 hours prior to surgery prevents the possibility that food retained in the stomach will obstruct the jejunojejunal anastomosis immediately after surgery; such obstruction is a potential cause of acute gastric distension.[14]

Bariatric patients are a moderate risk for perioperative venous thromboembolism.[15] Prophylaxis in the form of mechanical means (sequential compression boots and early ambulation) and pharmacologic means (subcutaneous fractionated or unfractionated heparin) is advised. Traditional parenteral antibiotic prophylaxis is standard.

The positioning of the patient in the operating room must include attention to the prevention of pressure sores and neuropathy. Dedicated operative tables must be weight-rated appropriately and have lateral extensions to accommodate the larger patients. Protocols for patient transfer and other safety issues should be included as part of a hospital-wide awareness program.

▶ SURGICAL PROCEDURE

Optimal port placement allows for dissection of the small bowel without compromising the exposure of the proximal stomach. Extremes of size can be challenging; adequate space to allow the formation of the Roux limb in smaller patients can be as problematic as the inadequate length of instrumentation and difficulties associated with visualizing the proximal stomach in the larger patients. It is interesting that authors describe various approaches and port locations to solve these issues while maintaining the critical nature of their particular port placement. We utilize five ports (Fig. 26-1). This arrangement also allows for concomitant cholecystectomy if it is indicated.

Initial entry is performed without insufflation utilizing a nonbladed optical trocar system. The camera is placed midline, 8 to 12 cm from the xiphoid, and other ports are placed to allow creation of the Roux limb, formation of the gastric pouch, and performance of the gastrojejunal anastomosis. Attention to the angle of entry of the port can reduce the resistance of the abdominal wall to the instrumentation, allowing for a more precise and less fatiguing operation. The ports can be redirected by creating a new fascial pathway, preserving the original skin entry site. These specific ports do not require fascial closure; this greatly improves operative efficiency and also reduces potential sources of postoperative pain.

The omentum is displaced cephalad to expose the ligament of Treitz. In patients whose omentum is adherent to pelvic structures or involved in an incarcerated ventral hernia, we prefer to incise the gastrocolic omentum and open the transverse mesocolon from above, thus exposing the ligament of Treitz directly. Ventral hernias are repaired at a later date when optimal weight loss and nutrition ensure a greater degree of primary success and the use of prosthetic mesh is not compromised by contamination by enteric contents.

The proximal jejunum is transected using a 2.5-mm linear stapler, and the mesentery is divided by another firing

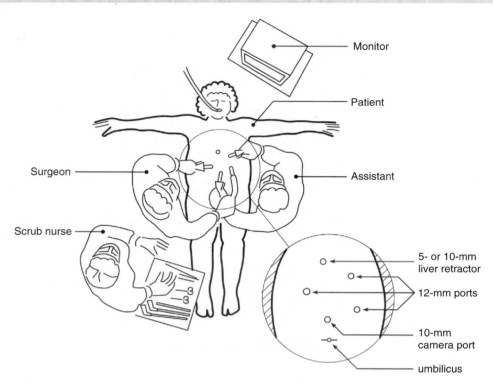

Monitor

Patient

Surgeon

Assistant

Scrub nurse

Figure 26-1. Position of patient and surgical team; port placement sites.

5- or 10-mm liver retractor

12-mm ports

10-mm camera port

umbilicus

of the instrument or by the harmonic scalpel. The Roux limb is measured, and a side-to-side linear anastomosis is performed (Fig. 26-2). Typically, the length of the Roux limb can be up to 150 cm without an associated increased incidence of malabsorptive complications.[16] The enterotomy is closed with a single layer of absorbable suture. The mesenteric defect must be closed with a continuous, nonabsorbable suture to limit the possibility of internal herniation.

The Roux limb is passed through a retrocolic tunnel and fixed to the transverse mesocolon with nonabsorbable sutures, which also includes closing the Petersen space, again to help prevent possible internal herniation. Alternatively, some surgeons prefer an antecolic route for the Roux limb, claiming a lower incidence of postoperative bowel obstructions.[17]

There are times when the mesocolon is uncomfortably short and does not allow for the safe passage of a retrocolic Roux limb. In these rare instances, the decision to route the Roux limb antecolic must be made prior to the transection of the jejunum. This site must be more distal from the ligament of Treitz, typically 50 to 100 cm, to limit the tension on the gastrojejunal anastomosis. By lengthening the biliopancreatic limb, iron and calcium absorption may be less efficient, and the incidence of these deficiencies may theoretically be increased or more difficult to manage with oral supplementation alone.

Controversy exists as to whether the large resultant Petersen space associated with an antecolic Roux limb requires closure. Clearly, these patients are still at risk for intestinal volvulous.[18] Therefore, our philosophy is to eliminate the risk of postoperative bowel obstruction rather than simply settling for a reduction in the incidence.

However, the long-term stability of suture closure of these defects is yet to be determined.

The liver retractor is now placed to allow dissection of the proximal stomach. Occasionally, a very large liver does not allow for sufficient visualization; this is an indication for open conversion. However, displacement of the liver to the right, rather than anterior, allows sufficient exposure in the largest of patients. Alternatively, the surgeon may decide to abort the procedure, evaluate the cause of hepatic enlargement (usually steatosis), and institute therapy (medical weight reduction) in anticipation of performing the procedure at a later time under more ideal circumstances. In this way, surgical restraint and proper judgment may reduce the morbidity associated with these operations.

Perigastric dissection along the lesser curve of the stomach is performed 3 to 5 cm distal to the gastroesophageal junction and continues until the retrogastric space is reached. At times, dense adhesions to the pancreas are encountered. Visualization is enhanced by opening a gastrocolic window and approaching this area from behind the stomach. Care is taken to avoid thermal injury to the adjacent viscera and vagus nerves.

A six-row, 3.5 mm, linear cutter stapler is used to form the lesser-curve-based, proximal gastric pouch. Four-row staplers have been unreliable, in our experience, without suture reinforcement to prevent failure.[10] It is essential to exclude the distensible gastric fundus in order to obtain optimal long-term weight management. This requires meticulous dissection behind the stomach at the level of the angle of His. This step also helps to prevent injury to the esophagus or spleen. A gastric pouch of no more than 20 ml is optimal.[19]

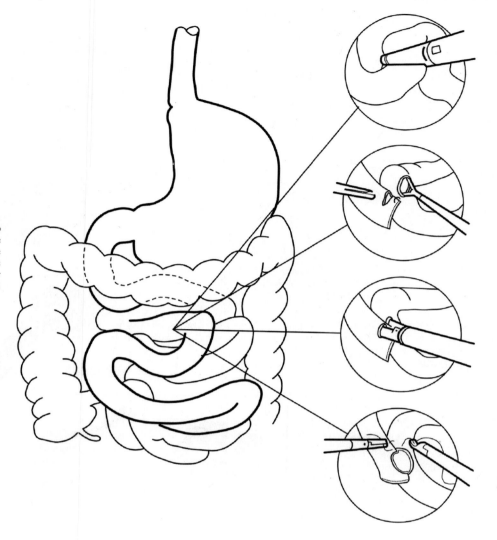

Figure 26-2. Formation of the Roux limb and jejunojejunostomy: measurement of the Roux limb; enterotomies for side-to-side anastomosis; construction of the anastomosis with the 2.5-mm linear stapler; enterotomy closure with a single layer of absorbable suture.

The inferior aspect of the pouch is determined, and the first horizontal stapler is brought in via the right upper quadrant port. All subsequent firings are vertically oriented through the left upper quadrant port. High subcostal placement of this port allows a standard-length stapling instrument to reach the angle of His in every instance. It is preferable to divide the fat pad at the hiatus so as to better visualize the gastroesophageal junction prior to stapling. Occasionally, a 4.5-mm stapler is required for exceptionally thick tissue.

A 34F orogastric tube is advanced into the stomach after the first horizontal stapling; it assists in the estimation of pouch size and prevents inadvertent transection of or the impingement of staples on the esophagus.

The retrocolic Roux limb is brought anterior to the gastric remnant to lie in close approximation to the newly formed gastric pouch. Although some surgeons prefer a retrogastric route, subsequent access and visualization of the anastomosis is more difficult if revisional surgery is necessary. A two-layer, hand-sewn anastomosis completes intestinal continuity.

The formation of the gastrojejunostomy begins with a running, posterior, exterior layer of 3-0 polyglactin (Vicryl) sutures. Beginning distally and sewing proximally, the antimesenteric side of the Roux limb is approximated to the inferior staple line of the gastric pouch, incorporating the staples in the suture line. Enterotomies are performed in the gastric pouch and the Roux limb adjacent to the suture line. A second posterior, full-thickness, running suture line is performed and continued anteriorly, beyond the termination of the first posterior suture (Fig. 26-3).

Two anterior suture lines are run from the distal anterior aspect of the enterotomy, the first being full thickness and the second seromuscular. Prior to completion of the anastomosis, the 34F tube is carefully inserted across the anastomosis to help calibrate the opening as well as to provide ensurance of a patent anastomosis. The anterior sutures are tied with their respective posterior counterparts.

The anastomosis and proximal staple lines can be tested with methyl blue dye, air insufflation via the orogastric tube, or operative endoscopy. However, we do not employ routine testing or drainage of the anastomosis unless dictated by clinical suspicion.

The port sites are inspected for bleeding upon withdrawal of the trocars, and the skin is closed with simple absorbable monofilament sutures.

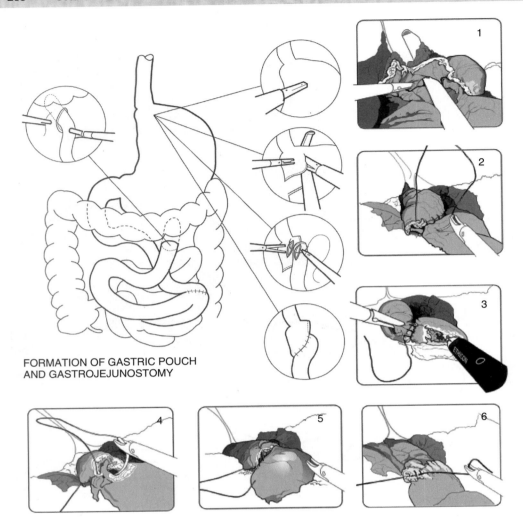

FORMATION OF GASTRIC POUCH
AND GASTROJEJUNOSTOMY

Figure 26-3. Formation of gastric pouch and gastrojejunostomy. Gastric pouch formation: first horizontal stapling to determine inferior aspect of pouch; subsequent vertical staplings to complete pouch division; side-to-side gastrojejunostomy; completed anastomosis. Hand-sewn gastrojejunostomy inserts: (1) retrocolic Roux limb brought anterior to the gastric remnant up to the gastric pouch; (2) running, posterior, exterior layer of 3-0 polyglactin suture, distal to proximal; (3) enterotomies performed; (4) second posterior, full-thickness running row of suture placed and continued beyond the termination of the first posterior suture; (5) first, full-thickness, running anterior row of sutures; (6) second, seromuscular, running anterior row of sutures. Both anterior sutures are tied with their respective posterior counterparts.

POSTOPERATIVE MANAGEMENT

Perioperative antibiotics are continued for 24 hours, and thromboembolism prophylaxis continues until the patient is discharged. Analgesia is in the form of patient-controlled narcotic delivery systems and intravenous ketoralac. Oral narcotics are offered when clear liquids are tolerated. Metoclopramide is administered routinely, and a variety of antiemetic pharmacologic agents are available for the nurses to use at their discretion.

Routine postoperative contrast studies add little to the management of these patients and serve only to delay discharge secondary to nausea.[20,21] A normal postoperative study should not preclude the surgeon from intervening based on clinical suspicion of a leak.[6]

The patients are started on clear liquids the day of surgery and are required to ambulate with assistance. Preoperative oral medications can be resumed as soon as the patient can tolerate clear liquids. Most patients are discharged by the second postoperative day.

Patients are continued on a clear liquid diet for 1 week and are slowly advanced to solids over a 3- to 4-week period. Patients are instructed to take either an H_2 blocker or proton pump inhibitor for 30 days. Routine follow-up visits are at 1 week, 3 weeks, and quarterly for the first year, then on a yearly basis. Ongoing nutritional, emotional, and exercise counseling and support groups are provided. Complete nutritional assessment occurs on a yearly basis or when symptoms or clinical suspicion dictates.

RESULTS

Wittgrove's 8-year data[5] suggest long-term weight loss equivalent to or better than the 5-year data for open gastric bypass reported by Maclean[22] and the 14-year data reported by Pories.[23] Our 5-year data suggest the same (Fig. 26-4). More important, reduction in comorbidities is quite remarkable, underscoring the impact and importance of surgical weight reduction on health care maintenance.

Early complication rates and operative times suffer from a very steep learning curve. This is dependent not only on the initial experience of the surgeon, but also on the surgeon's ability to organize a systematic method of approaching this complex operation. Efficiency resulting from the preparedness of the operative team is critical. Our data suggest that more than 100 procedures as primary

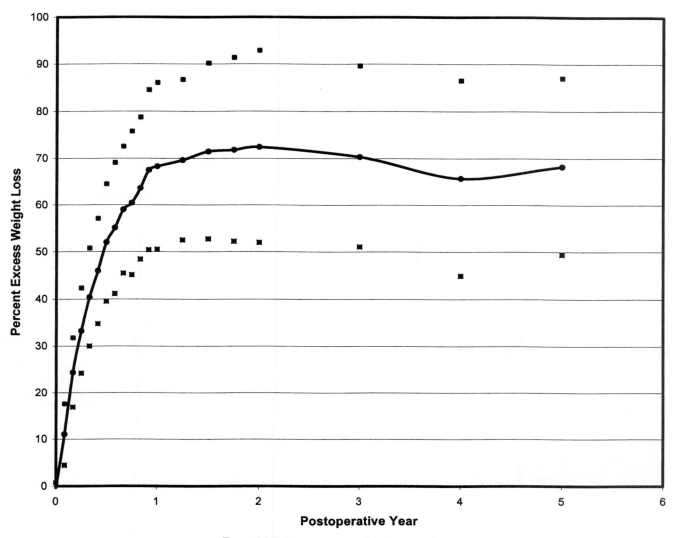

Figure 26-4. Percent excess weight loss over time.

surgeon may be necessary for this process (Fig. 26-5); this finding correlates with the experience of others.[24]

Short-term percentage of excess weight loss, reduction in medical comorbidities, and improvement in quality of life have been well documented for the open as well as the laparoscopic gastric bypass. However, and just as important, definitive 5- to 10-year data are lacking for but a few selective series. It is interesting that short-term laparoscopic data appear to indicate that it is superior to open standard gastric bypass, suggesting a subtle difference in the anatomic construct in the laparoscopic procedures.

▶ MANAGEMENT OF EARLY COMPLICATIONS

The most common complication in our series is stenosis of the gastrojejunal anastomosis (Table 26-3). This has remained constant at 4.9% to 5.21% and responds well to endoscopic balloon dilation. Patients complain of regression or intolerance of diet advancement at about the third postoperative week. The cause of this phenomenon is unclear and appears unrelated to the method of gastrojejunostomy (Table 26-4). Rarely does it occur at the level of the mesocolon or jejunojejunosomy. These locations do not respond to endoscopic dilation and must be repaired operatively. At times, a recurrent gastrojejunal stenosis also requires operative attention.

The second most common complication in our series is that of internal hernias and bowel obstructions (see Tables 26-3 and 26-5). They may occur immediately postoperatively or many years after the procedure. Caused primarily by migration of bowel through an open mesenteric defect, this phenomenon can be very difficult to detect in the absence of overt bowel obstruction. Patients commonly complain of intermittent, severe, postprandial abdominal pain, but noninvasive radiographic studies are completely normal in at least 50% of cases. Diagnostic laparoscopy must be performed on the basis of clinical suspicion; reduction and repair of the defects are straightforward.[25]

The prevention of internal hernias requires meticulous closure of all potential defects with nonabsorbable

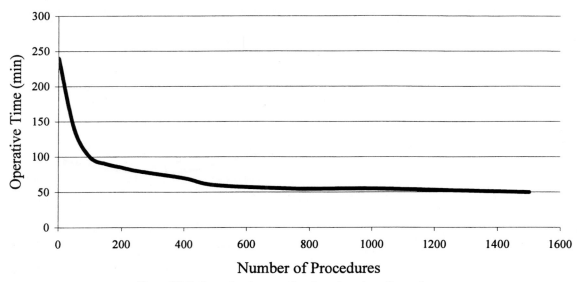

Figure 26-5. Operative time as a function of number of procedures.

suture material. Some surgeons have brought the Roux limb antecolic in the hope that the most common cause of small bowel obstruction, transmesocolic herniation, would be eliminated. However, the large resulting Petersen space and the jejunal mesentery defects are still potential sites that must be addressed.[7] We have not observed an internal hernia since we adopted the mesenteric closure techniques suggested by Schweitzer and colleagues.[26]

Proximal anastomotic leaks or staple line disruptions are tolerated poorly by the bariatric patient. Leaks are often subtle in their initial presentation; the only indication may be sustained tachycardia (>120/min). The typical

Table 26-3	COMPLICATIONS (2805 PATIENTS)				
TYPE	COMPLICATION	N	M	F	%
Anastomotic stenosis	Gastrojejunostomy	146	33	113	5.21
	Mesocolon	15	1	14	0.53
	Jejunojejunostomy	2	0	2	0.07
Total					5.81
Hernia	Trocar	4	3	1	0.14
	Internal	128			4.60
Total					4.7
Leaks	Staple line	21	9	12	0.75
	Gastrojejunostomy	2	0	2	0.07
	Jejunojejunostomy	1	0	1	0.04
Total					0.86
Infection (nonleak)	Wound	3	1	2	0.11
	Pneumonia	2	1	1	0.07
	Hepatic abscess	1	1	0	0.04
Total					0.21
Bleeding	Intervention required	13	7	6	0.46
	Transfusion only	11	1	10	0.39
	Observation	7	1	6	0.25
Total					1.1
Thrombo-embolic	Pulmonary embolism	5	0	5	0.18
	Deep venous thrombosis	2	1	1	0.07
Total					0.25
Biliary	Gallstones	77	7	70	2.75
	Acalculous cholecystitis	5	0	5	0.18
Total					2.92
Marginal Ulcer	Treated medically	17	3	14	0.61
	Perforation	9	0	9	0.32
	Revision required	3	0	3	0.11
TOTAL:					1.03
Death	Perioperative	4	1	3	0.14
Total: 478 of 2805; 17%					

N, number; M, male patients; F, female patients.

Table 26-4	INCIDENCE OF GASTROJEJUNAL STENOSIS	
AUTHOR	N	STENOSIS N (%)
Wittgrove et al[5] (2002)	1000	40 (4.0%)
Schauer et al[7] (2000)	275	13 (4.7%)
Higa et al[30] (2001)	1500	73 (4.9%)
Champion et al[31] (1999)	63	4 (6.3%)
DeMaria et al[32] (2002)	281	18 (6.6%)

N, number.

symptoms of abdominal pain, fever, or leukocytosis can be indistinguishable from cardiac events, pulmonary embolism, acute gastric distension, or hemorrhagic shock. Morbidly obese patients have little cardiopulmonary reserve; therefore, time to treatment is critical. Workup and evaluation must be expeditious and directed by clinical suspicion. If a leak is suspected, reexploration, usually laparoscopically, is the only definitive method to rule out this entity.

At surgery, there should be an attempt to identify and repair the defect, knowing that a secondary repair sometimes fails. Operative endoscopy is often helpful in identifying the leak and evaluating the repair. Drainage is essential, and enteric access via a gastrostomy tube in the gastric remnant can be established at this time. This will prevent gastric distension and can later be used as a conduit for nutritional support.

Venous thromboembolism and pulmonary emboli are the primary cause of death in most series. It is surprising that, given the physical attributes of the patient population, the presence of comorbid conditions, and the nature of the operation (position, prolonged operative times, etc.), they are rare occurrences. The use of both mechanical and pharmacologic prophylaxis along with early mobilization made possible by the elimination of incisional pain probably contribute to prevent this outcome. The use of prophylactic vena cava filters should be limited to patients with previous pulmonary embolism or significant pulmonary hypertension.

▶ MANAGEMENT OF LATE COMPLICATIONS

The use of tobacco or nonsteroidal analgesic agents contributes to marginal ulceration. Patients present with abdominal pain, dyspepsia and, occasionally, bleeding. The diagnosis can be made radiographically, but endoscopy is

Table 26-5	INTERNAL HERNIA DATA (2805 PATIENTS)	
LOCATION	N	(%)
Mesocolon	61	2.1
Jejunojejunostomy	41	1.5
Petersen	13	0.5
Multiple sites	13	0.5
Total	128	4.6

often required for the evaluation and treatment of an associated gastrojejunal stenosis or for control of bleeding.

Perforated marginal ulcers are amenable to laparoscopic intervention. The absence of significant intraabdominal adhesions and the anterior location of the anastomosis allow for a relatively simple closure and omental patch. Operative endoscopy is helpful in these cases to rule out gastrogastric fistulas and to evaluate the gastrojejunal anastomosis and repair.

Protein malabsorption/malnutrition is uncommon in proximal gastric bypass procedures. Still, patients should consume between 60 and 80 g of protein daily and have their albumin levels monitored appropriately. Often, patients do not tolerate meat initially and tend to avoid it. Rarely, protein supplementation is necessary.

Vitamin and mineral deficiency can occur in up to 30% of patients.[27] Ongoing nutritional evaluation and counseling along with oral multivitamins and calcium and B_{12} supplementation are recommended.[28]

Our data do not support routine cholecystectomy. However, no complications were observed as a result of removing the gallbladder at the time of the gastric bypass. Still, our approach is to consider concomitant cholecystectomy for known gallstones, but only if technically straightforward, given the patient's individual anatomy. In other words, if the dissection or identification of the cystic duct-common bile duct junction appears to be problematic, then it is advisable to wait until the patient has lost significant weight after gastric bypass before advising cholecystectomy. This approach helps to ensure more favorable anatomy and lowers the risk of bile duct injury. The trocar sites of the gastric bypass can be used for the subsequent cholecystectomy because adhesions are rarely encountered.

The causes of inadequate initial weight loss and of weight regain are multifactorial. It has been observed that participation in support groups by patients and follow-up with the surgeon may yield superior results. However, as the pathophysiology of surgical weight loss is poorly understood, patients themselves are often blamed for poor performance. This adds to the frustration shared by the patient and physician.

Clearly, the concept of obesity as a chronic disease should mandate a multidisciplinary and life-long approach to therapy. This includes the possibility of secondary surgical procedures for selected patients who do not achieve correction or stabilization of medical comorbid conditions. These considerations would take the form of a higher degree of restriction or malabsorption or both. Unfortunately, revision procedures are associated with at least double the morbidity of the primary operation and with unknown long-term results. Therefore, they must be performed only by surgeons with considerable experience and interest in this area.

▶ COMMENTS

The laparoscopic gastric bypass is one of the most challenging surgical procedures performed today. The distortion and obscuration of anatomy by intraabdominal fat in combination with the limitations of instrumentation have led to many ingenious solutions in attempts to emulate proven, standard open techniques. Although current endo-mechanical staplers have proven to be reliable, initial designs were less forgiving. Despite reliable anastomotic stapling techniques, experts agree that advanced laparoscopic suturing skills are required in order to perform this operation safely. In this respect, laparoscopic Roux-en-Y gastric bypass with a hand-sewn gastrojejunostomy has proven itself to be efficacious.

Current procedural refinements have allowed for laparoscopic operative efficiencies that surpass the open gastric bypass. The benefits patients find in minimally invasive surgery in terms of wound morbidity, cardiovascular compromise, and immune function have been demonstrated.[28,29] However, the learning curve for the surgeon is a long and tedious endeavor. In addition, bariatric patients present more than just a technical challenge. Ultimately, the treatment of obesity requires a multidisciplinary team dedicated to life-long management of this serious disease process. Morbid obesity, unlike its associated comorbidities, cannot be cured, only controlled. Surgeons unable to appreciate the management of obesity beyond the surgical procedure should not venture into this specialty.

▶ REFERENCES

1. Health Care Advisory Board, Marketing and Planning Leadership Council: Bariatric surgery programs: clinical innovation profile. Washington D.C., Health Care Advisory Board, 2002.
2. Wittgrove AC, Clark GW, Tremblay LJ: Laparoscopic gastric bypass, Roux-en-Y: preliminary report of five cases. Obes Surg 1994;4:353-357.
3. Wittgrove AC, Clark GW: Laparoscopic gastric bypass: a five-year prospective study of 500 patients followed from 3-60 months. Obes Surg 1999;9:123-143.
4. Wittgrove AC, Clark GW, Schubert KR: Laparoscopic gastric bypass, Roux-en-Y: technique and results in 75 patients with 3-30 month follow-up. Obes Surg 1996;6:500-504.
5. Wittgrove AC, Endres JE, Davis M, et al: Perioperative complications in a single surgeon's experience with 1,000 consecutive laparoscopic Roux-en-Y gastric bypass operations for morbid obesity. Obes Surg 2002;12:457-458 (abstract, L4).
6. de la Torre RA, Scott JS: Laparoscopic Roux-en-Y gastric bypass: a totally intra-abdominal approach: technique and preliminary report. Obes Surg 1999;9:492-498.
7. Schauer PR, Ikramuddin S, Gourash W, et al: Outcomes after laparoscopic Roux-en-Y gastric bypass for morbid obesity. Ann Surg 2000;232:515-529.
8. Higa KD, Boone KB, Ho T, et al: Laparoscopic Roux-en-Y gastric bypass for morbid obesity: technique and preliminary results of our first 400 patients. Arch Surg 2000;9:1029-1033.
9. Mason EE, Maher JW, Scott DH, et al: Ten years of vertical banded gastroplasty for severe obesity. In Mason EE (guest ed), Nyhus LM (ed): Surgical Treatment of Morbid Obesity, vol 9, pp. 280-289. Philadelphia, JB Lippincott, 1992.
10. MacLean LD, Rhode BM, Forse RA: Surgery for obesity: an update of a randomized trial. Obes Surg 1995;5:145-150.
11. National Institutes of Health Consensus Development Conference Draft Statement: Gastrointestinal surgery for severe obesity. Obes Surg 1991;1:257-266.
12. Buchwald H, American Society for Bariatric Surgery, Consensus Conference Panel: Bariatric surgery for morbid obesity: health implications for patients, health professionals, and third-party payers. J Am Coll Surg 2005;200:593-604.
13. Capella RF: Bariatric surgery in adolescents: is this the best age to operate? Obes Surg 2002;12:196 (abstract 13).
14. Higa KD, Boone KB, Ho T: Complications of the laparoscopic Roux-en-Y gastric bypass:1,040 patients—what have we learned? Obes Surg 2000;10:509-513.
15. Westling A, Bergvist D, Bostrom A, et al: Incidence of deep venous thrombosis in patients undergoing obesity surgery. World J Surg 2000;26:470-473.
16. Brolin RE, Kenler HA, Gorman JH, et al: Long-limb gastric bypass in the superobese: a prospective randomized trial. Ann Surg 1991; 215:387-395.
17. Champion JK: Small bowel obstruction after laparoscopic Roux-en-Y gastric bypass. Obes Surg 2002;12:197-198 (abstract 17).
18. Khanna A, Newman B, Reyes J, et al: Internal hernia and volvulus of the small bowel following liver transplantation. Transpl Int 1997;10: 133-136.
19. MacLean LD, Rhode BM, Nohr CW: Late outcome of isolated gastric bypass. Ann Surg 2000;231:524-528.
20. Singh R, Fisher B: Sensitivity and specificity of postoperative upper GI series following gastric bypass. Obes Surg 2003;13:73-75.
21. Sims TL, Mullican MA, Hamilton EC, et al: Routine upper gastrointestinal Gastrografin swallow after laparoscopic Roux-en-Y gastric bypass. Obes Surg 2003;13:66-72.
22. MacLean LD, Rhode BM, Forse RA: Results of the surgical treatment of obesity. Am J Surg 1993; 165:155-162.
23. Poires WJ, Swanson MS, MacDonald KG: Who would have thought it? An operation proves to be the most effective therapy for adult-onset diabetes mellitus. Ann Surg 1995;222:339-352.
24. Schauer PR, Ikramuddin S, Hammad G, et al: The learning curve for laparoscopic Roux-en-Y gastric bypass in 100 cases. Surg Endosc 2003;17:212-215.
25. Higa K, Ho T, Boone K: Internal hernias after laparoscopic Roux-en-Y gastric bypass: incidence, treatment and prevention. (in press).
26. Schweitzer MA, DeMaria EJ, Broderick TJ, et al: Laparoscopic closure of mesenteric defects after Roux-en-Y gastric bypass. J Laparoendosc Adv Surg Tech A 2000;10:173-175.
27. Rhode BM, MacLean LD: Vitamin and mineral supplementation after gastric bypass. In Deitel M, Cowan G (eds): Update: Surgery for the Morbidly Obese Patient, pp. 161-170. Toronto, FD-Communications, 2000.
28. Schauer PR: Physiologic consequences of laparoscopic surgery. In Eubanks WS, Soper NJ, Swanstrom LL (eds): Mastery of Endoscopic Surgery and Laparoscopic Surgery, pp. 22-38. Philadelphia, Lippincott Williams and Wilkins, 2000.
29. Nguyen NT, Lee SL, Goldman C, et al: Comparison of pulmonary function and postoperative pain after laparoscopic vs open gastric bypass: a randomized trial. J Am Coll Surg 2001;192:469-476.
30. Higa K, Ho T, Boone K: Laparoscopic Roux-en-Y gastric bypass: technique and 3-year follow-up. J Laparoendosc Adv Surg Tech 2001;11:377-382.
31. Champion JK, Hunt T, DeLisle N: Laparoscopic vertical banded gastroplasty and Roux-en-Y gastric bypass in morbid obesity. Obes Surg 1999;9:123-144.
32. DeMaria EJ, Sugerman HJ, Kellum JM, et al: Results of 281 consecutive total laparoscopic Roux-en-Y gastric bypasses to treat morbid obesity. Ann Surg 2002;235:640-647.

27

BANDED GASTRIC BYPASS

M.A.L. Fobi, M.D., Hoil Lee, M.D., Basil Felahy, M.D., Peter Ako, M.D., Nicole N. Fobi, M.D., and Martin Sanguinette, M.D.

The banded Roux-en-Y gastric bypass is composed of a small (20 ml or less) lesser-curvature, isolated pouch with a Silastic ring band around the lower third of the pouch. This band serves as a reinforced stoma. The transected edge of the pouch is covered by the antimesenteric border of the Roux limb, which is brought up for the establishment of bowel continuity. The gastrojejunostomy consists of a large, tangential anastomosis made end-to-side with a two-layer closure. The biliopancreatic and enteric limbs are both relatively short—about 60 cm each (Fig. 27-1).

This operation evolved from the observation that some patients experienced inadequate weight loss after anatomically precise and surgically intact vertical banded gastroplasties. When the gastroplasty was converted to gastric bypass, with the gastroenterostomy anastomosis just distal to the band, patients experienced better and more sustained weight loss, and this result occurred more often than it did in patients who had undergone nonbanded gastric bypass.[1] The band was left in place serendipitously because a Marlex band was used (as described by Mason[2]), and it would have been technically difficult to remove the band at the time of the conversion operation.

The first primary banded gastric bypasses were performed using a 5-cm Silastic band, just as in the Silastic ring vertical gastroplasty operation described by Laws.[3] The pouch was formed by stapling in continuity. This restrictive banded pouch resulted in a relatively high rate of intolerance of solid food[4] and a high incidence of staple-line breakdown and marginal ulcerations.[5,6] This problem was solved by using a 6-cm band in women and a 6.5-cm band in men. The pouch was also transected to minimize the incidence of staple-line breakdown.[6] Further, the transected edge of the pouch was covered with the antimesenteric border of the jejunal limb brought up for the gastrojejunostomy so as to minimize the incidence of gastrogastric fistula formation. Finally, to address the problem of access to the bypassed gastrointestinal segment, a temporary gastrostomy tube was placed in the bypassed stomach and a radiopaque marker was placed around this site to facilitate subsequent radiologic percutaneous access

to the bypassed gastric segment. This composite operation is popularly called the Fobi pouch gastric bypass operation for obesity[7] (see Fig. 27-1).

▶ SURGICAL TECHNIQUE

Creation of the Pouch

A Thompson retractor provides for good exposure of the gastroesophageal junction with retraction of both subcostal margins and the left lobe of the liver. Initially the bare area

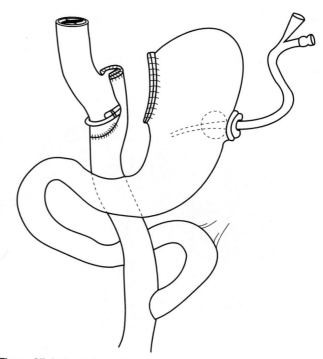

Figure 27-1. Banded gastric bypass with a temporary gastrostomy and gastrostomy site marker.

of the lesser omentum is entered. This is usually just overlying the caudate lobe of the liver. A window is made just to the left of the gastroesophageal junction. The gastroesophageal junction is mobilized by passing the hand through the defect overlying the caudate lobe and, with blunt dissection, bringing the middle finger through the window to the left of the gastroesophageal junction. This is done carefully in order to avoid any trauma to the liver, esophagus, diaphragm, pancreas, spleen, or proximal stomach. Rarely are any short gastric vessels ligated in this maneuver. Any adhesions to the spleen are lysed to prevent incidental avulsion of the splenic capsule and bleeding, which may necessitate transfusion and or an incidental splenectomy. A laparotomy pad is used to pack the spleen away from the operative site.

A nasogastric (NG) tube is inserted into the stomach by the anesthesiologist, and the stomach is decompressed. A defect is then made at a point 4 to 5 cm from the gastroesophageal junction on the lesser curvature, between the gastric serosa and the neurovascular bundle, with a blunt right-angle clamp. A ¼-inch wide Penrose drain is passed through this window, and the proximal stomach is retracted caudally stretching the 4- to 5-cm pouch to about 7 to 8 cm. The anvil of a 100-mm linear cutter stapler is inserted into this window and bought out just to the left of the gastroesophageal junction. The NG tube is held close to the lesser curvature of the proximal stomach as the other half of the stapler is engaged and placed on the anterior aspect of the stomach. The stomach is then pulled through the aperture of the stapler to leave as small a gastric pouch as possible. The stapling device is closed as the NG tube is withdrawn past the aperture of the stapling instrument. The proposed pouch is examined visually and manually to make sure it is not more than 25 ml in volume. The proximal pouch, from the lesser curvature to the left of the gastroesophageal junction, should be completely encompassed within the stapler (Fig. 27-2A, B). The NG tube should be withdrawn and reinserted into the proximal pouch to ensure that the tube is not stapled and that there is a patent pouch attached to the esophagus. The firing of

the stapler transects and staples both segments of the stomach. The pouch is again examined on both its anterior and its posterior surfaces to make certain that an acceptably small pouch has been formed. If the pouch is deemed to be too large, another application of the stapler is made to reduce the pouch to the desired size. The diaphragm, esophagus, stomach, and pancreas are carefully examined to make sure there are no tears or avulsed vessels that may bleed later. The cut edges of both the pouch and the bypassed stomach are imbricated with 3-0 Vicryl running sutures to reinforce the staple lines and ensure hemostasis (Fig. 27-3A, B).

A Silastic tube with two strands of 2-0 Prolene suture in it is passed through a window on the lesser curvature 2 to 2.5 cm from the caudal tip of the pouch and sutured to itself. A 7-cm tube is used in female patients, and a 7.5-cm tube is used in male patients. They are tied with a 1-cm overlap, leaving 6- and 6.5-cm functional circumferential lengths (Fig. 27-4A, B, C). This band provides for an outlet stoma that does not dilate (Fig. 27-5). The pouch between the esophagus and the band is about 15 to 20 ml in volume. The retrogastric space of the bypassed stomach is mobilized to provide a clear space through which the Roux limb can be brought.

Formation of the Roux-en Y Limb

A good vascular arcade is found between 30 and 75 cm from the ligament of Treitz, and the jejunum is transected at that point. The biliopancreatic limb is then fashioned by anastomosing the proximal divided jejunum side-to-side to the Roux limb about 60 cm from its cut edge. The mesenteric space between the Roux limb and the biliopancreatic limb is closed using nonabsorbable 3-0 sutures to minimize the occurrence of an internal hernia.

The Gastrojejunal Anastomosis

Once the Roux limb has been created and the mesenteric space closed, a window is made in the mesocolon into the

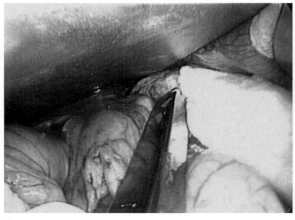
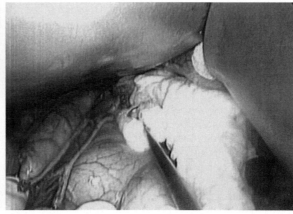

A   B

Figure 27-2. A. A 100-mm linear cutter stapler is passed through the window and completely encompasses the proximal pouch, which has an estimated volume of 25 ml. **B.** The transected proximal pouch.

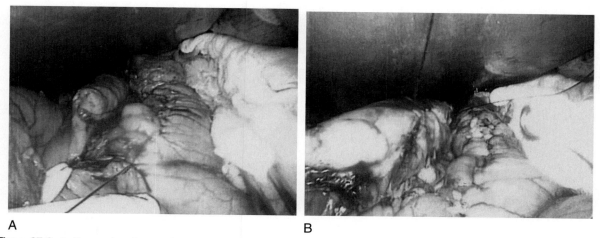

Figure 27-3. A. Oversewing the cut edge of the bypassed segment with absorbable sutures. **B.** Oversewing the cut edge of the pouch.

retrogastric space, just superior to the ligament of Treitz. Between 20 and 40 cm of the Roux limb are then passed into the retrogastric space. At this point, attention is directed to the pouch and the transected, bypassed stomach. The Roux limb in the retrogastric space is retrieved, brought up and out, and placed between the pouch and the

bypassed stomach (Fig. 27-6). The proximal segment of this limb is used to cover the cut-stapled edge of the pouch from the gastroesophageal junction to the band.

At least 0.5 cm distal to the band, a gastrojejunostomy is formed between the pouch and the jejunal limb. This consists of a tangential end-to-side anastomosis using 3-0 silk

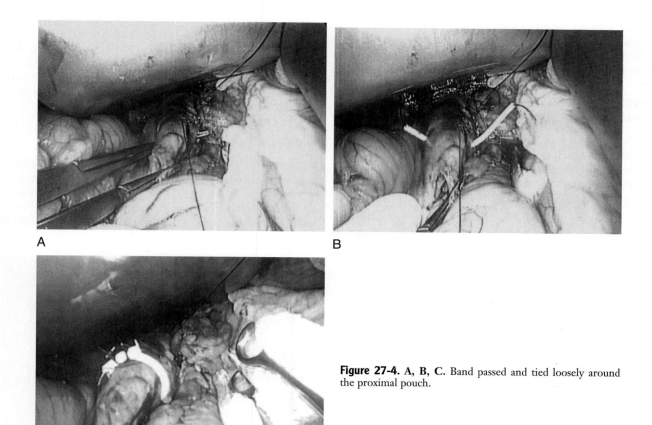

Figure 27-4. A, B, C. Band passed and tied loosely around the proximal pouch.

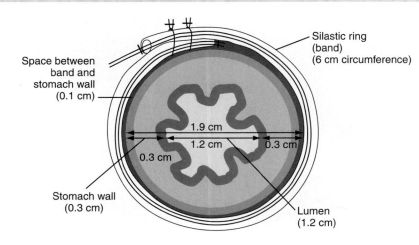

Figure 27-5. Transverse section through the banded stoma.

for the serosal layer and 3-0 Vicryl for the mucosal layer (Fig. 27-7). The staple line of the pouch is incorporated in the posterior suture line of the gastrojejunostomy. An 18F NG tube is advanced through the banded stoma, through the gastrojejunostomy, and into the Roux limb.

Once the gastrojejunal anastomosis is completed, the omentum and colon are retracted to expose the Roux limb as it passes through the mesocolon. This limb is then pulled down so that no redundant small bowel remains in the retrogastric space. The Roux limb is tagged to the mesocolon to prevent its prolapse into the retrogastric space. The space between the Roux limb and the retroperitonium is closed with 3-0 silk sutures to minimize internal herniation or volvulus formation. The previously made enteroenterostomy is reexamined for bleeding, patency, and kinking.

Placement of the Gastrostomy Tube and Marker Plus Closure

A site is chosen on the anterior wall of the bypassed stomach that will reach the abdominoperitoneal wall without tension, about three fingerbreadths below the left costal margin. Two purse-string sutures are placed concentrically, and a 16F gastrostomy tube is brought through the skin at a point at least three fingerbreadths below the left costal margin. The tube is inserted into a gastrostomy made in the middle of the purse-string sutures. The purse-string sutures are tied to prevent or minimize leakage around the tube. The tube, with the balloon inflated, is pulled up against the abdominal wall. Silk sutures are used to tack the gastrostomy site to the abdominal wall, causing a seal between the gastric and abdominal walls. An 8-cm Silastic ring tube is placed around the gastrostomy site. This is a radiopaque ring that acts as a marker for the gastrostomy site (Fig. 27-8). This marker is placed to assist radiologic visualization of the bypassed gastrointestinal segment for radiologic and endoscopic evaluation at any time after the operation (Fig. 27-9).[8]

The operation is completed by closure of the abdominal fascia with a double stranded Vicryl running suture. The subcutaneous layer is irrigated copiously with an antibiotic solution. The skin can be closed with either skin staples or subcuticular sutures and Steri-Strips.

Concurrent Operations

Concurrent operations include but are not limited to cholecystectomy, panniculectomy, herniorraphy, ovarian cystectomy, bilateral tubal ligation, hysterectomy, and oophorectomy. Any other surgical pathology may be addressed at the time of the primary procedure, as indicated.[9]

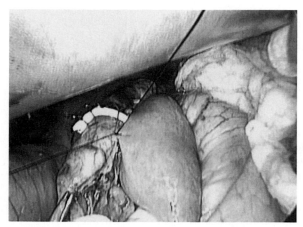

Figure 27-6. The efferent limb is brought up from the retrogastric space and used to plicate the edge of the pouch from the gastroesophageal junction to just after the band.

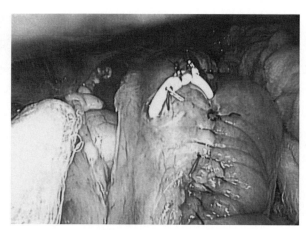

Figure 27-7. Gastrojejunostomy.

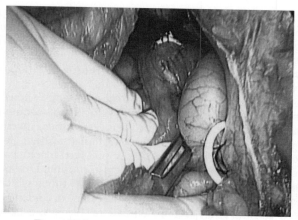

Figure 27-8. Gastrostomy site marker placement.

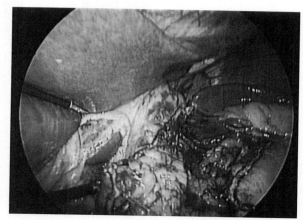

Figure 27-10. Laparoscopic transection of the proximal gastric pouch.

Laparoscopic Technique

This operation is currently being performed laparoscopically, preserving all of the details of the open approach. Six ports are usually necessary to perform the banded gastric bypass laparoscopically.

As in the open approach, once the exposure with insufflation and liver retraction has been made, the bare area of the lesser omentum is entered and the retrogastric space is mobilized with sharp and blunt dissection. There is usually a fat pad at the esophagogastrolienal junction just to the left of the esophagus. This area is mobilized, and an esophageal blade is passed through the bare area in the lesser omentum and brought out through the defect created at the esophagogastrolienial junction.

At this point, another window is made through the lesser omentum between the stomach and the neurovascular bundle at a point about 4 to 5cm from the gastrointestinal junction. An endosurgical three-row stapler is used to transect the stomach at a 45- to 60-degree angle (Fig. 27-10). The esophageal retractor is then passed through the space created by this transection. It is brought out at the gastroesophageal junction and used to expose the stomach for further transection. The endosurgical stapler is then placed to transect the pouch vertically. This maneuver is repeated to complete the transection of the pouch up to the angle of His. It usually entails two, and occasionally three, applications of the endosurgical stapler. The cut edge of both the pouch and the bypassed stomach are oversewn, just as in the open approach. The Silastic band is placed just as in the open approach (Fig. 27-11). The retrogastric space is then mobilized to provide for passage of the Roux limb once it is formed; again, just as in the open approach.

With the patient in the Trendelenburg position, the colon and omentum are retracted and the Roux limb fashioned. The only difference in forming the Roux limb

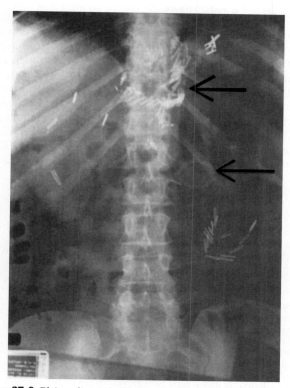

Figure 27-9. Plain radiograph showing the Silastic band and gastrostomy site marker.

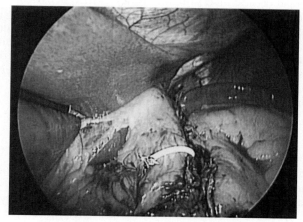

Figure 27-11. The placement of the Silastic band.

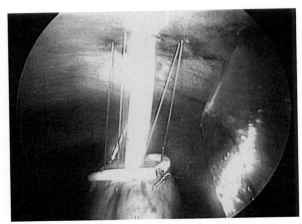

Figure 27-12. The placement of the gastrostomy site marker laparoscopically.

laparoscopically is that in the open approach, the entero-enterostomy opening is closed using a stapler, but in the laparoscopic approach, it is hand sewn. The mesenteric gap between the small bowel limbs is also closed, and through a window in the mesocolon, the Roux limb is passed into the retrogastric space. The plication with the proximal jejunal limb of the gastric pouch, the hand-sewn two-layer gastrojejunostomy, the reduction of the Roux limb from the retrogastric space, the suturing of the limb to the mesocolon and, finally, the closure of the retroperitoneal space are all done as in the open approach.

The gastrostomy tube and gastrostomy site marker are placed by passing the tube through the preformed ring into the stomach and then tying the purse-string sutures. The gastrostomy site of the stomach is sutured to the peritoneal surface of the abdominal wall with three equidistant sutures within the radiopaque marker ring and tied on the outside of the abdomen. (Fig. 27-12). Unlike the open procedure, a drain is routinely used in the laparoscopic approach.

Secondary Operations

Secondary operations are banded gastric bypass operations in patients with previous bariatric operations, such as jejunoileal bypass, gastric banding, various gastroplasties, biliopancreatic diversion, and other gastric bypass operations. These reoperations account for about 7% of all the banded gastric bypass operations we perform. A banded gastric bypass operation after a previous bariatric operation should be undertaken only if a vertical pouch on the lesser curvature can be formed safely. Secondary operations carry a higher incidence of complications than do primary operations.[10]

▶ PERIOPERATIVE CARE

Patient selection, with a few exceptions, follows the guidelines of the 1991 National Institutes of Health Consensus Statement on gastrointestinal surgery for obesity.[11] Preoperative evaluation entails a complete history and physical examination, including a detailed dietary history and listing of prior efforts at weight loss. All patients are seen by a multidisciplinary team that includes the surgeon, cardiologist, pulmonologist, psychologist/psychiatrist, patient counselor, and nutritionist. Other consultants are used as necessary. All patients have thorough laboratory screening evaluations.

Perioperative antibiotics, subcutaneous heparin, thromboembolic disease (TED) stockings, sequential compression devices for the lower extremities, incentive spirometers and, as indicated, continuous positive airway pressure or bilevel positive airway pressure machines are used routinely. Early ambulation is also routine. Drains are removed as indicated. The gastrostomy tube, which is connected to gravity drainage, becomes occluded after 36 to 48 hours and is removed in 7 to 10 days, usually in the office. Patients are started on ice chips 4 hours after returning from the operating room. A prescribed liquid diet is started on day 2 after operation, and the patient's diet is progressed on an outpatient basis. Contrast studies of the gastric pouch and outlet prior to discharge from the hospital are routine.

Perioperative Complications

The perioperative complications after the banded gastric bypass are the same as with other short-limb gastric bypass operations. They include intraoperative complications, atelectasis, wound problems, obstruction, leaks, deep vein thrombosis, pulmonary embolization, nausea, vomiting, mood swings, and depression (Table 27-1). It should be noted that the band markedly reduces the incidence of outlet stenosis requiring endoscopic dilation.

Long-Term Complications

Long-term complications after the banded gastric bypass are similar to those of most short-limb gastric bypass operations except that they demonstrate a lower incidence of inadequate weight loss as well as a lower incidence and magnitude of weight regain (Table 27-2). Complications include transient hair loss, marginal ulcers, diarrhea, hypoglycemia, dumping syndrome, and deficiency syndromes in vitamins A, D, and E and in calcium and iron. Band complications are seen in less than 3% of patients.[11] They consist mostly of band erosion and gastrojejunal or gastric fistulas.

Table 27-1	PERIOPERATIVE COMPLICATIONS OF THE BANDED GASTRIC BYPASS
Wound problems/infection/seroma	9.0%
Severe nausea	9.0%
Respiratory problems/atelectasis	3.0%
Leaks: pouch/anastomoses	0.8%
Pulmonary embolus	2.0%
Deep venous thrombosis	4.0%
Gastric ileus	3.0%
Depression/mood swings	5.0%
Death	0.4%

Table 27-2	LATE COMPLICATIONS OF BANDED GASTRIC BYPASS

Malnutrition
Vitamin and mineral deficiencies
Weight-loss failure
Excessive weight loss
Anorexia
Dehydration
Anemia
Osteoporosis
Constipation
Vomiting
Diarrhea
Nausea
Marginal ulcers
Incisional hernias
Small-bowel obstruction
Band erosion

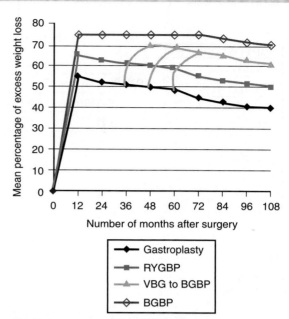

Figure 27-13. Long-term weight loss with various procedures evolving to the banded gastric bypass. RYGB, Roux-en-Y gastric bypass; VBG, vertical banded gastroplasty; BGBP, banded gastric bypass.

Revision/Conversion/Reversal Operations

The common indications for revision of the banded gastric bypass are inadequate weight loss, weight regain, excessive weight loss, and mechanical failures of the operation, such as outlet stenosis or obstruction, band erosion, and gastrogastric fistula with marginal ulceration and pain. Other (rare) indications include intractable diarrhea, intractable nausea, recurrent marginal ulcers, intractable anemia, and patient intolerance of the procedure.

The most common revision procedure after the banded gastric bypass is the shortening of the common channel to effect more weight loss.[12] When weight regain or inadequate weight loss is not caused by any mechanical or anatomic dysfunction associated with the operation, the banded gastric bypass is revised to effect more weight loss by increasing the malabsorptive component. The shortening of the common channel is also indicated in patients with significant weight regain following band removal for one reason or another. Occasionally, shortening is performed at the patient's request to maximize weight loss, in conjunction with another planned procedure. The degree of shortening of the common channel depends on how much weight the patient needs to lose as well as the patient's current bowel habits. Most commonly, the enteroenteric anastomosis that forms the Roux alimentary limb is equal in length to the Roux limb plus the common channel. Because this revision usually produces increased stool frequency with a watery consistency, it should not be done in a patient who already has more than six watery stools a day. Patients with increased malabsorption due to this reoperative procedure have been documented to have lowered their BMIs by 7 kg per m², or 60 lb. This occurs at the cost of an increased incidence of protein malnutrition, foul flatus and stool odor, and the need for more frequent biochemical monitoring.[13]

A few revision operations have been performed to take down gastrogastric or gastrojejunal fistulas. There have also been operations for conversion to vertical banded gastroplasty because of excessive weight loss, intractable nausea, intractable diarrhea, or intractable marginal ulceration not responsive to medication. Two of our cases were converted

9Y PEWL

TIME POST-OP	PEWL
0M	0.0
3M	37.2
6M	56.4
1Y	74.0
2Y	77.0
3Y	75.5
4Y	76.0
5Y	73.2
6Y	71.6
7Y	71.6
8Y	71.3
9Y	69.8

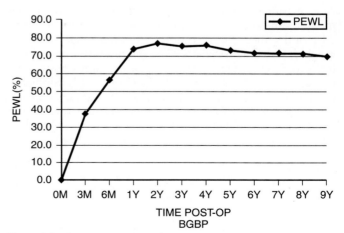

Figure 27-14. Excess weight loss with the banded gastric bypass after 9 years' follow-up. PEWL, percentage of excess weight loss.

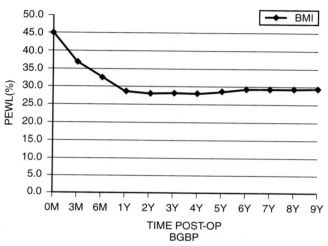

9Y BMI

TIME POST-OP	BMI
0M	44.7
3M	36.9
6M	32.8
1Y	28.8
2Y	28.0
3Y	28.2
4Y	28.1
5Y	28.7
6Y	29.2
7Y	29.1
8Y	29.1
9Y	29.3

IN BIM	
RANGE	35.6–64.6
AVE	44.7

Figure 27-15. BMI after nine years' follow-up after the banded gastric bypass. BMI, body mass index.

to banded gastroplasty because of short-bowel syndrome. Anatomic reversals of these operations have been performed because of recurrent marginal ulcers, patient intolerance, and anorexia. All reversal operations have, as a rule, resulted in rapid regain of the lost weight.

Weight Loss

After a banded gastric bypass, weight loss is rapid during the first 6 months and continues at a slower pace for up to 18 months after the operation. The percentage of excess weight loss in the first year is 77%, and this rate is maintained for 3 to 5 years (Fig. 27-13).[14-16] By the ninth postoperative year, it averages around 69.8% (Fig. 27-14). Similarly, the average BMI is maintained below 29.3kg per m², even after 9 years (Fig. 27-15). The success rate—that is, the percentage of patients with at least 50% excess weight loss after the banded gastric bypass—is 90% at 9 years.

▶ CONCLUSION

The banded gastric bypass operation enhances the restrictive component of the nonbanded short-limb gastric bypass. The augmented benefit of the increased percentage of weight loss, a lower incidence of outlet stenosis requiring endoscopic dilatation, and the increased weight-loss maintenance observed with the banded gastric bypass justifies the 3% incidence of band-related complications, which are usually inconsequential. Fisher summarized the effectiveness of the banded gastric bypass when he wrote "... adding the band to the gastric bypass results in more weight loss in more patients that is maintained over a longer period of time."[17]

▶ REFERENCES

1. Fobi MAL, Lee H, Fleming A: Surgical technique of the banded R-Y gastric bypass. J Obes 1989;8:99-103.
2. Mason EE: Vertical banded gastroplasty for morbid obesity. Arch Surg 1982;117:701-706.
3. Laws HL, Piantadosi S: Superior gastric reduction procedure for morbid obesity. Am J Surg 1981;193:334-340.
4. Crampton NA, Izvomikov V, Stubbs RS: Silastic ring gastric bypass: a comparison of two ring sizes: a preliminary report. Obes Surg1997;7:495-499.
5. Fobi MAL: Marginal ulcer after gastric bypass. Probl Gen Surg 1991;9:345-352.
6. Capella JF, Capella RF: Staple line disruption and marginal ulceration in gastric bypass procedures for weight reduction. Obes Surg 1996;6:44-49.
7. Fobi MAL, Lee H: The surgical technique of Fobi-pouch operation for obesity (the transected Silastic vertical gastric bypass). Obes Surg 1998;8:283-288.
8. Fobi MAL, Chicola K, Lee H: Access to the bypassed stomach after gastric bypass. Obes Surg1998;8:289-295.
9. Igwe D, Fobi M, Lee H: Panniculectomy: an adjuvant to obesity surgery. Obes Surg 2000;10:530-539.
10. Fobi MAL, Lee H, Holness R, et al: Gastric bypass operation for obesity. World J Surg 1998;22:925-935.
11. Fobi MAL, Lee H, Igwe D, et al: Band erosion: etiology, management and outcome after banded vertical gastric bypass. Obes Surg 2001;11:699-707.
12. Fobi MAL, Lee H, Igwe D Jr, et al: Revision of failed gastric bypass to distal Roux-en-Y gastric bypass: review of 65 cases. Obes Surg 2001;11:190-195.
13. Scopinaro N, Gianetta E, Adami GF, et al: Biliopancreatic diversion for obesity at eighteen years. Surgery 1996;119:261-268.
14. Fobi MAL, Lee H, Igwe D, et al: Transected Silastic ring vertical gastric bypass with jejunal interposition: a gastrostomy and a gastrostomy site marker (Fobi pouch operation for obesity). In Deitel M, Cowan GSM (eds): Update: Surgery for the Morbidly Obese Patient, pp. 203-226. Toronto, FD Communications, 2000.
15. Howard L, Malone M, Michalek A, et al: Gastric bypass and vertical banded gastroplasty: a prospective randomized comparison and 5-year follow-up. Obes Surg 1995;5:55-60.
16. Fobi MAL, Lee H, Igwe D Jr, et al: Prospective comparative evaluation of stapled versus transected Silastic ring gastric bypass: 6-year follow-up. Obes Surg 2001;11:18-24.
17. Fisher BL, Barber AE: Gastric bypass procedures. Eur J Gastroenterol Hepatol 1999;11:93-97.

28

Long-Limb Roux Gastric Bypass

Robert E. Brolin, M.D.

The concept of superobesity was introduced by Mason in 1987 after recognizing that the heaviest patients commonly failed to achieve satisfactory weight loss after vertical banded gastroplasty.[1] In that report, Mason and colleagues arbitrarily defined superobesity as being more than 225% above ideal weight. Mason noted that the mean percentage of excess weight loss (%EWL) in the heaviest patients was approximately 40%, in comparison with approximately 60% in the remaining, less obese patients. They concluded that "superobese patients are sufficiently different that they require separate analysis in any study of operations for the treatment of obesity." He also asserted that "they (the superobese) are the patients who are most resistant to treatment." The latter statement has subsequently been supported in virtually every published report of weight-loss outcomes following bariatric operations.

At about the same time, we arbitrarily defined super-obesity as being more than 200 lb above ideal weight.[2] Our definition was chosen to reflect a minimum weight limit that corresponded to twice the minimum weight criterion (>100 lb overweight) that was used at that time to define morbid obesity. Subsequent reports of weight loss after gastric bariatric operations have defined superobesity as a BMI greater than 50 kg per m².[3,4] It should be noted, however, that superobesity is not recognized as a distinct weight category by classification systems that have been designed to stratify various weight-loss treatment regimens.[5] Recently, bariatric surgeons have amplified the concept of superobesity by contributing new names such as "supra super" obesity and "mega" obesity to patients with BMIs greater than 60 kg per m² and 70 kg per m², respectively.[6,7]

There is sufficient justification for making a distinction between morbid obesity and superobesity. First, the prevalence of coexisting medical problems is considerably greater in the superobese, which implies a greater overall health risk.[8] Second, a host of bariatric surgeons have independently reported that the likelihood of successful weight loss in the superobese is substantially lower than in less obese patients after conventional bariatric restrictive operations.[1,2,9] It seems obvious that the heaviest patients must lose more weight to reach a level that would represent a valid reduction in their actuarial mortality risk.

▶ HISTORY OF LONG-LIMB ROUX GASTRIC BYPASS

Relatively few reports have focused on the effect of Roux limb length on postoperative weight loss. Our group was the first to publish a prospective randomized comparison of Roux limb length in bariatric surgical patients. This study was undertaken because we recognized that conventional Roux-en-Y gastric bypass (RYGB) did not consistently provide sufficient long-term weight loss in a substantial number of superobese patients. Hence, it seemed logical to add malabsorption to an operation that is primarily oriented toward restricting calorie intake. Our 1992 prospective randomized study showed that Roux limb length had a significant impact on weight loss in superobese patients after gastric bypass.[2] In that report, patients who had 150-cm Roux limbs experienced significantly greater weight loss than did patients who had 75-cm Roux limbs. There was no difference in the postoperative complication rate between the two groups.

In 1997, Freeman and colleagues reported a series of 55 patients that included 23 who had had RYGB with 90-cm Roux limbs and 32 patients who had had RYGB with 45-cm Roux limbs.[10] Although these patients were matched for age and gender, this series was not randomized. Nonetheless, mean EWL in the group with the longer Roux limb was approximately 6% greater 24 months postoperatively, with no difference in the incidence of metabolic sequelae or diarrhea in the two groups.

Sugerman and colleagues were the first to prospectively compare a small-pouch (30 ml) biliopancreatic diversion (BPD) procedure with conventional RYGB in superobese patients.[11] Although weight loss at 1 year was significantly greater in those with the small-pouch BPDs than in those with conventional RYGBs, Sugerman's small-pouch BPD patients had a greater than 50% incidence of serious postoperative complications and metabolic sequelae, including two deaths resulting from hepatic failure. Sugerman and colleagues concluded that the incidence and severity of metabolic complications after their modification of the BPD, which included a 50-cm common channel, was too great to justify its use as a primary operation for treatment of patients with superobesity. In the same report, Sugerman and colleagues described a series of 22 superobese patients who, after failing conventional RYGB, had a distal modification of the gastric bypass that incorporated a 150-cm common channel and a 30-ml-capacity gastric pouch. Of these 22 patients, 4 (18%) had subsequent surgical procedures (three reductions of bypassed bowel, one tube gastrostomy) to correct protein-calorie malnutrition. The mean %EWL in these patients was 67% at 3 years and 69% at 5 years. There was a high incidence of metabolic sequelae despite aggressive prophylaxis by means of multivitamins, calcium, and additional supplements of vitamins A, D, E, and B_{12}.

The Mayo Clinic group was the first to publish a series using a very, very long Roux limb.[12] Weight loss with this procedure, which was performed in 26 superobese patients, was compared with weight loss in 11 patients who had had the Scopinaro BPD. Weight loss in the group with the very, very long limbs was less than in the group with the BPDs at 2 years postoperatively (57% vs. 68% mean %EWL), and there was a comparable early morbidity rate. Unfortunately, the incidence of late metabolic sequelae was not included in the Mayo report. However, one patient who had BPD subsequently died of liver failure.

In 2000, MacLean and colleagues reported a significant difference in successful weight loss between patients with BMIs of less than 50 kg per m^2 in comparison with the heavier superobese patients who underwent isolated RYGBs.[13] In that series of 274 patients, the final mean BMI in 96 superobese patients was 35 + 7 kg per m^2 as opposed to 29 + 4 kg per m^2 for the less overweight group. Although the reduction in mean BMI was greater in the superobese group (21 kg/m^2 vs. 18 kg/m^2 in the less obese), MacLean classified 43% of the superobese group as "failures" because they did not lose 50% of their excess body weight or achieve BMIs of less than 35 kg per m^2.

One year later, MacLean and colleagues reported the results of a comparison of Roux limb lengths in the same group of 274 patients, with a mean follow-up interval of $5\frac{1}{2}$ years.[14] MacLean's short-limb group had 40-cm Roux limbs and 10-cm afferent limbs, whereas both the Roux limbs and afferent limbs were 100 cm in length in the long-limb patients. In superobese patients there was a significant difference in final mean BMI between the short-limb and the long-limb groups (35.8 kg/m^2 vs. 32.7 kg/m^2; $P = 0.049$). MacLean also observed that "a subgroup of patients, all of whom had a BMI greater than 60 kg/m^2, benefited most from long limb bypass."[14] Conversely, in the less obese group, the difference in final BMI among those with the different limb lengths was not significant. There was no difference in the incidence of nutrition problems in the groups with the different limb lengths.

Choban and Flancbaum performed a prospective randomized comparison of three Roux limb lengths in a group of 133 patients.[15] Patients with BMIs less than 50 kg per m^2 had Roux limbs that measured 75 cm and 150 cm, whereas the heavier patients had Roux limbs of 150 cm and 250 cm, respectively. In patients with BMIs of less than 50 kg per m^2, there was no difference in weight loss between the groups. However, in the superobese group, the patients who had Roux limbs of 250 cm had significantly greater weight loss at 18 months than did patients

who had 150-cm Roux limbs. This difference appeared to persist beyond 18 months, though statistical significance was lost due to the small number of patients followed at 2 years and beyond. There was no mention of the incidence of nutrition complications in that study.

The Mount Sinai group compared multiple Roux limb lengths in 58 patients who had laparoscopic RYGB.[16] These 58 patients collectively were not superobese, having mean BMIs of 44 kg per m^2. The short-limb group was composed of patients with limb lengths ranging from 45 to 100 cm; whereas the measurement in the long-limb group was constant at 150 cm. Limb lengths for individual patients were chosen on the basis of preoperative BMIs, with additional length added in increments as small as 5.0 cm! Although there was no significant difference in weight loss among the patients with the various Roux limb lengths, the authors noted that "a trend toward an increased portion of patients with more than 50% excess weight loss ($P = 0.07$) was observed in the group with the longer Roux limbs."

Although our 150-cm limb gastric bypass improved weight loss in superobese patients, we noted that recidivism was common 4 to 5 years postoperatively. On the basis of that observation, we decided to study a more malabsorptive modification of RYGB in which the enteroenterostomy was performed 75 cm proximal to the ileocecal junction. This distal modification of RYGB (D-RYGB) differs substantially from both BPD and the duodenal switch in that only 15 to 25 cm of the proximal jejunum is totally excluded from digestive continuity. We hypothesized that using a short afferent limb in D-RYGB would enhance malabsorption of dietary fat without producing the manifestations of protein malabsorption or clinically overt malnutrition that were associated with BPD. The first malabsorptive D-RYGB was performed by us in 1988. The results of our D-RYGB over the ensuing 10-year period were then retrospectively compared with those of superobese patients who underwent RYGB using two shorter Roux limb lengths.[8] Roux limb measurements in the short-limb group ranged from 50 to 75 cm in length. These procedures were generally performed prior to 1990. Conversely, most of the 150-cm Roux limb operations were performed following the conclusion of our 1992 prospective randomized study. In the short and the 150-cm Roux limb groups the length of bowel below the jejunojejunostomy was not measured. Conversely, in patients who underwent D-RYGB, the common channel measurement below the jejunoileostomy was constant at 75 cm above the ileocecal junction, with Roux limb measurements ranging from 265 to 570 cm. The gastric restrictive parameters and the lengths of the afferent (bypassed) jejunum were the same for all patients. Examples of these techniques are illustrated in Figure 28-1.

The preoperative characteristics of the patients in our 2002 report are shown in Table 28-1. All patients were more than 200 lb overweight preoperatively, and all but one had BMIs of more than 50 kg per m^2. There was no difference in mean age or gender distribution among the three groups. However, the mean weights and BMIs of patients undergoing D-RYGB were significantly greater than those of patients in the two shorter-Roux-limb groups. Table 28-2 and Table 28-3 show the obesity-related

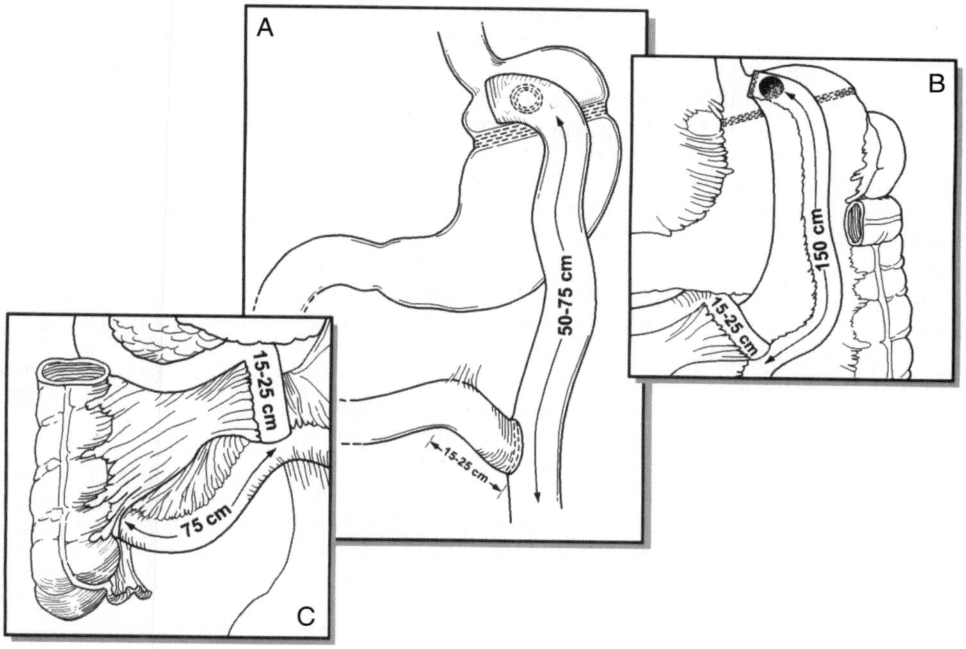

Figure 28-1. Roux-en-Y gastric bypass in each of the three limb-length groups was performed using the TA-90-B stapler (U.S. Surgical Corp., Norwalk, Conn.) to partition the cardia of the stomach, creating a 20 + 5 ml upper pouch. The jejunum is divided approximately 15 to 25 cm distal to the ligament of Treitz, with the distal end anastomosed to the upper stomach using a circular stapler to create a 1.1-cm-diameter anastomosis. The proximal end of jejunum is then anastomosed to the jejunum (**A** and **B**) or the ileum (**C**).

comorbidities in the study cohort. Only 35 patients (12%) in this study did not have at least one comorbidity. All but two of the patients without comorbidities were under the age of 40. There were significant differences in the incidence of comorbidities among the three operative groups, with sleep apnea, cardiac disease, and venous stasis being more prevalent in D-RYGB patients.

Follow-up in this report ranged from 6 months to 16 years. Mean follow-up was 60 + 46 months in the short-limb group, 37 + 34 months in 150-cm patients, and 46 + 25 months in the D-RYGB group. The follow-up rate at 3 years was 80% in the short-limb group, 68% in 150-cm patients, and 85% in D-RYGB patients. At 5 years, the follow-up rate was 66% of 88 available patients in the

Table 28-1	PREOPERATIVE PATIENT CHARACTERISTICS			
OPERATIVE GROUP	WEIGHT	BMI	AGE	GENDER (M/F)
Short limb	331±54	56.9±7	38.4±10	17/82
150 cm	356±57	55.3±7	39.4±9	35/117
D-RYGB	*448±76	*67.5±8	37.6±9	20/27

Data expressed as mean ± SD. Weight in pounds; body mass index (BMI) in kg/m²; age in years. The * indicates a significant difference between distal Roux-en-Y gastric bypass (D-RYGB) patients versus the other two groups ($P<0.05$ by ANOVA with Student-Neuman-Keuls test). (Reproduced courtesy of Elsevier Science Inc., New York.)

Table 28-2	MEDICAL COMORBIDITIES		
	SHORT (N = 99)	150 CM (N = 152)	D-RYGB (N = 47)
Hypertension	61 (62%)	78 (51%)	32 (68%)
Arthritis	45 (45%)	53 (35%)	20 (43%)
Asthma	22 (22%)	25 (16%)	6 (13%)
Hyperlipidemia	18 (18%)	29 (19%)	6 (13%)
Diabetes	9 (9%)	31 (21%)	8 (17%)
Cardiac disease*	13 (13%)	15 (10%)	12 (26%)*
Sleep apnea*	5 (5%)	30 (20%)	22 (47%)*
Venous stasis*	12 (12%)	12 (8%)	15 (32%)*

The number and percentage of patients with each comorbidity is listed for each group. The * indicates significantly greater prevalence of a comorbidity in distal Roux-en-Y gastric bypass (D-RYGB) patients versus the other groups ($P<0.02$ by chi square test). (Reproduced courtesy of Elsevier Science Inc., New York.)

Table 28-3	IMPROVEMENT OF COMORBIDITIES ANALYZED AT 3 YEARS POSTOPERATIVELY		
	RESOLVED	IMPROVED	UNCHANGED
Hypertension	74	56	5
Arthritis	4	81	4
Asthma	6	31	2
Hyperlipidemia	22	15	3
Diabetes	32	6	—
Cardiac disease	7	26	1
Sleep apnea	21	26	1
Venous stasis	5	20	3
	167(38%)	261(58%)	19(4%)

Comorbidities were considered resolved after normalization without the need for medication; they were considered improved when controlled by lower doses of medication than required preoperatively.

short-limb group, 64% of 56 available patients in the 150-cm group, and 78% of 22 available patients in the D-RYGB group.

Figure 28-2 and Figure 28-3 show postoperative weight loss expressed in pounds and as reduction in BMI units. Weight loss typically stabilized at 12 to 18 months after the shorter Roux-limb-length procedures. Weight loss after D-RYGB tended to last longer, with many patients reaching their nadirs between 24 and 36 months postoperatively. The lowest mean BMIs in the short-Roux-limb group was noted at 18 months postoperatively, whereas the lowest mean BMIs observed after the 150-cm and D-RYGB procedures were observed at 2 and 3 years, respectively. There were significant differences in weight loss among the three groups that favored the longer Roux limb lengths. These differences were apparent as early as 6 months postoperatively between D-RYGB and the shorter Roux limb lengths. The significantly greater weight loss provided by D-RYGB persisted through 5 years. Significant differences in weight loss between the short-limb D-RYGB group and the 150-cm group were apparent at 12 months postoperatively and persisted beyond that point. Some recidivism after 3 years was noted in all groups; the greatest weight regain was observed in the short-Roux-limb group.

The greatest mean %EWL in the short-limb patients was 56% at 18 months postoperatively as compared with 61% at 24 months postoperatively in the 150-cm group and 64% at 3 years in the D-RYGB patients. The number of patients who achieved more than a 50% loss of excess weight at some point during the study was 65 (65%) in the short-limb group, 114 (76%) in the 150-cm group, and 36 (80%) in the D-RYGB group. However, mean %EWL had declined to 45% by 5 years after short-limb RYGB and to 51% at 5 years in the 150-cm group. There was a lesser decline in mean EWL after D-RYGB, with maintenance in the range of 60% through 5 years postoperatively.

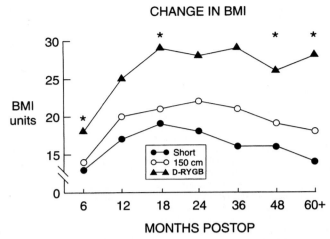

Figure 28-3. Change in body mass index (BMI) through 5 years postoperatively. There were significant differences among the groups at 12, 24, and 36 months postoperatively. The * indicates a significant difference between the distal Roux-en-Y gastric bypass (D-RYGB) patients and the short-limb groups. The difference was noted at 6, 18, 48, and 60 months (P<0.05 by ANOVA with Student-Newman-Keuls test). (Reproduced courtesy of Elsevier Science Inc., New York).

However, the difference in mean EWL at 5 years between the 150-cm and the D-RYGB groups was not significant.

Early postoperative complications in the three groups are shown in Table 28-4. There were minimal differences in the incidence of early complications among the three procedures. The overall incidence of early complications was 6.4%. The one perioperative death occurred in a 50-year-old, 354-lb woman whose BMI was 65.0 kg per m² and who had an uncomplicated 5-day postoperative course. She was readmitted 12 days later with pulmonary embolism and died 2 days after that admission as a result of cardiac arrest secondary to another embolus.

Late complications (30 days postoperatively) are shown in Table 28-5 and Table 28-6. There was a similar

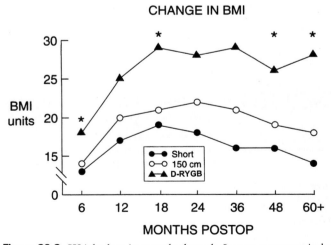

Figure 28-2. Weight loss in pounds through 5 years postoperatively. There were significant differences among each of the three groups at more than 1 year postoperatively. The * indicates a significant difference among the short-limb group as opposed to the distal Roux-en-Y gastric bypass (D-RYGB) group and the 150-cm patients at 6 months postoperatively. (P<0.05 by ANOVA with Student-Newman-Keuls test). (Reproduced courtesy of Elsevier Science Inc., New York).

Table 28-4	**EARLY COMPLICATIONS**		
COMPLICATION	SHORT (N = 99)	150 CM (N = 152)	D-RYGB (N = 47)
Wound infection	—	1	2
Leaks	1	2	1
Pulmonary embolism	—	3*	—
SBO	—	2	—
GI bleeding	—	1	—
Wound dehiscence	1	1	1
Bowel fistula	—	3	—
Total	2 (2%)	13 (8%)	4 (9%)

The leaks included three acute disruptions of the stapled gastric partition that were caused by violent retching and one esophageal perforation. The two cases of bowel obstruction were treated successfully by tube decompression. The dehiscences included two in the midline fascial closure and one major skin-level disruption. There were two small-bowel fistulae related to erosion of the polypropylene mesh used in prior hernia repairs; there was one jejunal perforation that occurred at a stay suture site at 3 weeks postoperatively.

D-RYGB, distal Roux-en-Y gastric bypass; SBO, small bowel obstruction; the * indicates that the one death in this series was caused by pulmonary embolism. (Reproduced courtesy of Elsevier Science Inc., New York.)

Table 28-5 LATE COMPLICATIONS

COMPLICATION	SHORT (N = 99)	150 CM (N = 152)	D-RYGB (N = 47)
Incisional hernia	14 (19%)	20 (13%)	7 (15%)
Marginal ulcer	4 (4%)	8 (5%)	5 (11%)
Staple disruption	2 (2%)	6 (4%)	2 (4%)
SBO	1 (2%)	6 (4%)	—
Stomal stenosis	2 (2%)	2 (1%)	1 (2%)
Liver failure	—	—	1 (2%)
Total	22 (22%)	41 (27%)	15 (32%)

All patients with stomal stenoses were hospitalized for intractable postprandial emesis. Patients with stomal stenoses who subsequently were found to have ulcers were included in the ulcer category. The ulcers associated with staple disruption were combined as one rather than considered as two separate complications in calculating the overall incidence of late complications in each group. D-RYGB, distal Roux-en-Y gastric bypass; SBO, small bowel obstruction. (Reproduced courtesy of Elsevier Science Inc., New York.)

incidence of specific complications among the three groups, except for marginal ulcer, which was more common in D-RYGB patients. Diarrhea, defined as three or more loose stools per day, was noted in 17 patients (36%) after D-RYGB; in 1 patient in the 150-cm group; and in none of the short-limb patients. The quality of loose stools in the D-RYGB patients was consistent with steatorrhea. All D-RYGB patients followed for at least 2 years had at least one metabolic abnormality. No deficiencies in protein or fat-soluble vitamins were noted in the shorter-limb groups. There were 5 late deaths. The 3 deaths in the short-limb group and the 1 death in the 150-cm group were not related to the operation. However, a 33-year-old man with preexisting cirrhosis died of hepatic failure 9 months after D-RYGB. It is possible that the operation played a role in this death.

There were 25 revision operations in this series of 298 patients (8.7%), including 12 in the short-limb group (12%); 11 of them were performed for unsatisfactory weight loss and 1 for a marginal ulcer. The 13 revision procedures in the 150-cm group (8.5%) included 7 for unsatisfactory weight loss and 6 for nonhealing marginal ulcers. There were no reoperations for unsatisfactory weight loss or nutritional complications in D-RYGB patients. However, one D-RYGB patient (2.1%) required reoperation for an intractable marginal ulcer. Of the patients (35%) who required reoperation, 9 had disruption of the stapled gastric partition, including 6 of the 9 patients who had intractable marginal ulcers. In addition, 35 patients in this series (12%) required repair of incisional hernias, and

14 subsequently underwent cholecystectomy for symptomatic gallstones.

MECHANISMS OF WEIGHT LOSS

Because of the high rate of recidivism with purely gastric restrictive operations, the pendulum in American bariatric surgery has clearly swung away from restriction towards malabsorption. Malabsorptive modifications of RYGB—Scopinaro's BPD and the so-called duodenal switch—are now being performed in large numbers in the United States. The driving forces behind lengthening the Roux limb, thereby adding malabsorption to the gastric restriction inherent in RYGB, have been unsatisfactory weight loss, recidivism, or both after RYGB performed with conventional limb lengths.

The precise mechanisms by which gastric bypass procedures produce weight loss have not been extensively studied. There have been virtually no animal studies that have measured the absorption of nutrients following gastric bariatric operations. In the mid-1970s, Scopinaro evaluated several modifications of BPD in dogs in order to determine a measurement for the common channel that would minimize diarrhea and electrolyte imbalance yet promote the fat excretion resulting from malabsorption.[17] These studies resulted in the 50-cm common channel length that has been used in Scopinaro's BPD during the past 25 years. Comparable studies in animals have not been performed using the duodenal switch or other malabsorptive modifications of RYGB.

Ghrelin is a recently identified hormone that has been associated with increased appetite in both animals and man. In 2002, Cummings showed that ghrelin levels were markedly reduced during the first few months after RYGB.[18] It is generally acknowledged that RYGB patients "lose their appetite" during the first few months postoperatively. However, appetite typically returns after the first year, which temporally coincides with cessation of weight loss. Although the role of ghrelin in this process is unknown, further studies may clarify the involvement of ghrelin in the mechanisms associated with weight loss following gastric bypass.

Remarkably, no clinical studies have carefully measured the absorption of macronutrients after any technique of RYGB. In 1992, our group showed that weight-loss maintenance after conventional RYGB is related to postoperative calorie intake, in that recidivism generally occurred when calorie intake exceeded 1500 calories per day

Table 28-6 POSTOPERATIVE METABOLIC DEFICIENCIES

OPERATION	IRON	B$_{12}$	ANEMIA	VIT A	VIT D	CALCIUM	ALBUMIN
Short (n = 80)	42 (52%)	30 (37%)	33 (41%)	—	—	—	—
150 cm (n = 102)	46 (45%)	34 (33%)	36 (35%)	—	—	—	—
D-RYGB (n = 39)	19 (49%)	3 (8%)*	29 (74%)*	4 (10%)	20 (51%)	4 (10%)	5 (13%)

n = the number of patients followed. Numbers and percentages corresponding to the incidence of deficiency are noted below each nutrient. Dashes indicate that these nutrients were not measured in the shorter limb groups. The * indicates a significant difference between distal Roux-en-Y gastric bypass (D-RYGB) patients and the other two groups ($P<0.003$ by chi square test). (Reproduced courtesy of Elsevier Science Inc., New York.)

in women and 1800 calories per day in men.[2] Patients who restricted their intake of high-calorie liquids and soft junk food invariably maintained their weight losses. Because mean calorie intake was consistently greater in the 150-cm than in the short-limb patients, the superior weight loss in the 150-cm group could be attributed to greater fat malabsorption resulting from more distal diversion of bile and pancreatic secretions in the functional digestive tract.

Our goal in comparing 75-cm to 150-cm Roux limbs was to see whether adding a relatively small increment of biliopancreatic diversion would improve weight loss. Because the total length of the small bowel (jejunum and ileum) is usually greater than 300 cm, we did not anticipate problems with electrolyte loss or protein-calorie malnutrition in our 150-cm patients. Conversely, we anticipated a greater number of metabolic complications after D-RYGB than after more conventional techniques of RYGB. However, we hoped to minimize hypoproteinemia and other serious nutrition problems by selecting patients who were committed to regular blood testing and long-term follow-up. We designed the D-RYGB with the hypothesis that the "passive" malabsorptive component might limit later weight regain and improve weight-loss maintenance. This hypothesis was based on the superlative weight maintenance reported in Scopinaro's series of BPD patients who were followed for 17 years.[19] Further support for the notion that a combination of restriction and malabsorption is more potent than either mechanism alone was provided by Scopinaro and colleagues when they modified the original BPD by reducing gastric capacity from 500 ml to 200 ml in superobese patients (the so-called very-little-stomach modification) in order to improve weight loss.[20] Remarkably, Scopinaro has not published results that show the long-term impact of gastric pouch volume on weight loss after BPD.

Other surgeon investigators have designed malabsorptive modifications of RYGB in order to improve long-term weight loss in superobese patients. The Mayo Clinic group's very-very-long-limb RYGB was remarkably similar to our D-RYGB, incorporating a 20- to 30-ml gastric pouch, a short afferent limb, and a 100-cm common channel.[12] The Medical College of Virginia group's distal RYGB incorporated a small gastric pouch, a 145-cm Roux limb, a 250- to 400-cm biliopancreatic limb, and a 150-cm common channel.[11] This "distal" RYGB more closely resembles BPD and the duodenal switch than our D-RYGB in that at least 50% of the small bowel is totally excluded from the functional digestive tract. Both BPD and the duodenal switch include transection of the small intestine near its midpoint and exclusion of nearly 50% of the small bowel from the functional digestive tract.[20,21]

The role of inadequate oral intake in the development of severe nutrition complications after combined restrictive-malabsorptive bariatric operations is generally acknowledged but poorly documented. There is solid evidence that both appetite and satiety are suppressed following jejunoileal bypass, suggesting that short-circuiting the bowel may trigger a variety of neural and endocrine signals that affect energy intake. Condon and colleagues noted a significant reduction in mean calorie intake compared to that of preoperative levels after jejunoileal bypass.[22] In fact, reduced intake, rather than malabsorption, accounted for nearly all of the observed weight loss in more than 40% of patients

in their series. Naslund and colleagues reported a decreased desire to eat after jejunoileal bypass in comparison with normal subjects. This reduction in desire to eat was associated with prolonged gastric emptying and decreased serum cholecystokinin levels.[23] Although it is generally believed that weight loss after BPD and the duodenal switch is due primarily to intestinal malabsorption rather than restriction of intake, Scopinaro has repeatedly described the "postcibal" effects of BPD, which can be summarized as protracted nausea. This nausea is occasionally severe enough to limit oral intake markedly. The author has observed a similar postcibal syndrome in a few patients who had D-RYGB. Unfortunately, there are no objective data that associate postoperative malnutrition with the postcibal syndrome that occasionally follows BPD. However, it seems clear that adding malabsorption to gastric restriction carries an increased metabolic price.

▶ RISK-BENEFIT ANALYSIS AND PATIENT SELECTION

Risk for Morbidity and Mortality

It is generally acknowledged that the rate of postoperative complications is increased in the heaviest bariatric surgical patients. In 1992, Sugerman and colleagues reported a 4.0% mortality rate in patients with sleep apnea as opposed to a 0.2% rate in the remaining patients who had undergone RYGB.[24] The patients with sleep apnea were also significantly heavier (mean weight = 164 kg vs. 135 kg; $P<0.0001$) than the remaining patients. In 2000, Sugerman and colleagues reported an 8% mortality rate in patients who had chronic venous insufficiency prior to undergoing RYGB.[25] Closer inspection of the patients who were the focus of that paper disclosed an older (mean age = 44 ± 10 years) and heavier (mean BMI = 61 ± 12 kg/m^2) group of patients with a significantly greater prevalence of other serious comorbidities. Our early complication rate in superobese patients is more than twice the morbidity rate previously reported in our lighter bariatric surgical patients.[26] In a recent retrospective study, Livingston and colleagues showed that weight (in pounds) was an independent predictor of "severe life-threatening adverse outcome," though BMI was not.[27]

Nutritional and Metabolic Risk

Several metabolic risks are inherent in RYGB. Unfortunately, the metabolic side effects of RYGB and BPD are grossly underinvestigated. I am unaware of any animal studies that have evaluated metabolic deficiencies in models of RYGB. The 30% to 40% incidence of postoperative vitamin and mineral deficiencies following the two shorter limb operations at our medical center is similar to the incidence of these deficiencies reported by other investigators after conventional RYGB with similar lengths of follow-up.[28-30] Our 20-year experience with 150-cm Roux limb procedures has shown no difference in the incidence of postoperative metabolic sequelae between 150-cm and shorter-Roux-limb patients. All postoperative vitamin and mineral deficiencies in our shorter-Roux-limb groups were managed on an outpatient basis. The great majority of metabolic sequelae in our D-RYGB patients were also managed in the outpatient setting. However, 2 of our 5 D-RYGB patients with low protein/albumin levels were hospitalized so they could receive parenteral nutritional support. Both patients had troublesome postprandial vomiting in addition to rapid weight loss. Of the two patients, one had the stigmata of zinc deficiency. Although the incidence of most metabolic sequelae after our D-RYGB is similar to that reported after BPD and the duodenal switch, the incidence and severity of protein-calorie malnutrition appear to be lower after D-RYGB.

Isolated cases of fatal hepatic failure are reported after various malabsorptive bariatric procedures, including distal modifications of RYGB.[11,12] Remarkably, Marceau and colleagues reported 11 cases of subsequently improved hepatic histopathology in patients with cirrhosis who had had the duodenal switch.[31] We were aware of Marceau's results, so the death from hepatic failure after D-RYGB in our series was unexpected, even in the setting of preexisting cirrhosis. On the basis of that negative experience, we do not perform D-RYGB in patients with cirrhosis. The virtual certainty of developing at least one metabolic deficiency coupled with the potential for developing diarrhea and protein-calorie malnutrition strongly suggest that D-RYGB should not be offered to patients who are not committed to long-term follow-up.

The prevention and control of metabolic deficiencies after RYGB should be easily accomplished in most patients. All patients should take a multivitamin supplement containing minerals postoperatively. Oral iron supplements containing at least 50 mg of elemental iron are recommended to all menstruating women. Many bariatric surgeons recommend prophylactic supplements of vitamin B_{12}. After short-limb RYGB, hemoglobin, hematocrit, and serum levels of iron/iron binding capacity and vitamin B_{12} should be measured at 6-month intervals during the first 2 years, then annually thereafter. Additional tests in patients who have D-RYGB or other malabsorptive modifications of RYGB should include serum electrolytes, albumin, total protein, calcium, bilirubin, serum glutamic-oxaloacetic transaminase, alkaline phosphatase, vitamin A, and vitamin D_{25}-OH. In patients who develop metabolic deficiencies, laboratory tests should be repeated at 3- to 6-month intervals until the deficiency has been corrected. Patient noncompliance in regularly taking vitamins and other nutritional supplements and in returning for follow-up blood tests is a primary cause of the development and progression of most metabolic deficiencies observed after RYGB.

Benefits

The primary goal of all bariatric operations is sustained weight loss sufficient to ameliorate obesity-related medical comorbidities. However, defining *successful* outcome after weight loss surgery is a complex issue. Loss of 50% of the excess weight has been used for many years as a minimum criterion to define successful weight loss following bariatric operations.[32,33] The mean BMI at the point of maximum weight loss among the superobese patients in our 2002 study was 37.3 kg per m^2 in short-limb patients; 35.8 kg per m^2 in RYGB 150-cm patients; and 38.6 kg per m^2 in D-RYGB patients. Calculated BMIs for patients who are approximately 50% overweight fall in the range of 34 kg per m^2 to 36.5 kg per m^2. The mean BMI of 42.0 kg per m^2, recorded in short-limb patients at 5 years postoperatively, corresponds to approximately 100% overweight and exceeds the BMI limit of 40 kg per m^2 that was established by the 1991 National Institutes of Health Consensus Development Panel as the minimum definition of morbid obesity.[34] Only 51 of the 298 superobese patients (17%) in our 2002 report stabilized at BMIs less than 30 kg per m^2 (approximately 20% overweight), and only 15 (6%) reached BMIs of less than 25 kg per m^2 (normal weight) at the nadir of weight loss. These BMI data provoke questions about the realistic and worthwhile weight-loss goals for superobese patients after bariatric operations. It is probably unrealistic to expect that most patients with preoperative BMIs exceeding 50 kg per m^2 will reach BMIs of less than 30 kg per m^2 after weight stabilization.

Although our 2002 report showed significantly greater weight loss after D-RYGB than after the two shorter Roux-limb lengths, this difference was confounded by the significant difference in both preoperative weight and BMI between the D-RYGB group and the shorter-Roux-limb patients. Conversely, the significant difference in both weight and BMI units lost between the short-limb and the 150-cm limb patients over a 5-year period provides solid evidence that adding even modest malabsorption in the form of longer Roux limb lengths results in superior long-term weight loss in superobese patients. However, lengthening the Roux limb to 150 cm did not prevent weight regain; the degree of recidivism in both our short-limb and 150-cm-limb patients was similar after 3 years. Conversely, recidivism was less after D-RYGB, suggesting that more malabsorption may provide better weight loss maintenance in the long term. This experience affirms the precept that in order to account for recidivism, a valid analysis of any obesity operation requires postoperative follow-up of at least 5 years.

Improvements in both coexisting medical problems and general lifestyle are dramatic among patients who lose substantial amounts of weight. The 96% incidence of improvement in or resolution of medical problems among patients in our 2002 report was substantially greater than the incidence of successful weight loss outcome, in that 28% of patients in that study did not lose at least 50% of their excess weight. Moreover, there is virtually no regression of improved or resolved medical problems in patients who maintain satisfactory weight loss. Conversely, improvement or resolution of medical problems is limited or transient in some patients who either do not lose 50% of their excess weight or regain a substantial portion of their lost weight.[33,35] The critical unanswered question is whether the greater weight loss and improvement of comorbidities that follow malabsorptive bariatric operations provide sufficient justification for the greater severity, prevalence, and cost of the anticipated metabolic sequelae.

Patient Selection

The great preponderance of data demonstrates that increasing the length of the Roux limb in RYGB produces significantly greater postoperative weight loss in superobese patients in comparison with conventional short-limb RYGB. Conversely, available data indicate no benefit of longer Roux limbs in bariatric patients with BMIs of less than 50 kg per m^2.[14-16] The 150-cm Roux limb has produced significantly better long-term weight loss than have the shorter Roux limb procedures during our 20-year experience with this technique. Moreover, there has been no difference in the incidence or severity of metabolic sequelae between the groups of patients who had 150-cm limbs or short limbs. Protein-calorie malnutrition has not been recognized in any of our patients with 150-cm limbs. Although the malabsorptive D-RYGB produced greater weight loss and better weight-loss maintenance than the two shorter limb-length procedures in our 2002 report, the higher incidence of metabolic complications in D-RYGB patients coupled with the unpredictability in postoperative follow-up mitigate against its routine use for all superobese patients. We currently offer D-RYGB to carefully screened patients with BMIs above 60 kg per m^2 who are committed to long-term follow-up. Compliance with follow-up is the key to minimizing the metabolic risks associated with malabsorptive modifications of RYGB.

▶ REFERENCES

1. Mason EE, Doherty C, Maher JW, et al: Super obesity and gastric reduction procedures. Gastroenterol Clin North Am 1987;16:495-502.
2. Brolin RE, Kenler HA, Gorman JG, et al: Long-limb gastric bypass in the super-obese: a prospective randomized study. Ann Surg 1992;215:387-395.
3. Benotti PN, Hollingsworth J, Mascioli EA, et al: Gastric restrictive operations for morbid obesity. Am J Surg 1989;157:150-155.
4. Yale CE: Gastric surgery for morbid obesity: complications and long-term weight control. Arch Surg 1989;124:941-947.
5. Bray GA: Definition, measurement and classification of the syndromes of obesity. Int J Obes 1978;2:99-112.
6. Higa KD, Boone KB, Ho T, et al: Laparoscopic Roux-en-Y gastric bypass for morbid obesity: technique and preliminary results of our first 400 patients. Arch Surg 2000;135:1029-1034.
7. Kreitz K, Rovito PF: Laparoscopic Roux-en-Y gastric bypass in the "megaobese." Arch Surg 2003;138:707-709.
8. Brolin RE, Lamarca LB, Kenler HA, et al: Malabsorptive gastric bypass in patients with super obesity. J Gastrointest Surg 2002,6:195-205.
9. MacLean LD, Rhode BM, Forse RA: Late results of vertical banded gastroplasty for morbid and super obesity. Surgery 1990;107:20-27.
10. Freeman JB, Kotlarewsky M, Phoenix C: Weight loss after extended gastric bypass. Obes Surg 1997;7:337-344.
11. Sugerman JH, Kellum JM, DeMaria EJ: Conversion of proximal to distal gastric bypass for failed gastric bypass for superobesity. J Gastrointest Surg 1997;1:517-525.
12. Murr MM, Balsiger BM, Kennedy FP, et al: Malabsorptive procedures for severe obesity: comparison of pancreaticobiliary bypass and very, very, long Roux-en-Y gastric bypass. J Gastrointest Surg 1998;3:607-612.
13. MacLean LD, Rhode BM, Nohr CW: Late outcome of isolated gastric bypass. Ann Surg 2000;231:524-528.
14. MacLean LD, Rhode BM, Nohr CW: Long-or short-limb gastric bypass? J Gastrointest Surg 2001;5:525-530.
15. Choban PS, Flancbaum LJ: The effect of Roux limb lengths on outcome after Roux-en-Y gastric bypass: a prospective randomized clinical trial. Obes Surg 2002;12:540-545.
16. Feng JJ, Gagner M, Pomp A, et al: Effect of standard vs extended Roux limb length on weight loss outcomes after laparoscopic Roux-en-Y gastric bypass. Surg Endosc 2003;17:1055-1060.
17. Scopinaro N, Gianetta E, Civalleri D, et al: Biliopancreatic bypass for obesity: an experimental study in dogs. Br J Surg 1979;66:613-617.
18. Cummings D, Weigle D, Frayo R, et al: Plasma ghrelin levels after diet-induced weight loss or gastric bypass surgery. N Engl J Med 2002;346:1623-1630.
19. Scopinaro N, Gianetta E, Adami GF, et al: Biliopancreatic diversion for obesity at eighteen years. Surg 1996;119:261-268.
20. Scopinaro N, Gianetta E, Friedman D, et al: Biliopancreatic diversion for obesity. Probl Gen Surg 1992;9:362-379.
21. Lagace M, Marceau P, Marceau S, et al: Biliopancreatic diversion with a new type of gastrectomy: some previous conclusions revisited. Obes Surg 1995;5:411-416.
22. Condon S, Janes N, Wise L, et al: Role of caloric intake in the weight loss after jejunoileal bypass for obesity. Gastroenterology 1978;74:34-37.
23. Naslund E, Melin I, Gryback P, et al: Reduced food intake after jejunoileal bypass: a possible association with prolonged gastric emptying and altered gut hormone patterns. Am J Clin Nutr 1997;65:26-32.
24. Sugerman HJ, Fairman RP, Sood PK: Long-term effects of gastric surgery for treating respiratory insufficiency of obesity. Am J Clin Nutr 1992;55(suppl):597-601.
25. Sugerman HJ, Sugerman EL, Wolfe L, et al: Risks/benefits of gastric bypass in morbidly obese patients with severe venous stasis disease. Ann Surg 2001;234:41-46.
26. Brolin RE, Robertson LB, Kenler HA, et al: Weight loss and dietary intake after vertical banded gastroplasty and Roux-en-Y gastric bypass. Ann Surg 1994;220:782-790.
27. Livingston EH, Huerta H, Arthur D, et al: Male gender is a predictor of morbidity and age a predictor of mortality for patients undergoing gastric bypass surgery. Ann Surg 2002;236:576-582.
28. Halverson JD, Zuckerman GR, Koehler RE, et al: Gastric bypass for morbid obesity: a medical-surgical assessment. Ann Surg 1981;194:152-160.
29. Brolin RE, Gorman JH, Gorman RC, et al: Are vitamin B$_{12}$ and folate deficiency clinically important after Roux-en-Y gastric bypass? J Gastrointest Surg 1998;2:436-442.
30. Amaral JF, Thompson WR, Caldwell MD, et al: prospective hematologic evaluation of gastric exclusion surgery for morbid obesity. Ann Surg 1985;201:186-193.
31. Marceau P, Biron S, Hould FS, et al: The metabolic syndrome as a risk for liver disease. Hepatology 1997;26:556A.
32. Halverson JD, Koehler RE: Gastric bypass: analysis of weight loss and factors determining success. Surgery 1981;90:446-455.
33. Brolin RE, Gorman RC, Kenler HK, et al: The dilemma of outcome assessment after operations for morbid obesity. Surgery 1989;105:337-346.
34. National Institutes of Health Consensus Development Panel: Gastrointestinal surgery for severe obesity. Am J Clin Nutr 1992;55(suppl): 615-619.
35. Carson JL, Ruddy ME, Duff AE, et al: The effect of gastric bypass surgery on hypertension in morbidly obese patients. Arch Int Med 1994;154:193-200.

29

Biliopancreatic Diversion

Nicola Scopinaro, M.D., Francesco Papadia, M.D., Giuseppe M. Marinari, M.D., and Giovanni Camerini, M.D.

Forty years of worldwide experience with surgical treatment of obesity have demonstrated that the more the success of a procedure depends on the patient's cooperation, the poorer the results are. This is why malabsorptive methods, which require minimal patient compliance, have always been the most effective obesity operations. The reduction of nutrient absorption was actually the first approach to the surgical treatment of obesity. The early weight-loss results with jejunoileal bypass (JIB) led to more than 100,000 of these operations' being performed in the United States through the 1960s and 1970s. However, analysis of late results and complications caused a drastic cooling of the initial enthusiasm associated with JIB. In addition to its complications, essentially due to indiscriminate malabsorption and the harmful effects of the long bypassed loop, the main problem with JIB was its narrow "therapeutic interval." In fact, the total length of the small bowel left in continuity was restrained to between 40 and 60 cm, a shorter or longer bypass resulting in life-threatening malabsorption or no weight reduction, respectively. The massive postoperative intestinal adaptation phenomena caused an increased absorptive surface that exceeded the upper limits of the effective therapeutic intestinal length, with ensuing substantial recovery of energy absorption capacity.[1] This, in addition to the frequent need for restoration of bowel continuity because of major complications following JIB, resulted in a high rate of failure with weight regain.[2,3] The high complication rate and the overall unsatisfactory weight-loss results of JIB led, around 1980, to a general abandonment of the malabsorptive approach to obesity surgery, and to the gastric restriction procedures' becoming those used most frequently.

Because of the absence of a bypassed loop and of the malabsorption essentially selective for fat and starch, biliopancreatic diversion (BPD) is free of the complications that result from JIB.[4,5] Moreover, BPD has a very wide therapeutic interval because, by varying the length of the intestinal limbs, selective fat, starch, and protein malabsorption can be created; thereby, the procedure is adaptive to the population's or even the patient's characteristics in order to obtain the best possible weight-loss results with the minimum of complications.[6] This extreme flexibility also allows us to neutralize the consequences of intestinal adaptation phenomena that are minimally present in BPD. These qualities of BPD have gradually led to reacceptance of malabsorption as a surgical approach to obesity therapy, a procedure with many versions that is performed increasingly in the Western world.

The results and complications of BPD, after nearly 30 years of clinical use, are well known to bariatric surgeons. Therefore, the main purpose of this chapter is to describe the physiology of the operation, of which knowledge has increased considerably in recent years. A full understanding of the mechanisms of action of BPD is of paramount clinical importance, as it enables each surgeon to exploit the flexibility of the procedure.[7]

▶ CASE MATERIAL

Of the 2645 patients operated on since May 1976, 1738 (562 men and 1176 women) underwent the "ad hoc stomach" (AHS) type of BPD, performed by the same surgical team between June 1984 and July 2003. Mean age was 37 years (11-70 years); mean weight was 128 kg (73-236 kg); and mean excess weight was 69 kg (20-156 kg), corresponding to 117% excess weight (41%-311%) and to a mean body mass index (BMI) of 47 kg per m² (29-87 kg/m²). Maximum follow-up was 19 years. The availability for follow-up evaluation was nearly total.

In the AHS BPD (Fig. 29-1), the gastric volume, which is the main determinant of the initial weight loss (temporary food intake limitation due to decrease of appetite and occurrence of the postcibal syndrome) and also influences the stabilization weight (see subsequent text), is adapted to the preoperative excess weight and other individual characteristics (e.g., sex, age, eating habits, socioeconomic status, and expected degree of compliance), with the aim of obtaining the best weight-loss results with the minimum of nutritional complications.[8] Intestinal lengths, which determine energy absorption and thus the weight of stabilization and its indefinite maintenance, were adapted to patient characteristics only in the past 11 years.

a considerable depth. The EEA can be done with any technique, bringing the BPL to the left side of the AL.

The distal gastrectomy is performed, the duodenal stump is closed, the gallbladder is removed, and a wedge liver biopsy is obtained. We are used to cutting the stomach on a TA-90 linear stapler placed as obliquely as possible so as to compensate for the shortness of the ileal mesentery. The gastric pouch should be measured in all instances; this is easily accomplished by filling the pouch with water via a condom that has been tied to the end of a nasogastric tube. Gastric volume should be measured until the surgeon becomes able to evaluate it by sight.

The mesocolon is incised and the AL is brought into the supramesocolic space, checking for possible torsion. Any technique can be used for the GEA. We prefer to do it end-to-side, by cutting away the left corner of the gastric pouch. The GEA is then anchored by two stitches to the mesocolic rent so as to avoid intestinal kinking and internal hernias. We always close the distal mesenteric defect and never the proximal. The last maneuver is the final intestinal check, starting from the ICV, for proper alignment.

Laparoscopic

The laparoscopic technique entails the use of five trocars, placed in the positions illustrated in Figure 29-2. The gastrocolic ligament is incised at about its midpoint and the dissection, carried out with a harmonic scalpel, is performed until the traction of the greater curvature allows for the mobilization of the gastric fundus, which implies

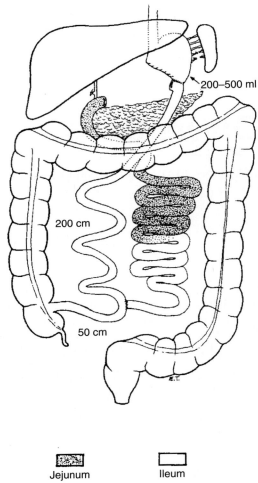

Jejunum   **Ileum**

Figure 29-1. Schematic representation of AHS BPD.

▶ SURGICAL TECHNIQUE

Open

The operation consists of a distal gastrectomy with closure of the duodenal stump and a long Roux-en-Y reconstruction, where the enteroenterostomy (EEA) is placed in the distal ileum 50 cm proximal to the ileocecal valve (ICV), and the gastroenterostomy (GEA) is at 250 cm. Three intestinal limbs can then be recognized: the alimentary limb (AL), from the GEA to the EEA (200 cm); the common limb (CL), from the EEA to the ICV (50 cm); and the biliopancreatic limb (BPL), from the ligament of Treitz to the EEA, which contains all the rest of the small bowel. A prophylactic cholecystectomy completes the operation.

After opening the abdomen through a midline supraumbilical incision, the first step is intestinal measurement. The small bowel is measured backward from the ICV to the ligament of Treitz, and marking stitches are placed at 50 cm and 250 cm. It is very important that the small bowel be measured fully stretched, so intestinal measurements are reproducible. The small bowel is then transected at the 250-cm level, and the ileal mesentery is sectioned to

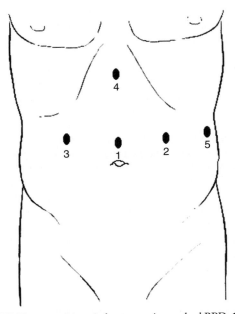

Figure 29-2. Trocar positions in laparoscopic standard BPD. **1.** supraumbilical (10-12 mm), on the midline, 3-4 cm above the superior margin of the umbilicus; **2.** left hypondriac (10-12 mm), along the left midclavicular line, about 6 cm below the costal margin; **3.** right hypondriac (10-12 mm), along the right midclavicular line, about 6 cm below the costal margin; **4.** xiphoid (10-12 mm), on the midline, 3 cm below the xiphoid; **5.** left subcostal (5 mm), on the left costal margin, along the left middle axillary line.

that the avascular area is always sectioned. The sectioning of the right gastroepiploic and the right gastric vessels completes the isolation of the duodenum, which is divided with single or double application of the endostapler. The lesser curvature is then isolated cranially with the ultrasound scissors, stopping 1 or 2 cm before the trunk of the left gastric artery, and the gastric resection is carried out by repeated firings of the endostapler. The gastric volume is measured by using the technique described earlier. A gastric sectioning from the greater curvature, moderately stretched, at approximately 15 cm from the cardia to the lesser curvature, at 5 cm from the cardia, corresponds to a gastric volume of about 300 ml. A distance of 20 cm along the greater curvature corresponds to a volume of about 400 ml.

After the cholecystectomy has been carried out, the patient is placed in a slight Trendelenburg position. The small bowel is measured backwards from the cecum, fully stretched, using two forceps marked at 10 cm in alternating movements. A mark is left at 50 cm, the ileum is divided at 250 cm by using the endostapler, and the mesentery is sectioned to a considerable depth with the ultrasonic scissors. The EEA is fashioned by a side-to-side technique, with an endostapler through two small enterotomies made by the harmonic scalpel. The conjoined defect is closed by a running seromuscular suture.

The left angle of the gastric stump is then pulled into the submesocolic space through an incision performed in the transverse mesocolon over the ligament of Treitz. The distal intestinal pouch is identified and perforated by the ultrasonic scissors at a distance from the suture line equal to the operative length of the endostapler. The latter is used to perform a side-to-side isoperistaltic GEA on the posterior wall of the stomach, as close as possible to the distal angle and midway between the suture line and the greater curve, with manual closure of the conjoined defect.

▶ EATING HABITS

During the first postoperative months, all patients undergoing BPD experience reduced appetite due to food's stimulation of the ileum,[9] and they have early satiety, occasionally in association with epigastric pain, vomiting, or both. These symptoms characterize the postcibal syndrome and are caused by rapid gastric emptying with subsequent distention of the postanastomotic loop. All of these symptoms, which are the more intense and lasting the smaller the gastric volume, rapidly regress with time, most likely due to intestinal adaptation. After 1 year, appetite and eating capacity are fully restored, and patients' mean self-reported food intake is 1.5 times as much as preoperatively, independent of gastric volume. Patients undergoing BPD must be aware that for the rest of their lives they will absorb minimal fat,[10,11] little starch, sufficient protein,[11,12] and nearly all mono- and disaccharides, short-chain triglycerides, and alcohol (i.e., the energy content of sugar, fruit, sweets, soft drinks, milk, and alcoholic beverages). They must also understand that when their body weights have reached the level of stabilization, the intake of these aliments may be varied as needed for individual weight adjustments.

▶ BOWEL HABITS

After full resumption of food intake, BPD subjects generally have two to four daily bowel movements of soft stools. Most have foul-smelling stools and flatulence. These phenomena, which can be reduced by the modification of eating habits or by the administration of neomycin, metronidazole, or pancreatic enzymes, tend to decrease with time, along with a reduction in the bowel movement frequency and increased stool consistency. Diarrhea usually appears only in the context of postcibal syndrome, and then it rapidly disappears, being practically absent by the fourth month.[6] Sporadic acute gastroenterocolitis, generally lasting not more than a few days, may be observed, especially during the summer. Plasma prothrombin should be checked in these instances, because colonic bacteria are the main source of vitamin K in BPD subjects. Because the colon is also the main site of protein digestion-absorption after BPD, a longer period of diarrhea may result in lower serum protein concentration, with spontaneous recovery after diarrhea has ceased.

The absence of diarrhea after BPD is easily explained, considering that, unlike the aftermath of JIB, the loss of bile salts into the colon was calibrated at about 750 mg per day by choosing the appropriate length for the common limb,[11] and that due to the lack of fat digestion, steatorrhea is essentially neutral, fecal pH being around 7. In fact, studies of intestinal transit time 1, 4, and 12 months after BPD showed, in comparison to the preoperative state, a transport time decreased by 50% in the small bowel but unchanged in the large bowel,[11,13] this being in keeping with the observed changes in gut hormone activity on intestinal motility.[14]

▶ WEIGHT LOSS

Weight reduction after AHS BPD in unrevised patients, when expressed as percentage of loss of the initial excess weight (IEW), was 72 ± 16 at 2 years (1555 cases); 73 ± 16 at 4 years (1423 cases); 73 ± 15 at 6 years (1347 cases); 74 ± 15 at 8 years (1280 cases); 74 ± 15 at 10 years (1120 cases); 75 ± 16 at 12 years (839 cases); 75 ± 16 at 14 years (417 cases); 76 ± 15 at 16 years (146 cases); and 77 ± 17 at 18 years (87 cases), with no differences between "morbidly obese" and "superobese" patients (IEW>120%).[6] At 10 years, 90% of the operated patients showed reduction of the IEW $\geq 50\%$. The failure rate (loss of less than 25% of the IEW) was 0.5%.

As noted, the initial weight loss is determined by the temporary forced food limitation that occurs immediately after operation. The weight stabilization, however, depends on the amount of daily energy absorption allowed by the BPD, which is the consequence of a mechanism that acts permanently. As a rule, the operated patient fully recovers appetite and eating capacity before the stabilization weight is attained, so that the final weight loss depends on the reduced intestinal absorption of energy. The stabilization weight is also influenced by the gastric volume, most likely because a smaller stomach with more rapid gastric emptying accelerates intestinal transit, thereby reducing absorption.[15]

▶ WEIGHT MAINTENANCE

The original philosophy for limitation of digestion in BPD was to delay the meeting between food and biliopancreatic juice in order to confine the digestion by pancreatic enzymes to a short segment of small bowel. In the first experimental model of BPD, the length of the BPL was only 30 cm, and the CL was equal to ⅐ to ⅒ of the small bowel's total length, that is, about 100 cm, so that the AL was about 7 m long. The analysis of changes in weight loss and in intestinal absorption of proteins in the BPD models that followed each other in the evolution of the operation[12,16-19] demonstrated that in the present model of BPD no pancreatic digestion occurs in the CL. Protein and starch digestion, which is due only to intestinal brush-border enzymes, occurs in the entire small bowel from the GEA to the ICV, whereas fat absorption, which needs the presence of bile salts, is confined to the CL.

The extraordinarily good weight maintenance that occurs after BPD is exemplified by a group of 40 patients who underwent the "half-half" (HH) type of operation, which differs from the AHS type only in that the stomach is larger and the alimentary limb is longer.[8] Comprehensibly, the weight reduction was smaller, but the weight attained was strictly maintained up to the twenty-fifth year of follow-up (Fig. 29-3). It is interesting that these data are the only 20-year results ever reported in obesity therapy.

Some clinical-statistical observations of the modalities of this very-long-term weight maintenance indicate that body weight after BPD is essentially independent of individual and interindividual variations in food intake. This prompted us to investigate the relationships between usual energy intake and intestinal absorption of energy.

An absorption study carried out (Table 29-1) demonstrated that the BPD digestive-absorptive apparatus has a maximum transport capacity for fat and starch and, thus, for energy.[20] Consequently, all of the energy intake that exceeds the maximum transport threshold is not absorbed; therefore, assuming that daily energy intake is much higher than the aforementioned threshold, daily energy absorption is constant in each subject. In conclusion, the original intestinal lengths and gastric volume being equal, the interindividual variability in weight stabilization in BPD subjects is accounted for by interindividual differences in (1) original energy intestinal digestive-absorptive capacity per unit

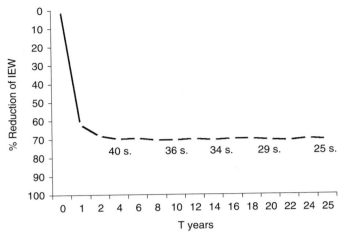

Figure 29-3. Changes in body weight after half-half BPD.

of surface; (2) intestinal adaptation phenomena; (3) intestinal transit time (which, in addition to gastric volume, can be influenced by the intake of fluids); (4) simple sugar intake; and (5) energy expenditure per unit of body mass. However, in each BPD individual, the weight of stabilization cannot be modified by any increase or decrease in fat-starch intake, provided the intake is greater than the maximum transport threshold. In reality, because the intestinal carrier becomes rapidly desaturated after the passage of food, an increased number of meals per day can also increase energy absorption, and this is confirmed by clinical experience.

The above results were confirmed by an overfeeding study in which 10 long-term BPD subjects kept a strictly stable body weight when fed their usual diets for 15 days and the same diet plus 2000 fat-starch kcal per day (without increasing the number of meals per day) for 15 more days (Table 29-2).

Although the preoperative energy intake in most of our patients was much higher than the mean energy absorption found in our study, the many obese women with preoperative energy intakes (confirmed by a measured total energy expenditure, TEE) lower than 1750 kcal per day lost weight after BPD. This can be explained only by an increase in energy expenditure per unit of body mass caused by the operation, as already suggested by three previous studies

Table 29-1	INTESTINAL ABSORPTION				
		ALIMENTARY INTAKE	FECAL LOSS	APPARENT ABSORPTION	APPARENT ABSORPTION (%)
Energy (kcal/24h)	Mean	3070	1329	1741	58
	Range	1840-4060	210-2590	1012-2827	32-71
Fat (g/24h)	Mean	130	89	39	28
	Range	88-185	22-251	13-94	12-59
Nitrogen (g/24h)	Mean	27	12	15	57
	Range	15-48	2.5-36	6.7-20	25-82
Calcium (mg/24h)	Mean	1994	1443	551	26
	Range	1037-3979	453-2565	251-1414	−24-69

Intestinal absorption of energy, fat, nitrogen, and calcium in 15 subjects (3 men) with stable body weight 2 to 3 years after biliopancreatic diversion (mean ± SD body weight: at the time of the operation, 119 ± 24 kg; at the time of the study, 75 ± 14 kg).

Table 29-2	STUDY OF OVERFEEDING AFTER BILIOPANCREATIC DIVERSION		
SUBJECT	INITIAL BW	BW ON USUAL FOOD INTAKE	BW AFTER OVERFEEDING
1	77.7	78.0	78.0
2	90.0	90.5	89.2
3	97.0	96.5	95.7
4	73.0	72.7	73.4
5	89.1	88.8	90.3
6	68.5	68.0	68.5
7	102.8	103.5	103.0
8	87.0	87.0	86.5
9	66.5	66.0	66.0
10	70.5	70.0	71.0

Overfeeding study in 10 subjects 3 to 9 years after biliopancreatic diversion. Individual data of body weight (BW, kg) at the beginning of the study; after a 15-day period on usual food intake (mean, ~3800 kcal/day); and after a 15-day period of overfeeding (usual food intake plus 2000 fat/starch kcal/day).

that demonstrated that after BPD, energy expenditure is greater than that which is, theoretically, expected after the observed weight reduction.[21-23]

A longitudinal study of resting energy expenditure (REE) in 53 subjects with stable body weight prior to operation and at 1, 2, and 3 years after BPD was then carried out; the results are reported in Table 29-3.[24] Although the mean body weight was reduced by about 50 kg, and the mean lean body mass by 8 kg, the mean REE at 1, 2, and 3 years was similar to the preoperative REE. (The difference between the mean postoperative TEE in this group calculated from REE with the 1.3 coefficient and the mean measured energy absorption [which corresponds to the mean TEE] in the absorption study group can be explained by considering the intergroup variability [mean REE was 1424 kcal per day in the absorption study group and around 1600 in the energy expenditure study group] and a possible underreporting of simple sugar intake in the alimentary diary of the absorption study group.) This means that, on average, after BPD, our patients absorbed as much energy as they were eating before, which raises obvious questions about the reason for the weight loss.

The weight reduction in our sample can be explained by considering the different energy expenditure of human body sectors. In fact, whereas adipose tissue consumes only about 5 kcal per kg per day,[25] the REE of muscle is about 18 kcal per kg per day, and the energy consumption of internal organs is as high as about 360 kcal per kg per day.[26] Therefore, if energy intake remains constant, a relatively small variation in internal organ mass must be balanced by a relatively large variation in the less-consuming body sectors, namely, adipose tissue and muscles, so that the overall energy expenditure, which must equal the energy intake, remains unchanged. Although the plasma levels of the gut hormones that stimulate intestinal adaptation changes were found to be greatly increased after both JIB and BPD,[14] after the latter, contrary to what happens following JIB, the entire bowel receives an intraluminal stimulus to adaptation,[27] which causes an increase in the size and functional activity of the whole intestinal tract.[28,29] This obviously results in increased energy consumption which, because daily energy absorption cannot be modified, must be balanced by a loss in the other body sectors such that it produces an identical decrease in energy consumption so that the eventual overall energy expenditure equals the intestinal absorption of energy. Actually, the increase in energy expenditure attributable to the augmented bowel-size function fully accounts for the corresponding decrease owing to the loss of adipose tissue, muscle mass, and nonbowel visceral mass in our sample of operated patients; the net increase of visceral mass corresponds to about 1 kg, or 360 kcal, per day.[30] Therefore, in our 53 BPD subjects, the average weight loss can be explained by the changes in body composition that follow the operation.

In conclusion, after BPD, weight maintenance is ensured by the existence of an intestinal energy transport threshold. The weight of stabilization depends partly on that threshold and partly on the changes in body composition consequent to the operation.

A final consideration concerning the differences existing in our population between men and women is that after weight stabilization, women weigh significantly less than men, and this means that they absorb less than men per unit of intestinal surface. The same applies to height (i.e., taller individuals absorb more per unit of intestinal surface).

▶ OTHER BENEFICIAL EFFECTS

The other benefits obtained after BPD are listed in Table 29-4. The percentage of changes observed after the operation was calculated for each benefit in patients by a minimum follow-up that corresponded to the postoperative time after which there was generally no further substantial modification. Recovery and improvement were considered only when favorable changes were essentially maintained at all subsequent reexaminations. The observed beneficial effects are obviously not attributable to the BPD itself but to the weight loss, the reduced nutrient absorption, or both, the only two exceptions being the effects on glucose and cholesterol metabolism.[31,32]

In fact, of the 2155 (total series) AHS BPD patients with a minimum follow-up of 1 year, not only the 302 (14%) with preoperative simple hyperglycemia, nor only the

Table 29-3	COMPARISON OF OBESE AND HEALTHY INDIVIDUALS			
	BW	BMI	FFM	REE
Prior to BPD	127.6 ± 26.9	47.4 ± 9.5	64.3 ± 12.9	1591 ± 638
At 1 year	83.0 ± 15.4*	30.8 ± 5.6*	55.5 ± 8.3*	1578 ± 305
At 2 years	78.0 ± 12.6*	28.9 ± 4.4*	54.2 ± 8.6*	1600 ± 310
At 3 years	79.4 ± 13.8*	29.4 ± 4.8*	55.8 ± 8.6*	1580 ± 229
Controls	77.2 ± 11.0*	28.5 ± 4.3*	53.9 ± 7.1*	1317 ± 199

One-way ANOVA: * $P < 0.0001$ vs. preoperative.

BW, body weight (kg); BMI, body mass index (kg/m²); FFM, fat free mass (kg); REE, resting energy expenditure (kcal/24h). These levels were found in 53 obese subjects (11 men) at various times relative to biliopancreatic diversion (BPD) and in 30 never-obese, healthy controls (mean ± SD).

Table 29-4	OTHER BENEFICIAL EFFECTS OF AD HOC STOMACH AND BILIOPANCREATIC DIVERSION				
	MINIMUM FOLLOW-UP (MO)	DISAPPEARED (%)	IMPROVED (%)	UNCHANGED (%)	IMPAIRED (%)
Pickwickian syndrome* (2%)	1	100	—	—	—
Somnolence† (7%)	1	100	—	—	—
Hypertension‡ (42%)	12	80	14	6	—
Fatty liver§ (52%)	24	87	9	4	—
Leg stasis• (32%)	12	44	40	16	—
Hypercholesterolemia¶ (54%)	1	100	—	—	—
Hypertriglyceridemia (35%)	12	94	6	—	—
Hyperglycemia (14%)	4	100	—	—	—
Diabetes mellitus (6%)	4	100	—	—	—
Diabetes mellitus requiring insulin (2%)	12	100	—	—	—
Hyperuricemia (17%)	4	94	—	4	2
Gout (2%)	4	100#	—	—	—

(%), percent of patients with condition; *, somnolence with cyanosis, polycythemia, and hypercapnia; † in absence of one or more characteristics of pickwickian syndrome; ‡ systolic ≥155, diastolic ≥95 mmHg, or both; §, more than 10%; •, moderate or severe; ¶, more than 200 mg/ml (21% more than 240 mg/ml); #, serum uric acid normalized, no more clinical symptoms. n = 53.

135 (6.3%) with type 2 diabetes mellitus manageable with oral hypoglycemics, but also the 38 (1.8%) patients with preoperative type 2 diabetes mellitus requiring insulin therapy, 1 year after BPD and permanently thereafter, had normal serum glucose levels without medication and on totally free diets. This was accompanied by normalization of serum insulin levels, as demonstrated in cross-sectional[33] and longitudinal studies (serum insulin [µg/ml] in 53 AHS BPD subjects: preoperative 18 ± 10 µg per ml; at 1 year 5.2 ± 2.3; at 2 years 4.6 ± 2.0; at 3 years 6.0 ± 3.1; controls 6.9 ± 2.6; ANOVA: each group versus preoperative $P<0.0001$), as well as in normalization of insulin sensitivity (Table 29-5). Considering that about 20% of type 2 diabetes mellitus patients are not obese, and about 20% of formerly obese patients with type 2 diabetes mellitus still require insulin therapy after weight normalization by dieting, it must be concluded that simple weight loss cannot account for the observed 100% recovery from type 2 diabetes mellitus after BPD.

The *primum movens* in the onset of type 2 diabetes mellitus in obesity could be, according to Randle,[34,35] an increased oxidation of free fatty acids which in turn inhibits glucose oxidation, thus causing insulin resistance. More recently, it was suggested that insulin resistance could be caused by hyperinsulinemia due to decreased hepatic clearance of insulin secondary to increased free fatty acid concentration in the portal blood.[36,37] In either case, the normalization of insulin sensitivity after BPD could be due to decreased lipid absorption, to reduction of intraabdominal adipose tissue, or to both. Therefore, it would not be a specific action of BPD, and it would not explain the serum glucose normalization seen in the 20% of obese patients with type 2 diabetes mellitus who would still require insulin therapy after weight normalization by dieting. After BPD, however, serum glucose in previously diabetic patients is generally normalized 1 month after operation, when overweight is still greater than 80%; this does suggest a specific action of BPD on glucose metabolism.

Now, if we consider that, independently of the *primum movens*, type 2 diabetes mellitus is characterized by a vicious circle in which the high serum insulin level increases insulin resistance and vice versa, it is reasonable that any factor resulting in reduction of insulin production would beneficially affect that vicious circle. An interruption of the enteroinsular axis would be such a factor, and this is what the specific action of BPD could be identified with. Indeed, the gastric inhibitory polypeptide level after BPD shows a substantially flat curve in response to the test meal, along with normalization of basal and meal-stimulated serum insulin levels.[13]

If this hypothesis is correct, BPD and reduction of insulin production should result in the worsening of type 1 diabetes mellitus. This occurred in two young women in our series who, after BPD, in spite of very good weight reduction, had to increase their insulin therapy by about 10 U per day.

Although reduction of fat intake, and thus absorption, is common to any weight-reduction method, the extreme and selective limitation of fat absorption consequent to BPD is not obtainable by any other means. This should also be considered a specific action of the operation.

There were four cases of late relapse of hyperglycemia in the 173 patients with preoperative type 2 diabetes mellitus,

Table 29-5	COMPARATIVE STUDY OF GLUCOSE AND INSULIN LEVELS			
		OBESE SUBJECTS	BPD SUBJECTS	LEAN CONTROLS
Number		9	6	6
Glycemia (mg/dl)	Mean	99.1*	74.6	86.6*
	Range	63-116	69-81	83-92
Insulinemia (µU/ml)	Mean	21.7	4.4§	10.3§
	Range	11-41	1-13	9-12
Glucose uptake (mg/kg/min)	Mean	2.9	9.3†	10.5†
	Range	1.7-7.2	6.8-11	8.5-12

Serum glucose and insulin concentrations plus insulin sensitivity (euglycemic hyperinsulinemic clamp) in obese patients; in subjects 2 to 4 years after biliopancreatic diversion (BPD); and in lean controls.
U-Mann Whitney test: *$P < 0.01$ vs. BPD subjects; §$P < 0.03$ vs. obese patients; †$P < 0.001$ vs. obese patients.

two at 5 years, one at 13 years, and one at 14 years. None of them needed any therapy, and none of them ever had serum glucose values higher than 150 mg per dl. One patient with severe preoperative diabetes never reached serum glucose normalization but kept values around 120 mg per dl for more than 10 years on a totally free diet and without any hypoglycemic therapy.

Two specific actions of BPD account for the permanent serum cholesterol normalization in 100% of operated patients. The first is the calibrated interruption of the enterohepatic bile salt circulation (bile acids are electively absorbed by the distal ileum) that causes enhanced synthesis of bile acids at the expense of the cholesterol pool. The second is the strongly reduced absorption of endogenous cholesterol consequent to the limitation of fat absorption.

The serum cholesterol level shows a stable mean reduction of approximately 30% in patients with normal preoperative values and 45% in patients who where hypercholesterolemic before the operation.[38] High-density lipoprotein (HDL) cholesterol remains unchanged, the reduction being entirely at the expense of low-density lipoprotein (LDL) and very-low-density lipoprotein cholesterol.[39] These results were maintained in the long term; the HDL cholesterol showed a significant increase in 51 BPD subjects at 6 years (total serum cholesterol: preoperative 210 ± 46 mg/dl, postoperative 124 ± 25 mg/dl, Student's t test, $P < 0.0001$; HDL cholesterol: preoperative 44 ± 12 mg/dl, postoperative 50 ± 15 mg/dl, Student's t test, $P < 0.03$) and at very long term in the 10 HH BPD subjects whose values were available 15 to 20 years after operation. With the U.S. National Institutes of Health criterion of 200 mg per dl as the upper recommended limit for serum cholesterol, of the 2635 (total series) obese patients submitted to BPD with a minimum follow-up of 1 month, 1397 had hypercholesterolemia (553 had values higher than 240 mg/dl, and 99 higher than 300 mg/dl). All of these patients had serum cholesterol values lower than 200 mg per dl 1 month after operation; the values remained below that level at all subsequent examinations.

Gasbarrini and colleagues[40] submitted to HH BPD a lean young woman with familial chylomicronemia (serum triglycerides: 4500 mg/dl; serum cholesterol: 502 mg/dl) and secondary type 2 diabetes mellitus (insulin 150 U/day to maintain serum glucose around 250 mg/dl). One year after operation she had gained 2 kg in weight; blood glucose, serum insulin, and insulin sensitivity were normal; serum triglycerides were 380 mg per dl, and serum cholesterol was 137 mg per dl on a totally free diet and without any medication. One year later, her younger sister, who had the same condition, underwent the same operation with similar results.[41] BPD, therefore, may be effective and safe in the treatment of severe type 2 diabetes mellitus and familial hyperlipidemia in lean subjects.

▶ NUTRITION

The easiest way to appraise nutritional status is to observe and talk to the subject. A person who looks well and exhibits complete well-being and the ability to work generally has good nutritional status. This has been the case for nearly all the AHS BPD patients once the early postoperative period has passed. Our studies on particular aspects of nutritional status showed normal immunologic status,[42] attainment of stable healthy body composition,[43] and the capacity to get pregnant, carry out a normal pregnancy, and deliver a healthy baby.[44]

▶ NONSPECIFIC COMPLICATIONS

Increasing practice and experience led us out of the learning curve with BPD as far as immediate complications are concerned. When the first 738 subjects, the subsequent 500 subjects, and the last 500 subjects undergoing AHS BPD are evaluated separately, a stable reduction of operative mortality to less than 0.5% and the near disappearance of general and intraabdominal complications are seen. Similarly, the incidence of wound complications appears to have been steadily reduced to approximately 1% (Table 29-6).

In contrast, the incidence of nonspecific late complications, around 15% for incisional hernia (≥3 cm)[45] and 1% for

Table 29-6	IMMEDIATE COMPLICATIONS FOLLOWING BILIOPANCREATIC DIVERSION		
	FIRST 738 SUBJECTS JUNE 1984-DECEMBER 1990	SUBSEQUENT 500 SUBJECTS DECEMBER 1990-OCTOBER 1999	LAST 500 SUBJECTS OCTOBER 1999-JULY 2003
Operative Mortality	1.1% 3 heart arrests 3 pulmonary embolisms 1 malignant hyperthermia 1 wound infection	0.4% 1 pulmonary embolism 1 GEA bleeding	0.4% 1 heart arrest 1 GEA leak and multiple organ failure
General Complications	1.2% 5 pulmonary embolisms 1 pneumonia 3 deep thrombophlebitis	0.2% 1 pulmonary embolism	0.4% 1 pulmonary embolism 1 deep thrombophlebitis
Surgical Complications	2.7% 2 GEA leaks 1 gastric perforation 2 intraperitoneal bleeding 6 wound dehiscences 9 wound infections	1.2% 3 wound infections 2 wound dehiscences 1 intraperitoneal bleeding	1.4% 2 intraperitoneal bleeding 2 wound dehiscences 3 wound infections

GEA, gastroenterostomy

intestinal obstruction, has not substantially changed throughout the years. Of note is the potential seriousness of biliopancreatic limb obstruction which, because of its particular anatomic-functional situation, does not cause any specific clinical or radiologic signs. However, it may lead to acute pancreatitis, which is more probable and more rapid in onset when the obstruction is more proximal. Any acute abdominal pain that raises suspicion for this complication should lead to an immediate search for duodenal and proximal jejunal distention (by computed tomography) and testing for abnormally high levels of serum amylase and bilirubin. If one or more of these signs are present, immediate laparotomy is mandatory.[46]

▶ SPECIFIC LATE COMPLICATIONS

Anemia

The exclusion of the primary site of iron absorption in the alimentary tract can cause iron deficiency anemia. More rarely, the anemia is due to folate deficiency and, exceptionally, to vitamin B_{12} deficiency (the Schilling test gives normal results in the short term after BPD[11,47]). Anemia, as a rule, appears in BPD patients with chronic physiologic (menstruation) or pathologic (hemorrhoids, stomal ulcer) bleeding. Most cases are microcytic, fewer are normocytic, and a few are macrocytic. The general incidence of anemia after BPD in our population would probably be around 40%, but supplementation with periodic iron, folate, or both can reduce its occurrence to less than 5%. Over time, less supplementation is required.

Stomal Ulcer

BPD is a potentially ulcerogenic procedure.[48] Since the beginning of experimental work in dogs,[4] distal gastrectomy has been preferred to gastric bypass[49] because it was thought to be more effective in preventing stomal ulcer[50] and because of concern for the fate of the bypassed stomach.[51]

The incidence of stomal ulcer was initially rather high (12.5% with the HH BPD) because of the large residual parietal cell mass. Considering only the ulcers diagnosed in the first 2 postoperative years in order to allow comparisons among groups, the incidence was successively reduced to 8.3% in the first 132 consecutive patients submitted to AHS BPD, simply due to the reduced stomach size.[52] Some changes in surgical technique, namely, preserving as much as possible of the gastrolienal ligament, with its sympathetic nerve fibers,[11] and shifting from end-to-end to end-to-side gastroenterostomy, the latter being better vascularized and less prone to stenosis,[53] led to further reduction (5.6% in the subsequent 650 cases). In the subsequent group of 640 AHS patients, operated on from January 1991 to March 1999, thanks to H_2-blocker oral prophylaxis[54] during the first postoperative year in patients at risk (see later text), the incidence of stomal ulcer in the first 2 years was further reduced to 3.4%.

When the totality of stomal ulcers in the first two groups is considered, it is clear that they were significantly more common in men (14.4%) than in women (5.2%).

As opposed to reports in previous articles,[6,7,51] the incidence of stomal ulcer appeared to be unaffected by alcohol consumption, increased in men (though not significantly) by cigarette smoking, and significantly increased (more in women than in men) by the association of alcohol and smoking. Stomal ulcers responded well to medical treatment (100% healing with H_2-blocker therapy), and they showed no tendency to recur, provided the patient refrained from smoking.

Endoscopic evidence of stomal ulcer was obtained in 52% of cases within the first postoperative year, in 26% of cases within the second year, and in 22% of cases, with progressively decreasing frequency, between the third and the tenth years. However, it must be considered that (1) most patients diagnosed in the second and the third years had already been symptomatic in the first one; (2) most patients diagnosed a longer time after the operation had been treated (one or more times) previously because of specific symptoms; (3) many patients once or repeatedly treated because of specific symptoms had refused endoscopy; (4) in some cases operated patients with no endoscopic diagnosis had received H_2-blocker therapy from their family doctors; and (5) with the exception of one man, all patients with specific symptoms who appeared after the second postoperative year were smokers or smokers and drinkers. The consideration of all the above facts leads to the conclusions that for BPD patients who are not smokers or smokers and drinkers, the risk for developing peptic ulcers is essentially confined to the first postoperative year, and that the real incidence of stomal ulcer after BPD is certainly higher than that reported in the data noted.

Oral prophylaxis with H2-blockers was started in 1991 because about one fifth of healed ulcers in patients in the first two groups had occurred with GEA stenosis requiring endoscopic dilation or surgical revision that involved a higher gastrectomy. Ranitidine was chosen because its intestinal absorption had proved to be normal.[54] In a previous analysis,[51] cigarette consumption appeared to increase the incidence of stomal ulcer in women more than in men, though not significantly, so oral prophylaxis was given to all men and all smoking women for the entire first postoperative year, and to nonsmoking women only for the first 2 months. The result of this prophylaxis was the reduction of stomal ulcer incidence in all the subgroups (men and women, with or without alcohol and/or smoking), which was statistically significant only for the nonsmoking men, in whom no ulcer appeared in 56 operated subjects during an overall 8-year follow-up period, whereas the incidence in nonsmoking women was unchanged. The differences present in the first two groups (men vs. women and smokers/drinkers vs. nonsmokers/nondrinkers) were still significant in the prophylaxis group, in which the difference between smoking and nonsmoking men became significant, evidently due to the disappearance of ulcers in the second subgroup. We concluded that oral H2-blocker (more recently, proton-pump inhibitor) prophylaxis should be given to all BPD subjects for the entire first postoperative year. In fact, no ulcers appeared in the 51 nonsmoking women operated on from March 1999, when all operated patients started receiving prophylaxis for the first postoperative year, to July 2001 (minimum follow-up of 2 years).

Bone Demineralization

The duodenum and proximal jejunum are selective sites for calcium absorption. However, our study of calcium intestinal absorption showed more than sufficient mean apparent absorption in the 15 subjects on free diets (see Table 29-1).[20] Moreover, intestinal absorption as an absolute value was positively correlated with the intake (Kendall rank test: $P < 0.03$), which means that, unlike fat and energy and similar to protein, the increase in calcium intake results in increased absorption. Therefore, all of our patients are encouraged to maintain an oral calcium intake of 2 g per day (with tablet supplementation, if needed), and intake of the daily requirements of vitamin D, as well as of all other vitamins and trace elements, is recommended for life. In old[55,56] and recent (unpublished data) studies, serum levels of vitamin D_2 and D_3 were found to be normal in nearly all our BPD subjects.

When the natural history of bone disease was investigated by us in obese patients and operated subjects not taking any supplements 1 to 10 years after BPD, histomorphologic signs of mild to severe bone demineralization (cross-sectional study on 252 transiliac bone biopsies after double-labeling with tetracycline, 58 of which were done preoperatively) were present in 28% of the obese patients and 62% of the operated subjects. Slightly low levels of serum calcium and high levels of alkaline phosphatase were found in about 20% of subjects in that study, with no significant differences between those of obese patients and operated subjects or between those of operated subjects with and without bone alterations. Serum magnesium, phosphorus, and 25-hydroxyvitamin D levels were essentially normal, both prior to and after operation. The prevalence and severity of metabolic bone disease (MBD) increased after BPD until the fourth year (prevalence: $16/58$ preoperatively, $15/21$ at 4 years, chi square test: $P < 0.001$; severity [subjects with moderate or severe MBD]: $7/58$ preoperatively, $8/21$ at 4 years; chi square test: $P < 0.01$), at which point they tended to regress. Long-term (6-10 years) mineralization status was not significantly worse than that observed before operation. Patients with the most severe preoperative alterations—the older and the heavier patients—showed sharp improvements in bone mineralization status compared to their preoperative statuses (prevalence of moderate or severe MBD in patients over 45 years old: 25% preoperatively, 29% at 1 to 2 years, 33% at 3 to 5 years, and 11% at 6 to 10 years; in patients with IEWs greater than 120%, these values were, respectively, 24%, 28%, 53%, and 14%).[11,55-57]

The histomorphology data were in total agreement with the clinical findings. Bone pain attributable to demineralization (with prompt regression after calcium, vitamin D only when needed, and diphosphonate therapy) was observed in 6% of patients, generally between the second and fifth postoperative years (maximum prevalence: 2.4% during the fourth year), and more rarely in the long term (10-20 years). Four cases of rib fractures and one case of vertebral collapse have been reported so far in patients undergoing AHS BPD.

The pathogenesis of bone demineralization in obese patients is unclear. The bone problems caused by BPD do not seem to differ substantially from those reported in 25% to 35% of postgastrectomy subjects with duodenal exclusion for peptic ulcer[58-60] and in one third of patients with gastric bypass for obesity.[61] The mechanism is very likely a decreased calcium absorption causing an augmented parathyroid hormone release, which is generally sufficient to normalize serum calcium level at the expense of bone calcium content. During the first postoperative years, the adverse effect of reduced calcium absorption seems to prevail over the beneficial effect of weight loss, whereas the opposite happens in the long term, this being more evident in the subjects with the most severe preoperative alterations. Recently, it has been suggested that a low albumin level is also implicated in the pathogenesis of MBD after BPD.[62]

In our experience, oral calcium supplementation seems to be able both to prevent and to cure bone alterations caused by BPD, as monitored by computerized bone mineralometry. Still, there are the observations that, on one hand, most of our operated patients do not take the recommended calcium supplementations but very few develop serious MBD; and, on the other hand, the bone problems caused by BPD seem to be more severe in the United States.[63,64] This suggests that great differences in calcium requirement and metabolism exist among populations and among individuals in the same population. Vitamin D synthesis in the skin at various latitudes probably also plays a major role. It is important to remember that parenteral vitamin D supplementation should not be used in the treatment of MBD unless low serum levels have been documented. In fact, an excess of vitamin D can cause bone damage similar to that caused by its deficiency.

Neurologic Complications

Peripheral neuropathy and Wernicke encephalopathy, early complications caused by excessive food limitation,[65] have now totally disappeared (none in the last consecutive 1703 operated subjects of the total series with a minimum follow-up of 1 year) because of prompt administration of large doses of thiamine to patients at risk, that is, those reporting very little food intake during the early postoperative weeks.

Protein Malnutrition

Characterized by hypoalbuminemia, anemia, edema, asthenia, and alopecia, protein malnutrition (PM) represents the most serious late specific complication of BPD, and its correction generally requires 2 to 3 weeks of parenteral feeding.

Our understanding of the pathogenesis of PM following BPD has considerably improved during recent years. Intestinal absorption of protein (measured by means of I-125 albumin) had been investigated at the beginning of the clinical experience,[12] and the study had been repeated after completion of the developmental phase[17] and again later,[18] with similar results. Still, the roughly 30% protein malabsorption that was observed did not seem to explain the occurrence of PM. A determinant contribution came from the more recent and complete study of intestinal absorption mentioned earlier.[20] In fact, the comparison between intestinal absorption of alimentary protein (73%) and apparent nitrogen absorption (see Table 29-1) revealed a mean loss of endogenous nitrogen of about 5 g per day, corresponding to a protein loss of about 30 g per day (i.e., approximately fivefold the normal value). The extra nitrogen lost, which, because of the length of the BPL, should not contain unreabsorbed pancreatic enzymes, could be represented by increased cell desquamation and, hypothetically, by active albumin secretion, both caused by the chronic irritation caused by malabsorption. Assuming that a 40 g per day protein requirement and a loss of about 6 g per day are normal, the average post-BPD protein requirement should be about 90 g per day, which is quite reasonable, considering that the 15 long-term subjects in our study had an average intake of about 170 g per day.

The increased loss of endogenous nitrogen, if confirmed in the short term, would result in a much greater impact in the first months following BPD, when the forced food limitation causes a negative balance for both energy and nitrogen, thus creating a condition of protein-energy malnutrition (PEM). For the latter, as is known, two subtypes can be identified: the marasmic form (MF) and the hypoalbuminemic form (HAF). In MF PEM, which represents effective metabolic adaptation to starvation, both energy and nitrogen deficits are present. The ensuing hypoinsulinemia allows lipolysis and proteolysis from skeletal muscles that supply amino acids for visceral pool preservation and hepatic synthesis of glucose necessary for brain, heart, and kidney metabolism and for the oxidation of fatty acids. This, in association with protein sparing due to negative energy balance, ensures both energy and protein homeostasis. The result is a loss of weight due to the reduction of adipose tissue and muscle mass in a state of complete well-being. In contrast, in HAF PEM, the nitrogen deficit is associated with a normal or near-normal energy (carbohydrate) supply. This causes hyperinsulinemia, which inhibits both lipolysis and skeletal muscle proteolysis. Not being able to draw on its protein stores, and in the absence of protein sparing, the organism reduces visceral protein synthesis, with consequent hypoalbuminemia, anemia, and immunodepression. The result is a severely ill person with body weight unchanged or increased, maintained adipose tissue size, and lean body composition pathologically altered, with decreased visceral cell mass and increased extracellular water.

During the early post-BPD period, preservation of protein homeostasis, already threatened by the negative energy-protein balance due to food limitation, would be made more difficult by the presence of an increased endogenous nitrogen loss. If operated patients devote the reduced eating capacity mainly to protein-rich foods, they would compensate for the loss and, like starving individuals, develop MF PEM, which is the goal of the procedure. If, on the contrary, they eat mainly carbohydrates, the nitrogen loss would make the HAF PEM even more severe than that found in cases of kwashiorkor. Paradoxically, starving patients are in a better metabolic situation because they can draw on their protein stores to try to satisfy the requirement and compensate for the loss. Therefore, HAF PEM is milder than that in carbohydrate-eaters. Between the two extremes, HAF PEM of varying severity can take place in patients with mixed intake, depending on

(1) how much smaller the protein intake is than the protein loss, and (2) how much the relatively excessive energy intake prevents skeletal muscle proteolysis and protein sparing.

The presence of increased endogenous nitrogen loss also explains late sporadic PM which, even if rarely, may occur at any length of time after the BPD and is caused by reduced food intake for any reason or by prolonged diarrhea due to nonspecific enterocolitis. PM is usually more severe in the latter situation because, the colon being an important site of protein digestion and absorption after BPD,[17] protein absorption may be more affected than carbohydrate absorption.

The goal of treatment of early PM, when significant excess weight is still present, is to change the PEM from HAF into MF, providing patients with the possibility of exploiting their energy and protein stores. This state is obtained by annulling alimentary carbohydrate intake and, taking into account the protein intake, administering intravenously only amino acids in amounts sufficient to compensate for the endogenous protein loss. In contrast, therapy for late PM, when body weight is normal or nearly normal, must be aimed at eliminating PEM and restoring normal nutritional status by means of parenteral feeding that includes both the nitrogen and the energy necessary to restore the amino acid pool, reestablishing the anabolic condition and resynthesizing deficient visceral protein.

The pathogenesis of PM after BPD is, then, multifactorial, depending on some operation-related (biologic) variables (gastric volume, intestinal limb lengths, individual capacity of intestinal absorption and adaptation, amount of endogenous nitrogen loss) and on some patient-related (psychological and environmental) variables (customary eating habits, ability to adapt them to the requirements, socioeconomic status). In most cases PM is limited to a single episode that occurs during the first or the second year because the patient-related factors are preeminent. Delayed appearance of sporadic PM is increasingly less common as time passes.[66] The operation-related factors are of greater importance in the recurrent form of PM, which is usually caused by excessive malabsorption and requires elongation of the common limb. Rarely, it is due to excessive duration of the food-limitation mechanism (permanent decrease of appetite and occurrence of the postcibal syndrome), generally in conjunction with poor protein intake, which may require restoration of intestinal continuity.[6,67]

In addition to the increased endogenous nitrogen loss, with its impact on daily protein requirements, another important phenomenon acting in the same direction is the overgrowth of colonic bacterial flora. The latter would not affect protein requirement if protein were not absorbed by the colonic mucosa. We demonstrated that in both BPD and intact subjects, the colon has the capacity of absorbing about 50% of a load of 10 g albumin directly instilled into the cecum.[17] This absorption capacity is considerable, and it is fully exploited in BPD. If we consider that in the above experiment albumin was given as a bolus, whereas in our absorption study the fraction of the 60-g protein meal not absorbed in the small bowel reached the cecum diluted by intestinal transit, we must conclude that the colon is a very important site for protein absorption in BPD.

Therefore, overgrown bacterial flora, the synthesis of which partially or totally occurs at the expense of alimentary protein escaped to absorption in the small bowel, reduces protein absorption by the colonic mucosa, thus increasing protein malabsorption and protein requirement.

It is interesting to note that there is in BPD a sort of counterbalance mechanism between increased endogenous nitrogen loss and bacterial overgrowth on one side, both caused by malabsorption and both increasing protein requirement, and food intake on the other side, which exerts a protective action against protein malnutrition. Actually, the BPD subjects who eat more, having a greater malabsorption, are likely to have greater endogenous nitrogen loss and greater colonic bacterial overgrowth, but this is compensated for by the greater protein intake. On the contrary, the BPD subjects who eat less are also likely to have less common occurrence of these two factors of increased protein requirement. Clearly, this phenomenon does not favor the subjects with greater intake of protein-poor food.

MINOR OR RARE LATE COMPLICATIONS

Among the 1555 AHS BPD patients with minimum follow-up of 2 years, the following minor or rare complications were observed or reported: 67 (4.3%) cases of hemorrhoids; 28 (1.8%) cases of anal fissures; 6 (0.4%) cases of perianal abscess; 53 (3.4%) cases of acne; 10 (0.6%) cases of inguinoperineal furunculosis; 41 (2.6%) cases of night blindness; 4 cases of lipothymia due to hypoglycemia; 2 cases of transient dumping syndrome; 1 case of bypass arthritis; and 1 case of gallstone ileus.

Halitosis after BPD could be due either to food stagnation in a virtually achloridic stomach, which can be avoided by correct execution of the gastroenterostomy; or to pulmonary expiration of ill-smelling substances resulting from malabsorption, which can be aided by oral administration of pancreatic enzymes. This unpleasant side effect has become less common in our series, currently affecting less than 5% of the operated patients.

BPD causes oxalate hyperabsorption, but not hyperoxaluria, though oxalate urinary excretion in the operated patients is significantly higher than in controls.[68] The procedure can then be considered a remote cause of kidney stone formation, keeping in mind that not even hyperoxaluria can cause this complication in the absence of cofactors, the first of which is decreased urinary volume resulting from dehydration. The incidence of kidney stones in our series (5 of 1555, or 0.3%) does not differ from that of the general population. We obtained 32 needle kidney biopsies at long-term relaparotomy in BPD patients and failed to demonstrate any microscopic or ultrastructural alterations (personal unpublished data: study in cooperation with Dr. Thomas Stanley, VA Hospital, Los Angeles, 1984).

LATE MORTALITY

Specific late mortality consisted of 3 cases of protein malnutrition (inadequately treated elsewhere) and 1 case of Wernicke encephalopathy. Semispecific mortality (i.e., the operation being a remote cause of death) included 6 cases of alcoholic cirrhosis (the pharmacologic effect of alcohol is enhanced by the distal gastrectomy due to more rapid intestinal absorption) and 4 cases of obstruction of the biliopancreatic limb (late or no diagnosis elsewhere).

ELONGATIONS AND RESTORATIONS

With the exception of 8 cases of higher gastrectomy required for GEA stenosis following stomal ulcer, nearly all specific late reoperations after BPD consisted of elongations of the common limb or restorations of intestinal continuity because of protein malnutrition (with or without additional problems). Because both reoperations are generally implemented to correct an excess effect of the original operation, and they entail permanent modifications of intestinal absorption, it is critical to ensure that intestinal adaptation mechanisms have been substantially completed, which requires at least 1 year. If the problems persist, reoperation is indicated, and the risk of reoperating prematurely, with resultant overcorrection and undue weight regain, is minimal.

The elongation of the common limb is indicated whenever a recurrent PM occurs in a BPD subject with normal food intake. In this case, PM is due to insufficient protein intestinal absorption, either absolute (insufficient absorption capacity per unit of intestinal length, too rapid intestinal transit due to excessively little stomach) or relative (insufficient protein content of ingested food, excessive loss of endogenous nitrogen). In both cases the aim of the surgical revision is to increase protein absorption. Because protein absorption after BPD depends substantially on the total intestinal length from the GEA to the ICV, the elongation of the common limb for correction of recurrent PM must be performed at the expense of the biliopancreatic limb. In our experience, the effective length in all cases is 150 cm, with the result of a total of 400 cm of small bowel in the food stream.

The total number of revisions in the 1639 AHS BPD subjects, with a minimum follow-up of 1 year, was 112, or 6.8%; 77 (4.7%) were elongation of the common limb, and 35 (2.1%) were restoration of intestinal continuity. When three groups earlier in the evolution of AHS BPD are considered, the revision rates in these three groups of 192, 430, and 429 patients were, respectively: 10.4% (elongations 8.3%, restorations 2.1%); 11.2% (elongations 7.9%, restorations 3.3%); and 8.1% (elongations 5.5%, restorations 2.6%).

EVALUATION

In order to assess BPD outcome according to the criteria of the Bariatric Analysis and Reporting Outcome System,[70] in December 2000 we sent out a questionnaire to the first consecutive 1800 AHS BPD subjects with a minimum follow-up of 2 years (maximum 16 years). The response rate was 51%. The mean total score was 5.1 ± 2.2, which represents a very good result; 3% of patients were classified as "failures," whereas results were "fair" in 11%, "good" in 23%, "very good" in 40%, and "excellent" in 23% of cases.

CONCLUSION

The studies carried out during recent years have greatly enlarged our knowledge of the physiology of BPD. Such knowledge has enabled us to make better use of the procedure, thereby improving its cost-benefit ratio considerably.

BPD is the most effective procedure for the surgical treatment of obesity. Like any other powerful weapon, it can be dangerous if used improperly. After 27 years of careful investigation and clinical experience, it has become, in our hands, a very safe operation. The learning curve has been very long, consisting of increasingly adapting the operation to the patient's individual characteristics, so that the best weight-loss results would be achieved in the subjects at low risk for nutritional complications, and so that there was acceptance of less weight reduction in the less compliant patients so as to minimize potential nutrition problems.

REFERENCES

1. Scopinaro N: Intervento in tavola rotonda su: trattamento medico-chirurgico della obesità grave. Accad Med 1974;88-89:215-234.
2. Halverson JD, Scheff RJ, Gentry K, et al: Jeunoileal bypass: late metabolic sequelae and weight gain. Am J Surg 1980;140:347-350.
3. MacLean LD, Rhode BM: Surgical treatment of obesity: metabolic implications. In Griffen WO, Printen KJ (eds): Surgical Management of Morbid Obesity, pp. 205-233. New York-Basel, Marcel Dekker, 1987.
4. Scopinaro N, Gianetta E, Civalleri D, et al: Bilio-pancreatic by-pass for obesity. I. An experimental study in dogs. Br J Surg 1979;66:613-617.
5. Scopinaro N, Gianetta E, Civalleri D, et al: Bilio-pancreatic by-pass for obesity. II. Initial experience in man. Br J Surg 1979;66:619-620.
6. Scopinaro N, Gianetta E, Adami GF, et al: Biliopancreatic diversion for obesity at eighteen years. Surgery 1996;119:261-268.
7. Scopinaro N, Adami GF, Marinari GM, et al: Biliopancreatic diversion. World J Surg 1998;22:936-946.
8. Scopinaro N, Gianetta E, Friedman D, et al: Evolution of biliopancreatic bypass. Clin Nutr 1986;5(suppl):137-146.
9. Koopmans HS, Sclafani A: Control of body weight by lower gut signals. Int J Obes 1981;5:491-494.
10. Gianetta E, Civalleri D, Bonalumi U, et al: Studio dell'assorbimento lipidico dopo bypass biliopancreatico per l'obesità. Min Diet e Gastr 1981;27:65-70.
11. Scopinaro N, Gianetta E, Civalleri D, et al: Biliopancreatic diversion. In Griffen WO, Printen KJ (eds): Surgical Management of Morbid Obesity, 93-162. New York-Basel, Marcel Dekker, 1987.
12. Gianetta E, Civalleri D, Bonalumi U, et al: Studio dell'assorbimento proteico dopo bypass bilio-pancreatico per l'obesità. Min Diet e Gastr 1980;26:251-256.
13. Bonalumi U, Moresco L, Gianetta E, et al: Il tempo di transito intestinale nel bypass biliopancreatico. Min Chir 1980;35:993-996.
14. Sarson DL, Scopinaro N, Bloom SR: Gut hormone changes after jeunoileal or biliopancreatic bypass surgery for morbid obesity. Int J Obes 1981;5:513-518.
15. Scopinaro N, Marinari GM, Adami GF, et al: The influence of gastric volume on energy and protein absorption after BPD. Obes Surg 1999;2:125-126.
16. Scopinaro N, Gianetta E, Civalleri D, et al: Two years of clinical experience with biliopancreatic bypass for obesity. Am J Clin Nutr 1980;33:506-514.
17. Bonalumi U, Cafiero F, Caponnetto A, et al: Protein absorption studies in biliopancreatic bypass patients. Int J Obes 1981;5:543.
18. Friedman D, Caponnetto A, Gianetta E, et al: Protein absorption (PA) and protein malnutrition (PM) after biliopancreatic diversion (BPD). Proceedings of the Third International Symposium on Obesity Surgery, Genoa, Italy, September 20-23, 1987:50.
19. Scopinaro N, Marinari GM, Gianetta E, et al: The respective importance of the alimentary limb (AL) and the common limb (CL) in protein absorption (PA) after BPD. Obes Surg 1997;7:108.
20. Scopinaro N, Marinari GM, Camerini G, et al: Energy and nitrogen absorption after biliopancreatic diversion. Obes Surg 2000;10:436-441.
21. Adami GF, Campostano A, Bessarione D, et al: Resting energy expenditure in long-term postobese subjects after weight normalization by dieting or biliopancreatic diversion. Obes Surg 1993;3:397-399.
22. Greco AV, Tataranni PA, Tacchino RM, et al: Daily energy expenditure in postobese patients. Int J Obes 1993;17:27.
23. Marinari G, Simonelli A, Friedman D, et al: Very long-term assessment of subjects with "half-half" biliopancreatic diversion. Obes Surg 1995;5:124.
24. Adami GF, Campostano A, Gandolfo P, et al: Body composition and energy expenditure in obese patients prior to and following biliopancreatic diversion for obesity. Eur Surg Res 1996;28:295-298.
25. Nelson KM, Weinsier RL, Long CL, et al: Prediction of resting energy expenditure from fat-free mass and fat mass. Am J Clin Nutr 1992;56:848-856.
26. Holliday MA: Metabolic rate and organ size during growth from infancy to adolescence and during late gestation and early infancy. Pediatrics 1971;47:101-117.
27. Dowling RH: Small bowel adaptation and its regulation. Scand J Gastroenterol 1982;74(suppl):53-75.
28. Stock-Damgé C, Aprahamian M, Raul F, et al: Small intestinal and colonic changes after biliopancreatic bypass for morbid obesity. Scand J Gastroenterol 1986;21:1115-1123.
29. Evrard S, Aprahamian M, Hoeltzel A, et al: Trophic and enzymatic adaptation of the intestine to biliopancreatic bypass in the rat. Int J Obes 1993;17:541-547.
30. Scopinaro N, Gianetta E, Adami GF, et al: Recenti acquisizioni fisiopatologiche e nuove strategie d'uso nella diversione biliopancreatica. Proceedings of the Novantottesimo Congresso della Società Italiana di Chirurgia, Rome, October 13-16, 1966;2:37-62.
31. Scopinaro N, Adami GF, Marinari G, et al: The effect of biliopancreatic diversion on glucose metabolism. Obes Surg 1997;7:296-297.
32. Marinari G, Adami GF, Camerini G, et al: The effect of biliopancreatic diversion on serum cholesterol. Obes Surg 1997;7:297.
33. Scopinaro N, Sarson DL, Civalleri D, et al: Changes in plasma gut hormones after biliopancreatic bypass for obesity: a preliminary report. Ital J Gastrenterol 1980;12:93-96.
34. Randle PJ, Newsholme EA, Garland PB: Regulation of glucose uptake by muscle. 8. Effects of fatty acids, ketone bodies and pyruvate, and of alloxan-diabetes and starvation, on the uptake and metabolic fate of glucose in rat heart and diaphragm muscles. Biochem J 1964;93:652-665.
35. Randle PJ, Garland PB, Newsholme EA, et al: The glucose fatty acid cycle in obesity and maturity onset diabetes mellitus. Ann N Y Acad Sci 1965;131:324-333.
36. Stromblad G, Bjorntorp P: Reduced hepatic insulin clearance in rats with dietary-induced obesity. Metabolism 1986;35:323-327.
37. Peiris AN, Mueller RA, Smith GA, et al: Splanchnic insulin metabolism in obesity: influence of body fat distribution. J Clin Invest 1986;78:1648-1657.
38. Gianetta E, Friedman D, Adami GF, et al: Effects of biliopancreatic bypass on hypercholesterolemia and hypertriglyceridemia. Proceedings of the Second Annual Meeting of the American Society for Bariatric Surgery, Iowa City, Iowa, June 13-14, 1985:138-142.
39. Montagna G, Gianetta E, Elicio N, et al: Plasma lipid and apoprotein pattern in patients with morbid obesity before and after biliopancreatic bypass. Atheroscl Cardiovasc Dis 1987;3:1069-1074.
40. Gasbarrini G, Mingrone G, Greco AV, et al: An 18-year-old woman with familial chylomicronaemia who would not stick to a diet. Lancet 1996;348:794.
41. Mingrone G, Henriksen FL, Greco AV, et al: Triglyceride-induced diabetes associated with familial lipoproteinlipase deficiency. Diabetes 1999;48:1258-1263.
42. Adami GF, Civalleri D, Gianetta E, et al: In vivo evaluation of immunological status after biliopancreatic bypass for obesity. Int J Obes 1985;9:171-175.
43. Adami GF, Barreca A, Gianetta E, et al: Body composition in subjects with surgically obtained stable body weight normalization. Int J Obes 1989;13:55-58.

44. Friedman D, Cuneo S, Valenzano M, et al: Pregnancies in an 18-year follow-up after biliopancreatic diversion. Obes Surg 1995;5:308-313.
45. Friedman D, Traverso E, Adami G, et al: Incisional hernias following biliopancreatic diversion (BPD). Obes Surg 1996;6:304.
46. Gianetta E, Friedman D, Traverso E, et al: Small bowel obstruction after biliopancreatic diversion. Probl Gen Surg 1992;9:386-389.
47. Civalleri D, Scopinaro G, Gianetta E, et al: Assorbimento della vitamina B_{12} dopo bypass biliopancreatico per l'obesità. Min Diet Gastroenterol 1982;28:181-188.
48. Mann FC, Williamson CS: The experimental production of peptic ulcer. Ann Surg 1923;77:409-422.
49. Mason EE, Ito C: Gastric bypass in obesity. Surg Clin North Am 1967;47:1345-1352.
50. Storer EH, Woodward ER, Dragstedt LR: The effect of vagotomy and antrum resection on the Mann-Williamson ulcer. Surgery 1950;27:526-530.
51. Scopinaro N, Gianetta E, Friedman D, et al: Biliopancreatic diversion for obesity. Probl Gen Surg 1992;9:362-379.
52. Civalleri D, Gianetta E, Friedman D, et al: Changes of gastric acid secretion after partial biliopancreatic bypass. Clin Nutr 1986;5(suppl):215-220.
53. Gianetta E, Friedman D, Adami GF, et al: Present status of biliopancreatic diversion (BPD). Proceedings of the Third International Symposium on Obesity Surgery, Genoa, Italy, September 20-23, 1987:11-13.
54. Adami GF, Gandolfo P, Esposito M, et al: Orally-administered serum ranitidine concentration after biliopancreatic diversion. Obes Surg 1991;1:293-294.
55. Compston JE, Vedi S, Gianetta E, et al: Bone histomorphometry and vitamin D status after biliopancreatic bypass for obesity. Gastroenterology 1984;87:350-356.
56. Compston JE, Vedi S, Watson GJ, et al: Metabolic bone disease in patients with biliopancreatic bypass. Clin Nutr 1986;5(suppl):221-224.
57. Adami GF, Compston JE, Gianetta E, et al: Changes in bone histomorphometry following biliopancreatic diversion. Proceedings of the Third International Symposium on Obesity Surgery, Genoa, Italy, September 20-23, 1987:46-47.
58. Williams JA: Effects of upper gastro-intestinal surgery on blood formation and bone metabolism. Br J Surg 1964;51:125-134.
59. Eddy RL: Metabolic bone disease after gastrectomy. Am J Med 1984;8:293-302.
60. Fisher AB: Twenty-five years after Billroth II gastrectomy for duodenal ulcer. World J Surg 1984;8:293-302.
61. Crowley LV, Seay J, Mullin Jr GT: Long-term hematopoietic and skeletal effects of gastric bypass. Clin Nutr 1986;5(suppl):185-187.
62. Marceau P, Biron S, Lebel S, et al: Does bone change after biliopancreatic diversion? J Gastrointest Surg 2002;6:690-698.
63. Fox SR: The use of biliopancreatic diversion as a treatment for failed gastric partitioning in the morbidly obese. Obes Surg 1991;1:89-93.
64. Chapin BL, LeMar HJ Jr, Knodel DH, et al: Secondary hyperparathyroidism following biliopancreatic diversion. Arch Surg 1996;1048-1053.
65. Primavera A, Schenone A, Simonetti S, et al: Neurological disorders following biliopancreatic diversion. Proceedings of the Third International Symposium on Obesity Surgery, Genoa, Italy, September 20-23, 1987:48-49.
66. Gianetta E, Friedman D, Adami GF, et al: Etiological factors of protein malnutrition after biliopancreatic diversion. Gastroenterol Clin North Am 1987;16:503-504.
67. Scopinaro N, Gianetta E, Friedman D, et al: Surgical revision of biliopancreatic bypass. Gastroenterol Clin North Am 1987;16:529-531.
68. Hofmann AF, Schnuck G, Scopinaro N, et al: Hyperoxaluria associated with intestinal bypass surgery for morbid obesity: occurrence, pathogenesis and approaches to treatment. Int J Obes 1981;5:513-518.
69. Oria HE, Moorehead MK: Bariatric analysis and reporting outcome system (BAROS). Obes Surg 1998;8:487-499.

30

Biliopancreatic Diversion with Duodenal Switch

Douglas S. Hess, M.D.

During the 1970s and 1980s, many purely restrictive operations were ultimately proving to be unsuccessful, as were the restrictive revisions and reoperations. Thus, the search began for a procedure that would produce better long-term results and fewer failures, that is, regain of weight. The biliopancreatic diversion with duodenal switch (BPD/DS) was first performed in 1988 as a reoperation in a patient with a failed restrictive procedure.[1] The BPD/DS incorporates two other distinct procedures: the biliopancreatic diversion (BPD) that has been well established since its introduction by Dr. Scopinaro in 1976[2] and the duodenal switch (DS), introduced by Dr. DeMeester in 1987.[3]

At first, Scopinaro's BPD was used only for reoperations on failed restrictive procedures, the expectation being better long-term results. The standard BPD was used, including a few cases without a distal gastrectomy. The BPD without gastrectomy resulted in ulcers and strictures, and most had to be taken down. The BPD with gastrectomy presented its own problems, stemming primarily from the distal gastrectomy component of that procedure. The dense adhesions found in the upper gastric area of previously stapled patients caused difficulty in placing the anastomosis, and marginal ulcers occasionally formed at the site of the anastomosis in the upper stomach. Further, it sometimes left the patient with an uncomfortable dumping syndrome. These problems prompted the search for a method that would anastomose the small bowel to the duodenum or lower stomach, away from the site of the previous surgery, to reduce the possibility of complications.

Review of the literature uncovered the article by DeMeester, describing the DS.[3] It was developed for the treatment of duodenogastric reflux, after experimental success in a group of 29 Mann-Williamson dogs. In that experiment, DeMeester found that by leaving a short portion of the proximal duodenum attached to the pylorus, the incidence of ulcer formation was significantly reduced. He compared two groups: those with direct anastomoses to the pylorus with two different jejunal lengths, and those with portions of the proximal duodenums left in place with

two different jejunal lengths. The groups with the proximal segment of the duodenum in place had a marked reduction of ulcers and ulcer perforations. Dr. DeMeester successfully applied this knowledge to his clinical practice in patients with duodenogastric reflux.

This same duodenal switch was incorporated into the BPD by Dr. Hess, creating a hybrid bariatric operation, the biliopancreatic diversion with duodenal switch. The expectation was that this new procedure would offer the benefits of both component procedures—the adequate long-term weight loss with the BPD and the reduction in marginal ulcers and dumping syndrome with the incorporation of the DS.

The first patient on whom the BPD/DS was performed was a 56-year-old man who had had a transverse gastroplasty 9 years earlier, in 1979, when he had weighed 166 kg (365 lb). In 1988 when the BPD/DS was performed, he had gained weight to the level of 206 kg (454 lb) and had a body mass index (BMI) of 61 kg per m². He was in early heart failure. A 70% vertical gastrectomy was performed to form a moderate gastric restriction with a stomach volume of 200 ml. The alimentary limb was 275 cm in total length, of which the distal 75 cm formed the common channel. At 17 years after the BPD/DS, he maintained a weight of 100 kg (220 lb), with a BMI of 29 kg per m².

After performing several of these reoperations with good weight loss and patient satisfaction, the BPD/DS became the procedure of choice for all of the bariatric patients, whether primary or reoperations. By November 2004, 1402 surgeries had been performed, of which 159 were reoperations. The surgical technique and parameters remain essentially the same today as in the first BPD/DS surgery.

▶ RATIONALE FOR THE DUODENAL SWITCH

The DS has now been established as a viable procedure to combat the relatively high rate of marginal ulcers after a more distal Roux-en-Y anastomosis. As in DeMeester's dogs, the BPD patients in whom the pylorus and a proximal segment of the duodenum was left in place have a lower incidence of ulcers. The rate of ulcer complications is 0.3%, compared with 3% for the standard BPD. The vertical gastrectomy performed in conjunction with the DS removes much of the acid-producing fundus of the stomach, thereby further reducing marginal ulcers.

With the pylorus and a short portion of the duodenum remaining in the food stream, the BPD/DS is also more functionally reversible than is the standard BPD. Further, the patient's own pylorus continues to control gastric emptying. This eliminates dumping syndrome, a problem often seen in bypass patients without the DS.

Reasoning Behind the Use of a Complex Procedure

Bariatric surgery can be separated into three general categories: restrictive, malabsorptive, and a combination thereof. Gastric bandings and staplings are restrictive; short-limb Roux-en-Y gastric bypasses are predominantly restrictive, with a negligible element of malabsorption; and the BPD/DS, BPD, and gastric bypass with long-limb Roux-en-Y are examples of combination procedures. The purely malabsorptive jejunoileal bypass is no longer performed today because of multiple documented complications and negative effects.

Bariatric surgery procedures can also be categorized as either simple or complex. In fact, no bariatric surgery is truly simple or without occasional complications. Nevertheless, the restrictive procedures are considered to be relatively simple, whereas the combination procedures, such as the BPD/DS, are considered to be complex.

Good long-term weight loss and reduction of the numerous comorbidities associated with serious obesity are important goals. The patient's initial surgical procedure for obesity presents a golden opportunity for success, and the procedure choice should be made carefully. The surgically more simple procedures may be easier to perform and have a relatively low rate of complications, but they commonly fail in the long term, requiring a higher number of reoperations, which are more difficult and riskier. A more complex and difficult procedure such as the BPD/DS may be the best choice for primary operations. This is true not only for the super morbidly obese patient, who is often in more extreme immediate danger and for whom sustained weight loss is vital, but also for the morbidly obese patient who might become super morbidly obese without the most effective, long-term surgical treatment (such as the patient discussed earlier).

The BPD/DS is a complex procedure, requiring close follow-up by the physician and willingness on the part of the patient to cooperate fully, including faithfully taking vitamins and other supplements for the rest of his or her life. However, with a committed physician and patient team, the advantages of the BPD/DS are numerous. If the gastrectomy is properly performed, there is seldom a need to operate on the difficult area of the stomach again, even in cases of later revisions or reversals. In addition, many comorbidities, such as hypertension, hypercholesterolemia, and arthritis in weight-bearing joints, are improved or cured at a higher rate than with less complex procedures. Current data for BPD/DS patients with type II diabetes show a 98% cure, that is, a euglycemia rate (Fig. 30-1). Sleep apnea and hypoventilation syndromes are also eliminated with the BPD/DS; and patients are generally more satisfied than they are after other procedures.

The malabsorption component of the BPD/DS relates primarily to lipid malabsorption and is dependent on the length of the common channel formed at the distal alimentary limb. The length of the alimentary limb affects primarily protein absorption and, to some degree,

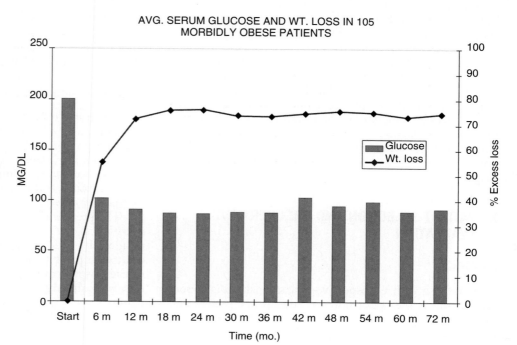

Figure 30-1. Average serum glucose and weight loss in 105 morbidly obese patients.

AVG. SERUM GLUCOSE AND WT. LOSS IN 105 MORBIDLY OBESE PATIENTS carbohydrate absorption. Both of these limbs are carefully constructed. Rather than using a standard measurement for all patients, the unique aspect of the BPD/DS is that it involves using a specific formula as well as considering individual patient factors in determining the lengths of the channels.

A vital distinction between the standard BPD and the BPD/DS is the surgical treatment of the patient's stomach. The BPD and other procedures involve a distal gastrectomy, whereas the restrictive component of the BPD/DS is achieved by the vertical gastrectomy. The newly formed stomach in a BPD/DS will continue to function normally because the pylorus remains intact. Although the removed portion of the stomach cannot be replaced, the remaining stomach is large enough to function essentially normally, even in the rare case when reversal of the small bowel is necessary.

The common channel is constructed to be 50, 75, or 100 cm. Age, sex, weight, and comorbidities are considered when determining which of the three figures to use when the actual measurement is in between these figures.

Protein deficiency may arise if the limbs are too short. The goal is to form an alimentary limb that is long enough for adequate protein absorption, but not so long as to impede satisfactory weight loss. Constructing appropriate limb lengths is paramount in the BPD/DS and, therefore, accurate measurements are necessary for good results.

When considering bariatric surgery, the long-term outcome, including possible reversals, revisions, and complications, should be the focus. The rate of revision after the BPD/DS is lower than that of many less complex procedures. Revisions that are performed are nearly always in the area of the small bowel, involving a simple shortening or lengthening of the distal Roux-en-Y. They do not involve the difficult area of the stomach between the liver, spleen, and diaphragm in the extreme left upper space of the abdomen. It is common for a previously operated stomach to have adhesions that can be severe, causing difficulties in later operations. Although rarely necessary, reversals of the bypass portion of the procedure are easily performed by a side-to-side anastomosis of the proximal small bowel.

The goal of complex bariatric surgery is to create a new gastrointestinal configuration with which the patient can live comfortably, while eliminating the debilitating and dangerous disease of obesity. The BPD/DS offers excellent long-term weight loss results, elimination of comorbidities, a relatively low rate of complications, and a high rate of patient satisfaction. Many surgeons agree that the favorable long-term outcome of a more complex procedure outweighs the risks and inconveniences of the more complex surgeries.

▶ PATIENT SELECTION AND PREOPERATIVE EVALUATION

First Visit

The first visit with a prospective bariatric patient is important, as this is the opportunity to educate the patient and assess his or her suitability for surgery. Generally, the prospective patient has already decided to have the surgery

Table 30-1	DEMOGRAPHICS OF PATIENTS UNDERGOING PRIMARY BARIATRIC SURGERY: AVERAGES BEFORE SURGERY
Male/female	310/932
Age in years	33.9 (14-65)
Starting weight (kg)	143 (89-303)
Percent ideal weight	226 (147-400)
Body mass index	50.9 (35-88)
Excess weight (kg)	79.7 (39-228)

n = 1243.

by the first visit. However, on rare occasions the person changes his or her mind or is found not to be a good candidate. All patients must meet the standard conditions of morbid obesity—45.5 kg (100 lb) over ideal weight-to be considered for bariatric surgery. As a rule, three times as many women as men are seen, and the average BMIs of the patients are greater than 50 kg per m^2 (Table 30-1).

The initial appointment is scheduled for the morning, and the patient is advised in advance that the initial screening process will consume most of the day. Upon the patient's arrival, the nurse weighs and measures the patient, takes a photograph, and obtains a medical history to be available to the physician later. The patient then views a 45-minute video explaining the surgical procedure, expected outcomes, risks, and possible complications. After the patient views the video, he or she meets with the surgeon who again reviews the procedure and answers questions. It is important that the surgeon explain to the patient all that is involved with the surgery, including the relative complexities of the procedure as well as the advantages. The patient should be made aware of the commitment and cooperation expected from him or her. If the parties agree that the surgery should be performed, the patient's name is placed on a surgery schedule. A letter is dictated to the insurance company and a copy of the letter is given to the patient. The patient is encouraged to attend monthly support meetings, both before and after surgery, to talk to other patients and ask questions of the surgeon. The initial consultation with the surgeon is videotaped and kept as a permanent record.

Hospital Introduction and Preoperative Tests

After the initial office visit, the patient obtains basic laboratory work, such as a complete blood count and chemistries, including thyroid and corticoid studies. A cardiac evaluation, including an electrocardiogram, is also performed. Chest radiographs, pulmonary function tests, and upper gastrointestinal and gallbladder radiographs are scheduled for another day.

The preoperative evaluation, including diagnostic tests, is critical in the screening process, as it is the opportunity to identify abnormalities and conditions that must be dealt with prior to surgery. Patients are usually admitted to the hospital on the day before surgery, at which time they will already have undergone most of their preoperative tests. Upon admission, they are seen by an anesthesiologist and an internist, and they receive bowel preparation.

Patients are given an anticoagulant (e.g., Lovenox) intramuscularly on the evening of admission and each evening thereafter during the hospital stay. It is given in the evening so that the coagulation capacity is relatively lower in the morning when the epidural catheter is inserted before surgery.

▶ DETAILS OF THE PROCEDURE

Under general anesthesia, a midline incision is made from the xyphoid to the umbilicus. A Gomez retractor is put in place, and the abdomen is explored. The procedure starts with a routine removal of the appendix. It is done first because it is convenient to do it while in the lower abdomen where the initial bowel measurements begin.

Next, the entire small bowel is measured along the antimesenteric border, with a full stretch between two Pennington clamps, from the cecum to the ligament of Treitz (Fig. 30-2). Using a metal ruler and calling out the measurement in centimeters, the scrub nurse keeps a running total of the measurements. Several silk sutures are placed in the margin of the bowel at the estimated location of the proximal common channel and the proximal alimentary limb. These measurements may be adjusted after the complete measurement of the bowel. The length of the alimentary limb is calculated by multiplying the total small bowel length by 40%. The common channel is the distal portion of the alimentary limb equal to 10% of the total small bowel length. The biliopancreatic limb is attached to the ileum by an end-to-side anastomosis at the proximal point of the common channel. The alimentary limb is constructed in increments of 25 cm, the final length generally being the point nearest to 40% of total length target. Most commonly, the alimentary canal will be 250, 275, 300, or 325 cm. Occasionally, 225 or 350 cm are used for patients with unusually short or long small bowels. The common channel is 50, 75, or 100 cm, whichever is closest to 10% of the total small bowel length. The epidural anesthesia is not used until after the measurements are completed because it may cause spasms of the small bowel.

The position of the table is changed from a flat or slight Trendelenburg position to a reverse Trendelenburg position for better access to the upper abdomen. The left triangular and falciform ligaments of the liver are incised to allow retraction of the liver away from the stomach. The liver is held with gauze and a liver retractor. By transecting a few short gastric vessels at the mid greater curvature of the stomach, the surgeon opens into the lesser sac. Using a cauterizing/cutting instrument, all of the short gastric vessels are transected, from the pylorus to the esophagus, freeing up the entire greater curvature portion and back wall of the stomach by dividing any adhesions in the area. Blood vessels are transected along the greater-curvature side of the duodenum for about 5 cm distal to the pylorus, and a Penrose drain is passed around the duodenum at this point. If a partial Kocher maneuver is performed, the area of the Penrose can be palpated to ensure that the drain is proximal to the common duct and the ampulla. In this area, the common duct must be carefully located and avoided because damage could lead to serious complications. The nasogastric tube is removed and a 40F dilator, to be used as a sizer, is passed into the stomach, along the lesser curvature, and through the pylorus into the duodenum. An assistant uses Babcock clamps to hold the greater curvature side of the stomach upward and to the left.

The new stomach is sized by vertically placing a 100-mm stapler along the right side of the dilator, at a distance of approximately 1 to 1½ finger breadths to the right of the dilator. Starting from the distal stomach, a few centimeters proximal to the pylorus, the stapling is repeated three to

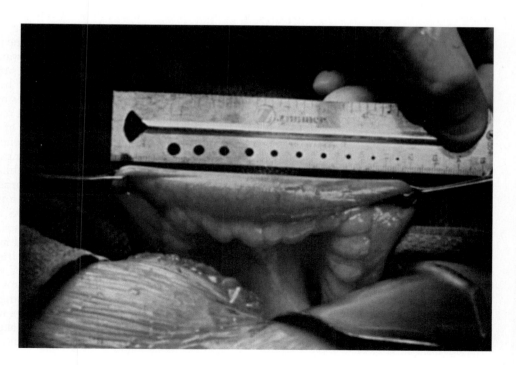

Figure 30-2. Measuring the small bowel.

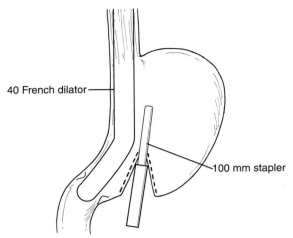

Figure 30-3. Stapling the stomach.

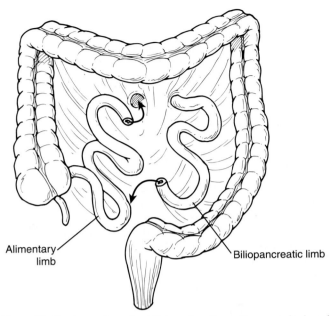

Figure 30-5. Transection of small bowel to form alimentary limb and biliopancreatic limb.

four times, as needed, to remove the entire greater-curvature side of the stomach. Care must be taken along the J-shaped part of the stomach because it can easily be made too narrow at this point. Bleeding points along the staple row are oversewn with figure-of-eight silk sutures. Then a continuous suture, using a running Lembert technique, inverts the staple row. The dilator is removed, and the duodenum is transected with a stapler at a point 4 to 5 cm distal to the pylorus (Figs. 30-3 and 30-4). The nasogastric tube is then reinserted into the stomach.

The volume of the stomach is measured by filling the stomach with saline and methylene blue dye. Pressing one hand against the esophagus prevents reflux of the saline. Dissection around the esophagus is not performed. When the stomach is fully distended, the saline is withdrawn and measured. This measurement, plus 10 ml, is considered to be the volume of the stomach. The surgeon is also able to check for any possible leaks.

The small bowel, which was previously marked for the alimentary limb, is transected by a stapler, and the mesentery

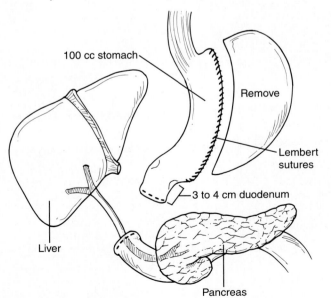

Figure 30-4. The stomach is removed and the duodenum transected. L, liver; P, pancreas.

is divided using a cauterizing/cutting instrument straight down until the distal ileum can be mobilized (Fig. 30-5). To avoid the possibility of connecting the wrong limb to the duodenum, both the proximal and distal transected edges should be marked in some consistent manner during every operation. The proximal end of the distal ileum is taken upward and retrocolic to the right of center to meet the remaining approximately 3 to 4 cm of duodenum that are still attached to the pylorus. It is anastomosed to the duodenum, end-to-end, using a Valtrac anastomosing ring (US Surgical, Norwalk, CT), generally a 1.5-mm gap with a 25-mm diameter. If the patient's duodenum is larger than usual, then a 2-mm gap and a 28-mm diameter Valtrac may be used. After forming the duodenoileal anastomosis, the surgeon must follow the ileum down to the cecum to ensure that the correct limb was connected to the duodenum. If it is discovered during surgery that the incorrect limb was mistakenly connected to the duodenum, it can be fairly easily corrected. If it is not discovered during surgery, serious complications will result.

The anastomosis of the duodenum and the ileum can also be formed by an end-to-end anastomosis, making it at least 25 mm to prevent a stricture. A stricture in this area reduces the patient's ability to eat protein and increases the possibility of ulcer formation, further increasing the stricture. Adequate protein intake is essential for the ultimate success of the BPD/DS, so it is important that the surgeon take steps to prevent stricture formation. Another possible complication to avoid at this point is a high small bowel obstruction resulting from accidentally twisting the ileum while it is being passed under the colon.

After the anastomosis of the distal ileum to the duodenum is complete, the mesentery is sutured to the posterior peritoneal wall to prevent internal hernias. The distal end of the proximal ileum is taken distally to the previously marked area on the distal ileum, and an end-to-side anastomosis is performed with a Valtrac anastomosing ring (1.5-mm gap and 25-mm diameter). Both anastomoses may be hand-sutured if the surgeon prefers that method. The remaining mesentery is closed with a running suture to the anastomosis. Then several interrupted silk sutures are taken on the other side to further support the distal small bowel mesentery and help prevent internal hernias. The abdomen is closed and a drain is placed in the general area of the gallbladder bed and duodenum.

Postoperative Diet

For a period of 3 to 4 weeks, patients are permitted only high-protein liquid diets so as to allow time for adequate healing. They gradually increase to a soft diet, then a regular diet. Patients must be advised that as they increase their solid food intake, they must use most of their stomach volume for protein foods, not the easily absorbed carbohydrates.

Concurrent Procedures

Many concurrent procedures have been performed during this surgery. A routine appendectomy is performed in each patient with an appendix. The practice prevents the need for any future operation for appendicitis and rules out the possibility that any future pain or problems stemming from a complication of the surgery could be mistaken for appendicitis. A cholecystectomy is also routinely performed in each patient who still has a gallbladder. This is done because there is a high risk for the development of gallstones in bariatric patients during the first postoperative year if the gallbladder is left in place. Other concurrent procedures may also be performed, as necessary.

▶ RESTRICTION AND MALABSORPTION: REASONS FOR PRECISE MEASUREMENTS

Lipid Malabsorption and Common Channel Length

Clinical evidence shows a direct relationship between the level of lipid malabsorption and the length of the common channel. The BPD/DS interferes with the absorption of lipids primarily by diverting the bile and pancreatic digestive enzymes to the relatively short distal portion of the alimentary limb known as the common channel. If the common channel is constructed so that it is too long, the reduction in absorption of fats will not be sufficient for adequate weight loss. If it is too short, the patient may lose too much weight and eventually require revision of the procedure.

For best results, the limb lengths should be calculated by using a percentage of the total small bowel length measured from the cecum to the ligament of Treitz. The correct length for the alimentary limb is 40% of the patient's total small bowel length; and the common channel should measure approximately 10% of the total bowel length. Percentage-based lengths have been found to provide more consistent and reliable weight loss than simple centimeter measurements because the total length of the small bowel varies considerably from patient to patient. Measurements of the total small bowel lengths in the

Table 30-2	TOTAL SMALL BOWEL LENGTHS			
	NUMBER OF PATIENTS	MAXIMUM LENGTH	MINIMUM LENGTH	AVERAGE LENGTH (cm)
Female	769	997	378	706
Male	237	1187	497	776
Both	1006	1187	378	718

n = 1006.

1006 patients illustrate the variation in small bowel lengths (Table 30-2). Figure 30-6 contains a graph showing seven different combinations of alimentary and common channel lengths in centimeters, all based on the 10% and 40% formula. It reveals good long-term weight loss results, nearly the same for all combinations.

Table 30-3 illustrates the significant variation in percentages of total bowel lengths that results from using a standard centimeter measurement to create the same limb length in all patients. The first three rows show the same limb lengths (100/250) with different total bowel lengths. The fourth row shows the most common small bowel length and limbs of 40% and 10%.

The first row shows an alimentary limb that is 50% and a common channel length of 16% of total small bowel length. Both are too long, and the patient may not lose weight satisfactorily.

The second row shows an alimentary limb of 33% and a common channel of 13% of the total small bowel length. This patient may have difficulty with low protein because the alimentary limb is too short. The length of the common channel may be acceptable.

The third row shows an alimentary limb of 25% and a common channel of 10%. This patient will have low protein levels and excess weight loss and will require a revision because only 25% of the small bowel is available for absorption.

The fourth row is an example of percentage-calculated limb lengths. The average of total small bowel length is 750 cm. The common channel is 75 cm, and the alimentary limb is 300 cm. Both are calculated by the 40% and 10% rule. This patient should lose weight without associated side effects or complications.

If a surgeon prefers to use common channels of the same length in all patients, a length of 75 cm should be effective in most cases. Table 30-4 illustrates the percentage of the total number of patients who received common channel lengths of 50, 75, or 100 cm. The table reveals that in the vast majority of patients, the common channel was constructed to be 75 cm long. The surgeon, however, must be aware of the risks of using the same channel lengths in all patients. In those with unusually short or long small bowels or with other relevant factors affecting weight loss, choosing the length automatically could lead to unpredictable long-term results that are less satisfactory than the results found in those with precisely determined channel lengths.

Protein Malabsorption

Although the BPD/DS affects primarily lipid absorption, it also decreases protein absorption. Protein deficiency may develop over time if there is too much protein malabsorption.

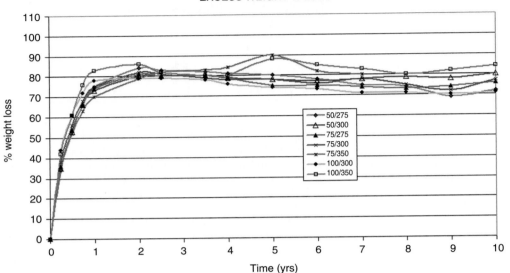

Figure 30-6. Seven different combinations of alimentary and common channel lengths in centimeters, based on the 10% and 40% formula. This graph shows similar weight loss results for all combinations.

To prevent protein deficiency, the alimentary limb must be constructed to be as long as possible without reaching the point at which it hinders adequate long-term weight loss. The formula of 40% of total length was determined with this in mind, and it has proven to be the appropriate formula in virtually all cases. There is a growing consensus on this point among bariatric surgeons performing this type of operation. It has been reported that the BPD/DS does not result in albumin/protein malnutrition if the common and alimentary channels are measured as a percentage of the total length of the small bowel.[4] The same report also revealed that albumin levels remained at the low to normal level, whether the patients were morbidly obese or super morbidly obese (Fig. 30-7). The surgeons writing the report also used the 40% and 10% formula. Nevertheless, rare cases of protein deficiency in BPD/DS patients do occur.

It has been proposed that a longer common channel might prevent the problem of protein deficiency. However, Dr. Scopinaro has reported that increasing the length of the common channel alone does not necessarily increase protein absorption, but it does have the negative effect of reducing fat malabsorption. He found that protein absorption increases significantly with the lengthening the alimentary limb. Accordingly, the ideal revision operation would increase only the alimentary limb so as to ensure protein absorption, while maintaining a relatively

short common channel so as to ensure continued weight loss. Unfortunately, this ideal revision is mechanically difficult to construct. An effective compromise that has been used for revision to correct protein deficiency is a procedure that simply advances the alimentary limb proximally on the biliopancreatic limb. This increases the lengths of both the common channel and the alimentary limb and has been successful in most cases (Fig. 30-8).

Table 30-4	COMMON CHANNEL LENGTHS	
NUMBER OF PATIENTS	LENGTH (cm)	PERCENTAGE
321	50	22.9
951	75	67.80
130	100	9.30

n = 1402.

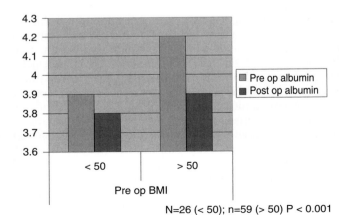

N=26 (< 50); n=59 (> 50) P < 0.001

Figure 30-7. Albumin levels remained low or normal in 26 patients with BMIs below 50 kg per m² and in 59 patients with BMIs above 50 kg per m²; P 0.001. BMI, body mass index.

Table 30-3	LIMB LENGTH BY PERCENTAGE			
SMALL BOWEL LENGTH (cm)	ALIMENTARY LENGTH (cm)	COMMON CHANNEL (cm)	PERCENT ALIMENTARY	PERCENT COMMON CHANNEL
500	250	100	50	16
750	250	100	33.30	13.30
1000	250	100	25	10
750	300	75	40	10

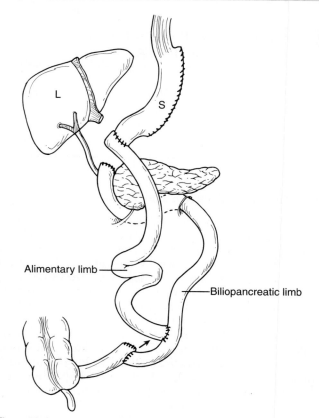

Figure 30-8. Revision: Advance alimentary limb upon biliopancreatic limb.

Carbohydrate Absorption

A restricted alimentary limb also affects carbohydrate absorption, but not to any detrimental degree. Because as much as 40% of the body's amylase is produced by the parotid and submandibular glands, carbohydrate digestion begins in the mouth. Therefore, more than enough absorption of carbohydrates is maintained, even with the restricted alimentary limb. In fact, if carbohydrate intake is excessive, weight loss will be inadequate. This is the reason for advising patients to eat a limited-carbohydrate diet. Increasing the alimentary limb length also increases the absorption of carbohydrates.

Stomach Volume

With the BPD/DS, a vertical gastrectomy is formed to restrict the patient's food intake.

The vertical gastrectomy, with its pylorus-saving feature, sets this operation apart from most other restrictive bariatric procedures, but the simple concept of restricted volume remains key in assisting patients to lose excess weight. Although reduced to a size that limits food intake, the stomach must be constructed so that it is large enough to allow consumption of sufficient protein and calories to prevent protein deficiency and excessive weight loss.

The stomachs in the early BPD/DS operations were conservatively constructed to have a volume of up to twice the volume of the stomachs in the current operations. It was later determined that the stomach could be made smaller without putting the patient at significant risk

for complications. The reduced stomach of 90 to 120 ml sufficiently restricts patients' intake of food while allowing them to eat more than is possible after other restrictive procedures. The stomach enlarges over time, however, and within approximately 2 years, once most of the excess weight has been lost, patients can then eat nearly normal amounts of food. Thus it is important to construct the stomach small enough so that it will not eventually dilatate to a size that allows the patient to gain weight.

▶ COMPLICATIONS

Gastric Leaks

The gastric leak is a life-threatening complication that can occur with any type of bariatric surgery. It may arise as early as the first or second postoperative day, or as late as a month or more after surgery. Most often it occurs within the first 1 to 3 weeks after surgery. Of 1402 patients who had undergone the BPD/DS, including reoperations, there were a total of 18 gastric leaks.

In the first 253 primary cases, a four-row stapler was used, and the staple row was sutured with an over-and-over suture. An unacceptable leak rate of 2.8% (7 leaks) developed in this group. The leak rate dropped dramatically in 1994 after the adoption of Baltasar's method of inverting the mucosal edge with a running Lembert suture.[5] Thereafter, a two-row staple line and inverted mucosa with a running Lembert suture was consistently used. There were 6 leaks (0.67%) in the 990 primary cases employing the mucosal inversion, none of which occurred in the 4-year period between the 2000 and late 2004. Changing to the two-row stapler and inverting the mucosa with a running Lembert suture was a major development in preventing gastric leaks.

Patients who are reoperated are at greater risk for development of gastric leaks due to the multiple adhesions and old staple rows from previous operations. Each additional bariatric surgery increases the possibility of complications, including gastric leaks (Table 30-5). In the 159 reoperations (conversions of failed restrictive procedures), there were 6 gastric leaks (3.77%). This computes to nearly five times the leak rate of the last 990 primary cases performed. Leaks developed in 2 of 9 patients (22.2%) who had had three previous bariatric restrictive procedures. All survived and lost weight but less weight than would be expected with a primary BPD/DS. In a group of

Table 30-5	**RESULTS AFTER PREVIOUS BARIATRIC SURGERIES**		
NUMBER OF PATIENTS	NUMBER OF LEAKS	NUMBER OF PREVIOUS SURGERIES	PERCENTAGE
9	2	3	22.20
38	3	2	7.89
112	1	1	0.89

n = 159 reoperations; leaks = 6; percentage of leaks after reoperation = 3.77.

38 patients who had had two previous bariatric surgeries, a leak rate of 7.89% was seen. The leak rate in 112 patients who had had only one previous bariatric surgery was .89%, slightly higher than the leak rate in primary BPD/DS patients. Although these figures represent three relatively small series, they distinctly reveal an increasing risk for developing gastric leaks with each successive bariatric surgery. It is vitally important to choose the most effective surgical procedure initially, so that the patient can expect the best long-term results with the lowest probability that a second surgery will be required.

Treatment of Gastric Leaks

All patients with gastric leaks are seriously ill and should be surgically explored as soon as stable. These patients are dehydrated, may be septic, and need IV fluids and antibiotics immediately while preparing for surgery. An upper gastrointestinal radiograph before surgery will help to locate the leak, which may not be easily located during surgery. Multiple drains should be placed near the leak and in the abscess during surgery. It is not necessary to find or suture the leak because the repair will ultimately fail. A feeding tube is placed in the jejunum on the biliopancreatic limb for future tube feedings. The duodenal and the distal Roux-en-Y anastomoses are checked to be certain there are no other leaks.

Postoperatively, the patient should be in the intensive care unit and on antibiotics and total parenteral nutrition. The patient may require a respirator. When stable (afebrile and with a functioning gastrointestinal tract, etc.), he or she may be started gradually on tube feedings. The feeding supplement should be a half-strength solution high in protein and low in carbohydrates; 1500 calories per day should be adequate for protein preservation. Using only half-strength solutions prevents the plugging of the feeding tube. The patient will be discharged on tube feedings, and the feedings may continue for several months.

Duodenoileostomy Leaks

The duodenoileostomy leak is unique to the BPD/DS and can occur in any patient. It is a difficult area of anastomosis because of the proximate position of vital ducts, vessels, and organs, such as the common duct, pancreas, portal vein, and multiple small arteries that are in the immediately surrounding area. The complexities of this area are magnified in morbidly obese patients because the area is deep in the abdomen, surrounded by adipose tissue, and often difficult to identify and isolate. Although a leak here is generally small, it can be large and critical. In the first 119 operations, the ileum was hand-sutured to the duodenum with an end-to-side anastomosis. There were two leaks (1.7%) and three strictures (2.5%) requiring reoperation. Beginning in 1994, the Valtrac anastomosing ring was used for all small bowel anastomoses. The ring simplified the process and resulted in better anastomoses and no strictures. The leak rate decreased to 1.2%. Minor changes in technique, including the use of double purse-string ties and fibrin glue around the anastomosis, have since been employed with the expectation that the leak rate will decrease (Table 30-6).

Table 30-6	DUODENOILEOSTOMY LEAKS AND STRICTURES	
PROCEDURE/NUMBER OF PATIENTS	**LEAKS (%)**	**STRICTURES**
End-to-side anastomosis/119	1.7	2.5%
Valtrac anastomosing ring/1283	1.2	None

Treatment of Duodenoileostomy Leaks

It is fortunate that most duodenoileostomy leaks are small and can be successfully treated without surgery. This is especially true if on radiograph there is no evidence of abscess formation, as shown by air-fluid levels near the leak area, and if the site is not septic. Conservative treatment entails nothing by mouth, total parenteral nutrition, antibiotics, and close observation. It is not usually necessary to use nasogastric suction.

If the leak is large and the site is septic, it is necessary to drain the area surgically. A jejunal feeding tube should be placed on the biliopancreatic limb for long-term nutritional support while the leak is closing. The feeding tube allows the patient to be discharged from the hospital prior to complete closure of the leak.

Distal Roux-en-Y Leaks

A leak at the site of a distal Roux-en-Y gastric bypass is life-threatening and difficult to diagnose. Because it is not common and because routine radiographs often do not reveal a distal Roux-en-Y leak, it can be easily overlooked. However, a Valtrac ring used in the anastomosis does show on a radiograph, allowing visualization of the leak. A vigilant surgeon will be alert to the possibility of such a leak. The author had one distal Roux-en-Y leak in 1402 cases. It was diagnosed during an exploratory laparotomy for sepsis in a patient who had had air escaping from around his Penrose drain. The leak was at a stapled anastomosis of the distal Roux-en-Y, which was treated by bringing the ends of the anastomosis out of the abdomen to form a controlled small bowel fistula. The patient was given antibiotics, intravenous fluids, and total parenteral nutrition. The controlled fistula was successfully closed later. If the distal Roux-en-Y leak is detected early when there is no more than minimal infection, it may be closed at the time of corrective surgery. In any event, the area must be drained.

Starting in 1994, the distal Roux-en-Y end-to-side anastomosis was created using a Valtrac anastomosing ring. This device was used in more than 1280 distal Roux-en-Y anastomoses, and thereafter there were no leaks or obstructions.

Other Complications

Various other complications may occur in a patient of any size who is undergoing surgery. However, the risk for complications is significantly greater when operating on patients with BMIs of 40 to 90 kg per m². There is the risk

Table 30-7	COMPLICATIONS	
COMPLICATIONS	NUMBER	PERCENTAGE
Atelectasis	187	13.3
Pneumonia	26	1.8
Pulmonary embolus	2 (fatal)	0.14
Nonfatal pulmonary embolus	3	0.21
ARDS	4	0.29
Thrombophlebitis	3	0.21
Gastric ulcer	3	0.21
Cystic duct leak	2	0.14
Marginal ulcer	4	0.29
Late complications		
Duodenoilium obstruction	3	0.21
Small bowel obstruction	14	1.03

n = 1402.
ARDS, acute respiratory distress syndrome.

for the usual surgical complications, as well as for those peculiar to the morbidly obese patient (Table 30-7).

Marginal ulcers at the site of the margin of the small bowel and the duodenum are a risk in BPD/DS surgery. The authors have treated one marginal ulcer in a BPD/DS patient. Three more patients were treated at other hospitals. Bleeding from these ulcers can be severe, and operating on these patients for bleeding ulcers is difficult because of adhesions in the gastric area.

In all bariatric surgeries that involve either a long- or a short-limb Roux-en-Y, including the BPD/DS, there is an increased incidence of small bowel obstruction. I operated on 11 of my BPD/DS patients for small bowel obstruction, and I know 3 of my patients were operated on at other centers. Most of the obstructions have been due to abdominal adhesions. Three were directly related to internal hernias and involved the biliopancreatic limb. Obstruction in the biliopancreatic limb portion does not show on the normal flat and upright film used to diagnose small bowel obstruction because there is no air-fluid level. A computed tomography scan may be required to make the diagnoses. The patient may have only minor abdominal complaints or may exhibit severe signs and symptoms. To decrease the chance of developing a small bowel obstruction, it is important to close the mesentery of the small bowel correctly at the time of the original surgery. Any patient with a Roux-en-Y gastric bypass who has severe abdominal pain should be taken to surgery without delay because it is commonly caused by internal hernia obstruction, which could easily lead to gangrene of the bowel without prompt surgical treatment.

Rhabdomyolysis is a newly mentioned complication in bariatric surgery. It involves necrosis of the gluteal muscles and renal failure, and it commonly leads to death. Although the condition is common in crush or reperfusion injuries, it now appears also to be a risk for super morbidly obese bariatric surgery patients. It was first reported as a risk in bariatric surgery at the American Surgical Association in April 2003.[6] The report discussed five patients who developed the condition, three of whom died. All the patients were male and super morbidly obese, and they all underwent unusually long operations. It now appears that a super morbidly obese patient lying in the same position for many hours during a lengthy surgery may be at risk for developing this serious condition.

Virtually all bariatric surgery patients are at risk for developing anemia. Because stomach acid and the intrinsic factor produced by the stomach are both decreased in restricted stomachs, iron absorption is also decreased. Dr. Brolin reported an anemia (<12 g/dl) rate of more than 40% in his bariatric subjects.[7] However, if the standards are more strictly applied, the anemia rates are much lower. Of my bariatric patients who were more than 1 year post surgery, 117 (8%) developed anemia, for which they were treated. However, many patients seek treatment from their family physicians for anemia and other minor complications, so it must be assumed that the actual level of treated anemia is probably somewhat higher than the 8% that is known. Occasionally, a patient develops anemia so severe that iron must be administered intramuscularly or intravenously, or blood transfusions must be performed.

At the 20th annual meeting of the American Society for Bariatric Surgery, it was reported that nearly all bariatric patients with anemia can be successfully treated by administering iron orally.[8] The patients discussed in that report maintained average iron levels of 11.6 mg per dl at 2 years postoperatively, and 11.8 mg per dl at 3 years, regardless of whether they had been treated for anemia. A recommendation was made for routine iron supplementation in all females during the menstruating years.

Hypoproteinemia can develop in any postoperative bariatric patient because both a restricted stomach and bypass of the small bowel hinder dietary protein absorption. For this reason all patients are expected to consume a high-protein diet, take supplements, and limit refined sugar and other carbohydrates in order to lose weight while maintaining normal albumin and other laboratory levels. Consuming adequate protein is vitally important. If the albumin drops to an abnormal level, the patient may be treated by taking albumin and oral pancreatic enzymes (Creon-10) with protein meals. If the problem persists, then a revision of the distal Roux-en-Y may be necessary.

Hypocalcemia may also occur after bariatric surgery. Calcium levels are related to protein and should be satisfactory if the patient eats well and takes absorbable calcium, such as calcium citrate (Citracal) or microcrystalline hydroxyapetite (Cal Apetite), which are 200 times more easily absorbed than calcium carbonate. A patient who takes only calcium carbonate will not be able to absorb adequate amounts of calcium.

Bariatric patients are at risk for developing vitamin deficiencies because of both the restrictive and the malabsorptive aspects of the surgery. This is especially true of the fat-soluble vitamins because the BPD/DS affects lipid absorption primarily. All patients must supplement their intake with water-miscible vitamins A and D.

The cohort used to evaluate laboratory findings comprises 110 patients, some with 8-year follow-up, others with 12-year follow-up. Of the 110 patients, 8 did not have complete reports. The majority of the group had 10-year follow-up and normal laboratory levels. All of the average laboratory results in the first 10-year cohort are within the normal range. However, a few of these patients had difficulty with low levels of protein, calcium, and

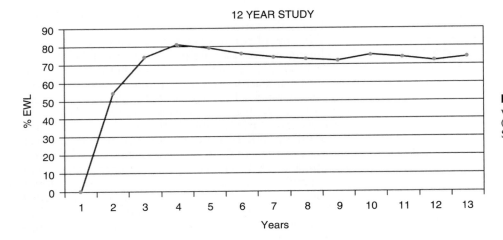

Figure 30-9. The study reveals a 72% excess weight loss at 12 years, with 75% follow-up. (Modified from Hess DS, Hess DW: Obes Surg 2005;3:408-416, by permission).

vitamins; most were treated medically, but some required revision of the distal Roux-en-Y. (See Revisions, later in this chapter.)

▶ RESULTS

Weight Loss

The weight loss results in the primary BPD/DS patients[9] are based on a 92% 10-year follow-up of a cohort of 182 consecutive patients, all of whom were at least 10 years postoperative, some of whom were 18 years postoperative. The average weight loss in this group of 167 patients peaked at 80% of excess weight loss at 4 years, dropped to 78% at 5 years (95% follow-up), and then leveled off at 75% of excess weight loss at 10 years (92% follow-up) (Fig. 30-9). The 12-year study indicates 72% excess weight loss at 12 years, with 75% follow-up. At 13 years, the number of follow-up patients was insignificant.

Weight loss results may be more appropriately studied by considering both average weight loss and individual results. When the same 167 patients are grouped by levels of success, 52% obtained excellent weight loss, and 33%

reached the level labeled good, for a total of 85% in the good and excellent categories (Tables 30-8 and 30-9). Another 9% obtained fair weight loss, with stable weight and cure of or reduction in comorbidities. This computes to 94% in the category labeled satisfactory and only 6% in the category labeled unsatisfactory.

Deaths

Overall, the death rate in patients in this practice after BPD/DS is 0.57% (Table 30-10). A higher death rate is seen in super morbidly obese patients (BMI >50 kg/m²); at 1.16%, it is eight times the death rate in morbidly obese patients who have BMIs less than 50, and it is more than twice the overall death rate. Seven of the eight deaths in this practice were patients categorized as super morbidly obese. There was only one death (0.13%) among the 796 patients who had BMIs less than 50. Not only do super morbidly obese patients suffer from a greater number and more

Table 30-8	INDIVIDUAL RESULTS IN EXCESS WEIGHT LOSS	
CLASSIFICATION	NUMBER OF PATIENTS	PERCENTAGE
Excellent	87	52
Good	55	33
Fair	15	9
Poor	7	4
Failure (absolute)	3	2
Good-excellent	142	85
Satisfactory	157	94
Unsatisfactory	10	6

n = 167; all follow-up was 10 years or more.
Grade determinants (all minimum values): excellent, 80% excess weight loss (EWL); good, 60% EWL; fair, 50% EWL; poor, 40% EWL; failure, <20% EWL; satisfactory, excellent, good, fair; unsatisfactory, poor, failure. (Modified from Hess DS, Hess DW: Obes Surg 2005;3:408-416, by permission.)

Table 30-9	INDIVIDUAL RESULTS IN EXCESS WEIGHT LOSS	
TEST PERFORMED	RESULTS	RANGE
Hemoglobin	12.2	12-16
WBC	6.7	4.8-1
Glucose	87.0	70-108
Calcium	8.7	8.7-10.5
Protein	6.6	6.1-8.0
Albumen	3.8	3.1-4.9
Bilirubin	0.59	0.2-1.1
Alkaline phosphatase	101	37-107
SGOT	24	12-45
SGPT	25	0-55
Triglyceride	95	0-199
Cholesterol	136	<200
HDL cholesterol	46	40-60
Vitamin A	46	
Vitamin D$_{25}$	20	
Vitamin D$_{125}$	74	

n = 110 (91% of cohort of 120).
HDL, high-density lipoprotein; SGOT, serum glutamic-oxaloacetic transaminase; SGPT, serum glutamic-pyruvic transaminase; wbc, white blood count.

Table 30-10	MORTALITY RATE DURING FIRST 60 DAYS POSTOPERATIVELY: 0.57%

BMI	CAUSE OF DEATH (ONE POINT EACH)
58	Pulmonary embolus
53	Pulmonary embolus
66	Leak, peritonitis
47	Diabetic, cardiac, multiple organ failure
74	Bilateral bronchial obstruction, sleep apnea
65	Hypoventilation syndrome, severe
54	Sepsis, negative exploration
61	Leak, sepsis, cardiac tamponade 2^0 to CVP line erosion

n = 1402; super morbid obese, n = 606; 7 cases in 606 = 1.16%.
1 case <50 kg/m^2 BMI in 796 = 0.13%.
BMI, body mass index; CVP, central venous pressure.

serious comorbidities, they also have a greater risk for death resulting from surgery related to these comorbidities.

OTHER BENEFICIAL EFFECTS OF BPD/DS

Pregnancy

A study of the effects of BPD/DS on pregnancies concluded that the surgery was beneficial to both mothers and babies, and that the children's growth and development were normal.[10] Of the patients who had been infertile prior to surgery, 50% became pregnant after surgery. There was no increase in the incidence of miscarriage or premature birth and no increased vomiting during pregnancy. Further, the patients had less difficulty following nutritious diets. The serum albumin, hemoglobin, and iron levels were not significantly different from the levels the patients had when not pregnant. The children over the age of 4 years who had been born after the mother's BPD/DS were found to be in good to excellent health.

The clinical evidence in my patients reveals similar outcomes regarding fertility and pregnancy after the BPD/DS. The handbook provided to every patient, however, includes a section on childbearing that advises against pregnancy in the early postoperative period, before the patient's weight stabilizes. During the initial postoperative period of rapid weight loss, the nutritional stress on the mother's body makes maintenance of sufficient nourishment for pregnancy more difficult. Nevertheless, there have been several pregnancies in the early post-BPD/DS period, and all have progressed normally and resulted in healthy offspring.

Effects on Liver

One of the most persistent erroneous claims regarding the BPD/DS is that the procedure increases or causes liver damage. The source of this misunderstanding may be the fact that liver disease did develop with jejunoileal bypasses. These bypasses are no longer performed today because of the numerous complications, including liver problems. The distinct and vital differences between the BPD/DS and the jejunoileal bypass must be appreciated.

The only functioning part of the small bowel after a jejunoileal bypass was a common channel approximately 2 feet long. The remaining bypassed part of the small bowel was completely unconnected to the alimentary system, with no bile salts or digestive enzymes passing through to clean the bowel and be reabsorbed in the natural manner. Bypassed bowel secretions often became inspissated and bacterially colonized. Infection probably traveled up through the portal vein to the liver. Likewise, extreme malabsorption led to serious nutrition (vitamin, mineral and protein) deficiencies, which also can cause liver disease.

Morbidly obese patients are commonly found to have related liver problems. In most cases, fatty metamorphosis is already present by the time the morbidly obese patient decides to have surgery. However, by 2 to 3 years after surgery, BPD/DS patients have been reported to have improvement in liver function on testing and reduction of liver steatosis on biopsy.[11] Also, I have had several patients with obesity-induced fatty livers who have experienced improvement after surgery, as indicated by liver function tests and occasional biopsies. There were no known cases of postoperative worsening of liver disease. Weight loss alone leads to improvement in liver steatosis, just as it improves other comorbidities of morbid obesity.

ADDITIONAL OPERATIONS

Revision or reversal should be considered for patients with persistent and serious low protein levels, excess weight loss, severe anemia, or hypocalcia. The causes of the deficiencies should be evaluated first. The patient simply may not be eating meals of sufficiently high protein content or may not be taking the prescribed vitamins and calcium. Aggressive medical management in a hospital setting, including intravenous fluids, vitamins, calcium, iron, and serum albumin, is necessary for patients with significant malnutrition. Oral multivitamins and calcium must also be given. Additionally, the patient's diet must consist of high-quality protein and pancreatic enzymes taken before, during, and after each meal. An upper gastrointestinal series with a small bowel follow-through should be performed to ensure that there are no strictures or other obstacles to the proper functioning of the gastrointestinal tract. With a partial stricture at the duodenal anastomosis, the patient's ability to consume enough protein and other nutrients is significantly reduced and can lead to malnutrition. Although aggressive medical treatment may lead to recovery without surgery, laboratory levels should continue to be closely monitored after discharge. In rare instances, revision or reversal may become necessary. The decision to reverse the operation should be made carefully because the patient may regain all the weight lost.

Reversals

Of a total 1243 primary BPD/DS patients, 19 (1.53%) have undergone reversals. The reasons are various but usually involved excessive weight loss and protein malnutrition. At least three of the reversals were performed in patients who cooperated poorly, not returning for follow-up for 4 to 5 years and probably not taking supplements as prescribed. One patient was a drug addict with poor compliance who was reversed at the first opportunity.

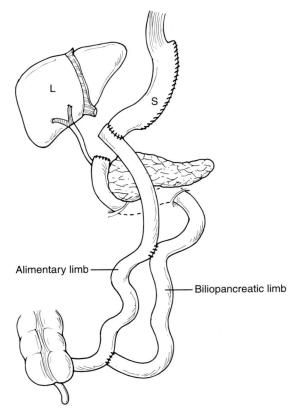

Figure 30-10. Reversal: Side to side anastomosis jejunum to ileum, close to ligament of Treitz.

Surgical reversal can be performed by creating a side-to-side anastomosis between the jejunum, just beyond the ligament of Treitz, and the proximal alimentary limb. This creates a crossover between the biliopancreatic limb and the alimentary limb, which reverses the malabsorption. If the patient is in a state of severe malnutrition, a jejunal feeding tube is inserted for use until the patient fully recovers (Fig. 30-10).

Other surgeons have performed 10 reversals. I know neither the reasons for these reversals nor the types of procedures used. Because of a general bias against partial-malabsorption procedures, the surgeons may have reversed the procedures rather than attempting revisions. Alternatively, those surgeons may have been among the many who simply do not understand the BPD/DS. In some cases the small bowel may have been reverted to a relatively normal configuration, essentially creating a gastric bypass. In two cases, and for unknown reasons, the distal stomach was actually removed (Table 30-11).

Revisions

In our group of 1243 primary patients, 55 revisions (4.4%) were performed (Table 30-12). Most of the revisions occurred between 1 and 2 years postoperatively and were performed along with other procedures, such as incisional hernia repairs or abdominal panniculectomies. Of the 55 revisions, 31 (2.5%) were performed because of excess weight loss or protein deficiency and 4 (0.32%) for frequent episodes of diarrhea not adequately controlled.

Table 30-11	REVERSALS		
#	PRIMARY REASON	TYPE OF REVERSAL	RESULTS
1	No follow-up available	Side to side	Weight regain
2	Diarrhea	Side to side	Weight gain
1	Low protein, malnutrition	Long revision	Stable weight
1	Low protein, malnutrition	Side to side	Stable weight
1	Low protein, malnutrition	Side to side	Stable weight
1	Excess weight protein loss	2 revisions	Weight gain
1	Cirrhosis, low prt, weight loss	Side to side	Weight gain
1	Ovarian malignancy	Side to side	Expired
10	Other	Unknown	

Reversals = 19 of 1243 operations (1.53%).

The treatment of choice in these two groups of patients was to lengthen both the common and the alimentary channels by advancing the alimentary limb proximally on the biliopancreatic limb.

Of the 55 revisions, 7 (0.56%) were performed because of inadequate weight loss. In those patients, only the common channel was shortened. The results were unsatisfactory because none of the patients lost more than 20 additional pounds. However, the revision did prevent further weight gain. Clinical evidence shows that some patients simply cease losing weight and level off at a weight that is higher than expected.

Of the patients with revisions, 5 (0.4%) had been in the early group of primary operations when the stomach sizes were constructed so as to be larger. In all 5 cases, the stomachs were reduced in size by removing more of the greater-curvature portion, and the revisions were effective. Reduction in stomach size is an effective revision in patients with the correct limb lengths but enlarged stomachs, who have stopped losing weight or have gained weight.

Revisions were performed elsewhere in 8 (0.64%) patients. I do not know the reasons for the revisions or the procedures employed.

Reoperations to Change the Procedure

Operating to change the configuration of the stomach and small bowel from that created during a previously performed bariatric operation to a BPD/DS presents unique challenges. In my experience, these procedures

Table 30-12	REVISIONS		
NUMBER	REASON FOR REVISION	PROCEDURE	PERCENTAGE
31	Excess weight loss, low protein	Advance alimentary onto biliopancreatic limb	2.49
4	Excess diarrhea	Advance alimentary onto biliopancreatic limb	0.32
7	Poor weight loss	Shorten common channel	0.56
5	Poor weight loss	Reduce stomach size	0.4
8	Unknown (elsewhere)	Unknown	0.64
55	Total revisions	3.9% (our) revisions	4.4

n = 1243.

were most commonly performed to modify a failed restrictive procedure.

Extensive adhesions are commonly found in the abdomen, especially between the stomach and the liver. These adhesions must be taken down first, before assessing whether and how the BPD/DS can be performed. If the old row of staples was placed vertically, as in the vertical banded gastroplasty, the new vertical staple line should be placed inside, on the lesser-curvature side of the old staple line. This placement allows for good blood supply and diminishes the chances for leak formation. The band is often eroded and must be dealt with as the surgeon determines. I usually open the stomach on the greater-curvature side and resect the eroded band, removing as much as possible, then oversuture the mucosa in that area.

With a transverse gastroplasty, the stomach is also opened on the greater-curvature side, and any of the old staple rows that remain are removed. The old staple line is oversewn inside the stomach to prevent bleeding. The dilator can then be brought down and the vertical gastrectomy performed as in a primary case.

If the prior surgery was a gastric bypass with a short-limb Roux-en-Y, the proximal gastric pouch may be very small because of having been transected near the esophagus. The opening on the anterior portion of the small pouch where the pouch and bowel had been connected must be closed or removed when reconnecting the stomach. The sutures should all be interrupted so that it will be possible to staple vertically across them without interfering with the anastomosis. In some cases the stomach pouch is very small and can be reattached to the lower stomach with an end-to-end anastomosis. Generally, the portion of the jejunum that is above the colon is removed, rather than trying to save that short piece of bowel. The removed portion of jejunum is measured and the measurement is added to the total bowel length when determining the limb lengths. The remainder of the bowel is attached back to its original connection. At this point, the BPD/DS can be performed.

Reoperations are complex and lengthy, especially reoperations on gastric bypasses. To reduce the chance of developing rhabdomyolysis, some surgeons recommend that the reoperation be done in two stages in super morbidly obese male patients. Both Anthone[6] and Gagner[12] make this recommendation.

When performing reoperations, surgeons may be reluctant to construct limbs as short as recommended in patients who may not be as obese as they were originally and seem not to have a great deal of weight to lose. However, limbs that are too long will not offer the same weight loss outcome and the patient may end up being as obese as before the first operation. The limbs should be made the proper length. It is not difficult to revise the small bowel in a patient who loses too much weight. A revision for poor weight loss is much more difficult and uncertain.

▶ BPD/DS FOR TEENAGE OBESITY

As teenage obesity rapidly increases, it has a devastating effect on more victims. Along with the negative effects on health, morbid obesity can also lead to life-long emotional effects. These teens are often bullied and ostracized by their peers precisely at a time in their lives when their peers are all-important.

I have used BPD/DS successfully to treat super morbidly obese teenage patients: 19 teenagers between the ages of 14 and 18 have had the operation. They all had BMIs greater than 50 kg per m². One was a reoperation on a failed restrictive procedure performed 6 years earlier, when the patient was 14 years old. Prior to the initial surgery, his parents had become concerned about possible suicide because of their son's withdrawal and depression. The patient lost his excess weight and maintained the weight loss until the staples failed and he began gaining weight during his first year of college. At that time the BPD/DS was performed. After 12 years, he was married and had two children and had maintained a normal weight (Fig. 30-11).

A 15-year-old female patient with a BMI of 50, hypertension, and type II diabetes had a primary BPD/DS. She successfully lost her excess weight and no longer suffered from hypertension or type II diabetes. She graduated from high school with a weight of 55 kg and attended college on a scholarship. Similarly, another patient who was 228 kg

Figure 30-11. Although only 21 patients (14 to 18 years of age) are referred to here, the graph follows the expected results for percentage of excess weight loss. Of the two 17-year-old patients, one had a medical problem during the ninth year that caused an increase in weight loss but returned to normal at years 10 and 11 without surgery. The other 17-year-old patient had undergone a conversion to a PBD/DS 7 years earlier. One postoperative patient, at 10 years, had undergone conversion from a restrictive procedure to a PBD/DS. The number of primary teenage patients was one 14-year-old, two 15-year-olds, four 16-year-olds, five 17-year-olds, seven 18-year-olds, and two conversions to PBD/DS.

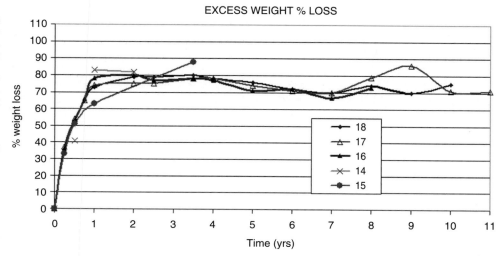

EXCESS WEIGHT % LOSS

% weight loss vs. Time (yrs)

Legend: 18, 17, 16, 14, 15

preoperatively was 100 kg and a mother of a 2-year-old child 10 years postoperatively.

One case was unsuccessful. The patient was noncompliant, and 10 years after surgery had gained back weight so that she was within 16 kg of her original weight.

For the teenage patient, there are several advantages to the BPD/DS. Revision is rarely necessary, unlike in some of the other procedures performed for obesity. Second, the BPD/DS results in the ability to eat normal small meals with few restrictions. The pylorus-saving feature of the BPD/DS allows for normal emptying of the stomach and prevents dumping syndrome. This ability to eat relatively normally permits the teenager to enjoy eating in social settings, as before the surgery. Another advantage for young female patients is that the BPD/DS has not been shown to have any detrimental effects on future pregnancies. These females may look forward to the possibility of normal pregnancies and childbirth, if desired. Finally, it is especially important for young patients to be able to plan for the future. The opportunity for sustained long-term weight loss is optimal with the BPD/DS.

▶ CONCLUSION

The BPD/DS has proven to be a safe and effective operation for the treatment of morbid obesity. It has low rates of complication, allows for excellent long-term weight loss, provides high levels of patient satisfaction, and is easy to revise or reverse. No foreign materials are used and the pylorus is retained. The BPD/DS is effective for all categories of morbidly obese patients, particularly the super morbidly obese patients who have far greater weight loss challenges than the average patient.

▶ REFERENCES

1. Hess DS, Hess DW: Biliopancreatic diversion with a duodenal switch. Obes Surg 1998;8:267-282.
2. Scopinaro N, Gianetta E, Civalleri D, et al: Biliopancreatic bypass for obesity: initial experience in man. Br J Surg 1979;66:618-620.
3. DeMeester TR, Fuchs KH, Ball CS, et al: Experimental and clinical results with proximal end-to-end duodenojejunostomy for pathologic duodenogastric reflux. Ann Surg 1987;206:414-424.
4. Keshishian A, Zahriya K: Percentage-based bypass of small bowel intestine results in exceptionally low protein malnutrition. American Society for Bariatric Surgery, 20th annual meeting; 2003 June 17-22,: Boston.
5. Baltasar A: Video presentation. American Society for Bariatric Surgery, 11th annual meeting; June 1994: Minneapolis.
6. Anthone G, Bostanjian D, Hamoui N, et al: Rhabdomyolysis of gluteal muscles leading to renal failure: a potentially fatal complication of surgery in the morbidly obese. Obes Surg 2003;13:302-305.
7. Brolin R, Leung M: Survey of vitamin and mineral supplementation after gastric bypass and biliopancreatic diversion for morbid obesity. Obes Surg 1999;9:150-154.
8. Rabkin RA, Rabkin JM, Metcalf B, et al: Nutritional markers following duodenal switch for morbid obesity. Obes Surg 2004;14:84-90.
9. Hess DS, Hess DW, Oakley RS: The biliopancreatic diversion with the duodenal switch: results beyond 10 years. Obes Surg 2005;3: 409-516.
10. Marceau P, Biron S, Kral JG, et al: Outcome of pregnancies after biliopancreatic diversion. American Society for Bariatric Surgery, 20th annual meeting; 2003 June 17-22,:Boston.
11. Biron S, Marceau S: Effects of weight loss after biliopancreatic diversion on liver morphology. Obes Surg 1996;6:121-125.
12. Gagner M: Complications: Intraoperative, post-op, long-term complications. Course presentation in Laparoscopic Surgery for Morbid Obesity, Mount Sinai School of Medicine; May 2003, New York.

31

Laparoscopic Duodenal Switch and Sleeve Gastrectomy Procedures

Crystine M. Lee, M.D., John J. Feng, M.D., F.A.C.S., Paul T. Cirangle, M.D., F.A.C.S., Janos Taller, M.D., and Gregg H. Jossart, M.D., F.A.C.S.

Bariatric surgery has evolved rapidly over the past decade. The laparoscopic technique, the adjustable gastric band, and a variety of modifications of the gastric bypass have been described. This chapter discusses adapting the laparoscopic approach to the duodenal switch operation, the staging of the duodenal switch operation, and the development of the vertical sleeve gastrectomy as a single-stage, purely restrictive procedure. At the time of preparation, extensive peer-reviewed data was still very limited; fortunately, abstract data, personal communications, personal experience, and our preliminary data have allowed us to produce this introduction to the evolution of the laparoscopic duodenal switch and the vertical gastrectomy.

▶ DUODENAL SWITCH OPERATION FOR MORBID OBESITY

The duodenal switch procedure (DS) as described by Hess and Hess is a complex weight-loss procedure that combines moderate restriction with moderate malabsorption to attain a high degree of weight loss.[1] The operation was originally performed with the open technique through an upper-midline incision. The essential components of the operation include gastric restriction via a pylorus-preserving sleeve, or vertical (parietal cell) gastrectomy, and malabsorption via a duodenal switch with functional shortening of the small intestine (Fig. 31-1). The duodenum is divided 4 cm distal to the pylorus and anastomosed to the distal 250 cm of ileum; then the biliopancreatic limb is anastomosed to the distal ileum to create a 100-cm common channel and a 150-cm enteric limb. Hess's modifications of Scopinaro's biliopancreatic diversion[2] conserved normal vagal and antropyloric anatomy, thereby eliminating dumping syndrome and marginal ulcers.

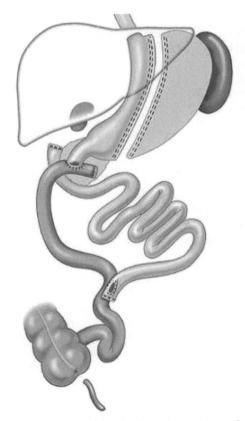

Figure 31-1. Schematic of the duodenal switch operation as described by Hess. The duodenal switch operation described by Hess consists of a sleeve gastrectomy along a 60F bougie, a duodenoenterostomy, a 250-cm enteric or alimentary limb, and a 100-cm common channel. Weight loss results from both the restrictive component of the tubularized stomach and the malabsorptive component of the functional shortening of the small intestine.

▶ EVOLUTION OF LAPAROSCOPIC BARIATRIC SURGERY

The most significant recent advance in bariatric surgery is the application of laparoscopic techniques. Cadiere pioneered the laparoscopic gastroplasty for obesity in 1994[3]; he and other authors found improved postoperative respiratory status, less postoperative pain, earlier mobilization, and shorter hospitalizations after laparoscopic vertical banded gastroplasty (VBG).[4,5] Laparoscopic Roux-en-Y gastric bypass (RYGB) feasibility studies in the porcine model were first performed in 1995[6] and were pioneered in human beings by Wittgrove and colleagues[7] and by Schauer and colleagues.[8]

The laparoscopic approach resulted in a significant reduction in morbidity and length of hospital stay.[9] Nguyen and colleagues demonstrated that laparoscopic RYGB can be performed with less blood loss, faster convalescence with less pain, fewer wound-related infections and hernias, and fewer anastomotic strictures.[10] Quality of life in the early postoperative period was superior, by SF-36 Health Survey and Bariatric Analysis of Reporting Outcome System measures but, in the long run, was equivalent in the laparoscopic and open groups. There were no differences in weight loss achieved, leak rates, or mortality, despite a longer mean operating room time.[10]

▶ EVOLUTION OF LAPAROSCOPIC DUODENAL SWITCH

Although the DS operation has been touted as one of the most effective procedures for weight loss,[11-13] the technical complexity and concerns about the long-term effects of malabsorption have limited its use. Even when performed open, the technically demanding and time-consuming procedures of a DS, with at least four staple lines and two anastomoses, are forbidding. Given the technical difficulty of the DS operation, laparoscopic-assisted and hand-assisted techniques have been performed in addition to the totally laparoscopic approach.[14]

Laparoscopy-Assisted Technique

With the laparoscopy-assisted approach, the gastrectomy and the duodenoenterostomy are performed laparoscopically. The pylorus is marked by a silk suture and a Kocher maneuver is performed. The duodenum is transected 4 cm distal to the pylorus by a linear stapler. A liver biopsy, cholecystectomy, and appendectomy can be performed. The greater curvature of the stomach is denuded, and a vertical sleeve gastrectomy is performed over a 52F bougie with linear staplers. The duodenum is then prepared by placing either a transoral or transabdominal circular anvil through the duodenal staple line. The periumbilical port site is then extended to 4 cm, allowing the stomach, gallbladder, and appendix to be removed. The entire small intestine is then measured extracorporeally and the distal anastomosis created. The circular stapler is placed into the lumen of the ileum, brought through the periumbilical incision, and docked to the anvil in the duodenum.

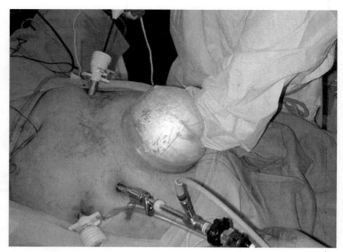

Figure 31-2. Port placement for hand-assisted duodenal switch. For the hand-assisted duodenal switch, an 8-cm periumbilical incision and three ports are used. The entire small intestine is measured and the distal anastomosis is created through the periumbilical incision. Then the Handport device is placed, and the surgeon's left hand is introduced and used to facilitate the remainder of the operation. A 10-mm camera port is placed in the right mid-quadrant, and 12-mm ports are placed in the right subcostal and left subcostal regions.

An antecolic or retrocolic proximal anastomosis is created, and the open end of the ileum is closed by a linear stapler. Methylene blue is introduced into the stomach via a nasogastric tube and, while clamping the ileum, the pouch and proximal anastomosis are checked for leakage, and measurement of the pouch volume is performed.

Hand-Assisted Technique

The hand-assisted technique is performed using an 8-cm periumbilical incision and three ports (Figs. 31-2 and 31-3). The entire small intestine is measured and the distal anastomosis is created through this incision. Using the Handport (Smith & Nephew, Andover, Mass.) or a similar device, the left hand is placed through the periumbilical

Hand-Assisted   **Totally Laparoscopic**

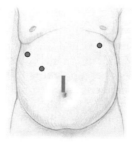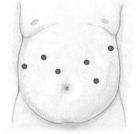

Figure 31-3. Schematic of port placement for hand-assisted and totally laparoscopic duodenal switch. This schematic compares the port placement for the hand-assisted duodenal switch and for the totally laparoscopic duodenal switch. For the hand-assisted operation, the operating surgeon stands on the patient's left, with the left hand in the Handport and the right hand working via the left upper quadrant trocar. The assistant holds the camera with the right hand and an instrument with the left hand. For the totally laparoscopic duodenal switch, the surgeon and assistant change positions several times during the operation, using different configurations of trocars for each portion of the operation.

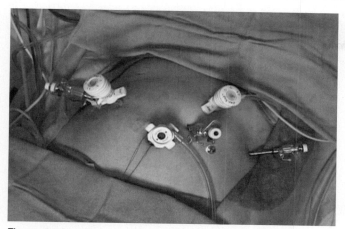

Figure 31-4. Port placement for the totally laparoscopic duodenal switch. Typically, six trocars are placed. Both the surgeon and the assistant start on the patient's left in order to create the distal anastomosis and the common channel. The assistant then moves to the patient's right in order to facilitate the passing of the small bowel through a retrocolic tunnel and the creation of the duodenoenterostomy. A pylorus-preserving greater-curvature gastrectomy along a bougie can be performed either before or after the duodenoenterostomy. Finally, if indicated, a cholecystectomy may be performed.

Table 31-1	VARIATIONS IN TECHNIQUE FOR THE TOTALLY LAPAROSCOPIC DUODENAL SWITCH

Surgical Approach
Hand-assisted: Rabkin RA, et al (Obes Surg 2003)[14]
Totally laparoscopic: Ren CJ, et al (Obes Surg 2000)[29]

Proximal Anastomosis (Duodenoenterostomy)
CEEA: Feng JJ, et al (Semin Laparosc Surg 2002)[30]
Flexible (SurgASSIST): Waage A, et al (Obes Surg 2003).[31]
  By Power Medical Interventions(r) (Pennsylvania, USA)
Hand-sewn: Baltasar A, et al (Obes Surg 2002)[19]

Antecolic vs. Retrocolic Roux
Antecolic: Feng JJ, et al (Semin Laparosc Surg 2002)[30]
Retrocolic: Camerini G, et al (Surg Lap Endosc Percut Tech 2003)[32]

Common Channel Length
100 cm: Lagace M, et al (Obes Surg 1995)[33]
50 cm: Marceau S, et al (Obes Surg 1995)[34]

Vertical Gastrectomy
60F bougie: Feng JJ, et al (Semin Laparosc Surg 2002)[30]
32F bougie: (unpublished data, Feng JJ, Cirangle PT, Jossart GH, 2006.)

incision and used to facilitate the remainder of the operation. A 10-mm camera port is placed in the right upper quadrant and 12-mm ports are placed in the right subcostal and left subcostal regions. The rest of the operation is performed in a fashion similar to that described above (Fig. 31-4).

The hand-assisted technique facilitated the transition from the laparoscopic-assisted to the totally laparoscopic approach. The operating-room time was significantly shorter for the hand-assisted technique(mean 191 minutes, range 105 to 360 minutes) than for the laparoscopic-assisted technique (mean 322 minutes, range 220 to 480 minutes). Furthermore, a decreased incidence of conversions was seen with the hand-assisted than with the laparoscopic-assisted technique (14.8% versus 9.4%).[14] Finally, surgery in patients of greater body mass index (BMI) was facilitated by employing the hand-assisted approach.

The hand-assisted technique is not without its problems. Wound complications occurred in as much as 15% of patients,[15] and in duodenal-switch patients who typically have higher BMIs and risk profiles, the complication rate can be higher. Unpublished data on 51 patients undergoing hand-assisted DS and 59 patients undergoing totally laparoscopic DS reveal that the incisional hernia rate was 31.4% as opposed to 0, respectively ($P < 0.05$), and the percentage of all complications that are wound-related is 56% as opposed to 17%, respectively ($P < 0.05$).

Totally Laparoscopic Technique

The totally laparoscopic DS is very technically challenging. The operation traverses the entire abdomen, with portions of the operation occurring in the left upper quadrant (vertical sleeve gastrectomy), the right upper quadrant (duodenal switch), and the right lower quadrant (creation of the common channel and distal anastomosis). Port placement is critical. Because of the multiple operative sites,

the ports' locations are not optimally situated for any portion of the operation, even when perfectly placed.

A feasibility study of the totally laparoscopic approach was pioneered in the porcine model by de Csepel and colleagues,[16] and despite two leaks in four animals, the study determined that the operation was technically possible. The first laparoscopic DS was subsequently reported by Ren and Gagner in a series of 40 patients.[29]

A number of variations in the totally laparoscopic approach have been described (Table 31-1), including how the duodenoenterostomy is performed (circular stapler, powered stapler, hand sewn), whether the duodenoenterostomy is ante- or retrocolic, the length of the common channel, and the sizing of the vertical gastrectomy.

▶ LAPAROSCOPIC SLEEVE GASTRECTOMY FOR MORBID OBESITY

The vertical gastrectomy procedure (also called vertical sleeve gastrectomy, sleeve gastrectomy, greater-curvature gastrectomy, parietal gastrectomy, gastric reduction, and even vertical gastroplasty) is a purely restrictive operation performed by approximately 20 surgeons worldwide. Historical data suggest that the DS operation achieves superior weight loss compared to the RYGB, and it has therefore been considered the most effective procedure for weight loss by superobese patients.[1,11] The disadvantages of the operation are its technically demanding nature and its significant morbidity rate, which have been reported to be as high as 23%[19-21] (Table 31-2). It is the superobese patients, who commonly have multiple comorbidities and carry the highest operative risks, who, paradoxically, most need this technically challenging operation so as to achieve adequate weight loss.

Performing just the restrictive component of the DS, an isolated laparoscopic vertical sleeve gastrectomy (VG),

Table 31-2	COMPLICATION RATES AFTER LAPAROSCOPIC DUODENAL SWITCH		
STUDY	NUMBER OF POINTS	AVERAGE PATIENT BMI (kg/m²)	MAJOR MORBIDITY
Ren et al, 2000[29]	40	60.0	6 (15.0%)
Baltasar et al, 2002[19]	16	>40	3 (18.8%)
Paiva et al, 2002[20]*	40	43.6	4 (12.5%)
Kim et al, 2003[21]	26	66.9	6 (23.0%)

*Paiva et al performed the Scopinaro biliopancreatic diversion.
  Due to the complexity of the operation, the incidence of complications after laparoscopic duodenal switch is high. Major complications can occur in as many as 13% to 23% of patients.
  BMI, body mass index.

is a lower risk option in this group of patients. In the United States and Germany, this procedure was first performed laparoscopically in patients with very high BMIs to try to reduce the overall risk of weight-loss surgery by staging the bariatric operations (Fig. 31-5). Particularly when a patient's BMI is above 60 kg per m², it is difficult to perform a laparoscopic RYGB or DS safely. In addition, a VG is a reasonable option for patients who have a contraindication to intestinal bypass (e.g., ulcer history, Crohn disease, renal failure, etc.).

The VG is a reasonable solution to this problem. It can usually be done laparoscopically, even in patients weighing more than 500 lb. The gastric restriction can allow these patients to lose more than 200 pounds and yields significant improvements in health and the resolution of associated medical problems, such as diabetes and sleep apnea, therefore effectively downstaging patients to a lower risk group. The patients can then return to the operating room for the second stage of the procedure, which can be the DS, the RYGB, or even laparoscopic adjustable gastric band (Band) placement.

Surgical Technique

Six trocars are placed in a configuration similar to that of the totally laparoscopic DS operation, as shown in Figure 31-3. Given the difficulties that can be experienced using the Veress needle in the morbidly obese patient, we advance a 12-mm Optiview trocar (Ethicon Endo-Surgery, Cincinnati, Ohio) under direct vision through the right rectus sheath. An epigastric Nathanson liver retractor can be used in lieu of a paddle or fan in the rightmost trocar for liver retraction.

After the greater curvature vessels are taken down using the LigaSure (ValleyLab, Boulder, Colo.), a transoral 32F esophageal dilator (Cook Medical, Bloomington, Ind.) is positioned along the lesser curvature. The rationale for using 32F sizing bougies was based on Johnston and colleagues' work with the magenstrasse and mill (MM) operation in which, between 1987 and 2003, he experimented with bougies of varying calibers, ranging from 40F down to 30F.[17] Johnston found that the 32F tube resulted in the best weight loss without any discernible increase in side effects. A comparison of abstract data from other groups performing the VG supports the concept that smaller sizing bougies result in better weight loss.

Starting at a point on the greater curvature, 3 to 6 cm from the pylorus, a greater-curvature gastrectomy is performed using sequential applications of linear 3.5- or 4.8-mm gastrointestinal staplers, thus creating a gastric tube that is 40 to 80 ml (Fig. 31-6). Bioabsorbable Seamguards (W.L. Gore, Flagstaff, Ariz.) are used selectively to buttress the staple line in diabetic patients and in those with staple-line bleeding. The vagus nerve remains intact, preserving the functions of the stomach, and the lack of intestinal bypass avoids complications such as marginal ulcers, vitamin deficiencies, and bowel obstructions.

A methylene blue leak test is performed to check staple-line integrity. Barium swallows are performed selectively on the first postoperative day if there are clinical concerns about a leak (Fig. 31-7).

A New Kind of Restrictive Operation?

Historically, restrictive bariatric operations have met with mixed success. The original horizontal gastroplasty introduced by Printen and Mason in 1973 utilized staplers to create a fundal pouch that emptied into the distal stomach via a stoma.[18] Unfortunately, the sizable pouch had a tendency to stretch and the stoma enlarge, resulting in arrested weight loss and often in weight regain. Reinforcement of the stoma was only partially successful.

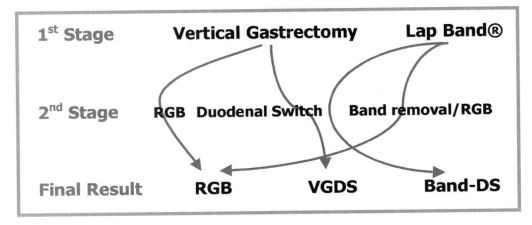

1st Stage Vertical Gastrectomy   Lap Band®

2nd Stage RGB Duodenal Switch   Band removal/RGB

Final Result   RGB   VGDS   Band-DS

Figure 31-5. Staged procedures for high-risk bariatric patients. The purpose of staged procedures for patients who have high BMIs or are at high risk is that of risk reduction. Rather than performing the definitive operation at the outset, a simpler and faster initial operation (e.g., vertical gastrectomy or Lap Band) is performed first. It results in interval weight loss, which reduces the patients' perioperative risk during the second-stage operation.

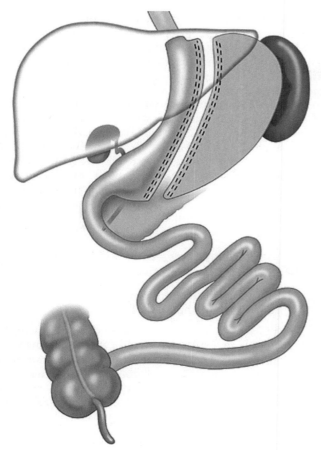

Figure 31-6. Laparoscopic vertical sleeve gastrectomy. A laparoscopic sleeve vertical gastrectomy is the restrictive part of the duodenal switch. It is performed by making multiple firings of linear staplers from the antrum to the angle of His, along a bougie. Port placement is similar to that in the totally laparoscopic duodenal switch operation shown in Figure 31-3, except that an epigastric Nathanson liver retractor may be used in lieu of a paddle or a fan in the rightmost port for liver retraction.

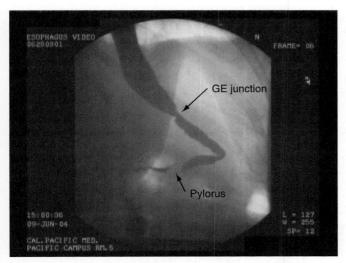

Figure 31-7. Barium swallow after vertical gastrectomy. This barium swallow was obtained on the first postoperative day after laparoscopic vertical gastrectomy. The tubularized stomach can be seen between the landmarks of the gastroesophageal (GE) junction and the pylorus (in spasm). The kink in the tubularized stomach is, in fact, the incisura of the stomach.

In 1982, Edward E. Mason attempted to improve on the operation by creating a vertical gastroplasty based on his observation that the thicker wall of the lesser curvature was less likely to stretch and distend.[22] He created a small, linear 14-ml pouch that was painstakingly measured under standardized hydrostatic pressure, because he thought that the decreased size also had less of a tendency to stretch. To prevent the stoma at the end of this pouch from stretching, he used a 5-cm strip of polypropylene mesh to create a ring around the pouch in this location. A variant of Mason's VBG utilizes a Silastic ring rather than polypropylene mesh and is appropriately called the Silastic ring vertical gastroplasty. These gastroplasty procedures all had promising 1- to 2-year weight-loss profiles with percentages of excess weight loss (%EWL) of 60% to 70% but with disappointing long-term weight loss (%EWL of 30% to 40% at 5 years). The reasons for the weight regain in many of these gastroplasty procedures were multifactorial and included staple-line disruption, pouch dilatation, and modification of diet to one high in liquid calories. In addition, these procedures also had complications specifically related to the restrictive mesh or ring, and they have nearly been abandoned. These procedures did yield a reasonable long-term weight loss for individuals with lower BMIs, suggesting that a purely restrictive procedure may be adequate for the lower-BMI group.

A recent development in restrictive bariatric surgery is laparoscopic Band placement, wherein an inflatable band is secured at the cardia, creating a 15- to 20-ml gastric pouch. Infusion of saline via a port narrows the internal diameter of the Band and can increase the degree of restriction. Weight loss occurs gradually over a 2- to 3-year period, with a %EWL of 48% at 1 year in one series.[23] Although recanalization is not a problem in this operation, the presence of the prosthesis introduces a host of its own problems, with slippage, erosions, infection, and port-related complications.[23]

Of all the existing purely restrictive operations, the MM operation most closely resembles the vertical gastrectomy and confers the advantage of the lack of a foreign body (Fig. 31-8). It was designed to be a more physiologically restrictive operation than the VBG because it preserves the antral "mill." The MM operation also uses a bougie placed along the lesser curvature to size and guide the creation of a vertical gastric tube.[17] An EEA stapler is then used to create a circular defect in the antrum, approximately 6 cm from the pylorus, which then allows linear staplers to be fired from the antrum up to the angle of His, creating the "magenstrasse," or "wide street of the stomach," while preserving the antral mill. The key difference between the MM and the VG is that the greater curvature of the stomach is entirely transected and removed in the VG, whereas in the MM, the greater curvature, though separated from the lesser curvature along much of its length, is still attached to the rest of the stomach at the antrum.

Results of Previous Restrictive Operations

All of the restrictive operations confer the benefit of weight loss without any malabsorptive component, so that vitamin deficiencies, calcium deficiency, and anemia are rare. However, long-term results after VBG are not

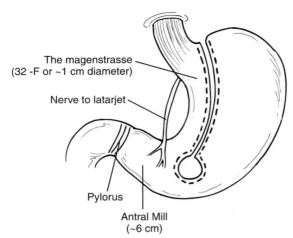

Figure 31-8. The magenstrasse and mill operation. The operation consists of a "magenstrasse," or "wide street," of a gastric tube along the lesser curvature, formed around a 3F bougie, and a preserved antral "mill" to maintain forward food flow. The major terminal branches of the nerve of Latarjet to the antrum are preserved. The secretions of the fundus and body of the stomach empty via a bridge of stomach at the antrum. (From Johnston D, Dachtler J, Sue-Ling HM, et al: The Magenstrasse and Mill operation for morbid obesity. Obes Surg 2003;13:10-16.)

impressive; a significant number of patients still meet the definition of obesity. Fobi reports an average %EWL after laparoscopic VBG at 10 years of 44% in 43 patients.[24] Other authors have found that patients with BMIs greater than 45 kg per m[2] fail to achieve BMIs of 35 kg per m[2], even at 5 years postoperatively.

Short-term data from multiple authors demonstrate a consistently good %EWL of 60% to 70% at 1 to 2 years postoperatively.[25,26] Long-term data, however, suggest a strong tendency toward weight regain. Salmon and McArdle[27] performed horizontal or vertical gastroplasties with varying sizes of gastric pouches (25 to 60 ml) and stomal diameters (3 to 20 mm) in 244 patients and found a superficial correlation in terms of stomal size. At a mean follow-up of 4.5 to 6 years, %EWL ranged from 28% to 40%, depending on gastric pouch size and stomal diameter. Ultimately, horizontal gastroplasty failed to achieve more

than 40% EWL in 84% to 89% of patients. Outcome was somewhat better after VBG, with failure rates from 73% to 81%. Unfortunately, weight loss with these restrictive gastroplasties has not been as effective as it has been with the RYGB and DS operations, perhaps because of hormonal mechanisms, lack of malabsorption, or less satiety.

The MM operation has enjoyed results superior to those of the other gastroplasties. Johnston's first 100 patients, who had average preoperative BMIs of 46.3 kg per m[2], saw mean weight losses of 84 ± 31 lb, and %EWL of 58% at 1 year. Now, with over 230 postoperative MM patients, Johnston has achieved a 5-year %EWL of 61%, with a stable weight generally achieved at 1 year postoperatively (Fig. 31-9). This has been achieved with no mortalities and a 4% rate of major complications.[17]

Vertical Gastrectomy Compared to Prior Gastroplasties and the Roux-en-Y Gastric Bypass

The VG is a significant improvement over prior gastroplasty procedures for a number of reasons:

1. The VG actually resects or removes the majority of the stomach. The explanted fundus of the stomach is responsible for secreting ghrelin, which is a hormone that is responsible for regulating hunger, satiety, and appetite. By removing this portion of the stomach rather than leaving it in place, the level of ghrelin may be reduced as it is after RYGB, causing loss of or a reduction in appetite.[28]
2. The residual tubularized lesser curvature of the stomach is the least compliant part of the stomach, which may therefore resist distension forces and may generate feelings of satiety with very small amounts of food.
3. Finally, by not having a foreign body wrapped around the stomach, the problems associated with these are eliminated.

The VG is a reasonable alternative to the RYGB for a number of reasons:

1. Because there is no intestinal bypass, there is no risk for malabsorptive complications, such as vitamin deficiency and protein deficiency.

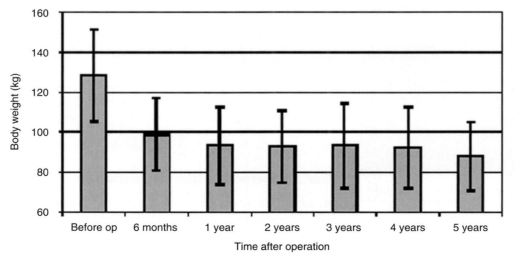

Figure 31-9. Long-term weight loss after the magenstrasse and mill operation. Durable long-term weight loss for up to at least 5 years can be achieved with the magenstrasse and mill operation. (From Johnston D, Dachtler J, Sue-Ling HM, et al: The Magenstrasse and Mill operation for morbid obesity. Obes Surg 2003; 13:10-16.)

Table 31-3	PREOPERATIVE VARIABLES IN PATIENTS UNDERGOING LAPAROSCOPIC TECHNIQUES				
	VG (N = 116)	BAND (N = 233)	RYGB (N = 279)	DS (N = 74)	P VALUES
Age (years)	44.6 ± 11.4	41.5 ± 11.1	43.8 ± 9.4	41.6 ± 7.7	NS
Male (%)	26 (22%)	29 (13%)	40 (14%)	6 (8%)	$P<0.05$ VG vs all
Preop weight (lb)	317 ± 85*	257 ± 43	282 ± 48	287 ± 48	$P<0.05$ VG vs all; $P<0.05$ Band vs RYGB, DS
Preop BMI (kg/m²)	51.2 ± 11.8	41.6 ± 5.5	45.9 ± 6.4	46.6 ± 6.0	$P<0.05$ VG vs all; $P<0.05$ Band vs RYGB, DS
Follow-up (days)	312 ± 217	410 ± 251	562 ± 266	692 ± 277	NS
OR time (mins)	101 ± 31	89 ± 25	144 ± 35	226 ± 43	$P<0.05$ vs RYGB, DS; $*P<0.05$ vs DS
EWL (ml)	43 ± 21	29 ± 15	57 ± 44	91 ± 48	$P<0.05$ Band vs DS
Length of stay (days)	3.7 ± 2.2	2.5 ± 0.6	3.9 ± 1.4	4.1 ± 2.2	$P<0.05$ Band vs all

Band, adjustable gastric band placement; BMI, body mass index; DS, vertical gastrectomy with duodenal switch; NS, not significant; OR, operating room; RYGB, Roux-en-Y gastric bypass; VG, vertical gastrectomy; EWL, excess weight loss.

2. There is no risk for marginal ulcer, which occurs in more than 2% of patients after RYGB.
3. There is no dumping syndrome.
4. There is no risk for intestinal obstruction because there is no intestinal bypass.
5. It is relatively easy to modify to an alternative procedure should weight loss be inadequate or weight regain occur.

Results After Vertical Gastrectomy

A comparative analysis was made of 776 primary bariatric operations performed at our institution. Of them, 145 were VG (16.8%); 223 were Band (32.2%); 279 were RYGB (40.3%); and 74 were DS (10.7%).

Preoperative variables are shown in Table 31-3. Key differences include: (1) the VG group included more men, who, empirically, have more intraabdominal fat and are thus technically more difficult to operate on; (2) VG patients were of greater preoperative weight and BMI because we encouraged superobese and high-risk patients to select this procedure; (3) the VG and Band operations took the shortest time to perform; and (4) lengths of stay were 1 to 2 days shorter after Band. Average age, duration of follow-up, and estimated blood loss were similar across all groups. Conversions to open procedures were not performed in any patient group.

Postoperative variables are shown in Figures 31-10, 31-11, and 31-12. Preoperatively, RYGB and DS patients were of similar weights and BMIs; VG patients were more

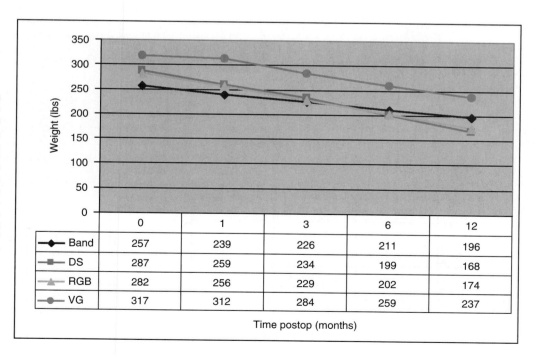

Figure 31-10. Weight in patients after undergoing laparoscopic vertical gastrectomy (VG), adjustable gastric band placement (Band), Roux-en-Y gastric bypass (RYGB), or vertical gastrectomy with duodenal switch (DS). Patients who have undergone VG are more obese than those who have undergone RYGB or DS, but they lose weight at similar rates (slope). After Band, patients are less obese and lose weight at approximately half the rate of patients who have undergone VG, RYGB, or DS.

	0	1	3	6	12
Band	257	239	226	211	196
DS	287	259	234	199	168
RGB	282	256	229	202	174
VG	317	312	284	259	237

Time postop (months)

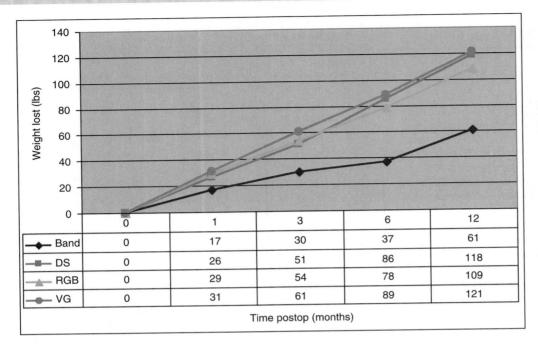

	0	1	3	6	12
Band	0	17	30	37	61
DS	0	26	51	86	118
RGB	0	29	54	78	109
VG	0	31	61	89	121

Time postop (months)

Figure 31-11. Postoperative weight loss in patients after undergoing laparoscopic vertical gastrectomy (VG), adjustable gastric band placement (Band), Roux-en-Y gastric bypass (RYGB), or vertical gastrectomy with duodenal switch (DS). Patients lost weight as effectively after VG as after RYGB and DS. After Band, patients lost half as much weight as patients in the other groups.

obese on average, and Band patients were less obese (see Table 31-3). The RYGB and DS patients were almost identical in their starting weights, postoperative weights, BMIs, rates of weight loss, and %EWL. They experienced approximately 110 to 120 lb of weight loss and a %EWL of 74% to 78% at 12 months (see Fig. 31-12). Band patients were less obese preoperatively but experienced a slower rate of weight loss (see Fig. 31-10). At 1 year, they had lost about half the amount of weight lost by the other three groups (approximate 60 lb versus 120 lb; see Fig. 31-11). Similarly, their %EWL was the lowest, only 47% at 1 year.

The VG patients have the highest preoperative weights and BMIs, but they experience similar rates of weight loss similar to the RYGB and DS groups. The %EWL is misleading lower in the VG group because for the same weight loss, a patient who is more obese preoperatively will have a lower %EWL than a less obese patient. This is because the calculation of %EWL = (weight lost)/(preoperative weight-ideal body weight) includes preoperative weight in the denominator, so %EWL is a dependent, not independent, variable of preoperative weight.

Complications, morbidity, and mortality are depicted in Table 31-4. VG and Band patients had the fewest

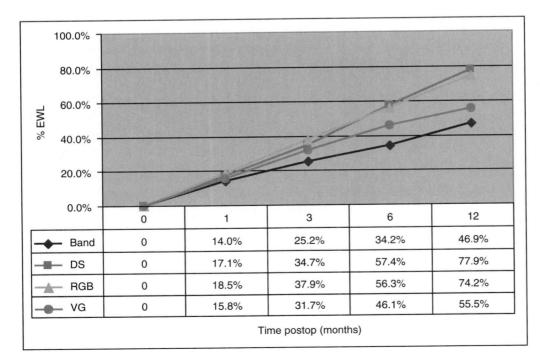

	0	1	3	6	12
Band	0	14.0%	25.2%	34.2%	46.9%
DS	0	17.1%	34.7%	57.4%	77.9%
RGB	0	18.5%	37.9%	56.3%	74.2%
VG	0	15.8%	31.7%	46.1%	55.5%

Time postop (months)

Figure 31-12. Percentage of excess weight loss (%EWL) in patients after undergoing laparoscopic vertical gastrectomy (VG), adjustable gastric band placement (Band), Roux-en-Y gastric bypass (RYGB), or vertical gastrectomy with duodenal switch (DS). The %EWL can be a deceptive parameter when comparing groups of patients who had differing preoperative weights. Even though patients lost similar amounts of weight after VG, RYBG, and DS, the %EWL in VG is misleadingly low because the preoperative weights of patients who underwent VG were significantly greater than those of the patients who underwent RYGB and DS.

Table 31-4	COMPLICATIONS IN PATIENTS UNDERGOING LAPAROSCOPIC TECHNIQUES				
	VG (N = 116)	BAND (N = 233)	RYGB (N = 279)	DS (N = 74)	*P* VALUES
Nonoperative readmissions (%)	1 (1.5%)	2 (1.3%)	8 (3.3%)	4 (6.1%)	NS
Reoperations (%)	0 (0)	4 (2.6%)	15 (6.4%)	11 (16.6%)	*P*<0.05 VG vs RYGB & DS; *P*<0.05 Band vs DS; *P*<0.05 RYGB vs DS
Deaths (%)	0 (0)	0 (0%)	0 (0%)	0 (0%)	NS
Minor complications (%)	3 (4.4%)	2 (1.3%)	21 (8.6%)	4 (6.1%)	*P*<0.05 Band vs RYGB, DS
Major complications (%)	1 (1.5%)	4 (2.6%)	16 (6.5%)	15 (22.7%)	*P*<0.05 VG vs DS; *P*<0.05 Band vs DS; *P*<0.05 RYGB vs DS
Total complications (%)	4 (5.9%)	6 (3.8%)	37 (15.1%)	19 (28.8%)	*P*<0.05 VG vs RYGB, DS; *P*<0.05 Band vs RYGB, DS; *P*<0.05 RYGB vs DS

Band, adjustable gastric band placement; DS, duodenal switch; NS, not significant; RYGB, Roux-en-Y gastric bypass; VG, vertical gastrectomy.

complications; DS had the most; and RYGB had an intermediate number of complications. VG patients had significantly fewer reoperations and major complications compared to the RYGB and DS groups.

Second-Stage Operation After Vertical Gastrectomy

Although we have not started doing the second-stage procedures, electing to wait until the rate of weight loss has reached a plateau, other groups such as Gagner's are performing second-stage operations after patients meet a criterion of weight loss of 100 lb or a time of 6 to 8 months after the initial operation. Weight-loss curves for individual patients after the staged operations are shown in Figure 31-13.

Gagner's group may be experiencing a plateau of weight loss because they perform their VG around a 60F bougie. Our group utilizes a 32F bougie, and it has thus far almost eliminated the need for a second-stage operation in

patients with BMIs of less than 50 kg per m². We found that many patients, even those who initially weigh more than 400 lb, lose significant weight and have not required second operations. At this time, statistical results of second-stage procedures are limited, but in our first 145 patients, we have performed second-stage procedures on only three patients.

Vertical Gastrectomy as the Only Operation for Patients With Low BMIs

Originally conceived as an operation for patients with high BMIs, the VG has proven to be quite safe and quite effective for individuals with BMIs in lower ranges. Johnston reported that after the MM operation, which is very similar to the VG, only 10% of his patients failed to achieve a BMI below 35 kg per m² at 5 years, and they tended to be very obese patients.[17] Our own data demonstrate that patients with BMIs of 55 kg per m² and below are able to achieve BMIs of less than 30 kg per m² within 9 to 12 months of their operations (Fig. 31-14), indicating that this may be the only bariatric procedure they need. Other patients with lower BMIs who should consider this procedure include:

1. Patients concerned about the potential long-term side effects of intestinal bypass, such as intestinal obstruction, ulcers, anemia, osteoporosis, protein deficiency, and vitamin deficiency;
2. Patients who are considering a Band but are concerned about a foreign body or who may not comply with frequent adjustments;
3. High-risk patients who have other medical problems that prevent them from having intestinal bypass, such as anemia, Crohn's disease, extensive prior surgery, severe asthma requiring frequent steroid use, and other complex medical conditions;
4. Patients who need to take antiinflammatory medications, because the VG is not associated with the higher risk of marginal ulcers that is associated with the RYGB; and
5. Patients who are on critical medications (e.g., cardiac medications or transplant medications) the absorption of which may be affected by intestinal bypass.

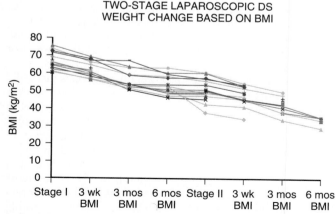

TWO-STAGE LAPAROSCOPIC DS WEIGHT CHANGE BASED ON BMI

Figure 31-13. Individual patient weights after staged laparoscopic vertical gastrectomy followed by completion duodenal switch (DS) after 6 to 12 months of initial weight loss. There is a plateau of weight loss following the first stage (the time scale is logarithmic); the second-stage operation results in ongoing weight loss. (Graph courtesy of Michel Gagner.) BMI, body mass index.

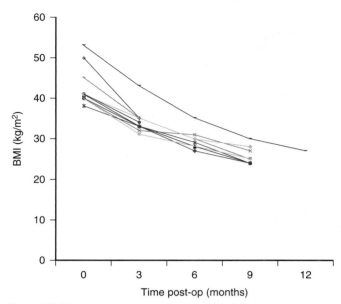

Figure 31-14. Individual patient weights after laparoscopic vertical gastrectomy alone in patients who had BMIs of 55 kg per m² or less. All patients achieved body mass indexes (BMIs) of less than 30 kg per m² within 9 to 12 months after surgery.

▶ ASSESSMENT

Our results have been quite surprising: we have several patients who lost more than 200 lb in 12 months. We did not expect to see such dramatic weight losses with this procedure, and we initially intended to perform the second-stage DS on these patients but have not had to. We also have a subgroup of patients with lower BMIs but higher risk factors (e.g., heart failure, prednisone therapy, history of cancer) who have achieved BMIs below 30 kg per m² in fewer than 12 months.

We have speculated that the main anatomic and physiologic benefits of this operation over other restrictive procedures are derived from the resection and removal of most of the stomach. This gastric reduction may eliminate most of the ghrelin-producing cells and alter the hunger and satiety pathways such that patients rarely experience significant hunger. Preservation of the pylorus probably leads to prolonged retention of food in the gastric pouch and thus creates a longer sense of satiety and an earlier sense of fullness. Last, reluctance to undergo a second-stage procedure may promote extreme patient compliance.

Another salient advantage of this procedure is that it is completely modifiable. In patients who do not have adequate weight loss or even, eventually, have weight gain, this procedure can be converted to an RYGB, a laparoscopic Band placement, or a DS. In addition, further gastric reduction is possible. This convertibility is an attractive feature when one considers that approximately 10% of RYGB patients will have weight regain and will need revisional surgery. Revising a divided gastric pouch after RYGB to another procedure is a technically much more difficult and risky operation. A VG revision would be much easier and safer.

Our main concerns about the safety and effectiveness of this procedure involve the risk for staple-line dehiscence. As a baseline in our practice, we have not had a single leak or staple-line dehiscence in more than 400 hand-sewn RYGBs. These patients did tend to have BMIs below 55 kg per m² and to be at lower risk because in our practice, the patients with higher BMIs and higher risk tend to undergo the VG or DS. The VG procedure has no anastomosis. It does, however, have a long vertical staple line, a narrow gastric pouch, and an intact pylorus that may yield unfavorable intragastric pressure dynamics and put the patient at risk for staple-line leak, especially the high-risk patients. Two patients experienced a staple-line leakage. One was 62 years old and had numerous severe comorbidities. Her stapling included buttress material, but it separated and the leak became apparent on the sixth postoperative day. We strongly suspect, given her comorbidities, that had we performed an RYGB, a similar complication would have occurred. The other patient had Crohn's disease. This underscores the fact that even with good technique, experience, buttressing, and a tension-free technique, staple line ischemia and disruption can occur.

This procedure may not eliminate leaks, but it does offer the benefit of avoiding many of the problems described in intestinal bypass, such as marginal ulcers, strictures, and bowel obstructions. It is extremely important to be aware of these problems because they always occur after patients have been discharged and usually months later when patients have recovered from the initial operation. Marginal ulcers occur in approximately 2% to 3% of patients and may lead to perforation, hemorrhage, and intractable pain. The VG is not an ulcerogenic procedure like the RYGB. By virtue of the gastrectomy, it is most likely an acid-reducing operation, and to date we have not seen any postoperative ulcers in our patients. Indeed, so few patients have needed endoscopy that we are not even aware of the occurrence of gastritis or esophagitis. Most patients report that their reflux symptoms have improved or resolved by the end of the first year after surgery. About 3% of RYGB patients develop strictures that require endoscopic dilation. This rate is most likely higher in the super morbidly obese patients because of anastomotic tension. To date, we have not seen any VG patients develop gastric strictures that require dilation. One patient did report vomiting, but the endoscope passed easily through the stomach and dilation was not required.

Theoretically, the risk for bowel obstruction is markedly reduced and can occur only because of an adhesion or a port-site hernia. It is impossible for a VG patient to develop a bowel obstruction due to an internal hernia because no intestinal bypass or mesenteric window is created. Numerous cases of bowel obstructions and internal hernias occurring after RYGB have been described, and they almost always require reoperation. Some patients have even died of a bowel obstruction related to an internal hernia. Thus, the VG effectively eliminates a possible source of death after weight-loss surgery and markedly reduces or eliminates other serious long-term complications, such as ulcers, strictures, obstructions, and metabolic deficiencies. The lack of an intestinal bypass in this procedure presumably helps to avoid long-term metabolic problems such as anemia, metabolic bone disease, and vitamin deficiencies.

We started doing this procedure for our high-risk and high-BMI patients approximately 4 years ago. We have been impressed by the level of patient satisfaction and the amount of weight loss. In our current series of more than 400 patients, there were no deaths, no conversions to open surgery, and only two leaks requiring reoperation. There was one pulmonary embolus. Our 2-year weight-loss results are similar to our results for the RYGB and the DS (81% to 86% EWL). We are cautiously optimistic about long-term weight loss and realize that weight regain is possible and may ultimately limit the widespread use of this procedure.

▶ CONCLUSION

In summary, both restriction and malabsorption are core modalities of bariatric surgery. They can be used in varying degrees to yield weight loss. The bulk of long-term metabolic complications occur in malabsorptive procedures, and it is avoidance of these complications that drives us to develop procedures that are limited to restriction only. Critics of restrictive-only procedures point out that long-term weight loss may be inadequate without malabsorption. We strongly believe there is a role for both purely restrictive procedures and combined procedures. Selection may depend on a patient's BMI, activity level, age, medical risk, personal preference, and so forth. The DS is an established procedure that is extremely effective in patients with high BMIs, and it can now be performed laparoscopically. We are certain that it will continue to evolve in terms of limb lengths and pouch sizes in the hope of attaining optimal weight loss while minimizing metabolic complications. The VG is gaining rapid acceptance as a first-stage procedure in the superobese and as a single-stage procedure in patients with higher risks and lower BMIs. The low morbidity and reasonable weight loss in higher risk patients is extremely appealing.

▶ REFERENCES

1. Hess DS, Hess DW: Biliopancreatic diversion with a duodenal switch. Obes Surg 1998;8:267-282.
2. Scopinaro N, Adami GF, Marinari GM, et al: Biliopancreatic diversion. World J Surg 1998;22:936-946.
3. Cadiere GB, Bruyns J, Himpens J, et al: Laparoscopic gastroplasty for morbid obesity. Br J Surg 1994;81:524.
4. Lonrith H, Dalenback J, Haglind E, et al: Vertical banded gastroplasty by laparoscopic technique in the treatment of morbid obesity. Surg Laparosc Endosc 1994;6:102-107.
5. Magnusson M, Freedman J, Jonas E, et al: Five-year results of laparoscopic vertical banded gastroplasty in the treatment of massive obesity. Obes Surg 2002;12:826-830.
6. Frantzides CT, Carlson MA, Schulte WJ: Laparoscopic gastric bypass in a porcine model. J Laparoendosc Surg 1995;5:97-100.
7. Wittgrove AC, Clark GW, Tremblay LJ: Laparoscopic Roux-en-Y gastric bypass: preliminary report of five cases. Obes Surg 1994;4:353-357.
8. Schauer PR, Ikramuddin S, Gourash WF: Laparoscopic Roux-en-Y gastric bypass: a case report at one-year follow-up. J Laparoendosc Adv Surg Tech A 1999;9:101-106.
9. Suter M, Giusti V, Heraief E, et al: Early results of laparoscopic gastric banding compared with open vertical banded gastroplasty. Obes Surg 1999;9:374-380.
10. Nguyen NT, Goldman C, Rosenquist CJ, et al: Laparoscopic versus open gastric bypass: a randomized study of outcomes, quality of life, and costs. Ann Surg 2001;234:279-289.
11. Marceau P, Hould FS, Simard S, et al: Biliopancreatic diversion with duodenal switch. World J Surg 1998;22:947-954.
12. Rabkin RA: Distal gastric bypass/duodenal switch, Roux-en-Y gastric bypass and biliopancreatic diversion in a community practice. Obes Surg 1998;8:53-59.
13. Baltasar A, Bou R, Bengochea M, et al: Duodenal switch: an effective therapy for morbid obesity, intermediate results. Obes Surg 2001;11:54-58.
14. Rabkin RA, Rabkin JM, Metcalf B, et al: Laparoscopic technique for performing duodenal switch with gastric reduction. Obes Surg 2003;13:263-268.
15. Derzie A, Silvestri F, Liriano E, et al: Wound closure technique and acute wound complications in gastric surgery for morbid obesity: a prospective randomized trial. J Am Coll Surg 2000;191:238-243.
16. de Csepel J, Burpee S, Jossart G, et al: Laparoscopic biliopancreatic diversion with a duodenal switch for morbid obesity: a feasibility study in pigs. J Laparoendosc Adv Surg Tech A 2001;11:79-83.
17. Johnston D, Dachtler J, Sue-Ling HM, et al: The magenstrasse and mill operation for morbid obesity. Obes Surg 2003;13:10-16.
18. Printen KJ, Mason EE: Gastric surgery for relief of morbid obesity. Arch Surg 1973;106:428-431.
19. Baltasar A, Bou R, Miro J, et al: Laparoscopic biliopancreatic diversion with duodenal switch and initial experience. Obes Surg 2002;12:245-248.
20. Paiva D, Bernardes L, Suretti L: Laparoscopic biliopancreatic diversion: technique and initial results. Obes Surg 2002;12:358-361.
21. Kim WW, Gagner M, Kini S, et al: Laparoscopic vs open biliopancreatic switch: a comparative study. J Gastrointest Surg 2003;7:552-557.
22. Mason EE: Vertical banded gastroplasty for morbid obesity. Arch Surg 1982;117:701-706.
23. Camerini G, Adami G, Marinari GM, et al: Thirteen years of follow-up in patients with adjustable silicone gastric banding for obesity: weight loss and constant rate of late specific complications. Obes Surg 2004;14:1343-1348.
24. Fobi MAL: Vertical banded gastroplasty vs gastric bypass: 10 years' follow-up. Obes Surg 1993;3:161-164.
25. Sugarman HJ, Londrey GL, Kellum JL, et al: Weight loss with vertical banded gastroplasty and Roux-en-Y gastric bypass for morbid obesity with selective versus random assignment. Am J Surg 1998;157:93-102.
26. Ismail T, Kirby RM, Growson MC, et al: Vertical Silastic ring gastroplasty: a 6-year experience. Br J Surg 1990;77:80-82.
27. Salmon PA, McArdle MO: Horizontal and vertical gastroplasties: extended follow-up and late results. Obes Surg 1992;2:51-59.
28. Langer FB, Reza Hoda MA, Bohdjalian A, et al: Sleeve gastrectomy and gastric banding: effects on plasma ghrelin levels. Obes Surg 2005;15:150-152.
29. Ren CJ, Patterson E, Gagner M: Early results of laparoscopic biliopancreatic diversion with duodenal switch: a case series of 40 consecutive patients. Obes Surg 2000;10:514-523.
30. Feng JJ, Gagner M: Laparoscopic biliopancreatic diversion with duodenal switch. Semin Laparosc Surg 2002;9:125-129.
31. Waage A, Gagner M, Biertho L, et al: Comparison between open hand-sewn, laparoscopic stapled and laparoscopic computer-mediated, circular stapled gastro-jejunostomies in Roux-en-Y gastric bypass in the porcine model. Obes Surg 2005;15:782-787.
32. Camerini G, Marinari GM, Scopinaro N: A new approach to the fashioning of the gastroenteroanastomosis in laparoscopic standard biliopancreatic diversion. Surg Laparosc Endosc Percutan Tech 2003;13:165-167.
33. Lagace M, Márceau P, Marceau S, et al: Biliopancreatic diversion with a new type of gastrectomy. Obes Surg 1995;5:411-418.
34. Márceau S, Biron S, Lagace M, et al: Biliopancreatic diversion with distal gastrectomy. Obes Surg 1995;5:303-307.

32

Implantable Gastric Stimulation for the Treatment of Morbid Obesity

Scott A. Shikora, M.D.

It is estimated that 64% of all adult Americans are overweight or obese.[1] Furthermore, 4.7% are extremely (morbidly) obese, which is defined as having a body mass index (BMI) greater than or equal to 40 kg per m[2]. Calculation suggests that the number of morbidly obese adults in the United States has reached a staggering 14 to 16 million people. These individuals suffer from a wide range of comorbidities and account for the second largest group of preventable deaths, after smoking (>300,000 yearly).[2] The cost of treating the obese is staggering, at approximately $70 billion yearly.[3] The impact of obesity is also not limited to the United States but is spreading worldwide. Globally, the prevalence of overweight and obesity was recently estimated to be 1.7 billion people.[4] Obesity accounts for more than 2.5 million deaths per year.[5] Not far behind the rate for adults is the growing epidemic of overweight adolescents. Currently, surgery is rarely offered to these patients for fear of operative complications and long-term compliance.

Bariatric surgery has, however, become a widely accepted treatment for morbid obesity. Numerous studies have demonstrated dramatic improvements in the obesity-associated comorbidities that result from the weight loss achieved by means of all of the procedures.[6-9] However, currently less than 1% of those who meet standard criteria for eligibility for surgical therapy undergo bariatric surgery in a given calendar year. Many potential candidates are denied surgery secondary to lack of medical insurance coverage or other disqualifications or do not seek out the surgery because they lack knowledge about the efficacy of these treatments, but a great number avoid surgery for fear of the potential operative complications and long-term consequences of the current operative procedures.

Implantable gastric stimulation for weight loss is an exciting new concept in the treatment of morbid obesity. It is unique in that it involves the least invasive surgery and does not alter the anatomy of the gastrointestinal tract. Since its inception in the mid 1990s, international investigations have demonstrated it to be the safest of all bariatric procedures in terms of both operative complications and

long-term consequences. In addition, advances in this technology have led to improving efficacy. This chapter reviews the theory and current experience with gastric implantable stimulation for weight loss.

▶ GASTRIC ELECTROPHYSIOLOGY AND MOTILITY

Motility is one of the most critical physiologic functions of the human gut. Without coordinated motility, digestion and absorption of dietary nutrients could not take place. To accomplish its functions effectively, the gut needs to generate contractions that are coordinated (peristalsis). This produces the transit of luminal contents to a position where the nutrients can be maximally absorbed. In addition, hypermotility must be avoided because it would negatively impact nutrient absorption by decreasing nutrients' exposure to the mucosa. In a similar fashion, the stomach requires coordinated gastric contractions for normal emptying.

Gastric contractions are regulated by the myoelectric activity of the stomach. Normal gastric myoelectric activity consists of two components: the slow wave and the spike potential.[10] The slow wave is omnipresent and occurs at regular intervals, whether or not the stomach contracts. It originates in the proximal stomach and propagates distally toward the pylorus (Fig. 32-1). The gastric slow wave determines the maximum frequency, propagation velocity, and propagation direction of gastric contractions. The normal frequency of the gastric slow wave is about 3 cycles per minute (cpm) in humans and 5 cpm in dogs. When a spike potential (similar to an action potential) is superimposed on the gastric slow wave, a strong lumen-occluding contraction occurs.

Gastric dysrhythmias represent aberrations from the normal gastric myoelectric activity. Similar to cardiac dysrhythmias, they include abnormally rapid contraction (tachygastria) and abnormally slow contraction (bradygastria). For example (Fig. 32-2), there can be an ectopic pacemaker in the distal stomach in addition to the normal pacemaker in the proximal stomach. The ectopic pacemaker generates

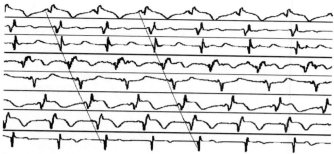

Figure 32-1. Normal gastric slow waves. Gastric slow waves recorded by electrodes implanted on the serosal surface of the stomach along the greater curvature in a healthy dog (1.5-min recording). The top tracing was obtained from a pair of electrodes 16 cm above the pylorus; the bottom tracing was obtained from the electrodes 2 cm above the pylorus. (Courtesy of Jiande Chen, Ph.D.)

slow waves with a higher frequency than normal (tachygastria), and with retrograde propagation toward the proximal stomach. These abnormal waves may interfere with the normal slow-wave propagation and possibly disrupt normal gastric contractions.

The prevalence and origin of various gastric dysrhythmias have been investigated.[11] It was found that the majority of bradygastria (80.5% ± 9.4%) originates in the proximal stomach (P < 0.04 vs. other locations) and propagates all the way to the distal antrum. That is, bradygastria is attributed to a decrease in the frequency of the normal pacemaker. In contrast, tachygastria originates primarily in the distal antrum (80.6% ± 8.8%; P < 0.04 vs. other locations) and propagates partially or all the way to the proximal stomach. During tachygastria, the normal pacemaker in the proximal stomach may still be present. That is, it is not uncommon for the proximal stomach to be dominated by normal slow waves and the distal stomach to be dominated by tachygastria. Overall, the prevalence of dysrhythmia was highest in the distal antrum and lowest in the proximal part of the stomach.

The patterns of gastric motility are different in the fed and the fasting states.[12] In the fed state, the human stomach contracts at its maximum frequency of 3 cpm. The contraction originates in the proximal stomach and propagates distally toward the pylorus. In healthy humans, 50% or more of the ingested food usually has been emptied from the stomach by 2 hours after the meal, and 95% or more has been emptied by 4 hours after the meal.[13] When the stomach has been emptied, the pattern of gastric motility changes. The gastric motility pattern in the fasting state (nonfed) undergoes a cycle of periodic fluctuation divided into three phases: phase I (no contractions, 40 to 60 minutes); phase II (intermittent contractions, 20 to 40 minutes); and phase III (regular rhythmic contractions, 2 to 10 minutes).

Gastric emptying plays an important role in regulating food intake. Several studies have shown that gastric distention acts as a satiety signal to inhibit food intake.[14] In addition, rapid gastric emptying is closely related to overeating and obesity. This is especially true for animals with lesions in the hypothalamic region of the brain.[15] In a study of 77 human subjects, composed of 46 obese and 31 age-, sex-, and race-matched nonobese individuals, obese subjects were found to have a more rapid gastric emptying rate than nonobese subjects.[16] The rate in obese men was found to be much more rapid than that of their nonobese counterparts. It was concluded that the rate of solid gastric emptying in the obese subjects was abnormally rapid. The significance and cause of this change in gastric emptying remain to be definitively established. However, on the basis of the work he performed at the University of Chicago in 1913, Carlson proposed that a relationship existed between the gastrointestinal tract and the hypothalamus and that that relationship regulated dietary intake.[17] It has been shown more recently that several peptides, including cholecystokinin (CCK) and corticotropin-releasing factor (CRF), suppress feeding and decrease gastric transit. Peripherally administered CCK-8 was found to decrease the rate of gastric emptying and food intake in various species.[18]

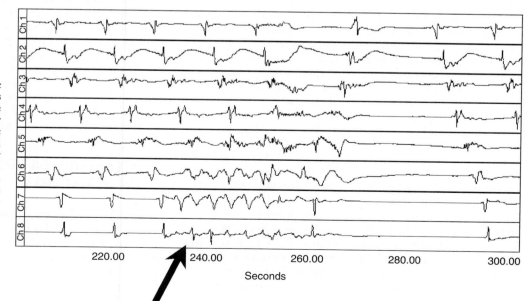

Figure 32-2. Tachygastria. Gastric slow waves recorded by electrodes implanted on the serosal surface of the stomach along the greater curvature, showing the ectopic tachygastrial activity in the distal stomach (arrow). The top tracing was obtained from a pair of electrodes 16 cm above the pylorus; the bottom tracing was obtained from the electrodes 2 cm above the pylorus. (Courtesy of Jiande Chen, Ph.D.)

CRF, when injected, has also been shown to decrease food intake and the rate of gastric emptying.[19] More recently, it was shown that in ob/ob mice (a genetic model of obesity), the rate of gastric emptying was accelerated compared with that in lean mice.[20] Urocortin, a 40-amino acid peptide member of the CRF family, dose-dependently and potently decreased food intake and body-weight gain as well as the rate of gastric emptying in ob/ob mice. This suggests that rapid gastric emptying may contribute to hyperphagia and obesity in ob/ob mice, and it opens new possibilities for the treatment of obesity.

▶ GASTRIC STIMULATION AND PACING

Gastric stimulation involves the application of an electric current to the stomach to alter its functioning. The utility of gastric pacing would be realized only if artificially generated electric current could entrain normal gastric pacesetter potentials. This, in fact, has been demonstrated in canines[21] and in humans.[22] The ways in which it affects gastric function are still to be determined.

Electric stimulation of the stomach can be directed from proximal to distal (antegrade pacing) or from distal to proximal (retrograde pacing). Although it would be attractive to assume that antegrade stimulation could improve normal gastric emptying, and retrograde stimulation would be utilized to retard or adversely impact normal gastric emptying, in human subjects these relationships have not been conclusively proven.

However, a number of papers have been published on gastrointestinal electric stimulation for the treatment of gastrointestinal motility disorders in both dogs and humans. These disorders are characterized by poor contractility and delayed emptying (in contrast with obesity), and the aim of electric stimulation in this setting is to normalize the underlying electric rhythm and improve these parameters. In general, it is done by antegrade, or forward, gastric (or intestinal) stimulation.

Previous work on antegrade gastrointestinal stimulation has been focused on its effects on (1) gastric myoelectric activity; (2) gastric motility; (3) gastric emptying; and (4) gastrointestinal symptoms.[23-30] These studies have shown that entrainment of gastric slow waves is possible by using an artificial pacemaker. Recent studies have indicated that such entrainment is dependent on certain critical parameters, including the width and frequency of the stimulation pulse.[23] Furthermore, antegrade intestinal electric stimulation can entrain intestinal slow waves using either serosal electrodes or intraluminal ring electrodes.[26,29] McCallum and coworkers demonstrated, in patients suffering from gastroparesis, that antegrade gastric pacing could entrain gastric slow waves in all 9 of their patients.[27] They paced the greater curvature of the stomach at frequencies approximately 10% higher than the slow wave frequencies measured. In 2 patients, it converted tachygastria to normal slow waves. In fact, electric pacing significantly improved gastric emptying and symptoms in these patients. In a case report, Familoni and colleagues also were able to improve gastric emptying and symptoms in a patient with severe diabetic gastroparesis by pacing the stomach at a high frequency (12 cpm).[31] In contrast, Hocking and colleagues were unable

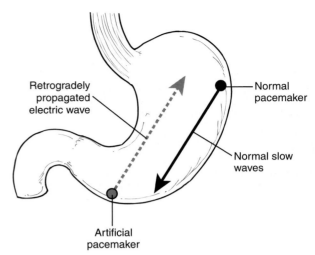

Figure 32-3. Retrograde gastric electric stimulation. Electric stimulation from an ectopic gastric pacemaker located in the distal stomach may.

to treat postgastrectomy gastric dysrhythmias by means of pacing in a patient who had undergone vagotomy and gastrojejunostomy for an obstructing duodenal ulcer.[32]

Retrograde pacing may be of benefit for patients with abnormally rapid gastric emptying, such as the morbidly obese and patients with dumping syndrome.[24] The principle of retrograde gastric electric stimulation is the opposite of the circumstances that have been described in patients with impaired gastric emptying. Retrograde gastric electric stimulation employs retrograde pacing (Fig. 32-3). As previously stated, the original working concept was that retrograde pacing might retard the propulsive activity of the stomach and slow down gastric emptying. This could be useful in the treatment of obesity, where it is postulated that a delay in gastric emptying would lead to early satiety and decreased food intake. Again, delayed gastric emptying as a mechanism of action of electric stimulation has not been proven in humans.

To accomplish retrograde gastric electric stimulation, an artificial pacemaker is connected to the distal stomach along the lesser curvature. This artificial pacemaker causes the electric waves to propagate from the distal to the proximal stomach. These waves conflict with the normal and physiologic electric waves that propagate from the proximal to the distal stomach. Consequently, gastric dysrhythmia is induced, and the regular propagation of gastric electric waves is impaired. The severity of impairment is determined by the strength of the electric stimulation.

▶ IMPLANTABLE GASTRIC STIMULATION FOR WEIGHT LOSS

Whether delayed gastric emptying can be accomplished by electric gastric stimulation or not, this modality has been shown to be safe and effective for the treatment of morbid obesity. The concept was first developed by an Italian surgeon, Valerio Cigaina, in the late 1980s. At that time, he hypothesized that exogenous electric impulses could be used to dysregulate normal gastric electromotor activity in obese patients, resulting in weight loss. Although the mechanism of action has still not been elucidated, gastric stimulation has been shown to achieve meaningful weight loss. A more current theory that also has been supported by animal study focuses on the effect of electric stimulation on fundic relaxation. This relaxation is seen in normal postprandial gastric distention and may result in satiety.[33]

Studies investigating the potential for gastric electric stimulation to induce weight loss were first reported by Cigaina and colleagues in 1992 in a porcine model.[34] The results showed that retrograde gastric electric stimulation was both safe and effective in moderating weight gain in growing swine. Animals were divided into three groups, two of which had electrodes implanted into the muscle layer of the distal antrum. Control animals received sham surgery. Implanted swine experienced either 3 or 8 months of electric antral stimulation at 5 or 100 Hz, respectively. All animals were fed ad libitum. As expected, immature swine in the control group progressively increased feeding and gained weight. Over the first 12 weeks of the study, there were no differences in animal feed intake or weight between the groups (both control and stimulated groups increased intake and weight). However, after 13 weeks, animals subjected to high-frequency stimulation decreased their feed intake relative to the control group, and then their weight decreased. After 8 months, the swine stimulated at 100 Hz weighed 10.5% less than the control animals. The overall feed intake in the group stimulated at 100 Hz was 12.8% lower than in the control group. However, animals in the group stimulated at the lower frequency (5 Hz) for only 3 months demonstrated dramatically less change than the control group.

Gastric peristalsis has also been studied in the swine model. Peristalsis was noted to be altered with electric stimulation. In a study in swine, those stimulated at 40 Hz were noted to have decreased peristalsis.[35] However, the exact mechanism of action was not elucidated, and gastric emptying was not evaluated.

As a consequence of the animal study results, initial human studies began in 1995.[36] Four women with BMIs of 40 kg per m² or greater were implanted and followed for up to 40 months. Via laparoscopy, platinum electrodes were implanted intramuscularly on the anterior gastric wall, adjacent to the lesser curve and proximal to the pes ancerinus. The system was bipolar in design, so two electrodes, one an anode and one a cathode, were inserted into the gastric muscle layer. A prototype electric stimulator was implanted in a subcutaneous pocket of the anterior abdominal wall. All four patients were permitted food and drink ad libitum. At 40 months after implantation, one patient had lost 32 kg and a second had lost 62 kg. Malfunctions in the stimulation systems were discovered in the other two patients. In one patient, a fracture in the lead was discovered; it compromised effectiveness. At 40 months after implantation, the patient had lost only two BMI units. Similarly, in a second patient there was also an apparent fracture of the lead, and that patient did not lose weight. In both of these patients, lead fracture led to unipolar pacing (only one electrode was presumed to be functional) rather than the intended bipolar stimulation. The two subjects who had no lead problems and received bipolar pacing had much better results. Therefore, it was concluded that bipolar electric stimulation was necessary. In addition, chronic gastric electric stimulation was considered safe because no side effects were reported.

In 1998, a second study was performed in human subjects to investigate the safety and efficacy of a first generation, dedicated gastric stimulator, the Prelude implantable gastric system.[37] All enrolled patients had BMIs of more than 40 kg per m², a history of unsuccessful weight loss, and an absence of serious cardiac, respiratory, or psychiatric problems. Patients with cardiac pacemakers were excluded for obvious reasons. Ten patients underwent a minimally invasive surgical procedure to implant the system. Stimulation was initiated 30 days after implantation. After implantation, all subjects were permitted food and drink ad libitum during three regular meals but were told not to eat between meals. Only sweet and alcoholic beverages were discouraged. Patients were followed at approximately monthly intervals. The stimulator was interrogated using transcutaneous radiofrequency telemetry, which linked the implanted device to a computerized programmer. Data collated included stimulation parameters, lead impedance, and residual battery charge.

This study demonstrated both safety and efficacy. There were no deaths or other significant medical problems during the study, no complications related to the procedure, and no long-term complications. Specifically, there were no lead fractures or failures of the electric components of the system. After receiving 51 months of stimulation, the mean weight loss was 23% of excess weight and appeared to be well maintained (Fig. 32-4). Not surprisingly, battery depletion led to weight regain and device replacement with a new battery resulted in renewed weight loss.

▶ CURRENT INTERNATIONAL EXPERIENCE WITH IMPLANTABLE GASTRIC STIMULATION FOR WEIGHT LOSS

The implantable gastric stimulator (IGS), a pacemaker-like device called Transcend (Transneuronix, Mt. Arlington, N.J.), includes a battery-operated pulse generator and a bipolar lead. The generator is similar to a heart pacemaker and about the size of a pocket watch. It is implanted under the skin in the left upper quadrant (Fig. 32-5). The system's lead is laparoscopically inserted into the seromuscular layer of the anterior stomach wall. In most cases, the operation can be performed in less than 1 hour. Most patients were discharged to home on the same day or the day following the procedure. The programmer is a standard computer connected to a wand. The programmer communicates via the computer and wand with the implanted IGS, using transcutaneous radiofrequency telemetry. The IGS can quickly and easily be interrogated or programmed in the clinic or office setting.

Currently, over 800 patients have been enrolled in research trials and had the IGS system implanted. There have been no deaths or major complications.

European Multicenter Study

After the pioneering work of Cigaina and colleagues, a multicenter trial was initiated in Europe. For the trial,

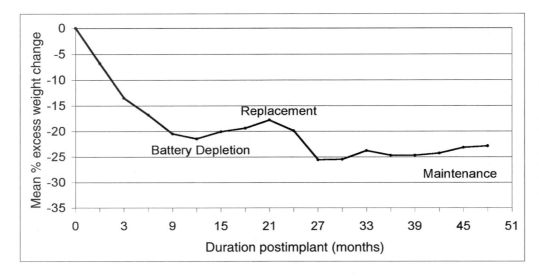

Figure 32-4. Long-term results from the preliminary pilot study of Cigaina et al. Ten patients were followed for more than 51 months. The patients achieved a mean of 23% excess weight loss. Also note that patients gained weight when there was battery depletion and lost weight once the devices were replaced.

50 patients were implanted at seven clinical centers, one each in Italy, France, Germany, Sweden, Greece, Austria, and Belgium. Although the study design varied somewhat at each of the clinical centers, most were open-labeled. There were no significant complications in any of the patients. Mean weight loss surpassed 40% of excess after a 2-year follow-up (Fig. 32-6).

Laparoscopic Obesity Stimulation Survey

More recently, a second multicenter investigation has been undertaken in Europe. This study, the Laparoscopic Obesity Stimulation Survey, enrolled 60 patients at eight participating sites. As in the previous study, there have been no significant complications. After a 10-month

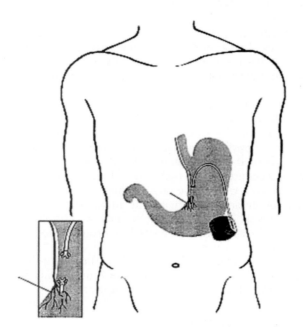

Figure 32-5. The implantable gastric stimulator system. The implantable gastric stimulator with the bipolar lead inserted into the muscular layer along the lesser curvature. The lead is placed close to the pes ancerinus.

period of follow-up, a mean excess weight loss of more than 20% had been achieved (Fig. 32-7).

U.S. O-01 Trial

In the United States, the first research investigation, the U.S. O-01 Trial was a multicenter, randomized, controlled, double-blinded trial developed to evaluate both the safety and the efficacy of the IGS system. It included 103 patients. The IGS lead was laparoscopically placed in 100 of the patients; in 3 patients it was placed via a small midline incision to assess the practicality of placing the device by traditional open surgery. After 1 month, patients were randomized to having the device activated or to having the devices remain in the *off* mode. After 7 months, the nonfunctioning devices were also activated. Device settings were universal for all patients. Patients were clinically evaluated monthly for 24 months and carefully monitored for complications and for weight loss. No dietary or behavioral counseling was provided.

No deaths or complications resulted from implantation. Although none of the patients experienced any untoward effects as a result of this procedure, 17 of the first 41 leads were discovered to have become dislodged from the stomach wall.[38] This occurrence led to an alteration in technique to ensure better lead security. However, lead dislodgment probably affected weight loss results. In addition, the lack of dietary and behavioral counseling, and the inclusion of patients with binge eating disorders may have also affected the weight-loss results. It is interesting that during the first 6 months, many patients admitted to having deliberately overeaten or experimented with their diets to discern whether their devices had been activated. Despite these issues, after 1 year of stimulation, 20% of the patients had lost more than 5% of their total body weights, and the mean total weight loss was 11%.

Dual-Lead Implantable Gastric Electric Stimulation Trial

In the hope of building on the lessons learned from the European and U.S. O-01 trials, a pilot study was designed for the United States to see whether the results could

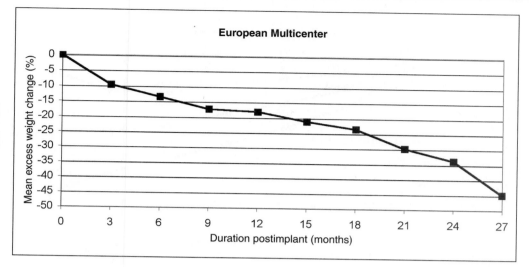

Figure 32-6. European multicenter study. Enrollment included 50 patients at seven clinical sites. Weight loss achieved was 40% of excess, with a mean follow-up of 27 months.

be improved. This open-label pilot trial, the Dual-Lead Implantable Gastric Electric Stimulation Trial, enrolled 30 patients at two clinical sites. The trial was unique for several reasons. First, binge eaters were excluded, as they had performed poorly in earlier trials. Second, behavioral support and dietary counseling were included. Third, the system included two leads (four electrodes) that could be programmed separately or together. Finally, the device was programmed individually for each patient.

A major clinical breakthrough was discovered early in this investigation. It was found that when programming high electric outputs, most patients immediately developed symptoms of bloating, nausea, retching, or abdominal pain. This finding may be similar to the capture of cardiac rhythm during heart pacing. The output was then reduced slightly. Patients who experienced symptoms have had dramatic reductions in appetite and most have achieved weight loss. Overall, there was a 15% excess weight loss at 38 weeks (Fig. 32-8). However, at our site, we have achieved a mean excess weight loss of 30.4% at a mean follow-up time of 9.5 months (8 to 14 months). Of our patients, 80% have lost weight, and 60% have lost more than 10% of

their excess weight (14.7% to 104% of excess weight loss). The dramatic differences between the results from the two investigative sites may reflect differences in patient selection and suggests the importance of this factor.

▶ NEED FOR CAREFUL PATIENT SELECTION

Thus far, the worldwide experience with the IGS system has proven that like all other surgical procedures for weight loss, no procedure is effective for all patients. This was recently validated when a simple screening tool (BaroScreen^M) was developed and retrospectively applied to approximately 250 IGS patients internationally. The screening tool is based on demographics and responses to questionnaire items, and it appeared to predict accurately both responders and nonresponders. Motivational factors seem to be most important. Applying this strategy retrospectively demonstrated that the patients who screened favorably for these motivational factors preformed significantly better than those who screened unfavorably. For both U.S. trials, its implementation would have eliminated approximately 75%

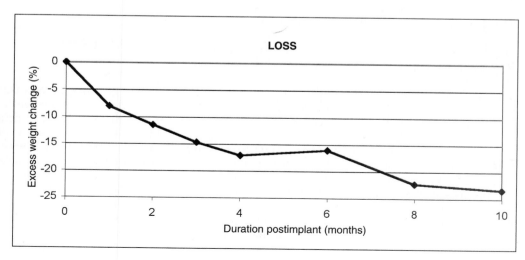

Figure 32-7. Laparoscopic Obesity Stimulation Survey (LOSS). Interim results from this multicenter European trial involving 60 patients at eight clinical centers. At a mean of 10 months of follow-up, patients lost more than 20% of their excess weight.

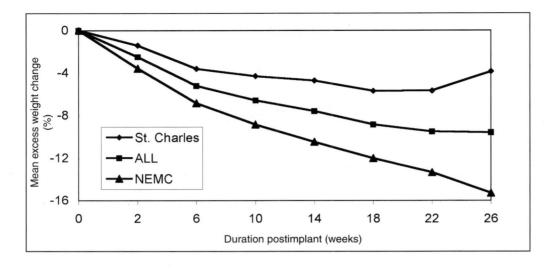

Figure 32-8. Dual-Lead Implantable Gastric Electric Stimulation Trial (DIGEST). Preliminary results for the 30 enrolled patients at two clinical centers (New England Medical Center and St. Charles Hospital).

of the participants. However, those who scored favorably had dramatic results (Fig. 32-9). Further prospective analysis is necessary to confirm these preliminary findings.

Superficially, screening out 75% of potential patients sounds like a problem for the future of this technology. However, it is important to remember that 25% of the tens of millions of potential patients who might benefit from this procedure is still a significant number of patients.

▶ FUTURE CONSIDERATIONS FOR THE IGS

Although the IGS system is an exciting new approach to the treatment of morbid obesity, there are still questions that need to be answered. Further animal and human research is needed to better clarify its mechanism of action, the selection of patients, and the proper application of the system.

Delayed gastric emptying was initially entertained as a potential mechanism of action, but this has not been demonstrated in a limited human investigation. Other causes are also being considered, such as the influence of gastric electric stimulation on the secretion of gastrointestinal hormones and on nerve function. In a preliminary study of 11 patients, Cigaina and colleagues found that IGS pacing resulted in meal-related responses by CKK and somatostatin, and basal levels of glucagon-like peptide-1 and leptin were significantly decreased as compared to controls.[39] Further studies of gastrointestinal hormones such as ghrelin are under way.

Appropriate patient selection also has to be better defined. The development of a simple patient-screening tool to segregate responders from nonresponders is a significant first step. As with electric stimulation for other conditions, such as epilepsy and urinary incontinence, avoiding implantation in patients not likely to respond would dramatically improve results. In addition, determining the best subgroups of obese patients for this technology

is also important. Obesity is a heterogeneous condition. For instance, this device may prove very effective for those with BMIs between 35 and 45 kg per m² but less so for those with BMIs greater than 60 kg per m². It may, indeed, be most effective for patients with BMIs between 30 and 40 kg per m². Approximately 50 million American adults have BMIs in this range and they generally are not considered for surgery and are poorly served by medical weight-loss strategies. The IGS may be attractive for the obese adolescent or could be used as a weight-maintenance strategy for patients who have lost weight by nonoperative means.

Further work must also be performed to refine the most appropriate setting parameters for the device, as well as the optimal locations for the leads in the stomach wall. Are two leads better than one, or should multiple leads be considered? Last, additional applications for the IGS can also be entertained. For example, the IGS may be considered for other gastrointestinal conditions such as severe gastrointestinal reflux. Preliminary work out of Germany found that the IGS improved lower esophageal pressures and lowered DeMeester scores in five patients with severe reflux.[40]

▶ CONCLUSION

Significant obesity is a major worldwide health concern that is growing in prevalence at alarming proportions. Although surgery currently offers the only therapeutic option that consistently achieves meaningful and sustained weight loss, the majority of eligible surgical candidates choose not to undergo surgery for fear of surgical complications or long-term sequelae. Implantable gastric stimulation is a new and unique surgical modality that may offer safe weight loss. There is still much to be learned about this technology, but it is clear that the IGS is introducing a paradigm shift in the surgical management of morbid obesity.

US TRIAL O-01

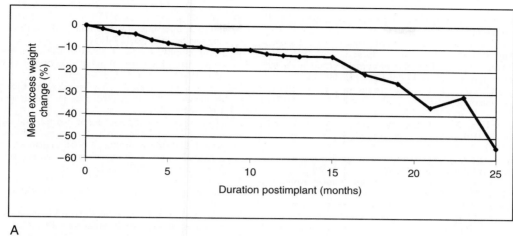

A

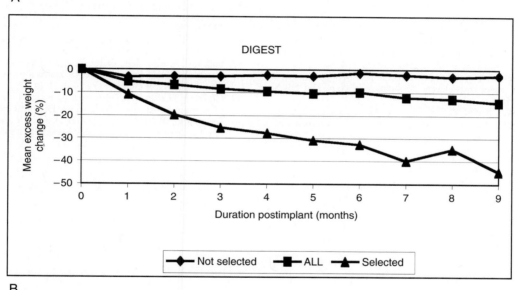

B

Figure 32-9 U.S. trial results with enhanced patient screening. A patient-screening tool was used to predict responders and nonresponders. These graphs depict the weight-loss results for both U.S. trials in selected responders. Dramatically improved weight loss was seen. **A.** U.S. Trial O-01. **B.** Dual-Lead Implantable Gastric Stimulation Trial (DIGEST).

▶ REFERENCES

1. Flegal KM, Carroll MD, Ogden CL, et al: Prevalence and trends in obesity among US adults, 1999-2000. JAMA 2002;288:1723-1727.
2. Mokdad AH, Ford ES, Bowman BA, et al: Prevalence of obesity, diabetes, and obesity-related health risk factors, 2001. JAMA 2003; 289:76-79.
3. Colditz GA: Economic costs of obesity and inactivity. Med Sports 1999;31:S663-S667.
4. Deitel M: Overweight and obesity worldwide now estimated at 1.7 billion people. Obes Surg 2003;13:329-330.
5. World Health Report 2002. *www.iotf.org. www.who.int/peh/burden/ globalestim.htm*
6. Schauer P, Ikramuddin S, Gourash W, et al: Outcomes after laparoscopic Roux-en-Y gastric bypass for severe obesity. Ann Surg 2000; 232:515-529.
7. Pories WJ, Swanson MS, MacDonald KG, et al: Who would have thought it? An operation proves to be the most effective therapy for adult-onset diabetes mellitus. Ann Surg 1995;222:339-352.
8. Dixon JB, O'Brien P: Health outcomes of morbidly obese type 2 diabetic subjects 1 year after laparoscopic adjustable silicone gastric banding. Diabetes Care 2002;25:358-363.
9. Buchwald H, Avidor Y, Braunwald E, et al: Bariatric surgery: a systematic review and meta-analysis. JAMA 2004;292: 1724-1737.
10. Chen JDZ, McCallum RW (eds): Electrogastrography: Principles and Applications. New York, Raven, 1995.
11. Qian LW, Pasricha PJ, Chen JDZ: Origins and patterns of spontaneous and drug-induced canine gastric myoelectric dysrhythmia. Dig Dis Sci 2003;48:508-515.
12. Hasler WL: The physiology of gastric motility and gastric emptying. In Yamada T, Alpers DH, Owyang C, et al (eds): Textbook of Gastroenterology, ed 2, pp. 181-206. Philadelphia, Lippincott, Williams & Wilkins, 1995.
13. Tougas G, Eaker EY, Abell TL, et al: Assessment of gastric emptying using a low fat meal: establishment of international control values. Am J Gastroenterol 2000;95:1456-1462.
14. Phillips RJ, Powley TL: Gastric volume rather than nutrient content inhibits food intake. Am J Physiol 1996;271:R766-R779.

15. Duggan JP, Booth DA: Obesity, overeating, and rapid gastric emptying in rats with ventromedial hypothalamic lesions. Science 1986; 231:609-611.

16. Wright RA, Krinsky S, Fleeman C, et al: Gastric emptying and obesity. Gastroenterology 1983;84:747-751.

17. Carlson AJ: The Control of Hunger in Health and Disease (Psychic Secretion in Man). Chicago, University of Chicago Press, 1916.

18. Moran TH, McHugh PR: Cholecystokinin suppresses food intake by inhibiting gastric emptying. Am J Physiol 1982;242:R491-R497.

19. Sheldon RJ, Qi JA, Porreca F, et al.: Gastrointestinal motor effects of corticotropic-releasing factor in mice. Regul Pept 1990;28: 137-151.

20. Asakawa A, Inui A, Ueno N, et al: Urocortin reduces food intake and gastric emptying in lean and ob/ob obese mice. Gastroenterology 1999;116:1287-1292.

21. Kelly KA: Differential responses of the canine gastric corpus and antrum to electric stimulation. Am J Physiol 1974;226:230-234.

22. Miedema BW, Sarr MG, Kelly KA: Pacing the human stomach. Surgery 1992;111:143-150.

23. Lin ZY, McCallum RW, Schirmer BD, et al: Effects of pacing parameters in the entrainment of gastric slow waves in patients with gastroparesis. Am J Physiol (Gastrointes Liver Physiol) 1998; 37:G186-G191.

24. Eagon JC, Kelly KA: Effects of gastric pacing on canine gastric motility and emptying. Am J Physiol 1993;265:G767-G774.

25. Hocking MP, Vogel SB, Sninsky CA: Human gastric myoelectric activity and gastric emptying following gastric surgery and with pacing. Gastroenterology 1992;103:1811-1816.

26. Lin XM, Peters LJ, Hayes J, et al: Entrainment of segmental small intestinal slow waves with electric stimulation in dogs. Dig Dis Sci 2000;45:652-656.

27. McCallum RW, Chen JDZ, Lin ZY, et al: Gastric pacing improves emptying and symptoms in patients with gastroparesis. Gastroenterology 1998;114:456-461.

28. Qian LW, Lin XM, Chen JDZ: Normalization of atropine-induced postprandial dysrhythmias with gastric pacing. Am J Physiol (Gastrointest Liver Physiol 39) 1999;276:G387-G392.

29. Abo M, Liang J, Qian LW, et al: Normalization of distention-induced intestinal dysrhythmia with intestinal pacing in dogs. Dig Dis Sci 2000;45:129-135.

30. Bellahsene BE, Lind CD, Schlimer BD, et al: Acceleration of gastric emptying with electric stimulation in canine model of gastroparesis. Am J Physiol 1992;262:G826-G834.

31. Familoni BO, Abell TL, Voeller G, et al: Electric stimulation at a frequency higher than usual rate in human stomach. Dig Dis Sci 1997;42:885-891.

32. Hocking MP: Postoperative gastroparesis and tachygastria: response to electric stimulation and erythromycin. Surgery 1993;114:538-542.

33. Xing JH, Brody F, Brodsky J et al: Gastric electrical stimulation of proximal stomach induces gastric relaxation in dogs. Neurogastroenterol Modif 2003;15:15-29.

34. Cigaina V, Saggioro A, Rigo V, et al: Long-term effects of gastric pacing to reduce feed intake in swine. Obes Surg 1996;6: 250-253.

35. Cigaina V: Gastric peristalsis control by mono situ electric stimulation: a preliminary study. Obes Surg 1996;6:247-249.

36. Cigaina V, Rigo V, Greenstein RJ: Gastric myo-electric pacing as therapy for morbid obesity: preliminary results. Obes Surg 1999;9:333.

37. Cigaina V: Gastric pacing as therapy for morbid obesity: preliminary results. Obes Surg 2002;12:12S-16S.

38. Shikora SA, Knox TA, Bailen L, et al: Successful use of endoscopic ultrasound (EU) to verify lead placement for the implantable gastric stimulator (IGS™). Obes Surg 2001;11:403.

39. Cigaina V, Hirshberg A: Gastric pacing for morbid obesity: plasma levels of gastrointestinal peptides and leptin. Obes Res 2003;11:1456-1462.

40. Knippig C, Wolff S, Weigt H, et al: Gastric pacing has a positive effect on gastrointestinal reflux disease. Obes Surg 2002;12:473.

33

Open Versus Laparoscopic Bariatric Surgery

Ninh T. Nguyen, M.D. and Bruce M. Wolfe, M.D.

Bariatric surgery began in the late 1950s with the introduction of the jejunoileal bypass and, in the 1960s, with the development of the Roux-en-Y gastric bypass (RYGB).[1] Recently, there have been increases in the demand for bariatric surgery and increases in the number of surgeons interested in learning the techniques of bariatric surgery. These increases in enthusiasm and the growth in the field are related, in large measure, to the development of minimally invasive surgical approaches to bariatric surgery. Although open bariatric surgery can be performed with relatively low morbidity and mortality rates, wound-related postoperative complications, such as infection and incisional hernia, are common. Wound infection can occur in as many as 25% of morbidly obese patients, and late incisional hernia can occur in as many as 16.7% of patients.[2,3] Laparoscopic bariatric surgery was initiated in an attempt to improve perioperative outcomes and reduce these common postoperative complications. Other possible advantages of laparoscopic bariatric surgery include less postoperative pain, shorter length of hospitalization, and faster recovery. These clinical advantages were observed after other laparoscopic operations such as cholecystectomy and Nissen fundoplication. Can we, however, attribute the benefits observed after laparoscopic cholecystectomy to laparoscopic bariatric surgery?

To answer this question, it is important to take into account that laparoscopic bariatric surgery is performed in the morbidly obese, a patient population with more preexisting medical conditions than are found in other populations, and the operation is technically more challenging than most other laparoscopic operations. Therefore, the debate about laparoscopic versus open bariatric surgery is important because the benefits observed after other laparoscopic operations do not necessarily apply to the morbidly obese undergoing laparoscopic bariatric surgery. Because RYGB is the most commonly performed bariatric operation in the United States, this chapter emphasizes the differences between the laparoscopic and open approaches to this procedure. This chapter examines the fundamental differences between laparoscopic and open bariatric surgery, reviews the important measures of outcome, stresses the importance of a valid comparison, discusses the physiologic mechanism of improved outcomes observed after laparoscopic bariatric surgery, examines the limitations of laparoscopic bariatric surgery, and summarizes the differences in clinical outcomes between laparoscopic and open RYGB.

▸ FUNDAMENTAL DIFFERENCES BETWEEN LAPAROSCOPIC AND OPEN BARIATRIC SURGERY

To understand the differences in clinical outcomes between laparoscopic and open RYGB, it is important to understand the fundamental differences between the two approaches, namely, the method of access and the method of exposure. The method of access in open RYGB is through an upper abdominal midline incision whereas the method of access in laparoscopic RYGB is through multiple small abdominal incisions. Hence, the laparoscopic approach reduces the injury associated with a large surgical incision. The methods of exposure during open RYGB include the use of abdominal wall retractors and mechanical retraction of the abdominal viscera. In contrast, the methods of exposure during laparoscopic RYGB include the use of pneumoperitoneum and gravity for displacement of the abdominal viscera. By reducing the length of the surgical incision and eliminating the need for mechanical retraction of the abdominal wall and viscera, the operative trauma after laparoscopic RYGB should be lower than after open RYGB. The reduction in surgical insult is believed to be the primary physiologic mechanism of the improved outcome after laparoscopic bariatric surgery.

▸ RATIONALE FOR OPEN VERSUS LAPAROSCOPIC BARIATRIC SURGERY

Surgeons opposed to the laparoscopic approach state that open RYGB can be performed through a relatively small upper abdominal incision, often in 1.5 hours, and the length of hospitalization is often less than 3 days. Then why should bariatric surgery be performed using the laparoscopic approach? Proponents of the laparoscopic approach, however, state that the benefits of laparoscopic RYGB should be similar to the benefits observed in other laparoscopic operations. Intuitively, the benefits of laparoscopy should apply to morbidly obese patients undergoing RYGB as long as the laparoscopic operation can be performed safely and the fundamentals of open surgery are adhered to. At the very least, laparoscopic bariatric surgery should reduce the risk of wound-related complications.

When comparing the outcomes of two different operations, it is important to understand what the important clinical outcomes are and how to measure these outcomes. From a surgeon's perspective, important outcomes tend to include operative time, length of stay in the intensive care unit and in the hospital, and morbidity and mortality rates. In contrast, from a patient's perspective, important outcomes include avoidance of postoperative complications, having minimal pain and discomfort, and having a quick recovery. Most patients do not care if the operation is performed in 1.5 hours, nor do they care if they are discharged in 3 days. What they do care about is the amount of postoperative pain they may experience and the time it takes for them to resume their normal daily function.

VALID COMPARISON

In order to ensure a valid comparison between two different surgical techniques, two important factors must be present. First, the technical aspects of the laparoscopic operation should be similar to those of the open operation. Initially, one of the criticisms of surgeons performing laparoscopic RYGB has been the omission of closing the mesenteric defects. By omitting this important step, late bowel obstruction was observed in the early series.[4,5] Second, the surgeon must pass the learning curve of the laparoscopic approach before performing a comparison between the two operations. Unlike medical trials, surgical trials rely heavily on the surgeon's knowledge and experience in both the conventional open operation and the laparoscopic operation. The development of any new laparoscopic operation has been shown to be associated with a learning curve, and adverse outcomes have been reported during this learning curve. Therefore, a valid comparison of laparoscopic and open bariatric surgery should take into account both of these factors. In a prospective randomized trial comparing laparoscopic and open RYGB, Westling and colleagues reported no significant differences between the two techniques in postoperative pain, length of hospital stay, and sick leave based on an intention-to-treat analysis.[6] In their trial of 51 patients (laparoscopic = 30, open = 21), conversion to laparotomy occurred in 7 (23%) of their 30 laparoscopic operations. The benefits of laparoscopic RYGB were not evident because almost one quarter of the patients who underwent laparoscopic RYGB required conversion to open RYGB. The results of the trial were derived during the learning curve of the laparoscopic technique.

PHYSIOLOGIC BASIS OF IMPROVED OUTCOME IN LAPAROSCOPIC BARIATRIC SURGERY

The basic mechanism of improved outcome after laparoscopic bariatric surgery is presumed from the overall reduced surgical insult to the host. Laparoscopic bariatric surgery is associated with a smaller access incision and reduced intraabdominal tissue injury and abdominal viscera manipulation. In addition, by avoiding the use of traumatic retraction devices, there should be less tissue injury to the abdominal wall. Nguyen and colleagues demonstrated that concentrations of creatine kinase increased significantly after both open and laparoscopic RYGB; however, creatine kinase levels were significantly lower after laparoscopic than after open RYGB.[7] An increase in creatine kinase concentrations and its levels represents the extent of musculoskeletal damage.

Surgical injury can also result in the accumulation of edema, known as third-space fluid, and the degree of edema is related to the extent of surgical trauma. The intraabdominal pressure indirectly measures the degree of postoperative tissue edema resulting from third-space fluid accumulation and bowel distention. An elevated intraabdominal pressure represents more third-space fluid accumulation and a greater degree of operative injury. Nguyen and colleagues reported that postoperative intraabdominal pressures were significantly higher after open RYGB than after the laparoscopic RYGB.[8] Another method of evaluating the degree of operative trauma is the measurement of the systemic stress response. The magnitude of the systemic stress response has been shown to be proportional to the degree of operative trauma. Interleukin-6 is a nonspecific cytokine, and its levels correlate with the degree of operative trauma. Interleukin-6 levels have been shown to be lower after laparoscopic RYGB than after open RYGB.[9]

These data demonstrate that laparoscopic RYGB causes less musculoskeletal injury, less third-space fluid accumulation, and a lower degree of systemic stress response. These data support the notion that laparoscopic RYGB is associated with reduced surgical insult compared to open RYGB, and this finding represents the physiologic basis of improved outcomes following the laparoscopic approach.

PHYSIOLOGIC ADVANTAGES OF LAPAROSCOPIC BARIATRIC SURGERY

Along with the clinical outcome, it is important to examine the potential physiologic advantages of laparoscopic bariatric surgery. Pulmonary function has been shown to be less impaired after laparoscopic cholecystectomy and colectomy.[10,11] Few studies, however, have evaluated the effects of laparoscopy on postoperative pulmonary function in morbidly obese patients. Joris and colleagues evaluated postoperative pulmonary function in 30 morbidly obese patients who underwent either laparoscopic or open gastroplasty.[12] Their study demonstrated less impairment of postoperative pulmonary function after laparoscopic than after open gastroplasty. Nguyen and colleagues demonstrated that pulmonary function was less impaired after laparoscopic than after open RYGB.[13] All respiratory flow parameters were decreased in both groups on the first postoperative day and persisted through the third postoperative day. However, pulmonary function parameters were less impaired after laparoscopic than after open RYGB. The levels of forced expiratory volume at 1 second were 38% higher on the first postoperative day after laparoscopic RYGB than after open RYGB. The advantages of laparoscopic RYGB also included less pulmonary atelectasis. Laparoscopic RYGB patients developed significantly less segmental atelectasis than did open patients.[13]

CLINICAL ADVANTAGES OF LAPAROSCOPIC BARIATRIC SURGERY

The objective clinical advantages of laparoscopic RYGB include the amount of postoperative pain and time for convalescence. Postoperative pain is an important measure of outcome because it can be measured objectively. The degree of postoperative pain after open RYGB is associated with the length of the surgical incision and the extent of operative dissection and operative trauma. Nguyen and colleagues reported that after laparoscopic RYGB, patients utilized significantly less intravenous morphine sulfate than did patients after open RYGB on the first postoperative day (46 ± 31 mg as opposed to 76 ± 39 mg, respectively).[13] Despite the greater amount of self-administered morphine sulfate after open RYGB, patients reported higher visual analog pain scores than did patients after laparoscopic RYGB.[13] After discharge, patients who had undergone open RYGB continued to report higher visual analog pain scores on postoperative day 7 than did patients who had undergone the laparoscopic surgery.

Recovery can be measured subjectively by inquiring into the amount of time before the patients returned to activities of daily living. Nguyen and colleagues reported that after laparoscopic RYGB, patients had more rapid return to activities of daily living than did patients after open RYGB.[14] In addition, time to recovery was examined on the basis of the patients' ability to return to physical, social, and sexual functioning and on their perception of their overall health. A health survey of 36 questions (Short-Form 36) was administered as an objective method of examining patients' physical and social functioning and their perception of their general health. The Moorehead-Ardelt Quality-of-Life questionnaire was used specifically to assess patients' sexual interest and activity. On the basis of the SF-36 survey of physical and social functioning, recovery was faster after laparoscopic RYGB than after open RYGB at 1 and 3 months postoperatively.[14] In addition, the score for the perception of overall health was higher after laparoscopic RYGB than after open RYGB when the health survey was taken at 1 month postoperatively. According to the Moorehead-Ardelt questionnaire, after laparoscopic RYGB, patients had more sexual interest than did patients after open RYGB at 3 months postoperatively.[14]

LIMITATIONS OF LAPAROSCOPIC BARIATRIC SURGERY

There has been only one randomized trial supporting the clinical benefits of laparoscopic RYGB.[14] However, there were limitations in this randomized trial. Because of the strict control in a randomized trial, the results of the trial often can be applied only to a subset of the patients who were examined in that trial. The trial reported by Nguyen and colleagues examined only patients with BMIs less than 60, with no prior upper abdominal operations, and with no hepatic, renal, cardiac, or pulmonary insufficiency. Therefore, there is minimal or no evidence-based data to support the use of laparoscopy in patients with BMIs of 60 kg per m²; in patients with prior bariatric surgery; or in patients with hepatic, renal, cardiac, or pulmonary insufficiency. In addition, the results of a randomized trial must be taken in the context of the surgeon's having passed the learning curve required by the laparoscopic operation.

CONCLUSIONS

The fundamental differences between laparoscopic and open RYGB are the method of access and the method of operative exposure. By reducing the size of the surgical incision and the trauma associated with the operative exposure, the surgical insult is less after laparoscopic than it is after open bariatric surgery. A review of evidence-based data shows that laparoscopic RYGB is associated with less operative trauma, including a reduction in musculoskeletal damage, less third-space fluid accumulation, and a lower systemic stress response than open RYGB. The reduction in surgical insult during laparoscopic RYGB is believed to be the physiologic basis for the observed clinical advantages of laparoscopic RYGB. The physiologic advantages of laparoscopic RYGB include less impairment of postoperative pulmonary function and less pulmonary atelectasis. The clinical advantages of laparoscopic RYGB include a reduction in postoperative pain and faster recovery. At the current time, there are ample evidence-based data to support the physiologic and clinical advantages of laparoscopic bariatric surgery. Therefore, laparoscopic bariatric surgery may represent the new standard for the treatment of morbid obesity, with the caveat that the surgeon has passed the learning curve for the laparoscopic approach.

REFERENCES

1. Buchwald H: Overview of bariatric surgery. J Am Coll Surg 2002;194:367-375.
2. See C, Carter PL, Elliott D, et al: An institutional experience with laparoscopic gastric bypass complications seen in the first year compared with open gastric bypass complications during the same period. Am J Surg 2002;183:533-538.
3. Balsiger BM, Kennedy FP, Abu-Lebdeh HS, et al: Prospective evaluation of Roux-en-Y gastric bypass as primary operation for medically complicated obesity. Mayo Clin Proc 2000;75:673-680.
4. Nguyen NT, Ho HS, Palmer LS, et al: A comparison study of laparoscopic versus open gastric bypass for morbid obesity. J Am Coll Surg 2000;191:149-157.

5. Schauer PR, Ikramuddin S, Gourash W, et al: Outcomes after laparoscopic Roux-en-Y gastric bypass for morbid obesity. Ann Surg 2000; 232:515-529.

6. Westling A, Gustavsson S: Laparoscopic vs open Roux-en-Y gastric bypass: a prospective, randomized trial. Obes Surg 2001;11:284-292.

7. Nguyen NT, Braley S, Fleming NW, et al: Comparison of postoperative hepatic function after laparoscopic versus open gastric bypass. Am J Surg 2003;186:40-44.

8. Nguyen NT, Lee SL, Anderson JT, et al: Evaluation of intraabdominal pressure after open and laparoscopic gastric bypass. Obes Surg 2001; 11:40-45.

9. Nguyen NT, Goldman CD, Ho HS, et al: Systemic stress response after laparoscopic and open gastric bypass. J Am Coll Surg 2002; 194:557-567.

10. Frazee RC, Roberts JW, Okeson GC, et al: Open versus laparoscopic cholecystectomy. Ann Surg 1991;213:651-654.

11. Schwenk W, Bohm B, Witt C, et al: Pulmonary function following laparoscopic or conventional colorectal resection. Arch Surg 1999; 134:6-12.

12. Joris JL, Hinque VL, Laurent PE, et al: Pulmonary function and pain after gastroplasty performed via laparotomy and laparoscopy in morbidly obese patients. Br J Anaesth 1998;80:283-288.

13. Nguyen NT, Lee SL, Goldman C, et al: Comparison of pulmonary function and postoperative pain after laparoscopic versus open gastric bypass: a randomized trial. J Am Coll Surg 2001;192:469-476.

14. Nguyen NT, Goldman C, Rosenquist CJ, et al: Laparoscopic versus open gastric bypass: a randomized study of outcomes, quality of life, and costs. Ann Surg 2001;234:279-289.

REOPERATIONS AND COMPLICATIONS

34

Principles of Revisional Bariatric Surgery

George S. M. Cowan, Jr., M.D.

Revisional bariatric surgery is employed to address certain chronic, subacute, or acute complications that occur at least 30 days after the primary surgery. The presentations for possible revision can, on the surface, appear anywhere from straightforward to frustrating and baffling.

Each candidate for revisional bariatric surgery needs a thorough work-up and surgery, where deemed appropriate, by an adequately experienced revisional bariatric surgeon[1] who employs sound principles pre-, intra- and postoperatively. These principles should be regarded, however, as merely guidelines, and they must allow for exceptions based upon the surgeon's experience and judgment.

▶ GENERAL PRINCIPLES OF REVISION

Unlike primary bariatric surgery,[2] there are no generally accepted guidelines for revisional bariatric surgical indications or procedures. Because candidates for revisional bariatric surgery present with a huge potential array of combinations and permutations of symptoms, signs, prior surgical procedures, findings, and diagnoses, they constitute an infinitely more complex population than their primary bariatric surgical counterparts. Therefore, specific guidelines akin to those agreed upon for primary bariatric surgery are not practicable. The understanding herein must be that the exception may more often prove the rule than any principle or guideline itself, and sound judgment by the experienced revisional bariatric surgeon is the first, and main, rule. Flexibility, including ability to revise previously set preoperative or intraoperative plans, based upon added information, is essential for success.

That not every bariatric surgery patient can achieve ideal weight or be free of problems must always be kept in mind. Current primary bariatric surgical modalities are highly effective, but they may not produce ideal body weight in all morbidly obese patients; that is, not everyone can become thin through bariatric surgery. Bariatric revisional surgery may not predictably provide complete, or even partial, relief from preexisting morbidities associated with previous bariatric surgery or obesity comorbidities.

Expect surprises and be prepared to handle them before, during, and after revisional bariatric surgery. Some patients who present for consideration for revisional bariatric surgery are not what they claim to be at their first clinic visit. For example, a patient's symptoms of intractable nausea, vomiting, and dysphagia following primary bariatric surgery may subsequently appear to be caused by the effects of chronic heavy alcohol intake not previously disclosed rather than by the referring physician's diagnosis of severe gastric inflammation secondary to prior gastric bypass.

On the other hand, relatively straightforward reasons for revision include gastroplasty band erosion, band migration, esophagitis, and staple-line disruption. Each may be treated successfully by, among other options, conversion to Roux-en-Y gastric bypass.[3-5] Failed vertical banded gastroplasty (VBG) conversion to gastric bypass Roux-en-Y produces more weight loss and less risk for reoperation failure than does repeat VBG.[6]

At surgery, unanticipated findings may also occur, sometimes in association with deficient or unavailable prior operative notes. Cancer, in all forms, has a higher incidence among the obese and, though rare, may appear unexpectedly.[7] Other surprise surgical findings may include intraabdominal tumor of the uterus or ovary, an internal hernia, or disease arising in the liver, gall bladder, kidney, or pancreas. Following revisional bariatric surgery, there may be other unusual and challenging developments, such as Guillain-Barré syndrome, recurrent volvulus, fistula formation, or the Munchausen syndrome.[8]

Revisional bariatric surgery is evolving into almost a subspeciality of bariatric surgery, wherein the most clinically skilled, valuable surgeons include those who are best informed of new developments in this area. They must also have a high volume of case experience.

▶ WORK-UP PRINCIPLES

Not all intractable nausea or vomiting necessarily requires revisional bariatric surgery. The presence of tinnitus or impaired hearing may provide support for a diagnosis of Meniere syndrome. Persistent early-morning, severe nausea may be associated with hypoglycemia developing during sleep; it responds to enteral or parenteral glucose given at bedtime until the condition spontaneously remits, sometimes in association with recommended treatment for reactive hypoglycemia. Rarely, preexisting bulimia-anorexia may not be detected in the preoperative evaluation and may prove to be responsible for postoperative nausea and vomiting. Undetected pregnancy also may explain complaints of nausea and vomiting.

A trial of 1 to 3 months of alternative weight-loss modalities unique to bariatric surgery patients experiencing weight loss "failures" may preclude the need for revisional weight-loss surgery. One or more years following bariatric surgery, some patients develop a sweets craving that may cause mild to severe weight increase. About two thirds of these patients may respond, in varying degrees, to an over-the-counter medication, 5-hydroxytryptamine. An alternative is ingesting a high-protein diet that may episodically dampen or abort the sweets craving. "Stuffing the pouch" with snacks of low-calorie foods, such as dry popcorn, rice cakes, celery, raw cauliflower, cantaloupe, cottage cheese, or carrots, is an ancillary strategy that can induce satiety.

Certain medications are known to affect weight loss adversely after bariatric surgery.[9] They include antidepressants, antihypertensives, antihistamines, hypoglycemic agents, hormone therapy (including birth-control medications), and steroids. If a patient is taking such medications and her or his chief complaint is weight regain or inadequate weight loss, a trial of alternative non-weight-gain-related medications might be worthwhile before committing to revisional surgery.

Not all cases of malnutrition, "dumping," or severe diarrhea following primary bariatric surgery require revision. During the early stages after gastric bypass surgery, the weight-loss curve resembles one that may occur with certain severe forms of short-bowel syndrome. However, once the massive weight-loss curve levels off at an acceptable weight, this pseudo-short-bowel syndrome is ameliorated when the patient reaches a new level of nutritional balance and is able to ingest and absorb sufficient nutrition to satisfactorily maintain her or his massively reduced weight.

Unfortunately, a minority of postoperative bariatric surgery patients are unable to absorb enterally sufficient nutrients to maintain a healthy state. This may be the result, for example, of preexisting but occult nutrient abnormalities, celiac sprue, sprue-like conditions, pancreatic exocrine insufficiency, or lactose intolerance. Correction of nutritional and fluid abnormalities by enteral or parenteral feeding, special dietary regimens with, for instance, oral or enteric pancreatic extract, atropine, Metamucil, cholestyramine, or lactase may be sufficient alone or in combination, without the need for revisional surgery.

Following work-up for *Clostridium difficile* or other alimentary tract infection, even if negative, empiric antimicrobial treatment may be effective for problems with diarrhea. Severe cases of diarrheal dumping may be effectively managed by parenteral correction of associated vitamin D deficiency, which may be involved in the cause of this problem.

Revisional bariatric surgery may be indicated when nonsurgical management of significant problems is either not practicable or fails to provide adequate relief. This decision depends upon a sufficiently thorough prior work-up to justify and guide the surgical approach, often being more thorough than far primary bariatric surgery. Where available, review of prior bariatric surgery records and other relevant accounts is most desirable and is important for revisional operative success.

Additional work-up may include cardiopulmonary, psychiatric, and nutritional evaluations; appropriate gastroenterologic, laboratory, and radiologic studies; and pregnancy testing in all potentially fertile female patients. Ensuring that Papanicolaou (PAP) smears and breast exams are current is also wise. It is important to study patients for possible cardiopulmonary damage resulting from prior phentermine-fenfluramine ("phen-fen") exposure, in addition to reviewing all prior prescription and nonprescription drugs.

Physical examination can sometimes be misleading. For example, avoid interpreting patient complaints of "obvious" severe abdominal pain as arising from *within* the abdomen. The pain source may, on closer examination, be found to be hyperesthesia or musculoskeletalchondral pains of the lower anterior thoracoabdominal wall. Hyperesthesia, xiphisternitis, and costochondritis are diagnosable by careful physical examination, and they may explain chronic pain in these areas without the need for revisional surgery.

It is a good practice to review all gastrointestinal radiographs with the radiologist. For example, complete or partial obstruction of the biliopancreatic (afferent) limb is a potentially lethal condition. This is particularly so because it may be overlooked by unsuspecting clinicians. The biliopancreatic limb represents the bypassed small intestine and, therefore, orally ingested contrast material ordinarily cannot reach it. In the presence of biliopancreatic limb obstruction, the marked distention of the bypassed stomach can displace, overstretch, and interrupt the mesenteric blood supply to an antecolic alimentary limb. This can result in limb gangrene as well as in perforation of the bypassed stomach or in stomal disruption.[10] A computed tomography scan of the abdomen usually detects a distended C-loop, an abnormally enlarged bypassed stomach and, sometimes, an abnormal alimentary limb. However, some radiologists, unfamiliar with this anatomy and potential problems, may not consider this appearance sufficiently abnormal as to merit the reporting of these findings.

Any significant nutritional problems should be corrected prior to revisional bariatric surgery.[11]

All postoperative bariatric surgery patients are at risk for developing malnutrition due to complications of the surgery. Such complications include but are not limited to these deficiencies in serum albumin, zinc, iron, vitamins A, D, and B_{12}, thiamine and folate, calcium, phosphate, and magnesium that usually result from inadequate nutritional intake or absorption. Some of the clinical manifestations include significant lower-extremity edema, beefy red tongue, cheilosis, pallor, esophageal monilia, weakness, tiredness, numbness, paralysis, confusion, hypohydration, and occult myocardial damage.

Avoid arriving prematurely at a psychiatric diagnosis to explain a patient's physical complaints following bariatric surgery. A patient may possess an affect, behavior pattern, or prior history that may sometimes tempt the surgeon to describe the physical complaints as psychiatric in origin without benefit of proper evaluation. Psychiatric diagnosis in such instances is, however, wisely regarded as a diagnosis of exclusion, appropriate only after properly ruling out all other diagnoses by means of a complete and thorough work-up.

It is wise to require a psychological evaluation as part of the revisional bariatric surgery work-up. Of patients presenting to our clinic as primary bariatric surgery candidates, 89% tested positive for depression,[12] and this is often worsened in patients presenting with significant problems following earlier bariatric surgery. In many, abdominal pain and other symptoms were considerably magnified by depression.

Provide informed consent at least as thorough as that for primary bariatric surgery patients. Most bariatric surgeons have a more or less standardized, thorough approach to providing primary bariatric surgery candidates with adequate, well-documented, informed consent. This is not usually the case with revisional bariatric surgery because it is less commonly performed, encompasses more variables and, in the past, lacked readily available informed consent models as compared with the primary surgery. We have published a method of documenting adequate patient education before revisional bariatric surgery; it is based upon a reasonably time-tested, preoperative, true/false examination model that has been used with primary bariatric surgery.[13-15] From a risk-management perspective, it would seem extremely difficult for patients to claim not to have understood the informed consent material when they have signed, and had witnessed, their correctly answered questions concerning the surgery.

DIFFICULT DECISION MAKING

Reversal of primary bariatric surgery is rarely in patients' long-term best interests. Patients' demand for reversal of primary bariatric surgery is rarely an appropriate answer to postprimary operative problems or frustrations. Patients who have reversal performed are left with scarring of the abdomen, at least two operative procedures, and usually the same obesity-related comorbidities and related risks that existed before the initial bariatric surgery—no net gain for the pain, risk, and expense.

A wise approach for the revisional bariatric surgeon is gently to insist that patients requesting reversal have a "time-out" lasting weeks or longer during which the patients may receive further work-ups, receive full and complete informed consent information concerning the consequences of reversal and, most important, have an opportunity to come to evaluate more thoroughly their feelings of "buyer's remorse." If at the end of this time, they still insist upon reversal and later regret the decision, they cannot credibly complain that they were not provided with adequate time to consider the consequences of their decisions or that they lacked adequate informed consent.

In patients with Crohn's disease or other autoimmune disorders in which intestinal involvement has occurred or may occur, revision of a bariatric procedure that is confined to the stomach, such as an inflatable gastric band or VBG procedure, ought to be strongly considered. The concern-worthy, potentially life-threatening risk for anemia or bleeding, acute or chronic, in Jehovah's Witness patients has

prompted many revisional bariatric surgeons to perform only simple restrictive procedures in these patients.

When in doubt, the revision should be done using the open technique. Because of the minimal adhesions following most laparoscopic bariatric surgeries, revisional surgery via the laparoscopic route is feasible and, perhaps, preferred by well-trained and experienced surgeons. Experience is necessary to determine which approach to use; the adage "when in doubt, do the case open" generally applies.

INTRAOPERATIVE PRINCIPLES

Pay careful attention to measuring and recording all small-intestine limb lengths when performing small-intestine revisional bariatric surgery. Failure to pay careful attention to revised or preexisting small-intestine limb lengths may have significant consequences such as biliary reflux into the gastric pouch, esophagus, or oral cavity. Ordinarily, a 40- to 45-cm alimentary limb length is sufficient to prevent biliary reflux. However, the small intestine is notoriously difficult to measure accurately, and it may contract to one half of its length with handling. Therefore, the use of at least a 90-cm alimentary limb length is advisable so that, even in the worst-case scenario, the gastroenterostomy stoma remains at least 45 cm from the enteroenterostomy.[16]

During revisional surgery, the bariatric surgeon may conclude that the prior bariatric surgeon's limb lengths, particularly the alimentary or common limbs, were too short or were inaccurately measured. However, excessive handling of the small intestine, particularly in the dissection of the extensive adhesions often accompanying revisional surgery, can itself cause considerable contraction and, hence, artefactually apparent shortening of the small intestine.

All abdominal hernias do not need simultaneous repair during revisional bariatric surgery. For example, massive ventral hernias existing at the time of revisional bariatric surgery may, if repaired, result in abdominal compartment syndrome, excessively prolonged surgery, or an unacceptable risk for herniorrhaphy implant infection. In these instances, it is wise to leave a large, widely open, hernia sac, which is unlikely to produce postoperative complications.

It is wise to consider insertion of a caval umbrella in a patient with a coagulopathy, prior deep venous thrombosis or pulmonary embolism, severe obstructive sleep apnea, or pulmonary hypertension.

When right-colon or distal ileal pathology exists, it is desirable, where feasible, to avoid ileocecal valve resection, particularly in the presence of a malabsorptive bariatric procedure. Such resection may result in unpredictably increased malabsorption with malnutrition or troublesome diarrhea due to retrograde bacterial overgrowth in the distal small intestine.

The presence of liver pathology may not be grossly or biochemically apparent at the time of revisional bariatric surgery.[17] Unfortunately, in some instances, this pathology may be progressive and may contribute to postoperative problems. Hence, obtaining a liver biopsy during revisional surgery may alert the surgeon to overlooked fibrosis, cirrhosis, hemochromatosis, or other findings before they present clinically.

Intestinal diverticula may result following functional end-to-side or end-to-end stapled anastomoses. These may, in time, enlarge considerably. When encountered during revisional bariatric surgery, careful dissection and resection of such enlarged enteric diverticula, especially when they are part of the biliopancreatic limb, may prevent subsequent problems involving blind-loop syndrome.

When in doubt, drain effectively and at a safe distance from staple or suture lines. Postoperative leakage occurs infrequently, but when it does, early warning may be demonstrated by bilious fluid drainage or by the presence of amylase in a sample of wound drainage or of swallowed fluid, colored dye or food emerging via the drain site. A drain can potentially, but not always reliably, channel any fistulous drainage externally as a "controlled leak."

No matter how thorough the preoperative work-up, unanticipated intraoperative findings are possible, and they occur not infrequently. For example, large diverticula of the enteroenterostomy, dense or absent intestinal adhesions, intestinal kinking, very long, thinned-out intestinal mesenteries, internal hernia, or limb lengths at variance with prior measurements may be encountered.

Avoid crossing prior gastric staple lines with additional rows of staples at an angle. Crossing prior gastric staple lines, such as is involved in converting a prior horizontally stapled pouch to a vertical one, involves a substantially increased risk for postoperative stenosis or leakage as compared with stapling across an area of previously unstapled stomach. Where horizontal-to-vertical pouch conversion appears to be of overriding importance, interposition of intestine between gastric pouch and distal stomach may reduce leakage.[18] If avoidance of crossing prior gastric staple lines is not feasible, it is important to invert the gastric-pouch staple line with nonabsorbable, interrupted Lembert sutures over an indwelling bougie in order to reduce risks for leakage and fistulas.[19]

Use limb tags to help prevent switched limbs. After dividing the small intestine distal to the ligament of Treitz, the proximal end of the divided intestine may be anastomosed to the gastric pouch instead of to the end-to-side enteroenterostomy. This can be avoided by taking just the small amount of extra time required to tag the most distal aspect of the divided small-bowel stapled ends.

Dissect out all small intestine in small-bowel obstruction. During exploratory surgery for possible obstruction, an "obvious" site of obstruction is sometimes apparent; however, other sites may also be involved or at risk for subsequent small-bowel obstruction. It is, therefore, wise to dissect out the full length of each small-intestine limb unless overriding reasons exist that preclude it. This should also disclose the presence of an internal herniation, particularly following laparoscopic gastric bypass procedures.[20] Potential sites for internal herniation include the enteroenterostomy mesenteric junction and the mesocolic opening for retrocolic alimentary limb passage.[21]

CONCLUSION

Revisional bariatric surgery occupies a unique and demanding place within the field of bariatric surgery. The demands for experience and current knowledge are mandated by the cadre of bariatric patients who develop highly challenging apparent or actual problems following their primary surgeries. These patients rely upon their revisional bariatric surgeons to steer a unique course for them, to make wise diagnoses, to operate skillfully on the basis of appropriate indications, and to manage and follow them for life.

REFERENCES

1. Cowan GSM Jr: The Cancun International Federation for the Surgery of Obesity (IFSO) statement on bariatric surgeon qualifications. Obes Surg 1998;8:86.
2. National Institutes of Health: NIH guidelines: gastrointestinal surgery for severe obesity. NIH Consensus Statement 1991;9:1-20.
3. Westling A, Ohrvall M, Gastavsson S: Roux-en-Y gastric bypass after previous unsuccessful gastric restrictive surgery. J Gastrointest Surg 2002;6:206-211.
4. Balsiger BM, Murr MM, Mai J, et al: Gastroesophageal reflux after intact vertical banded gastroplasty: correction by conversion to Roux-en-Y gastric bypass. J Gastrointest Surg 2000;4:276-281.
5. Macgregor AM, Rand CS: Revision of staple line failure following Roux-en-Y gastric bypass for obesity: a follow-up of weight loss. Obes Surg 1991;1:151-154.
6. van Gemert WG, van Wersch MM, Greve JW, et al: Revisional surgery after failed vertical banded gastroplasty: restoration of vertical banded gastroplasty or conversion to gastric bypass. Obes Surg 1998;8:21-28.
7. Sweet WA: Linitis plastica presenting as pouch outlet stenosis 13 years after vertical banded gastroplasty. Obes Surg 1996;6:66-70.
8. Cowan GSM Jr, Battle AO, Buffington C, et al: Munchausen's syndrome in postoperative bariatric surgical patients. Obes Surg 1997;7:98-99
9. Aronne LJ, Bray GA, Pi-Sunyer FX, et al: Management of Drug-Induced Weight Gain: A Continuing Education Monograph for Physicians. Madison, WI, University of Wisconsin Medical School, 2002.
10. Keysser EJ, Ahmed NA, Mott BD, et al: Double closed loop obstruction and perforation in a previous Roux-en-Y gastric bypass. Obes Surg 1998;8:475-479.
11. Kushner R: Managing the obese patient after bariatric surgery: a case report of severe malnutrition and review of the literature. J Parenter Enteral Nutr 2000;24:126-132.
12. Cowan GSM III, Buffington CK, Vickerstaff S, et al: Psychological status of the morbidly obese. Obes Surg 1996;6:107-108.
13. Cowan GSM Jr: Informed consent in bariatric surgery. In Deitel M (ed): Obesity Surgery, pp. 327-337. Lea & Febiger, Philadelphia, 1989.
14. Cowan GM Jr, Hiler ML, Martin LF: Reoperative obesity surgery. In Martin LF (ed): Obesity Surgery, pp. 301-334, New York, McGraw-Hill, 2004.
15. Cowan GSM: Informed consent in bariatric surgery and anaesthesia. In Alvarez A, Brodsky A, Cowan GSM, et al (eds): Morbid Obesity, Intra-Operative Management, pp. 27-42. Cambridge, U.K., Cambridge University Press, 2004.
16. Cowan GSM Jr, Buffington CK, Hiler ML: Enteric limb lengths in bariatric surgery. In Deitel M, Cowan GSM Jr (eds): Update: Obesity Surgery for the Morbidly Obese Patient, pp. 267-276. Toronto, FD Publications, 2000.
17. Gholam PM, Kotler DP, Flancbaum LJ: Liver pathology in morbidly obese patients undergoing Roux-en-Y gastric bypass surgery. Obes Surg 2002;12:49-51.
18. Capella JF, Capella RF: Staple disruption and marginal ulceration in gastric bypass procedures for weight reduction. Obes Surg 1996;6:44-49.
19. Cucchi SG, Pories WJ, MacDonald KG, et al: Gastrogastric fistulas: a complication of divided gastric bypass surgery. Ann Surg 1995;221:387-391.
20. Schweitzer MA, DeMaria EJ, Broderick TJ, et al: Laparoscopic closure of mesenteric defects after Roux-en-Y gastric bypass. J Laparoendosc Adv Surg Tech A 2000;10:173-175.
21. Serra C, Baltasar A, Bou R, et al: Internal hernias and gastric perforation after a laparoscopic gastric bypass. Obes Surg 1999;9:546-549.

35

Strictures and Marginal Ulcers in Bariatric Surgery

Bruce David Schirmer, M.D.

Stricture after bariatric surgical operations is generally defined as a stricture of the proximal anastomosis, or gastric outflow channel, of the operation. In Roux-en-Y gastric bypass (RYGB), strictures occur at the gastrojejunostomy. In gastroplasties, in particular in vertical banded gastroplasties (VBG), they occur at the gastric pouch outflow site. Stricture of the distal bowel, distal anastomosis of the RYGB, or other areas of the gastrointestinal tract after a bariatric operation is generally considered to be a form of postoperative bowel obstruction and is so addressed in the literature. Therefore, this chapter confines itself to the subject of stricture as defined above. In this chapter, the words *stricture* and *stenosis* have identical meaning.

Generally, strictures that are postoperative complications of bariatric surgery are not life threatening unless neglected and the patient suffers subsequent metabolic or nutritional deficiencies. Strictures can, however, be sources of considerable debility and may at times lead to the need for reoperative surgery to repair, revise, resect, or bypass the stricture, as the situation dictates.

Because marginal ulcers are closely related to stricture formation after RYGB, that topic will also be considered in this chapter.

STRICTURES AFTER ROUX-EN-Y GASTRIC BYPASS

Etiology and Incidence

Following RYGB, one of the potential complications that may occur at the proximal anastomosis is stricture, or stenosis. The causes of such strictures are multifactorial. Thus the reason for any individual stricture may not be readily apparent on the basis of its clinical presentation. It is fortunate that in most situations, with the exception of stricture associated with marginal ulcer or stricture associated with ischemia, the cause of the stricture does not always dictate the course of typical diagnosis and treatment. Patients who present with stricture following RYGB are usually diagnosed and treated similarly, whatever the cause of the stricture.

Table 35-1 shows the most common causes of stricture of the gastrojejunostomy after RYGB. Strictures that occur as a result of the presence of a marginal ulcer may be more difficult to treat and have a higher incidence of reoperative surgery. The topic of marginal ulcers is discussed separately later in the chapter. Strictures that occur as a result of ischemia may not be as amenable to dilatation as are those resulting from other causes, and they may be more likely to require reoperation. Although this is true elsewhere in the gastrointestinal tract, data to confirm it in bariatric surgery do not exist. However, the analogous situations elsewhere in the gastrointestinal tract suggest that this is the case.

The incidence of stricture after RYGB varies widely as reported in the bariatric surgery literature. Some reviews of large institutional series do not even include stricture or stenosis as a complication of the procedure. Reports that describe the incidence of this complication give figures that typically range from 6% to 15%.[1,2] The reported incidence of the complication is likely to be a product of several factors, which are listed in Table 35-2.

The reported incidence of stricture is almost certainly proportional to the percentage of patient follow-up the surgeon has and to the accurate recording of stricture or stenosis in a database for long-term data storage. Similarly, the degree to which the surgeon pursues patient complaints of obstructive symptoms suggesting a possible stricture, in terms of performing postoperative studies to document

Table 35-1	ETIOLOGIES FOR STRICTURE AFTER GASTRIC BYPASS

Tension on the anastomosis
Foreign body reaction
Technical error in creation
Marginal ulcer
Ischemia
Leak with associated scarring
Idiopathic

Table 35-2	FACTORS CONTRIBUTING TO THE REPORTED INCIDENCE OF STRICTURE FOLLOWING ROUX-EN-Y GASTRIC BYPASS

Surgeon/author recording it as a complication/event
Degree to which surgeon/author follows patients
Surgeon/author is an endoscopist
Patient returns to surgeon with symptoms
Type of anastomosis (stapled versus sewn)
Type of suture material
Intention to limit anastomosis size
Degree to which complaints are assessed with endoscopy and radiology
Foreign body used to band anastomosis

stenosis if present, certainly influences the documented incidence of stenosis. Surgeons who practice flexible upper endoscopy are much more likely to investigate symptoms of obstruction using endoscopy and hence are more likely to diagnose strictures correctly postoperatively. In our experience, the incidence of actual stricture, based on the symptoms and clinical pictures, is correct in only approximately 75% of cases when endoscopy is performed. Therefore, the combination of close follow-up and investigation of obstructive symptoms will yield a greater incidence of stricture in any cohort of patients following RYGB.

Techniques of anastomosis also are likely to be important in the generation of postoperative stricture. We witnessed an increased incidence of stricture that approached 20% during a brief time when a 21-mm circular stapler was used to create the gastrojejunostomy. We then used a 25-mm end-to-end anastomosis (EEA) device for RYGB, which returned the stenosis rate to the 10% range. Since using a linear stapler, our incidence of strictures has fallen to under 3% for the past 3 years. Nguyen and colleagues observed a stricture rate of 8.8% using a 25-mm circular stapler, whereas the rate was 14.4% when using a 21-mm circular stapler.[3] A stricture rate of 27% was reported by Matthews and colleagues following laparoscopic RYGB.[4] Gonzalez and colleagues conducted an analysis of three techniques of performing gastrojejunostomy after laparoscopic RYGB.[5] They found the incidence of stricture after circular stapling to be 31%, whereas the stricture rate after hand-sewn operations was significantly lower, at 3%, and was 0 for patients in whom linear stapling was used. One criticism of this study is that the groups in which linear stapling and circular stapling were used had small numbers of patients (8 and 13, respectively). Other authors, such as Capella and Capella,[6] have reported a decrease in postoperative marginal ulcers and, hence, in strictures since they began performing hand-sewn anastomoses using only absorbable suture.

Results of large series of laparoscopic RYGB procedures have similarly reported variable rates of stricture. Higa and colleagues reported 21 of 400, or a 5.25% incidence of postoperative anastomotic stenosis in their initial series,[7] and a 4.9% incidence in a follow-up report of 1500 cases.[8] Goitein and colleagues reported an incidence of 5.1% strictures following laparoscopic RYGB in 369 patients.[9] Our initial experience with laparoscopic RYGB, when we used an EEA-type anastomosis for the gastrojejunostomy, produced approximately a 9% incidence of postoperative stenosis requiring dilation. We have now adopted the use of a gastrointestinal anastomosis (GIA) stapler for the proximal anastomosis and have witnessed a decrease to less than 3% in the past 500 cases in the incidence of stenosis. Ahmad and colleagues reported a similarly low incidence of postoperative stricture after laparoscopic RYGB.[10] In their series of 450 patients, they had a 3.1% incidence of stricture in the gastrojejunostomy. Go and colleagues reported a 6.8% incidence of stricture in a population of 562 patients undergoing laparoscopic RYGB when they used a 25-mm circular stapler for the gastrojejunostomy.[11] The 38 patients requiring dilation in this group presented at 7.7 weeks postoperatively and required an average of 2.1 dilations to be successfully treated. Two required surgery, one for a complication of a dilation.

Presentation

Patients with postoperative proximal anastomotic strictures normally describe symptom patterns of intolerance to ingestion of soft or solid food, which they had been ingesting without difficulty the previous week. The intolerance is at first to solids but then progresses to include larger volumes of liquids. The typical history describes a rapid evolution to tolerance of only sips of fluids. The typical time frame in which this symptom pattern occurs is 3.5 to 8 weeks after surgery. Goitein and colleagues found an average time of 45 days after surgery until the appearance of symptoms.[9] Ahmad and colleagues reported an average time of 2.7 months after surgery.[10] However, stricture may on occasion present as long as 12 weeks after surgery without accompanying marginal ulcer, and even later if a marginal ulcer has developed. Marginal ulcers cause edema and scarring at the anastomosis, resulting in stricture in a high percentage of cases where the ulcer is severe. Persistence of a severe ulcer significantly increases the difficulty in simple treatment of the stricture.

Diagnosis

An excellent screening test for diagnosing stricture is a barium swallow. This usually shows the narrowing quite clearly. However, care must be taken to have the patient's anastomosis viewed on two planes in order to have an accurate idea of the true severity of the stricture. A barium swallow is most appropriately done if the index of suspicion for a stricture is low or moderate or if the surgeon or a competent endoscopist is not readily available to perform a flexible upper endoscopy. Flexible endoscopy is the definitive test to determine the severity of a stricture. The endoscopist also obtains other important information about the potential or likely causes of the stricture and about the overall picture of the upper gastrointestinal anatomy after the RYGB. The other main advantage of performing an endoscopy as the diagnostic procedure is that therapy may be performed in the same setting. Figure 35-1 illustrates a stenosis after RYGB.

The argument for using a barium study as the initial procedure is that the accuracy of determining stenosis based on clinical symptoms is far from 100%. In our series it is actually close to 75% for patients presenting in the

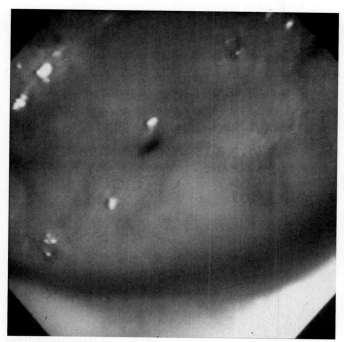

Figure 35-1. Endoscopic view of a stenosis of a gastrojejunostomy after gastric bypass. (Copyright © 2006, Bruce David Schirmer, M.D.)

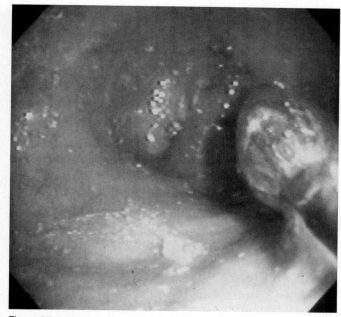

Figure 35-2. Balloon dilation of the stenosis in Figure 35-1. (Copyright © 2006, Bruce David Schirmer, M.D.)

1- to 3-month period after surgery, but it drops off to approximately 50% for delayed symptoms, giving an overall accuracy of 66% in correctly diagnosing anastomotic stenosis based on clinical symptoms. Because a barium swallow is significantly less costly than an upper endoscopy, it may be a preferable screening tool. Other arguments for using endoscopy as the initial diagnostic test include the potential for treatment in the same setting and the additional information obtained at the time of the procedure. A patient's preference is governed largely by his or her relative experience with each procedure. A barium swallow alone is quite benign. When it is associated with fluoroscopically directed anastomotic dilation, especially when such dilation is done with low levels of sedation, the patient may find the entire procedure uncomfortable and objectionable. Alternatively, when an endoscopy is performed with adequate levels of conscious sedation, the patient is often willing to have another such procedure if it is indicated.

Strictures reinforce how important it is that a surgeon who performs bariatric surgery perform flexible upper endoscopy too, whenever possible. The surgeon is in the best position, has the best knowledge of the operation, and can render the most accurate decision as to the best course of action based on endoscopic findings of symptoms after a bariatric operation. The complete bariatric surgeon should perform flexible upper endoscopy for his or her patients in order to optimize efficient care.

Treatment

Balloon dilation is the treatment of choice for stricture following RYGB or laparoscopic RYGB. It may be done either endoscopically or fluoroscopically. The advantages of the endoscopic approach are that the diagnosis can be confirmed and the lesion treated in one session. Figure 35-2 illustrates the performance of an endoscopic balloon dilation for stenosis following RYGB. The endoscopist-surgeon can also appreciate pouch size, the presence of any other lesions, the presence of marginal ulcers, and so forth. Patients often prefer the heavier sedation associated with upper endoscopy to the lesser sedation of fluoroscopic dilation. The disadvantages of the endoscopic approach are that typically the largest balloon that can be easily passed via the therapeutic upper scope channel is an 18F or a 20F balloon.

Fluoroscopic dilation, on the other hand, may be performed with a much larger balloon. Consequently the dilation will be greater. The other advantage of the fluoroscopic approach is that the patient avoids the risks, though small, of sedation. The disadvantage of the fluoroscopic approach is that the patients find the procedure uncomfortable. Another disadvantage of fluoroscopy is that the stenosis may be too narrow to allow easy passage of a guide wire through the anastomosis. In such cases, endoscopy is required to pass the guide wire. We have found that for such tight stenoses, a subsequently planned combined endoscopic and fluoroscopic approach has worked well. A diagnostic endoscopy with placement of a guide wire through the narrow stricture is followed by a fluoroscopic dilation using the guide wire to pass the dilating balloon into the correct position. Endoscopy is also more likely to succeed in dilating very tight strictures in which direct visualization of placement of the dilating balloon into the tight stricture is necessary for success. Table 35-3 summarizes the relative advantages of endoscopic versus fluoroscopic balloon dilation of stenosis after RYGB.

When performing endoscopic balloon dilation of a stricture following RYGB, the endoscopist must follow certain general principles. The indications for endoscopy should include symptoms of nausea, vomiting, and food

Table 35-3	ADVANTAGES OF ENDOSCOPIC VERSUS FLUOROSCOPIC BALLOON DIATION OF STRICTURE AFTER ROUX-EN-Y GASTRIC BYPASS

ENDOSCOPIC
Most accurate for determining stricture diameter
Combined diagnostic and therapeutic procedures in one
Best for very narrow strictures
Direct visualization of the dilatation process
Determination of other upper gastrointestinal anatomy and pathology
Patient preference for sedation

FLUOROSCOPIC
Dilating balloon size larger allowing larger dialatation
Slightly less cost
Avoids excess sedation

intolerance. Such symptoms occurring up to 6 months after surgery are most likely to yield the diagnosis of stricture. Appropriate conscious-sedation guidelines must be followed, and the endoscopist must be familiar with the anatomy to be expected after RYGB.

If the anastomotic stricture is very tight, it may be initially hard to locate and even more difficult to dilate. The endoscopist is cautioned to perform the initial dilation of tight strictures with only a small distal portion of the balloon catheter. The balloon catheter does have a rigid enough tip that blind passage of the majority of the balloon through a stricture when the lumen beyond cannot be visualized is risking a significant potential for perforation of the jejunum beyond the anastomosis.

Many gastrojejunostomies during RYGB, especially those created using a linear stapling technique or a hand-sewn technique, are created in an end-to-side or side-to-side fashion. The back wall of the jejunum lies directly in the path beyond the anastomosis in such situations, and perforation by aggressive insertion of the balloon dilator is quite possible. Instead, it is recommended that the initial dilation be done by inserting only 1 to 2 cm of the balloon into the stricture. This usually allows the endoscope to then be passed into, if not through, the anastomotic stricture, from where direct visualization of the subsequent balloon advancement is possible. The balloon, thus safely passed into the jejunal lumen, is then withdrawn back under endoscopic guidance to lie across the anastomosis before insufflation is performed.

During the postdilation period, if the patient experiences ongoing severe abdominal pain, a water-soluble contrast study is indicated to rule out a perforation. The treatment for perforation is operative, should it occur. Bleeding is extremely rare after anastomotic dilation following RYGB.

After balloon dilation, patients should be observed and monitored as they would after any therapeutic endoscopic procedure. The postprocedure diet consists of liquids, advancing to solids at the discretion of the surgeon or endoscopist (optimally, the same person) and based on the anatomy and clinical picture.

Depending on the severity of the nutrition and fluid depletion the patient has experienced during the time of symptomatic anastomotic stricture, hospitalization for administration of intravenous fluids, electrolytes, vitamins, and nutrition may be indicated, based on the severity of the patient's condition. However, this circumstance is rare, and most patients are able to be treated on an outpatient basis with balloon dilation. A patient who has experienced days of severe vomiting is at risk for thiamine deficiency and must be given thiamine intramuscularly or intravenously to ensure prevention of neurologic deficits resulting from an acute lack of this vitamin.

Surgery for anastomotic stricture following RYGB is required only in a minority of cases. Many of them, in our experience, are associated with marginal ulcer (see subsequent text).

Results

In an early series of 411 of our patients undergoing open RYGB, 58 (14.1%) developed anastomotic stricture or stenosis. The incidence was considerably higher with the EEA stapled technique (19.0%) than with the hand-sewn technique (8.8%, $P<0.05$) when creating the gastrojejunostomy. The efficacy of treatment for either endoscopic or fluoroscopic dilation was good. In our series of balloon dilations, 38 patients required only one procedure; 10 required two, 5 required three, and 5 required more than three dilations. Most of the group requiring more than three procedures (4 of the 5) had scarring from associated marginal ulcer and subsequently underwent reoperative therapy.[12] Thus, in the setting of no associated marginal ulcer, the vast majority of patients were successfully treated with one or two balloon dilations for this problem. There have been few severe complications associated with this series. One patient developed methemoglobinemia due to benzocaine spray. There was one perforation requiring emergent surgery in a patient for whom surgery was planned imminently, had dilation not succeeded.

Others have had similarly good success using balloon dilation for stricture or stenosis following RYGB. Wolper and colleagues[13] reported that 13 of 16 patients had been successfully dilated. Kretzschmar and colleagues[14] reported that 10 of 14 patients were successfully treated using balloon dilation after RYGB. One endoscopic balloon dilation was therapeutic for 9 of 14 patients in the report by Ahmad and colleagues.[10] Goitein and colleagues[9] reported 20 patients, 18 of whom were successfully endoscopically dilated, using 62 dilations. In their experience, only 22% of patients were successfully treated with one dilation, whereas 39% required two and 35% more than two dilations. One patient suffered perforation, and two of the patients, both having had reoperations, required 7 and 10 dilations, respectively. Higa and colleagues[8] reported successful balloon dilation in 72 of 73 patients with stricture following laparoscopic RYGB.

▶ MARGINAL ULCERS

Marginal ulcers are not uncommon following RYGB.[1] The incidence reported in the literature varies from 2% to 12%. Undoubtedly, the degree of suspicion and the aggressiveness of endoscopic investigation of symptoms accounts for some of the variability in the incidence, as with the variability in reported incidence of strictures after this procedure. Empiric treatment of suspected ulcers by medication rather than by performing diagnostic endoscopy would result in a significantly lower reported incidence of this problem than would routine endoscopy for symptoms suspicious for marginal ulcer. Percentage of patient follow-up also contributes to the true incidence of the problem. As noted earlier for stricture, the technique of performing the anastomosis has also been shown to correlate with the incidence of postoperative marginal ulcer formation.[6] The creation of a larger gastric pouch, with increased parietal cell mass and potential for acid secretion, is associated with a higher incidence of postoperative marginal ulcer. Foreign body reaction may also be a nidus for ulcer formation. Also, the presence of *Helicobacter pylori* has been shown to be associated with an increased incidence of marginal ulcer after RYGB (see later text).

Presentation

Patients with marginal ulcer following RYGB generally present with one of three symptom complexes. They may present with the same symptoms as patients with stenosis; in these cases, it is the ulcer that is causing the stenosis. This presentation usually occurs at a later time after surgery than simple stenosis unassociated with marginal ulcer. The second symptom complex is simply persistent stabbing, burning pain in the epigastric region. Commonly, this pain is unaffected by eating and is fairly constant in nature. Severity may vary. The third symptom complex is that of upper gastrointestinal bleeding, with or without associated pain. Of these presentations, the second one, that of persistent epigastric pain, is the most common.

Diagnosis

Flexible upper endoscopy is the best and only indicated procedure if a patient is suspected of having a marginal ulcer following laparoscopic RYGB. An upper gastrointestinal (GI) series is much less accurate in diagnosing marginal ulcers because marginal ulcers are often superficial and are not always apparent on GI contrast studies. Properly performed endoscopy should approach 100% accuracy in diagnosing marginal ulcers. Figure 35-3 illustrates a typical marginal ulcer seen after laparoscopic RYGB. If bleeding is the presenting symptom, upper endoscopy would be used to diagnose and usually also simultaneously to treat the bleeding problem.

A marginal ulcer that is deeper or more chronic or presents late following surgery and is associated with obstructive symptoms and persistent severe abdominal pain should raise the concern that a gastrogastric fistula has been created by the ulcer. An upper GI series should be performed if such an ulcer is found and should always be performed if an ulcer persists despite maximal medical therapy. The contrast study usually but not always reveals the fistula. A strong index of suspicion for such a problem must remain in the surgeon's mind if a persistent marginal ulcer does not respond to therapy.

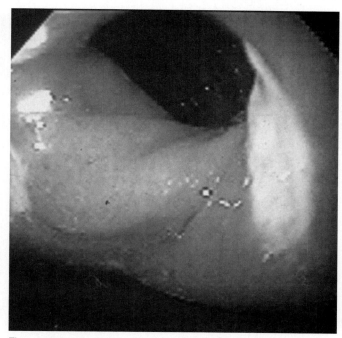

Figure 35-3. Endoscopic view of a marginal ulcer after gastric bypass. (Copyright © 2006, Bruce David Schirmer, M.D.)

Treatment

The treatment of marginal ulcer following RYGB is primarily medical. Patients should be empirically treated by triple therapy (i.e., chlorythromycin, metronidazole, and proton pump inhibitor), whether or not a urease slide test is positive for *H. pylori*. Once the full 2-week course of triple therapy is finished, the continuation of the proton pump inhibitor for 6 months is indicated. Response to medical therapy is quite high—more than 90%.

Failure of medical therapy usually can be attributed to the patient's ongoing ingestion of steroids, aspirin, or nonsteroidal antiinflammatory drugs or to the presence of a ruptured gastric pouch staple line and a gastrogastric fistula. Smoking may decrease successful ulcer healing.

The most difficult situation associated with marginal ulcer occurs when the ulcer has fistulized to the distal stomach following a RYGB in which the stomach had been completely divided by stapling. We have had two such patients in our experience. Once a marginal ulcer has created a gastrogastric fistula, or a gastrogastric fistula exists (resulting from a ruptured staple line) and causes a marginal ulceration, the patient will require reoperative therapy for treatment. If the inflammation is not severe, simple redivision of the stomach is usually feasible and is not associated with an excessive complication rate. Simultaneous decrease in the size of the gastric pouch, if it is excessively large, is indicated. Preservation of the original gastrojejunostomy is appropriate if that anastomosis is not strictured. These procedures can be difficult if the marginal ulcer is long-standing and has produced an intense inflammatory reaction. The best means of preventing such a situation is maintaining follow-up of patients and promptly addressing symptoms of marginal ulcer, including prompt reoperation should the presence of a gastrogastric fistula be clearly documented.

Results

Our experience with marginal ulcer following RYGB has been an observed incidence of 24 of 354 of our RYGB patients developing marginal ulcers postoperatively, for an incidence of 6.8%. This was prior to our performing testing for the presence of *H. pylori*. We subsequently performed such testing using preoperative endoscopic biopsies for our next 166 patients undergoing RYGB, and we found that the incidence of marginal ulcer postoperatively had fallen significantly, to 3.0%.[12] We now perform either routine preoperative endoscopic or serum testing for *H. pylori* in all patients planning to undergo RYGB.

Since beginning to perform laparoscopic RYGB, our method of performing the proximal anastomosis has changed. During the series of patients undergoing laparoscopic RYGB with the use of an EEA stapling approach to the gastrojejunostomy, the incidence of marginal ulcer was low, approximating the open series. Since adopting the GIA type of approach to create the gastrojejunostomy, the incidence of marginal ulcer has been just over 1%. However, for many of these patients less than 1 year has passed since surgery, and they are still potentially at risk for this problem. Still, these data suggest that we will see a very low incidence of this problem because of having used the combination of preoperative testing for *H. pylori* and the technique of GIA stapling to create the gastrojejunostomy for laparoscopic RYGB.

▶ STRICTURES FOLLOWING VERTICAL BANDED GASTROPLASTY

Mason first published his description of VBG in 1982.[15] During the next decade, it was the most popular bariatric operation performed in the United States. However, reports of poor maintenance of lost weight on long-term follow-up[16] and the tendency of patients to adopt a high-calorie liquid and dairy diet, with subsequent weight regain,[17] led many surgeons to abandon the procedure in favor of RYGB. Currently, VBG is performed in less than 5% of bariatric surgeries performed in the United States. As such, it is presented here only to provide the reader with background and with the knowledge that strictures may continue to form in patients who have undergone this procedure in the past. Fortunately, the 21st century replacement for the VBG in the United States, the laparoscopic adjustable gastric banding procedure, has been shown to produce an extremely low incidence of stricture formation.

Postoperative stricture and stenosis after VBG occur at the outlet site of the gastric pouch. It is almost uniformly associated with the presence of the band itself, which is commonly made of a nonabsorbable material capable of inciting a significant foreign-body scar reaction over time. Because this is the cause of the stenosis in most cases that occur after VBG, the progressive scarring at the site is much more difficult to successfully treat than is anastomotic stricture after RYGB.

The incidence of gastric outlet obstruction after VBG has been variably reported in the literature in the past. We reviewed our own experience with VBG and found an incidence of 17% stenosis after the procedure. The element that was of most concern in this group of patients, however, was that the mean time to presentation was more than 1 year after the initial operation. Our success rate with a combination of endoscopic and subsequent fluoroscopic dilation has been poor. Our institution's overall success with dilation of upper gastrointestinal anastomotic strictures fluoroscopically is excellent, but patients who had had bariatric surgery, including those with outflow stenosis after VBG, had only a 50% overall success rate.[18] Because the success rate for fluoroscopic or endoscopic dilation or a combination of the two approaches after RYGB in our series was 91%, most of the failures after balloon dilation for morbid obesity involved patients with VBG or patients who had marginal ulcers associated with RYGB. Thus, the success rate of balloon dilation for patients with VBG was under 50%. Reoperation involving a variety of approaches was used. Although the series was relatively small, the best results were obtained when we converted a VBG to an RYGB, rather than performing an operative procedure to remove the band, dilate the band tract, or create a gastrogastrostomy.

Conversion of VBG to RYGB because of a variety of symptoms, most commonly weight regain, has been reported in the literature with some frequency. Most series do not include stenosis as a common indication for this conversion, but many indicate it as a symptom requiring such surgery in a minority of the patients in the series. Overall, the incidence of postoperative complications following revisional surgery such as VBG to RYGB is higher than it is following the initial bariatric operation. Despite this increased complication rate, the failure of a VBG has most often been treated successfully by using surgical intervention to convert to an RYGB. Excision of the band during this procedure is not necessary, but it is often done to prevent potential postoperative complications of band erosion or ulceration of the distal stomach, which is an area difficult to access for diagnostic endoscopic examination after RYGB. Sugerman and colleagues[19] performed conversions of 53 VBG procedures with complications to RYGB, achieving 67% excess weight loss. The complication rate was approximately 50% for the series, including 20 marginal ulcers.

▶ STRICTURE AFTER MALABSORPTIVE OPERATIONS

Malabsorptive operations, defined as biliopancreatic diversion (BPD) and biliopancreatic diversion with duodenal switch (BPD-DS), represent less than 10% of bariatric operations performed in the United States today. Stricture after BPD is not commonly described, whereas marginal ulcer was reported in 12.5% of the initial patient group treated by Scopinaro and colleagues.[20] They were able to reduce that incidence to 3.2% by changes in the technique of gastrojejunostomy and by the use of H_2 blockers; the overall incidence was 5.6%. Most marginal ulcers appeared within 1 year of surgery, and 75% were successfully treated by medical therapy. There was a reported 20% incidence of stenosis during healing, requiring subsequent endoscopic dilation or surgical revision.

One of the main reasons that Marceau, Hess, and other pioneers of the use of the duodenal switch modification of the BPD adopted that procedure was to decrease the incidence of marginal ulcers after BPD. The BPD-DS has no gastrojejunostomy, and hence no marginal ulcers. The duodenoileostomy is a technically difficult anastomosis to perform as part of the BPD-DS. Although there is the potential for stricture of this anastomosis, the incidence is not well documented in the literature to date.

▶ SUMMARY

Stricture following bariatric surgical procedures is most commonly described after RYGB, with an incidence varying from 2% to 27%. Stricture usually presents within 3 to 13 weeks after surgery and is manifested by progressive intolerance to solid food and then to liquid food intake. Diagnosis is made by means of an upper GI series or a flexible upper endoscopy. Treatment is performed by means of balloon dilation, performed either endoscopically or fluoroscopically. Success is excellent with balloon dilation, and reoperative rates are low. Marginal ulcers may cause or be associated with strictures. Such strictures tend to present later and are more difficult to treat successfully by means of endoscopy. If the marginal ulcer is associated with a connection to the distal stomach, reoperation is indicated. Simple marginal ulcers after RYGB are treated medically, and resolution occurs in more than 90% of cases. Their incidence can be decreased by preoperative treatment for *H. pylori*. Stenosis after VBG consists of a progressive narrowing of the gastric outlet tract, which usually presents late after surgery. Endoscopic dilation has less long-term success in these patients, and surgical revision of RYGB is commonly necessary. Marginal ulcers occur in at least 5% of patients undergoing BPD, but usually they are amenable to medical therapy.

▶ REFERENCES

1. Sanyal AJ, Sugerman HJ, Kellum JM, et al: Stomal complications of gastric bypass: incidence and outcome of therapy. Am J Gastroenterol 1992;87:1165-1169.
2. Pope GD, Goodney PP, Burchard KW, et al: Peptic ulcer/stricture after gastric bypass: a comparison of technique and acid suppression variables. Obes Surg 2002;12:30-33.
3. Nguyen NT, Stevens CM, Wolfe BM: Incidence and outcome of anastomotic stricture after laparoscopic gastric bypass. J Gastrointest Surg 2003;7:997-1003.
4. Matthews BD, Sing RF, DeLegge MH, et al: Initial results with a stapled gastrojejunostomy for the laparoscopic isolated Roux-en-Y gastric bypass. Am J Surg 2000;179:476-481.
5. Gonzalez R, Lin E, Venkatesh KR, et al: Gastrojejunostomy during laparoscopic gastric bypass: analysis of 3 techniques. Arch Surg 2003;138:181-184.
6. Capella JF, Capella RF: Gastro-gastric fistulas and marginal ulcers in gastric bypass procedures for weight reduction. Obes Surg 1999;9:22-28.
7. Higa KD, Boone KB, Ho T, et al: Laparoscopic Roux-en-Y gastric bypass for morbid obesity: technique and preliminary results of our first 400 patients. Arch Surg 2000;135:1029-1034.
8. Higa KD, Ho T, Boone KB: Laparoscopic Roux-en-Y gastric bypass: technique and 3-year follow-up. J Laparoendosc Adv Surg Tech A 2001;11:377-382.
9. Goitein D, Papasavas PK, Gagne D, et al: Gastrojejunal strictures following laparoscopic Roux-en-Y gastric bypass for morbid obesity. Surg Endosc 2005;19:628-632.
10. Ahmad J, Martin J, Ikramuddin S, et al: Endoscopic balloon dilation of gastroenteric anastomotic stricture following laparoscopic gastric bypass. Endoscopy 2003;35:725-728.
11. Go MR, Muscarella P, Needleman BJ, et al: Endoscopic management of stomal stenosis after Roux-en-Y gastric bypass. Surg Endosc 2004;18:56-59.
12. Erenoglu C, Schirmer BD, Miller A: Flexible endoscopy in the management of patients undergoing Roux-en-Y gastric bypass. Obes Surg 2002;12:634-638.
13. Wolper JC, Messmer JM, Turner MA, et al: Endoscopic balloon dilation of late stomal stenosis: its use following gastric surgery for morbid obesity. Arch Surg 1984;119:836-837.
14. Kretzschmar CS, Hamilton JW, Wissler DW, et al: Balloon dilation for the treatment of stomal stenosis complicating gastric surgery for morbid obesity. Surgery 1987;102:443-446.
15. Mason E:. Vertical banded gastroplasty. Arch Surg 1982:117;701-706.
16. Balsinger BM, Poggio JL, Mai J, et al: Ten and more years after vertical banded gastroplasty as primary operation for morbid obesity. J Gastrointest Surg 2000;4:598-605.
17. Brolin RE, Robertson LB, Kenler HA, et al: Weight loss and dietary intake after vertical banded gastroplasty and Roux-en-Y gastric bypass. Ann Surg 1994;220:782-790.
18. Vance PL, de Lange EE, Shaffer HA Jr, et al: Gastric outlet obstruction following surgery for morbid obesity: efficacy of fluoroscopically guided balloon dilation. Radiology 2002;222:70-72.
19. Sugerman HJ, Kellum JM, DeMaria EJ, et al: Conversion of failed or complicated vertical banded gastroplasty to gastric bypass in morbid obesity. Am J Surg 1996;171:263-269.
20. Scopinaro N, Adami GF, Marinari GM, et al: Biliopancreatic diversion. World J Surg 1998;22:936-946.

36

Leaks and Gastric Disruption in Bariatric Surgery

S. Ross Fox, M.D. and Myur S. Srikanth, M.D.

The main themes of this chapter are as follows:

1. The best treatment of a leak following bariatric surgery is its prevention.
2. All bariatric surgeons, irrespective of their skill and experience, will encounter leaks.
3. The ability to manage leaks effectively is the mark of a fully competent bariatric surgeon.
4. Failure to manage such leaks properly places the bariatric surgical patient at risk for severe infection and possible death.
5. Recognition of a leak is the main challenge.
6. Once a leak is identified, the therapy is relatively straightforward.

Significance of Leaks

Various life-threatening complications can occur, both intraoperatively and postoperatively, in a bariatric surgery patient, the most serious of which is pulmonary embolism.[1] Other serious, potentially life-threatening complications include anastomotic and staple line leaks, respiratory arrest, wound infection, subphrenic abscess, gastrointestinal bleeding, fascial dehiscence, gastroenteric obstruction, peptic ulceration, and pancreatitis. Since the introduction of the gastric bypass procedure in the late 1960s,[2] a leak from the stomach or the anastomosis has been considered one of the most serious complications. After pulmonary embolism, the most seriously life-threatening complication is intraabdominal sepsis. The sepsis usually arises when the leak from an anastomosis or a staple line has not been detected early enough or treated appropriately.[1]

Incidence of Leaks

It is difficult to generalize the incidence of anastomotic and other leaks because numerous factors are involved. Leakage rates for the various types of bariatric surgery procedures have been published (Table 36-1). The learning curve, as for any surgical procedure, must also be taken into account, because operative times and leakage rates decrease with experience and improved techniques.[3]

Nguyen and colleagues found, in a randomized study of laparoscopic versus open gastric bypass, that the rates of postoperative anastomotic leak were similar.[4]

The weight of the patient[5] and the presence of a complicating condition such as severe venous stasis[6] can influence the likelihood that a leak may occur. Body configuration (i.e., android vs. gynecoid) is another important predisposing factor. The study design, with respect to variables, such as prospective versus retrospective analysis, the age of the patients,[7] and the number of patients per group, might be expected to have a bearing on the findings. Because gastroenterostomy leaks are more common than enteroenterostomy leaks, it is useful to determine the incidences separately by location; however, not all reports differentiate among types of anastomotic leaks. Finally, the leakage rate, as for other complications, is higher for revisions than for primary surgery. Notwithstanding the various complicating factors, the leak rates published in the medical literature generally lie within the range of 0.4% to 5.1% for primary gastric bypass procedures.

In the large series of bariatric surgical procedures described by Fobi,[1] a total of 1756 patients underwent the Fobi pouch operation; of them 2.6% had documented leaks but only 0.4% required surgical intervention because of the routine use of drains in all secondary operations. In Fobi's experience, the incidence of leaks following secondary operations was 15 times that of primary procedures.

Detection and Treatment of Leaks

The recognition of leaks, together with the risk that they may develop into intraabdominal sepsis, present the greatest challenge for a bariatric surgeon. Whatever methodology is employed, the timely diagnosis of leaks and sepsis in the bariatric surgical patient is of paramount importance.

The challenge for the bariatric surgeon is to intervene before a leak causes a systemic inflammation response syndrome and to keep such a response from progressing to sepsis, severe sepsis, and septic shock. Also to be avoided is the end-organ dysfunction caused by the cytokine cascade generated by the sepsis; the sequelae being adult respiratory

Table 36-1	PUBLISHED INCIDENCES OF LEAKS IN BARIATRIC SURGERY PROCEDURES		
STUDY	PROCEDURE	TYPE OF LEAK	INCIDENCE (%)
Fobi, 2000[1]	FPO/primary	Anastomosis	15/1371 (1.1)
	FPO/revision	Anastomosis	9/97 (9.3)
	Transected Silastic ring vertical GB	Anastomosis	22/288 (7.6)
DeMaria et al, 2002[3]	RYGB initial (LS)	Anastomosis with peritonitis	14/281 (5.1)
	RYGB LS (recent; 2-layer anastomosis)	Anastomosis	3/164 (1.8)
Murr et al, 1995[7]	VBG (n = 23); RYGB (n = 43); biliopancreatic diversion (n = 2)	Gastric anastomosis (overall)	2/68 (2.9)
Schauer et al, 2000[13]	RYGB (LS) primary	Anastomosis	13/1264 (1.0)
		Pouch/distal stomach	10/1264 (0.08)
Toppino et al, 2001[17]	VBG	Gastric leak	3/327 (0.9)
	RYGB	Anastomosis	2/55 (3.6)
Koehler, Halverson, 1982[18]	RYGB	Staple-line dehiscence	5/72 (6.9)
		Proximal gastric pouch	2/72 (2.8)
Schwartz et al, 1988[19]	RYGB	Staple-line breakdown	6/920 (0.7)
		Anastomosis	4/920 (0.4)
Fox et al, 1996[20]	Distal RYGB	Staple line	1/81 (1.2)
	VBG	No leaks	0 (0)
Sugerman et al, 1996[21]	VBG to RYGB conversion	VBG: staple-line disruption	15/58 (26.0)
		Conversion: staple-line disruption	3/58 (5.2)
		VBG: anastomosis with peritonitis	2/58 (3.4)
		Conversion: anastomosis with wound infection	2/58 (3.4)
Curry et al, 1998[22]	Resectional RYGB (primary, n = 47)	Anastomosis	1/85 (1.2)
Matthews et al, 2000[23]	RYGB/LS	Gastrojejunal anastomosis	1/48 (2.1)
Balsiger et al, 2000[24]	RYGB (primary)	Partial staple-line disruption	2/191 (1.0)
		Anastomosis	1/191 (0.5)
Gould et al, 2002[25]	RYGB (HALS)	Anastomosis	1/81 (1.2)
	RYGB fully LS	Anastomosis	4/223 (1.8)
Oh, Srikanth, 2003[26]	AGB	Posterior pouch	3/130 (2.3)

AGB, adjustable gastric band; FPO, Fobi pouch operation; GB, gastric bypass; HALS, hand-assisted laparoscopic; LS, fully laparoscopic surgery; RYGB, Roux-en-Y gastric bypass; VBG, vertical banded gastroplasty.

distress syndrome (ARDS), acute respiratory failure, disseminated intravascular clotting, septic shock, and death.[8]

▶ DEALING WITH LEAKS

Locating Leaks

As stated earlier, leaks usually occur at anastomoses, with gastroenterostomy leaks being more common than those at the enteroenterostomy.

Causes of Leaks

ORIGIN OF LEAKS

The origin of leaks is commonly multifactorial. Fernandez and colleagues evaluated 3073 consecutive bariatric surgical patients and reported a leak rate of 3.2% (mortality 1.5%).[9] Independent factors for leak included hypertension, diabetes mellitus, sleep apnea, age, gender, body mass index, and surgery type. Sugerman and colleagues include venous stasis disease and abdominal compartment syndrome as contributing factors.[6]

TENSION ON THE ANASTOMOSIS

The mobility or elasticity of the small bowel is often reduced in bariatric surgical patients due to the amount of fat in the mesentery. As a result of the decrease in mobility and elasticity, the creation of a tension-free anastomosis

between the gastric pouch and the small intestine may often be difficult. If there is any significant tension on a completed anastomosis, the chances of a leak are markedly increased.

STAPLE OR STAPLER MALFUNCTION

Occasionally, leaks can occur due to malfunction of either the stapling device or a staple. At one time or another, every bariatric surgeon will experience malfunctioning equipment and he or she must always be alert to this possibility. This is an important reason for checking the integrity of every anastomosis before closing the abdomen. Anastomoses should be carefully inspected and pressure-tested with air, methylene blue, or succus entericus, as appropriate.

SUTURE OR STAPLE-LINE SEEPAGE

Oozing can occur through sutures or staple lines and is a likely source of small anastomotic self-draining abscesses that are seen from time to time. These self-draining abscesses can, of course, develop into major abscesses or abdominal sepsis.

SURGICAL TECHNIQUE

Poor surgical technique, such as lack of finesse in handling tissues and the use of traumatizing instruments, contributes to leakage. Failure to irrigate the peritoneal cavity at the conclusion of the procedure increases the likelihood of the development of intraabdominal sepsis.

OBSTRUCTION

Increased intraluminal pressure resulting from obstruction secondary to adhesions distal to anastomoses is another cause of leaks. Even though the anastomosis may be carefully inspected to ascertain adequate integrity, should there be a partial or complete obstruction distal to that anastomosis, it may break down.

HYPOVASCULARIZATION

A leak can occur due to hypovascularization of the tissues at the site of the anastomosis. Therefore, all tissues must be checked for adequate circulation.

ADHESIOLYSIS

Care must be taken to ascertain the integrity of the gastrointestinal serosa in patients who have undergone adhesiolysis; there is a possibility of leaks related to bowel denudation.

MICROHEMATOMATA

Microhematomata can also contribute to leakage at an anastomosis, especially with the prophylactic use of anticoagulants and the simultaneous administration of other medications that inhibit coagulation (e.g., ketorolac tromethamine [Toradol] injection). The hematoma forms within the staple line and, as it grows, it spreads apart the edges of the anastomosis and, thus, creates a leak. This type of leak may take several days to make itself evident.

PANCREATIC ENZYMES AND BILE

Peritonitis caused by bile or pancreatic enzyme spillage can precipitate the breakdown of an anastomosis and cause a leak.

SEPSIS UNRELATED TO LEAK

Sepsis that is not primarily related to a leak can also cause the disruption of an anastomosis.

Frequency of Leaks

In our series of 1541 consecutive bariatric surgical patients, 19 had leaks (1.2%). There were no leaks among 242 primary vertical banded gastroplasty procedures. In 868 primary gastric bypass (Roux-en-Y [RYGB]-type) procedures, there were 7 leaks (0.8%). In 431 revisions of RYGB procedures (including secondary procedures after primary operations that had been performed at other centers), 12 had leaks (2.5%). Jones reports a leak rate in revisions of 4.9%.[10] These results emphasize the fact that revisions result in a higher incidence of leaks (threefold higher in our series) than occur in primary operations (see Table 36-1). This is, in part, due to the greater complexity of the secondary surgical procedures and to poor healing at the anastomosis site. Clearly, a leak becomes even more likely with two or more revisions in a single patient.

In our series, two leaks resolved by spontaneous development of fistulas; the remaining 17 required subsequent laparotomy. In 62% of patients, the second leak occurred at the original site, despite repair and the application of omental or serosal patches when that could be done. A summary of leakage in our series is shown in Table 36-2. In primary RYGB procedures performed laparoscopically,

Table 36-2	**BREAKDOWN OF 19 LEAKS IN 1541 CONSECUTIVE BARIATRIC SURGICAL PATIENTS (FOX SERIES)**		
ANASTOMOSIS	N (% OF TOTAL CASES)	NO ANASTOMOSIS	N (% OF TOTAL CASES)
Gastroenterostomy	7 (0.45%)	Gastric staple line; proximal pouch	5 (0.32%)
Enteroenterostomy	5 (0.32%)	Distal stomach staple line	1 (0.06%)
		Liver capsule tear, 2° to adhesiolysis (bile leak and severe bile peritonitis)	1 (0.06%)
Total anastomotic	12 (0.77%)	Total nonanastomotic	7 (0.45%)

a leak rate of 6.2% is reported by Blachar and Federle,[11] though the rate is considerably lower in other series (see Table 36-1). Leaks can occur up to 10 days after surgery, but usually they occur within 48 hours.

Android (Central) Obesity and Gynecoid (Peripheral) Obesity

In our experience, leaks occur more commonly in android patients because bariatric surgical procedures in patients with extensive intraabdominal adiposity are technically more difficult, and the anastomoses are more likely to be performed under tension. Another factor is that central obesity leaves less working space in the abdomen than is available in gynecoid patients, with their characteristic pattern of peripheral obesity. Mesenteries are less pliant in the presence of excess fatty tissue. Livers are commonly enlarged due to hepatosteatosis. Another important factor is that intraabdominal pressure is higher in central obesity.[12] This makes the deployment of instruments and the manipulation of the tissues difficult.

Self-Draining Leaks

Self-draining leaks are currently being recognized more often because, in general, surgeons are aggressively looking for leaks. However, many self-draining leaks remain undiagnosed because they rarely cause symptoms. The only times these leaks need to be drained is when the sinus tract draining them becomes plugged and when septic material escapes from the site. These self-contained leaks can be quite large and can represent major disruptions of the anastomosis. We have seen them as small as 2 mm in diameter, in juxtaposition to the anastomosis, and as large as 3 × 5 cm. In the latter case, a wide neck was seen on endoscopy. The defect ultimately granulated in from the bottom and required no surgical intervention.

Diagnosis of Intraabdominal Sepsis

Detection of intraabdominal sepsis in the bariatric surgical patient presents one of the most challenging diagnoses for a surgeon. Although straightforward on some occasions, often the diagnosis can be made only on the basis of unusual signs or symptoms or even of intuition on the part of the experienced surgeon. This is because morbidly obese patients do not always display the usual signs and symptoms characteristic of abdominal sepsis in the nonobese patient. A surgeon cannot depend on physical examination alone in such cases. Unfortunately, laboratory studies, along with radiologic evaluations, are also at times nondiagnostic in these situations.

Symptoms of Leakage

In our experience, leaks that contain only gastric contents are usually slower to cause symptoms than those that contain intestinal contents, because saliva is far less irritating to peritoneal tissues than is succus entericus, with its bile and pancreatic enzyme content.

FAILURE TO THRIVE

A surgeon, after performing a large number of bariatric procedures, develops a sense of how patients should be faring postoperatively if they have no complications. A postoperative course that is not going according to plan raises the possibility of intraabdominal sepsis.

POSTOPERATIVE NAUSEA

Nausea can arise for a host of reasons, including a leak. If the nausea is more than transient, studies to identify a leak may have to be initiated.

ABDOMINAL PAIN

Pain is an unreliable symptom because it commonly occurs postoperatively without the presence of a leak. Also, obese patients with advanced intraabdominal sepsis can be ambulating and yet complain of little or no abdominal discomfort.

SHOULDER PAIN

Shoulder pain is commonly present in patients with leaks. This symptom is due to diaphragmatic irritation. The pain is more common on the left side because the gastric contents tend to flow to the left when a leak occurs. Even blood beneath the diaphragm can be sufficiently irritating to cause shoulder pain. Working on or near the diaphragm can provide enough irritation to cause the discomfort. All shoulder pain, however, should be assumed to be due to a leak until proven otherwise.

SHORTNESS OF BREATH

Commonly occurring with abdominal sepsis, shortness of breath is usually related to diaphragmatic irritation, diaphragmatic splinting, or sepsis syndrome. A pleural effusion (usually on the left side) develops because of the subdiaphragmatic process, and the pleural effusion decreases the pulmonary tidal volume.

BLOATING SENSATIONS

Abdominal distention results from the sepsis and the serosal irritation and ileus that accompanies it, causing the sensation of bloating, which can range from minimal to severe, depending on the relative dissemination of the abdominal sepsis and the degree of ileus that occurs.

GRUNTING RESPIRATIONS

Grunting respirations are virtually pathognomonic of intraabdominal sepsis and their presence requires immediate confirmation of a leak by appropriate diagnostic tests and surgical intervention. The "Buddha position" describes a patient who is observed sitting cross-legged on the bed, leaning forward, and having grunting respirations. This combination is pathognomonic of diffuse abdominal sepsis with peritoneal irritation. Commonly these patients are significantly bloated as well.

Signs of Leak and Sepsis

TACHYCARDIA

Tachycardia is one of the most dependable signs of problems developing intraabdominally. It is caused by the systemic inflammation response. A pulse rate of 120 or greater is assumed to be due to a leak until proven otherwise and should trigger a leak workup. Of course, other events can cause tachycardia: hypovolemia, atelectasis, pneumonia, pulmonary embolus, anxiety, and fever. Nonetheless, intraabdominal sepsis should always be considered first when tachycardia is present.

FEVER

Patients with leaks often become febrile over a 24- to 48-hour period. The leak can be quite advanced before the febrile response becomes pronounced. Occasionally, a patient will remain afebrile in spite of serious intraabdominal sepsis.

TACHYPNEA

Tachypnea, particularly in conjunction with tachycardia, should lead the surgeon to suspect intraabdominal sepsis. The cardinal earliest signs of leak are tachycardia, tachypnea, and fever. Whenever this triad occurs, a leak study should always be undertaken.

PLEURAL EFFUSION

Pleural effusion is usually associated with subdiaphragmatic irritation and commonly occurs on the left side. This irritation commonly causes left shoulder pain. This type of discomfort should also trigger a complete leak workup. Often, microorganisms present beneath the diaphragm can be cultured from the pleural fluid.

OLIGURIA

Oliguria results from third-spacing or prerenal failure. It is an ominous sign. Sepsis must be suspected and vigorous fluid resuscitation should be initiated.

SENSE OF IMPENDING DOOM

The patient may well report a sense of impending doom that is nonspecific and difficult to define but is highly diagnostic of an intraabdominal catastrophe.

Leak Studies

COMPLETE BLOOD COUNT AND METABOLIC PANEL

A complete blood count and a complete metabolic panel should be done immediately when intraabdominal sepsis is suspected and daily thereafter, until the issue of sepsis has been resolved. Some surgeons repeat the white blood count every 12 hours. Leukocytosis is a fairly dependable sign, although leukocytopenia can occur late in the progress of abdominal sepsis. However, bandemia usually persists and becomes more pronounced, even with a decreasing white blood count.

ABDOMINAL SCAN WITH ORAL AND INTRAVENOUS CONTRAST

Whenever a surgeon thinks that there is even the remote possibility of a leak, a computed tomography (CT) scan with oral and intravenous contrast media should be performed. Many (but not all) gastroenterostomy leaks, as well as leaks from the staple line along the gastric transection site, will be detected by this procedure. A CT scan will often identify enteroenterostomy leaks if they are present. Both the size of the leak and the volume of the leak can at times be estimated during this process. If a patient is too large for the CT scanner, laparotomy is the best diagnostic test for a leak.

CT (or upper gastrointestinal x-rays) is always part of the leak workup. When the results are positive, the CT is the most effective diagnostic tool at the disposal of the surgeon. However, a negative result does not necessarily mean the patient is leak-free. Some leaks have a propensity for self-healing, and the septic material may be extraluminal. An abscess may already be developing by the time the leak has sealed. The signs and symptoms that originally alerted the surgeon to the possibility of a leak should continue to be followed closely. Unless the patient shows early improvement with the therapy that has been initiated, a CT scan should be carried out every 48 hours until satisfactory improvement is realized or leak intervention has been performed.

CHEST RADIOGRAPH

A radiograph of the chest should be requested to rule out pleural effusion and pneumonia. By this means, it is possible to detect significant atelectasis which, if present, might explain a febrile response in the absence of a leak. Radiographs should be repeated as often as daily until the patient is improving.

GLUCOSE AND ALBUMIN

Serum glucose, prealbumin, and albumin levels should be carefully monitored because they are very sensitive indicators of progressive sepsis, especially in morbidly obese patients. Hyperglycemia occurs in many patients whether or not they have documented diabetes. The degree of elevation of the serum glucose concentration is often indicative of the severity of the septic process. Hypoalbuminemia is a sensitive indicator of sepsis, not just of intraperitoneal sepsis, but also of infection anywhere in the body.

URINALYSIS

Urinalysis is required to exclude urinary tract infection. These infections are not common in bariatric surgical patients, but if the patient has an indwelling catheter, the possibility of a urinary tract infection must be considered.

DEEP VEIN THROMBOSIS AND PULMONARY EMBOLUS STUDIES

If there are indications of phlebitis, deep vein thrombosis is a possibility, and appropriate tests should be performed to investigate it. A pulmonary embolus can mimic some of the signs and symptoms of intraabdominal sepsis, such as shortness of breath, tachycardia, tachypnea, upper abdominal or lower chest pain, and a sense of impending doom. A spiral CT is appropriate to rule out a pulmonary embolus.

INTRAPERITONEAL CYTOKINE LEVELS

Abdominal sepsis causes an elevation of the peritoneal cytokines. Increased levels are probably the earliest warning of serious sepsis. As more is learned about cytokines, and as physicians are better able to measure their intraabdominal levels, it is likely cytokines will help us diagnose leaks significantly earlier than is now possible. Determining peritoneal cytokine levels requires that an intraabdominal drain be left in place or that a peritoneal tap be performed.

Treatment of Leaks With or Without Intraabdominal Sepsis

An algorithm for leak and intraabdominal sepsis management is given in Figure 36-1.

IDENTIFICATION OF LEAK SITE

If not documented by the CT scan, a leak site can be identified laparoscopically or by open laparotomy. Until recent years, therapy has almost invariably required open laparotomy. Our experience in performing laparotomy on the majority of patients with leaks has taught us that sepsis is often localized following a leak, but the infection can be spread significantly at the time of laparotomy. According to Schauer and colleagues, almost all leaks can be managed laparoscopically.[13] Currently, in a high percentage of cases, the interventional radiologist can drain percutaneously many intraabdominal septic processes without the need for a laparotomy (open or closed). If laparotomy can be avoided, the hospital stay is often considerably shortened.

Some leaks are difficult to diagnose, so the surgeon must weigh the risks of reoperation against the benefits, considering the degree of suspicion that a leak or abscess exists and the clinical condition of the patient.

The medicolegal ramifications of a leak are significant. Attorneys will usually not fault a surgeon for an early exploration of a patient in the case of a suspected leak. However, delayed drainage will always be faulted by attorneys, even when that criticism is not warranted.

LAPAROTOMY: USE OF TUBE GASTROSTOMY

A tube gastrostomy is often done during laparotomy because of a leak. This provides the surgeon with an opportunity to provide tube feedings as well as the ability to decompress the small bowel when necessary. In our practice, we do not always place a gastrostomy tube, even though many bariatric surgeons do.

REPAIR OF THE LEAK

The leak should be repaired, if feasible. However, in many cases the tissue is too friable and indurated to justify an attempt to suture the leak. Often an omental or serosal

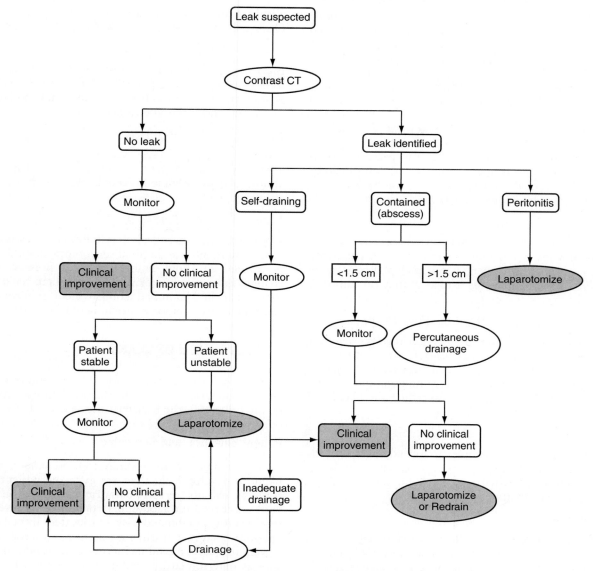

Figure 36-1. Algorithm for intraabdominal leaks and sepsis.

patch can be applied to the leak, or a fibrin sealant can be applied. This can sometimes shorten the convalescence, even if a releak occurs. Releak is common following repair. In our series of 19 patients with intraabdominal sepsis, the releakage rate was 62%, and fistula development was common. This is why adequate drainage is so important. With appropriate use of antibiotics and provision of adequate nutrition, most upper gastrointestinal, low-output fistulas close nonsurgically.

ABDOMINAL DRAINAGE

As indicated earlier, percutaneous drainage without laparotomy is currently a common form of treatment. When it is used, the patient must be followed carefully so the surgeon can be certain that adequate drainage has been established. Adequate drainage is more important than repairing the leak. If laparoscopic or open drainage is required, any

transudate on the peritoneal surfaces, or as much of it as possible, should be removed. Multiple abdominal drains should be placed after thorough irrigation of the peritoneal cavity. A large drain should be used at the site of the leak and wherever significant amounts of septic material have been removed. Smaller drains can be placed in quadrants where there is minimal peritoneal contamination, but all quadrants should be drained. The patient must be carefully monitored with serial CT scans, leukocyte counts, and blood chemistry tests, particularly glucose and albumin tests.

ABDOMINAL CLOSURE

If, after identification and treatment of a leak by laparotomy (open or closed), there is significant edema of the tissues or unresolved dilatation of the loops of bowel, closure of the incision may cause dangerous increases in intraabdominal pressure. This will result in abdominal compartment syndrome, with decreased visceral arterial perfusion, venous stasis, upward displacement of the diaphragm, decreased tidal volumes, and ultimately, multiple organ failure.[14] When a surgeon determines that a patient is at risk for abdominal compartment syndrome, the incision should not be closed until the edema and intestinal dilation have subsided. If the leak intervention has been performed laparoscopically, an abdomen-relaxing incision may have to be made.

After open laparotomy, whether the fascia has been left open or not, the subcutaneous tissue and skin should be left open. The wound can be allowed to heal by secondary intention or may be treated by secondary closure.

How to Treat Fistulas

Gastrocutaneous or enterocutaneous fistulas sometimes develop following either a laparotomy or a transcutaneous drainage of an abscess. Upper gastrointestinal fistulas rarely fail to close. Enterocutaneous fistulas, if they remain open for several months, will require surgical intervention.

Total Parenteral Nutrition or Tube Feeding

Either total parenteral nutrition or gastrostomy/jejunostomy tube feeding is always necessary because nutrition is markedly compromised in the face of intraabdominal sepsis. Tube feeding has the advantage of stimulating the production of gut hormones. This tends to reduce the likelihood of the development of ARDS.

Antibiotics

Administration of the appropriate antibiotics is exceedingly important in the management of patients with leaks. Periodic bacterial sensitivity testing should be carried out over the course of treatment.

Cytokine Management

Altering the progression of the intraabdominal cytokine cascade, as yet imperfectly understood, will most likely diminish the morbidity and mortality of leak-induced sepsis.[15] The earlier such therapy is initiated, the better the outcome is in leak patients.[16] Early recognition of a leak in a young adult is imperative because an exaggerated cytokine response, mediated by the immune system, may occur, leading to death. This type of response is less likely to occur in an older person.

Serial Laboratory Testing

Laboratory testing should be performed regularly (commonly, daily) to maintain surveillance of the body's responses to the septic process and of the effectiveness of the therapy being administered.

Deep Vein Thrombosis and Pulmonary Embolism

Routine precautions against deep vein thrombosis and pulmonary embolism should be taken. Additionally, care should be taken to avoid ischemic cutaneous ulcers, which are particularly serious in very heavy patients.

Pleural Effusions

Pleural effusions occur fairly commonly and may necessitate tube thoracostomy. The chest tube, in a patient with a leak, is not usually required to be left in place for long. Ordinarily, it can be removed within a few days.

Albumin Infusion

Intravenous albumin is administered if the serum albumin level falls below 2.0 g per 100 ml so as to (1) reduce the possibility of ARDS and (2) minimize the possibility of peripheral and cerebral edema.

Intraabdominal Hematoma

If they are large, peritoneal hematomas should be removed surgically. In our experience, intraabdominal hematomas almost always become infected, even with the use of antibiotics.

Intraabdominal Pressure

In patients with increased intraabdominal pressure after a leak, emergency abdominal decompression should be performed to avoid potentially fatal pressure-induced changes in vascular, cardiac, pulmonary, and renal systems that occur in abdominal compartment syndrome. The abdominal fascial closure should be undone.[14]

▶ PREVENTION OF LEAKS

Even though this section is placed at the end of the chapter, we emphasized at the start that preventing leaks should be the priority of the bariatric surgeon.

Patient Selection and Screening

As indicated previously, severely android patients are more likely to develop leaks than are gynecoid patients. Many surgeons will not perform bariatric procedures on patients with increased intraabdominal pressure because of the significantly heightened risk.[12] Elevated intraabdominal pressure is suggested when a patient has a tense abdomen or venous stasis or exhibits increased intraabdominal pressure as determined by bladder manometry with a Foley catheter in place. In such cases, leaks might be avoided by requiring that the patient lose some weight prior to the operation. If the patient is able to lose 35 lb or more, the bariatric surgical procedure becomes technically easier and usually there is less risk for a leak.

Good Surgical Technique

In addition to the previous remarks concerning the factors that contribute to leaks, it must be stated that careful handling of tissues and avoidance of traumatizing instrumentation help to prevent leakage. We have noted leaks at sites of instrumentation. The surgeon should avoid or minimize tension at suture and staple lines and should carefully check anastomoses for patency. In particular, anastomoses should be checked for leakage before the abdomen is closed. One or more drains should be placed if circumstances so indicate, or even if circumstances merely suggest the need. We recommend erring on the side of caution. However, one should always consider drains in revisions. As previously stated, good surgical practice requires that the abdomen be thoroughly irrigated before closure.

Testing the Gastroenterostomy

One method of determining the integrity of staple and suture lines is by air insufflation of the small gastric pouch via the nasogastric tube. This is performed readily by the anesthesiologist at the completion of the procedure. Sterile saline is placed in the abdomen. Any leaks can easily be detected by the presence of bubbling. With gentle distension of the gastric pouch, the size of the pouch can be estimated fairly accurately while the integrity of the gastroenterostomy and of the staple lines is being checked. Another time-honored technique is the placement of methylene blue into the stomach. We find the use of methylene blue more difficult and less tidy than air.

Testing the Enteroenterostomy

Enteroenterostomies can be tested by gently squeezing succus entericus into the area of the enteroenterostomy while looking for bile leaks.

Staple Lines

It is our opinion, and that of many other bariatric surgeons, that it is important to oversew staple lines wherever possible so as to prevent staple-line leaks. Also, stapling across existing staple lines should be avoided. There is always the possibility of devascularization of the tissue at the intersection of the staple lines, with the resulting necrosis liable to precipitate a leak.[10] Rather than cross a staple line, the surgeon should resect the old staple line and use fresh tissues for stapling if possible.

Tissue Vascularity

The vascularity of the tissues in the vicinity of an anastomosis should always be determined. If tissues appear cyanotic, the anastomosis should be redone. Sometimes adhesions contribute to hypovascularization of tissues at or near an anastomosis, especially in revisions. Breakdown may occur, resulting in a leak. This is probably the reason leaks are more common in revisional bariatric surgical procedures than in primary cases.

Secondary Procedures and Revisions

Some particular requirements for secondary or revisional procedures include the following: oversew all anastomoses; be certain there are no obstructions (complete or partial) distal to the anastomoses; place at least one drain in the abdomen; leave the nasogastric tube in place until there are good bowel sounds; always administer antibiotics, including antifungals (a high percentage of bypassed stomachs have resident yeast forms).

SUMMARY

Intraabdominal leaks are usually caused by anastomotic disruption or staple-line problems. The incidence of such leaks is much higher in revisionary procedures. The diagnostic triad of tachycardia, tachypnea, and fever are usually present with intraabdominal sepsis, but they cannot be depended upon entirely to make the diagnosis. Abdominal pain is often present. Rebound tenderness, shoulder pain, leukocytosis, pleural effusion, and bloating also occur commonly but again, these signs and symptoms cannot be depended upon entirely. An abdominal CT scan, with intravenous and oral contrast media, is the best tool for making the diagnosis of a leak with secondary intraabdominal sepsis. However, even the CT scan cannot be depended upon for the diagnosis in all cases, because sepsis can often be present in the absence of a positive CT scan. Therefore a high degree of suspicion must be maintained if the patient is not faring well postoperatively. Detecting leaks can be very difficult in the early stages. The surgeon is well advised to continue careful vigilance and testing, even in the presence of negative preliminary findings.

Treatment involves either percutaneous drainage of the localized septic process or early laparotomy, either open or laparoscopic. Repair of the leak and thorough irrigation of the peritoneal cavity should be carried out if a laparotomy is undertaken. A tube gastrostomy can be placed (although it is not mandatory), and multiple drains should always be placed. Antibiotics are necessary; as we learn more about altering the peritoneal cytokine cascade, whatever can be done to interrupt it should be done. Either total parenteral nutrition or gastrostomy/jejunostomy tube feedings are almost always needed. When early diagnosis is made and appropriate therapy initiated aggressively, morbidity and mortality can be greatly reduced.

REFERENCES

1. Fobi MAL, Lee A, Igwe D, et al: Transected Silastic ring vertical gastric bypass with jejunal interposition, a gastrostomy, and a gastrostomy site marker. In Deitel M, Cowan GSM Jr (eds): Update: Surgery for the Morbidly Obese Patient, pp. 215-218. Toronto, Canada, FD Communications Inc. 2000.
2. Mason EE, Ito C: Gastric bypass in obesity. Surg Clin North Am 1967;4:1345-1351.
3. DeMaria EG, Sugerman HJ, Kellum JM, et al: Results of 281 consecutive total laparoscopic Roux-en-Y gastric bypasses to treat morbidity. Ann Surg 2002;235:640-645.
4. Nguyen NT, Goldman C, Rosenquist CJ, et al: Laparoscopic versus open gastric bypass: a randomized study of outcomes, quality of life, and costs. Ann Surg 2001;234:289-291.
5. Oliak D, Ballantyne GH, Davies RJ, et al: Short-term results of laparoscopic gastric bypass in patients with BMI = 60. Obes Surg 2002;12:643-647.
6. Sugerman HJ, Sugerman EL, Wolfe L, et al: Risks and benefits of gastric bypass in morbidly obese patients with severe venous stasis. Ann Surg 2001;234:41-46.
7. Murr MM, Siadati MR, Sarr MG: Results of bariatric surgery for morbid obesity in patients older than 50 years. Obes Surg 1995;5:399-402.
8. Hotchkiss RS, Karl E: The pathophysiology and treatment of sepsis. N Engl J Med 2003;348:138-150.
9. Fernandez AZ: Experience with over 3000 open and laparoscopic bariatric procedures: multivariate analysis of factors related to leak and resultant mortality. Surg Endosc 2004;18:193-197.
10. Jones KB: Revisional bariatric surgery—safe and effective. Obes Surg 2001;11:183-189.
11. Blachar A, Federle MP, Pealer KM, et al: Gastrointestinal complications of laparoscopic Roux-en-Y gastric bypass surgery: clinical and imaging findings. Radiology 2002;223:625-632.
12. Sugerman HJ: Effects of increased intra-abdominal pressure in severe obesity. Surg Clin North Am 2001;81:1063-1075.

13. Schauer PR, Ikramuddin S, Gourash W, et al: Complication of bariatric surgery. Ann Surg 2000; 232:415-429.
14. Saggi BH, Sugerman HJ, Ivaturi RR, et al: Abdominal compartment syndrome. J Trauma 1998;45:597-609.
15. Sharma S, Kumar A: Septic shock, multiple organ failure, and acute respiratory distress syndrome. Curr Opin Pulm Med 2003; 9:199-209.
16. van Berge Henegouwen MI, van der Poll T, van Deventer SJ, et al: Peritoneal cytokine release after elective gastrointestinal surgery and postoperative complications. Am J Surg 1998;174:311-316.
17. Toppino M, Cesarini F, Comba A, et al: The role of early radiological studies after gastric bariatric surgery. Obes Surg 2001;11:447-454.
18. Koehler RE, Halverson JD: Radiographic abnormalities after gastric bypass. Am J Roentgenol 1982;138:267-270.
19. Schwartz RW, Strodel WE, Simpson WS, et al: Gastric bypass revision: lessons learned from 920 cases. Surgery 1988;104:806-812.
20. Fox SR, Oh KH, Fox K: Vertical banded gastroplasty and distal gastric bypass as primary procedures: a comparison. Obes Surg 1996; 6:421-425.
21. Sugerman HJ, Kellum JM Jr, DeMaria EJ, et al: Conversion of failed or complicated vertical banded gastroplasty to gastric bypass in morbid obesity. Am J Surg 1996;171:263-269.
22. Curry TK, Carter PL, Porter CA, et al: Resectional gastric bypass is a new alternative in morbid obesity. Am J Surg 1998;175: 367-370.
23. Matthews BD, Sing RF, DeLegge MH, et al: Initial results with a stapled gastrojejunostomy for the laparoscopic isolated Roux-en-Y gastric bypass. Am J Surg 2000;179:476-481.
24. Balsiger BM, Kennedy FP, Abu-Lebdeh HS, et al: Prospective evaluation of Roux-en-Y gastric bypass as primary operation for medically complicated obesity. Mayo Clin Proc 2000;75:673-680.
25. Gould JC, Needleman BJ, Elison EC, et al: Evolution of minimally invasive bariatric surgery. Surgery 2002;132:565-571.
26. Oh KH, Srikanth MS: Personal communication, 2003.

section VII

SPECIAL CONSIDERATIONS

37

Adolescent Bariatric Surgery

Victor F. Garcia, M.D.

The arguments in support of bariatric surgery for obese adolescents appear to be compelling and almost self-evident. The epidemic of pediatric obesity has been unabated.[1] Consequently, an increasing number of adolescents present with premature onset of adult disease. The related increases in health care costs are staggering.[2] Moreover, adolescent obesity is a risk factor for adult morbidity and premature mortality.[3-5] Behavioral approaches to prevention and treatment are found wanting. They may be effective in the short term,[6] but there are limited studies of the long-term outcomes of these approaches, particularly among severely obese patients. Surgical weight loss results in amelioration if not resolution of most obesity-related comorbidities; however, the gaps in our knowledge about long-term efficacy and potential adverse consequences related to decreased absorption of nutrients are substantive and warrant a deliberate and closely measured use of bariatric surgery in adolescence. Indeed, the long-term consequences in adolescence of the most popular bariatric procedures are unknown.

There are no prospective evaluations of the efficacy or safety of bariatric surgery performed in adolescence, which makes the arguments in favor of adolescent bariatric surgery far from incontrovertible. The possibility of significant recidivism suggested by the Richmond experience with bariatric surgery in adolescents[7] is at once sobering and anticipated.[8] Obesity in adolescents may also be more virulent and more difficult to manage surgically than obesity in adults.[3] Only the development of the fetus approaches the scope, magnitude, and rapidity of physiologic changes that occur in adolescence. This fact serves to underscore the importance of developing a detailed understanding of the consequences of surgical interventions in this group of young patients. The vagaries and vicissitudes of the adolescent's intellectual and cognitive development make comprehension of and compliance with bariatric surgery challenging at best.

This chapter suggests a context, given the best available evidence, within which adolescent bariatric surgery programs and centers can identify and meet the unique physiologic, cognitive, and psychosocial needs of the adolescent; the ultimate goal is to offer the highest likelihood of long-term success in the management of body weight and of the devastating comorbidities of severe overweight in adolescence. The approach offered borrows heavily from "best practices" in treating adolescents who have other chronic diseases, such as cystic fibrosis, asthma, and cancer, so as to include family-centered, behavior-based interventions, regionalization of care, and the use of a national patient database and a national collaborative effort to study adolescents who undergo bariatric surgery. A national collaborative effort may greatly accelerate the refinement of current approaches and our understanding of the most effective and safest approaches to bariatric surgery in the adolescent.

▶ DEFINITIONS

At risk for overweight, *overweight*, and *obesity* are all terms that have been used in various contexts to refer to the increasing weight problem in children. *Overweight* is a term that can be used to refer to children who have excess fat or other body tissues that contribute to their weight. Obesity, however, is a term that more specifically refers to that condition of having excess body fat. Of the various methods used to define obesity, the body mass index (BMI; kg/m^2) is preferred in children because this measure is reasonably accurate for predicting adiposity, is reproducible in the clinical setting, and can easily be used as a screening tool.[9,10] Just as stature increases during childhood, BMI also increases as a function of age, as lean mass and fat mass are acquired.[11,12] For instance, the average BMI for a 12-year-old boy is nearly 18 kg per m^2, whereas the average BMI for a 20-year-old young man is 23 kg per m^2. The World Health Organization has defined obesity in adults as a BMI of 30 kg per m^2,[13] but the extrapolation of this definition to the younger age groups is difficult, and no specific definition of obesity in children and adolescents has been firmly established. A cut-off point related to age is certainly needed to define childhood obesity, based on the same principle at different ages. In this regard, the 85th and 95th percentiles of BMI for age and sex (based on nationally representative survey data) have been recommended to define overweight and obesity.[14] The 85th and 95th percentiles of BMI for age were chosen in large part

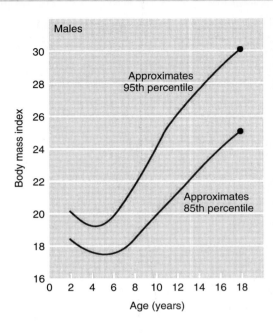
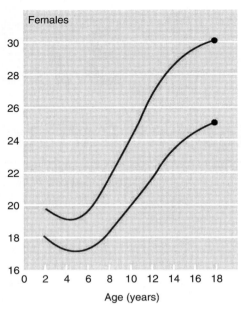

Figure 37-1. Body mass index for age curves to define obesity and overweight in adolescence.

because these percentile boundaries approximate a BMI in young adults of 25 kg per m² (overweight) and 30 kg per m² (obese), respectively (Fig. 37-1).

▶ RISK FACTORS FOR ADOLESCENT OBESITY

An informed approach to adolescent bariatric surgery requires the ability to recognize populations and individuals at risk. The risk associated with obesity accumulates with age and is influenced by genetic, biologic, psychological, sociocultural, and environmental factors acting at all stages of the life span. Recent insights into the fetal, neonatal, and developmental origins of obesity have implications for clinical evaluation of the adolescent candidate for bariatric surgery.[15] There are critical phases in the development of adolescent obesity within the period between preconception and adolescence. Neonatally, there is epidemiologic evidence linking birth weight and later BMI in childhood with adult BMI.[15,16] Lower birth weight elevates the risk for central obesity and insulin resistance.[16,17] The mechanism of this association is unknown but may be related to the "thrifty genotype or phenotype."[18] Childhood obesity risks are higher for offspring of mothers with diabetes mellitus.[19] Postnatally, longer duration of breast feeding[20] and later onset of adiposity[21] reduce the risk for adolescent overweight. Of all the aforementioned risk factors, low birth weight and high BMI of the adolescent confer the highest risk for chronic obesity.[22]

Obesity in family members is an additional risk factor for adolescent obesity. The odds ratio for the persistence of childhood obesity into adulthood is about 3 if one parent is obese and 10 if two parents are obese.[22] Puberty also is a critical period for the development of obesity.[23] Earlier menarche is seen in obese children. A BMI greater than the 85th percentile is associated with a twofold increase in rate of early menarche.[24] The risk that obesity will persist into adulthood is far higher among obese adolescents than it is among overweight younger children.[22]

There is a preexisting racial-ethnic disparity in the risk for obesity.[25] Lower socioeconomic groups may be especially vulnerable because of poor diet and limited opportunity for physical activity.[26] In the aggregate, these characteristics may offer considerable insight as to the phenotype of an individual who might be least able to manage obesity with conventional measures and one who may benefit most from surgical therapy.

▶ COMPLICATIONS OF ADOLESCENT OBESITY

Adolescent obesity is a multisystem disease with potentially devastating consequences (Table 37-1).[27] Associated with the remarkable increase in the prevalence and severity of pediatric obesity in the United States,[28] there is a parallel increase in obesity-related chronic diseases,[29] onset at a younger age,[30] and increased risk for adult morbidity and mortality.[31] Childhood obesity also has adverse social and economic consequences.[32] The persistence of obesity,[22] with approximately 70% to 80% of overweight children becoming obese adults,[22] is of particular concern in certain complications.

The clustering of hypertension, dyslipidemia, chronic inflammation, hypercoagulability, endothelial dysfunction, and hyperinsulinemia (known as insulin resistance syndrome[33]) has been identified in children as young as 5 years of age.[34] The Bogalusa Heart Study noted the correlation between cardiovascular-disease risk factors with asymptomatic coronary atherosclerosis, and the more severely obese individuals had more advanced lesions.[35]

A prediabetic state, consisting of glucose intolerance and insulin resistance, is highly prevalent among severely obese children, even before clinical diabetes has been diagnosed.[36] Even though formerly considered an

Table 37-1	COMPLICATIONS OF ADOLESCENT OBESITY
Psychosocial	Poor self-esteem
	Depression
	Eating disorders
Neurologic	Pseudotumor cerebri
Pulmonary	Sleep apnea
	Asthma, exercise intolerance
Cardiovascular	Dyslipidemia
	Hypertension
	Chronic inflammation
	Endothelial dysfunction
Gastrointestinal	Gallstones
	Steatohepatitis
Renal	Glomerulosclerosis
Endocrine	Type 2 diabetes mellitus
	Insulin resistance
	Precocious puberty
	Polycystic ovary syndrome
	Hypogonadism (boys)
Musculoskeletal	Slipped capital femoral epiphysis
	Blount disease
	Forearm fractures
	Flat feet

"adult-onset" disease, type 2 diabetes mellitus now accounts for nearly half of all new pediatric diagnoses of diabetes[37,38] and is thought to be largely the result of the pediatric obesity epidemic. Of particular concern are data from the Centers for Disease Control and Prevention that suggest that one third of all Americans born in the year 2001 will develop diabetes, and this number rises to nearly one half when one looks at blacks and Hispanics separately.[39] There are also compelling data suggesting that a decline in pancreatic β-cell function begins as early as 12 years prior to the diagnosis of diabetes[40]; the work clearly supports the hypothesis that type 2 diabetes, which develops in childhood or early adulthood, is more virulent than diabetes that develops later in adulthood.[41]

Nonalcoholic steatohepatitis is recognized as a common cause of chronic liver disease in children. This condition is commonly associated with obesity; 25% of overweight children in one report had abnormally elevated liver-function tests.[42] It has been suggested that obesity-related pediatric, nonalcoholic steatohepatitis may become a leading indication for liver transplantation in decades to come.[43,44]

Exercise intolerance, sleep-disordered breathing, and asthma are common pulmonary complications of adolescent obesity.[45] Asthma and exercise intolerance can also limit physical activity and contribute to further increases in weight.[46] Obstructive sleep apnea (OSA), the most severe manifestation of sleep-disordered breathing, can significantly impair obese adolescents' health-related quality of life,[47] result in abnormal left ventricular geometry,[48] and put them at increased risk for hyperactivity and learning difficulties.[49] Studies have also documented decreased somatic growth and systemic hypertension in children with OSA.[50] However, although we feel that OSA is a clinically significant problem that correlates directly with BMI, neither the prevalence of OSA in obese children nor the absolute risk for growth and cardiovascular problems has been accurately quantified in the published literature. Some work has suggested that obesity in childhood elevates the risk

for OSA four to five times above that seen in nonobese children. Anecdotally, in our clinically severely obese adolescent patients with OSA, gastric bypass has allowed them to avoid unnecessary tracheostomy, and within 6 months of surgery, no evidence of sleep apnea or sleep-disordered breathing is seen on polysomnograms.[51]

Arguably, the most prevalent and debilitating consequences of adolescent obesity are psychosocial. The psychological stress of social stigmatization imposed on obese children may be as damaging as the medical morbidities. Many obese adolescents have low self-esteem associated with sadness and high-risk behavior. A recent inventory of the health-related quality of life of obese adolescents compared obese adolescents with normal adolescents and adolescents with chronic diseases of childhood. Obese adolescents had significantly lower quality-of-life scores than normal children—scores that were comparable to those of adolescents diagnosed with cancer.[52]

ADOLESCENT COGNITIVE DEVELOPMENT

Concepts and Principles Relevant to Adolescent Bariatric Surgery

Cognitive development refers to the development of the ability to think concretely. Children (typically between 6 and 12 years of age) develop the ability to think concretely. Adolescence marks the beginning of more complex thinking. Adolescence includes three distinct developmental stages: early, middle, and late adolescence. At any given age, adolescents are at varying stages of cognitive, psychosocial, and biologic maturity. The development of cognition, psychosocial functioning, and several somatic organ systems more closely correlates with pubertal status than with chronologic age.[53] In addition, there are gender differences in the attainment of formal mental operations and identity formation that enable new levels of intellectual functioning, abstract thinking,[54] and cognitive skills that are critical to providing assent to, and compliance with, postoperative guidelines after bariatric surgery. Prior to the attainment of formal operations, the adolescent functions and reasons in concrete operations. Problems involve identifiable objects that are either directly perceived or imagined. Mental operations are possible only when they are applied to information from direct experience. In acquiring formal operations, the adolescent acquires the ability to reason, think abstractly and logically, form hypotheses, and consider various consequences. Examples of formal operations include thinking about possibilities, hypothetical reasoning, anticipating events that have not yet happened, thinking about conventional limits, and thinking about thought. The adolescent who has acquired these abilities is better able to consider the consequences of taking or not taking nutritional supplements or of following and adhering to the prescribed protein-sparing diet. Only about one third of high school graduates have attained the ability to perform formal operations.

Adolescence is generally regarded as a period of social experimentation, limit testing, and risk taking. Egocentrism develops in concert with the attainment of formal operations and predictably adds to the challenge of adolescent compliance with desired health behaviors. The mental constructs of egocentrism include the "imaginary audience," resulting in heightened self-consciousness, and the "personal fable," resulting in a sense of invulnerability.

The postoperative management of the adolescent bariatric patient requires an assessment of the level of intellectual functioning, an understanding of the risk-taking propensity of the adolescent, and the role played by the mental constructs that appear once the adolescent attains formal operations.[55] It is also important to note that the level of cognitive sophistication differs from adolescent to adolescent and may be independent of chronologic age.[56] The attainment of new mental abilities does not carry with it immediate proficiency in their use, nor does education alone counter the adolescent's construct of personal fable or imaginary audience.[57,58] Enhanced compliance with a vigorous nutritional and lifestyle regimen requires not only effective education that applies cognitive development theory but also inputs from peers that help the adolescent attain a more realistic appreciation of both the imaginary audience and his or her own special nature and vulnerability.

Compliance

Long-term therapeutic success with bariatric surgery is dependent upon compliance with the prescribed dietary, lifestyle, and nutritional-supplement regimen. Adolescence is generally viewed as a time of increased experimentation with a variety of health-related behaviors such as diet and exercise. Expertise in enhancing adherence to preventive health practices and compliance with treatment regimens is critical. This is especially germane in the context of bariatric surgery, given that compliance with health recommendations in this population is disappointingly low, estimated at 40% to 50% in adolescents with chronic medical conditions, such as cystic fibrosis, diabetes, and asthma.[59,60] In fact, Rand and McGregor found that after bypass surgery, less than 20% of adolescents demonstrated good compliance with regimes of vitamin and mineral supplementation.[61] Careful study has revealed that for adolescents with chronic medical conditions, adherence to rigorous medical and dietary regimens is substantially improved by the use of behavioral therapy.[62-64] That there is no clear profile of the psychosocial factors consistently associated with the compliant patient precludes a prescribed solution for the prevention and management of poor compliance in the adolescent who has undergone bariatric surgery.[65] To effectively aid the adolescent patient in postoperative compliance, comprehensive adolescent bariatric surgery programs and centers should include individuals capable of assessing levels of cognitive development, ethnically-specific variables, and personality characteristics such as self-esteem and locus of control, as well as family variables such as cohesiveness and level of effective communication.[56] Prior knowledge of these factors may greatly enhance the ability of the bariatric team and the primary care physician to offer useful anticipatory guidance postoperatively; for instance, it can be very useful to know when and with whom most nonnutritive calories are consumed so that the team is aware of the times and the people that may create dangerous situations postoperatively wherein the patient is vulnerable to maladaptive eating habits.

Adolescent compliance is enhanced by: (1) visual aids; (2) focus on the immediate benefits of treatment; (3) participation in self-management; (4) self-monitoring; and (5) self-reinforcement.[66,67] Adolescent self-management and related strategies encourage independence from the family, an important developmental task of adolescence. With the alterations in eating patterns that are required after bariatric surgery, repetitive reinforcement is needed to facilitate the formation of life-long health-promoting habits. Patients and their families require counseling and close follow-up that is designed to promote their physical and emotional well-being. The adolescent bariatric surgery program should build on the best practices of management programs for other adolescent diseases[68] and thus be based on the premise that sustained weight control by the adolescent requires structured family involvement and continued support.

Specific strategies to increase adolescent compliance include education, treatment regimen modification within the social-cultural context of the patient, and enlisting family and peer support. Some adolescents respond to formalized modes of reinforcement such as contracting. In the event of a dysfunctional family, enlisting their support may be counterproductive. An alternative approach is enlisting the support of a trusted adult counselor or confidant, a peer, or a peer support group.

▶ GUIDELINES FOR PERFORMING BARIATRIC SURGERY IN ADOLESCENTS

The impetus for performing bariatric surgery on severely obese adolescents is to prevent, ameliorate, or resolve the adverse consequences of obesity and potentially prevent obesity-related premature mortality. The health benefits of bariatric surgery seen in adults will most likely be observed among adolescents. Bariatric surgery is reasonable for selected adolescents with severe obesity who are unable to achieve and maintain a healthy weight with conventional measures. The published guidelines for adolescent bariatric surgery reflect a divergence of opinion over the appropriate BMI threshold for adolescent bariatric surgery.[69-71] Offering weight loss surgery to only adolescents with severe comorbidities or severe obesity may result in higher procedure-related complications and potentially less weight loss for those patients.[72,73]

Figure 37-2 outlines a suggested algorithm for management. For highly motivated adolescents who have undergone organized attempts at weight loss over a 6-month period without success, bariatric surgery should be considered an option.

Overweight adolescents with obesity-related health complications in whom bariatric surgery is being considered should be referred to specialized centers that offer bariatric surgery within the context of a multidisciplinary team capable of providing long-term follow-up and of managing the unique challenges posed by those in the adolescent age group. Consistent with the guidelines established by the American Bariatric Surgical Association,[74] these teams should include specialists with expertise in adolescent obesity evaluation and management, psychology, nutrition, physical activity instruction, and bariatric surgery.

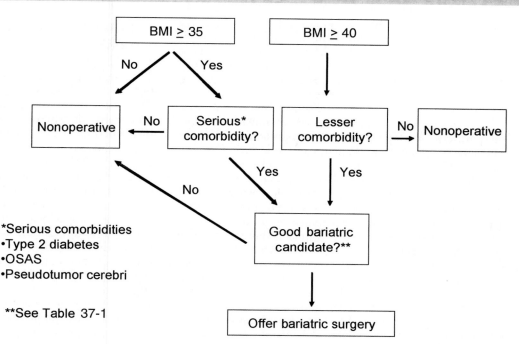

Figure 37-2. Algorithm for management of the obese adolescent after completion of growth.

*Serious comorbidities
•Type 2 diabetes
•OSAS
•Pseudotumor cerebri

**See Table 37-1

Depending on individual needs, additional expertise in adolescent medicine, endocrinology, pulmonology, gastroenterology, cardiology, orthopedics, and ethics should be readily available. The team approach should include a review process similar to that used in multidisciplinary oncology and transplant programs. This review should result in specific treatment recommendations for individual patients, including the appropriateness and timing of possible operative intervention.

The timing of surgical treatment for overweight children and adolescents is controversial and depends, in many cases, upon the compelling health needs of the patient. However, there are certain physiologic factors that need to be considered in planning an essentially elective operation. Physiologic maturation is generally complete by the time of sexual maturation (Tanner stage 3 or 4).[75] Skeletal maturation (adult stature) is normally attained by girls by the age of 13 to 14 and by boys by the age of 15 to 16. Overweight children generally experience accelerated onset of puberty. As a result, they are likely to be taller and have more advanced bone age than age-matched nonoverweight children. If there is uncertainty about whether adult stature has been attained, skeletal maturation (bone age) can be objectively assessed by a radiograph of the hand and wrist. If an individual has attained more than 95% of adult stature, there should be little concern that a bariatric procedure would significantly impair the completion of linear growth.

Before any decision to perform surgery is made, all candidates should undergo a comprehensive psychological evaluation. The goals of this evaluation are (1) to identify psychological stressors or conflicts within the family and to identify past and present psychiatric, emotional, behavioral, or eating disorders; (2) to define potential supports and barriers to patient adherence and to ascertain family readiness for the surgery and the required lifestyle changes it entails (particularly if one or both parents are obese); (3) to assess whether there are reasonable outcome expectations; and (4) to determine the level of cognitive and psychosocial development of the adolescent. With the alterations in eating patterns that are required after bariatric surgery, repetitive reinforcement is needed to facilitate the formation of life-long health-promoting habits. Bariatric surgical programs for this age group should be based on the premise that sustained weight control by the adolescent requires intensive and regular postoperative psychological support. The role of the behavioral therapist depends on the level of intellectual functioning of the adolescent and includes behavioral rehearsal of regimen components prior to surgery, the use of behavioral contracts to outline regimen requirements and document the patient's agreement to adhere, a plan for patient and parental monitoring of adherence, and contingency reinforcement for adherence. The therapist plays a central role in developing parent-adolescent communication and conflict-resolution skills and in creating empirically-based behavioral and family interventions that facilitate the family's management of the patient's new lifestyle.

▶ CLINICAL PATHWAY FOR THE MANAGEMENT OF THE ADOLESCENT UNDERGOING BARIATRIC SURGERY

Bariatric surgery reduces the intake of and decreases the absorption of food items rich in essential fatty acids, vitamins, and other specific nutrients; the long-term results of such reduction are unknown and are of legitimate concern.[76-80] Insufficient nutrition during fetal development can result in obesity, as suggested by the Dutch famine cohort.[80,81] Success in adolescent bariatric surgery requires an expanded definition of success so that it includes not only sustained weight loss but also subsequent normal progression through the remainder of adolescence into adulthood and, eventually, uncomplicated reproduction and normal offspring.

Because the long-term consequences of bariatric surgery performed in adolescents are unknown, the clinical pathway developed by the Comprehensive Weight Management Center at Cincinnati Children's Hospital Medical Center is designed to better characterize the prevalence and resolution of obesity-related complications among adolescents who undergo bariatric surgery, as well as to provide surveillance for the known and potential consequences of the more popular bariatric surgical procedures performed in patients who are comparatively young. The goals of adolescent bariatric surgery centers and programs should be not only to achieve dramatic and sustained weight loss but also to contribute to the understanding of the most effective operations, the risk factors for recidivism, and the long-term outcomes of undergoing bariatric surgery, particularly as they pertain to bone mineral density and the ramifications of life-long decreased vitamin and nutrient absorption for the adolescents and, particularly relevant to young women after bariatric surgery, for their offspring. The potential benefits of regionalizing selected complex surgical procedures have been recognized for at least 2 decades.[82,83]

Toward this end, adolescent bariatric surgery should be concentrated in programs and centers that are willing and able to provide comprehensive and extended pre- and postoperative investigations, including laboratory and diagnostic evaluations. Our preoperative panel includes the following profiles: serum electrolytes, albumin, calcium, uric acid, transferrin, homocysteine, iron, folate, vitamins A, B_1, B_6, B_{12}, D, E, K, lipids, urinalysis, chest radiograph, electrocardiogram, cell blood count, hemoglobin A_{1C}, fasting blood glucose and fasting insulin levels, thyroid-stimulating hormone, and a pregnancy test for females. Nondiabetics receive a 2-hour glucose-tolerance test. With the exception of the glucose-tolerance test, the aforementioned laboratory and diagnostic panels are repeated 3, 6, 9, and 12 months postoperatively, then yearly. Body composition is assessed by either bioelectric impedance (for patients weighing in excess of 300 lb) or dual energy x-ray absorptiometry analysis (DEXA; for patients weighing less than 300 lb) preoperatively and 3, 6, and 12 months postoperatively. DEXA not only allows for the measurement of the rate and relative amounts of fat and lean body mass loss but also provides a quantitative assessment of changes in bone mineral density. This body composition analysis is used to modify dietary plans intended to preserve lean body mass during the period of dramatic weight loss. Evidence suggesting that even as little as a two-standard-deviation change in bone mineral content in an adolescent can significantly increase the risk for osteoporosis and bone fractures in later life underscores the importance of meticulous and extended monitoring of nutrient, vitamin, and mineral absorption.[84] Because of the increased prevalence of abnormal heart geometry[85] and sleep disorders among obese adolescents compared to nonobese adolescents, candidates for bariatric surgery undergo echocardiography and pediatric-specific polysomnography.

▶ NUTRITIONAL AND METABOLIC CONSEQUENCES

The nutritional and metabolic consequences of bariatric surgery have been well delineated.[86] There is impaired absorption of iron, folate, calcium, and vitamin B_{12} after all procedures that bypass the lower stomach and proximal small intestine. Even with supplementation, iron, vitamin B_{12}, folate, and calcium deficiencies may occur. But given the disappointingly poor compliance among adolescents, certain nutrients, such as folate and calcium, warrant special consideration because of the adverse ramifications for the patient and the potential offspring.

Folate is specifically needed for the synthesis of DNA and RNA and for amino acid interconversion, particularly methylation reactions in the methionine-homocysteine cycle. It is essential for growth, cell differentiation, gene regulation, repair, and host defense.[87] Folic acid deficiency, suggested by elevated plasma homocysteine, is associated with cardiovascular diseases, increased risk for dysplasias, and the subsequent development of cancer. In the adolescent who undergoes bariatric surgery, taking folic acid supplementation as prescribed may not provide adequate folate levels;[87] measurement of serum homocysteine may allow identification of those with inadequate supplementation.[85]

Adolescence is a period of enormous skeletal growth and peak skeletal mineral accretion; it is, therefore, a window of opportunity to influence life-long bone health, both positively and negatively. Variations in calcium nutrition in adolescence may account for as much as 50% of the difference in hip fracture rates in postmenopausal years.[89] It is generally assumed that the obese adolescent has greater than normal bone mass and is not operating at a disadvantage for calcium absorption and risk for fracture or later osteoporosis. However, on the contrary, Goulding and colleagues have demonstrated that the obese adolescent may have less than normal bone mineral density and content, thus being at greater risk for fractures.[90] Furthermore, impaired accretion of bone mineral content in adolescence increases the risk for osteoporosis and results in a twofold greater risk for fractures in later life.[84] Given the impaired absorption of both vitamin D and calcium following bariatric surgery and the large individual variation in calcium accretion, it is essential to monitor closely bone mineral density in adolescents undergoing bariatric surgery, particularly gastric bypass and biliopancreatic diversion.

▶ SURGICAL OPTIONS

At the National Institutes of Health Bariatric Consensus Development Conference in 1991, participants concluded that insufficient data existed to recommend bariatric surgery for patients younger than 18 years of age.[91] More than a decade later, data are still limited regarding the safety and efficacy of bariatric procedures in adolescence, and no operation has been studied in a controlled fashion. Results of both Roux-en-Y gastric bypass[7,92-95] and adjustable gastric banding[96,97] have been retrospectively reviewed in small series of adolescents. None of the adolescents who have undergone adjustable gastric banding have been followed for more than 4 years. The median excess weight loss was 35 kg at 2 years. The band was judged to be safe and effective in this short-term study.

The largest and most lengthy follow-up comes from Richmond, Virginia.[78] Sugerman and colleagues reported a career-long series of 33 adolescents (mean preoperative BMI = 52 kg/m²) who underwent bariatric procedures, primarily gastric bypass. This group experienced an excess weight loss of 63% (mean BMI = 33 kg/m²) at 5 years and of 56% (mean BMI = 34 kg/m²) at 10 years after operation. Despite extensive efforts to locate and interview all patients in this series, only six patients could be found of the nine for whom 14 years had passed since operation; these six maintained only 33% excess weight loss (mean BMI = 38 kg/m²).[78] This suggests a high potential for late weight regain, perhaps higher than that seen in adults.

▶ BARIATRIC SURGERY IN A CHILDREN'S MEDICAL CENTER

The first comprehensive weight management program in a children's hospital was established in Cincinnati in 2001.[98] Over 70 adolescents, mean age 17 years, have undergone laparoscopic Roux-en-Y gastric bypass at Cincinnati Children's Hospital. Mean BMIs were 57 kg per m². There have been no deaths and no anastomotic leaks. All patients had comorbidities of obesity. More than 50% had obstructive sleep apnea.[51] After 1 year, the mean BMI was 35 kg/m². Excess weight loss has been 65%. Preoperative comorbidities of obesity have largely been reversed after gastric bypass. There has been a dramatic reduction in the severity of OSA in all patients and complete resolution in 90%.[51] Complete resolution of diabetes mellitus has occurred in all 6 patients who presented with the diagnosis.

Because adolescent obesity may represent a disease that is more serious and more difficult to manage surgically than it is in adults, and because we lack an understanding of the long-term outcomes (both positive and negative) of bariatric procedures in this population, centers offering bariatric care to adolescents should consider the feasibility of a controlled clinical trial to determine the best method of managing adolescent obesity. At the very least, centers offering this care should be regionalized to ensure high volume, and should be obligated prospectively to collect outcomes data (see Fig. 37-2; Table 37-2).

▶ SUMMARY

The obesity epidemic in this country has generated a population of adolescents with premature onset of adult comorbid diseases. Clinical and epidemiologic studies have elucidated some of the life-course risk factors for the development of childhood and adolescent obesity. Adolescent bariatric surgery programs and centers should have expertise that enables them to assess and meet the unique medical, cognitive, physiologic, and psychosocial needs of the adolescent. In the absence of robust evidence of long-term outcomes of bariatric surgery in adolescents,

Table 37-2	SUGGESTED ATTRIBUTES OF A "GOOD" ADOLESCENT BARIATRIC CANDIDATE

Patient is motivated and has good insight.
Patient has realistic expectations.
Family support and commitment are present.
Patient is compliant with health care commitments.
Family and patient understand that long-term lifestyle changes are needed.
Patient agrees to long-term follow-up.
Decisional capacity is present.
Patient has well-documented weight loss attempts.
There is no presence of major psychiatric disorders that may complicate postoperative regimen adherence.
There are no major conduct or behavioral problems.
There has been no substance abuse in the preceding year.
There are no plans for pregnancy in upcoming 2 years.

criteria for surgery should be conservative; the surgery should be performed in centers committed to clinical research and capable of long-term, detailed follow-up and data collection.

▶ REFERENCES

1. Flegal KM, Ogden CL, Wei R, et al: Prevalence of overweight in US children: comparison of US growth charts from the Centers for Disease Control and Prevention with other reference values for body mass index. Am J Clin Nutr 2001;76:1086-1093.
2. Wang G, Dietz WH: Economic burden of obesity in youths aged 6 to 17 years: 1979-1999. Pediatrics 2002;109:E81-81.
3. Freedman DS, Dietz WH, Srinivasan SR, Berenson GS: The relation of overweight to cardiovascular risk factors among children and adolescents: the Bogalusa Heart Study. Pediatrics 1999;103: 1175-1182.
4. Must A, Jacques PF, Dallal GE, et al: Long-term morbidity and mortality of overweight adolescents. A follow-up of the Harvard Growth Study of 1922 to 1935. N Engl J Med 1992;327:1350-1355.
5. Fontaine KR, Redden DT, Wang C, et al: Years of life lost due to obesity. JAMA 2003; 289:187-193.
6. Epstein LH, Roemmich JN, Raynor HA: Behavioral therapy in the treatment of pediatric obesity. Pediatr Clin North Am 2001;48: 981-993.
7. Sugerman HJ, Sugerman EL, DeMaria EJ, et al: Bariatric surgery for severely obese adolescents. J Gastrointest Surg 2003;7:102-108.
8. Rapoff MA: Commentary: pushing the envelope: furthering research on improving adherence to chronic pediatric disease regimens. J Pediatr Psychol 2001;26:277-278.
9. Dietz WH, Robinson TN: Use of the body mass index (BMI) as a measure of overweight in children and adolescents. J Pediatr 1998; 132:191-193.
10. Pietrobelli A, Faith MS, Allison DB, et al: Body mass index as a measure of adiposity among children and adolescents: a validation study. J Pediatr1998;132:204-210.
11. Cole TJ, Bellizzi MC, Flegal KM, Dietz WH: Establishing a standard definition for child overweight and obesity worldwide: international survey. BMJ 2000;320:1240-1243.
12. Rolland-Cachera MF, Sempe M, Guilloud-Bataille M, et al: Adiposity indices in children. Am J Clin Nutr 1982;36:178-184.
13. de Onis M, Blossner M: Prevalence and trends of overweight among preschool children in developing countries. 2000;72:1032-1039.
14. Barlow SE, Dietz WH: Obesity evaluation and treatment: Expert Committee recommendations. The Maternal and Child Health Bureau, Health Resources and Services Administration and the Department of Health and Human Services. Pediatrics 1998;102:E29.
15. Oken E, Gillman MW: Fetal origins of obesity. Obes Res 2003; 11:496-506.
16. Parsons TJ, Power C, Logan S, Summerbell CD: Childhood predictors of adult obesity: a systematic review. Int J Obes Relat Metab Disord 1999;23 Suppl 8:S1-107.

17. Bavdekar A, Yajnik CS, Fall CH, et al: Insulin resistance syndrome in 8-year-old Indian children: small at birth, big at 8 years, or both? Diabetes 1999;48:2422-2429.

18. Flodmark CE: Thrifty genotypes and phenotypes in the pathogenesis of early-onset obesity. Acta Paediatr 2002;91:737-738.

19. Silverman BL, Rizzo TA, Cho NH, Metzger BE: Long-term effects of the intrauterine environment. The Northwestern University Diabetes in Pregnancy Center. Diabetes Care 1998;21 (Suppl 2): B142-149.

20. Gillman MW: Breast-feeding and obesity. J Pediatr 2002;141:749-757.

21. Whitaker RC, Pepe MS, Wright JA, et al: Early adiposity rebound and the risk of adult obesity. Pediatrics 1998;101:E5.

22. Whitaker RC, Wright JA, Pepe MS, et al: Predicting obesity in young adulthood from childhood and parental obesity. N Engl J Med 1997;337:869-873.

23. Karlberg J: Secular trends in pubertal development. 2002;57 Suppl 2:19-30.

24. Wattigney WA, Srinivasan SR, Chen W, et al: Secular trend of earlier onset of menarche with increasing obesity in black and white girls: the Bogalusa Heart Study. Ethn Dis 1999;9:181-189.

25. Strauss RS, Pollack HA: Epidemic increase in childhood overweight, 1986-1998. JAMA 2001;286:2845-2848.

26. Gordon-Larsen P, Adair LS, Popkin BM: Ethnic differences in physical activity and inactivity patterns and overweight status. Obes Res 2002;10:141-149.

27. Dietz WH: Health consequences of obesity in youth: childhood predictors of adult disease. Pediatrics 1998;101(3 Pt 2):518-525.

28. Flegal KM, Troiano RP: Changes in the distribution of body mass index of adults and children in the US population. Int J Obes Relat Metab Disord 2000;24:807-818.

29. Dietz W: Overweight in childhood and adolescence. N Engl J Med 2004;350:855-857.

30. Dietz W: Current trends in obesity: clinical impact and interventions that work. Ethn Dis 2002;12:S2-17-20.

31. Dietz WH: Childhood weight affects adult morbidity and mortality. J Nutr 1998;128(2 Suppl):411S-414S.

32. Gortmaker SL, Must A, Perrin JM, et al: Social and economic consequences of overweight in adolescence and young adulthood. N Engl J Med 1993;329:1008-1012.

33. Srinivasan SR, Myers L, Berenson GS: Predictability of childhood adiposity and insulin for developing insulin resistance syndrome (syndrome X) in young adulthood: the Bogalusa Heart Study. Diabetes 2002;51:204-209.

34. Young-Hyman D, Schlundt DG, Herman L, et al: Evaluation of the insulin resistance syndrome in 5- to 10-year-old overweight/obese African-American children. Diabetes Care 2001;24:1359-1364.

35. Gidding SS, Bao W, Srinivasan SR, Berenson GS: Effects of secular trends in obesity on coronary risk factors in children: the Bogalusa Heart Study. J Pediatr 1995;127:868-874.

36. Sinha R, Fisch G, Teague B, et al: Prevalence of impaired glucose tolerance among children and adolescents with marked obesity. N Engl J Med 2002;346:802-810.

37. Fagot-Campagna A: Emergence of type 2 diabetes mellitus in children: epidemiological evidence. J Pediatr Endocrinol Metab 2000;13 Suppl 6:1395-1402.

38. Pinhas-Hamiel O, Dolan LM, Daniels SR, et al: Increased incidence of non-insulin-dependent diabetes mellitus among adolescents. J Pediatr 1996;128(5 Pt 1):608-615.

39. Narayan KMV: Lifetime Risk for Diabetes Mellitus in the United States. American Diabetes Association 63rd Annual Scientific Sessions, 2003.

40. UK Prospective Diabetes Study (UKPDS) Group: Effect of intensive blood-glucose control with metformin on complications in overweight patients with type 2 diabetes (UKPDS 34). Lancet 1998; 352:854-865.

41. Dean HFB: Natural history of the 2 diabetes mellitus diagnosed in childhood: long term follow-up in young adults. Diabetes 2002; 51(A24).

42. Franzese A, Vajro P, Argenziano A, et al: Liver involvement in obese chidren. Ultrasonography and liver enzyme levels at diagnosis and during follow-up in an Italian population. Dig Dis Sci 1997;42:1428-1432.

43. Rashid M, Roberts EA: Nonalcoholic steatohepatitis in children. J Pediatr Gastroenterol Nutr 2000;30:48-53.

44. Roberts EA: Nonalcoholic steatohepatitis in children. Curr Gastroenterol Rep 2003;5:253-259.

45. Gidding SS, Nehgme R, Heise C, et al: Severse obesity associated with cardiovascular deconditioning, high prevalence of cardiovascular risk factors, diabetes mellitus/hyperinsulinemia, and respiratory compromise. J Pediatr 2004;144:766-769.

46. Ebbeling CB, Pawlak DB, Ludwig DS: Childhood obesity: public-health crisis, common sense cure. Lancet 2002;360:473-482.

47. Schwimmer JB, Burwinkle TM, Varni JW: Health-related quality of life of severely obese children and adolescents. JAMA 2003;289:1813-1819.

48. Amin RS, Kimball TR, Bean JA, et al: Left ventricular hypertrophy and abnormal geometry in children and adolescents with obstructive sleep apnea. Am J Respir Crit Care Med 2002; 165:1395-1399.

49. Sterni LM, Tunkel DE: Obstructive sleep apnea in children: an update. Pediatr Clin North Am 2003;50:427-443.

50. Marcus CL, Greene MG, Carroll JL: Blood pressure in children with obstructive sleep apnea. Am J Respir Crit Care Med 1998;157(4 Pt 1): 1098-1103.

51. Kalra M, Inge T, Garcia V, et al: Obstructive sleep apnea in extremly overweight adolescents undergoing bariatric surgery. Obes Res 2005; 13:1175-1179.

52. Schwimmer JB, Burwinkle TM, Varni JW: Health-related quality of life of severely obese children and adolescents. JAMA 2003;289:1813-1819.

53. Taranger JEI, Lichenstein H, Svennberg-Redegren I: Somatic pubertal development. Acta Paediatr Scand Suppl 1976;258S: 121-135.

54. Piaget JIB: The Growth of Logical Thinking from Childhood to Adolescence. New York, Basic Books, 1958.

55. Elkind D: Cognitive Development. In Stanford Friedman MF, Schonberg SK, Alderman E (eds). Comprehensive Adolescent Health Care. St. Louis, Mosby-Year Book 1998, pp. 34-37.

56. Cromer B: Compliance with health recommendations. In Stanford Friedman MF, Schonberg SK, Alderman E (eds). Comprehensive Adolescent Health Care. St. Louis, Mosby-Year Book, 1998, pp. 104-108.

57. Elkind D: Egocentrism in adolescence. Child Dev 1967;38: 1025-1034.

58. Quadrel MJ, Fischhoff B, Davis W: Adolescent (in)vulnerability. Am Psychol 1993;48:102-116.

59. Phipps S, DeCuir-Whalley S: Adherence issues in pediatric bone marrow transplantation 1990;15:459-475.

60. Borowitz D, Wegman T, Harris M: Preventive care for patients with chronic illness. Multivitamin use in patients with cystic fibrosis. Clin Pediatr 1994;33:720-725.

61. Rand CS, Macgregor AM: Adolescents having obesity surgery: a 6-year follow-up. South Med J 1994;87:1208-1213.

62. Wysocki T, Greco P, Harris MS, et al: Behavior therapy for families of adolescents with diabetes: maintenance of treatment effects. Diabetes Care 2001; 24:441-446.

63. Delamater AM, Jacobson AM, Anderson B, et al: Psychosocial therapies in diabetes: report of the Psychosocial Therapies Working Group. 2001;24:1286-1292.

64. Wysocki T, Harris MA, Greco P, et al: Randomized, controlled trial of behavior therapy for families of adolescents with insulin-dependent diabetes mellitus. 2000;25:23-33.

65. Dunbar JWL: Patient compliance: pediatric and adolescent populations. In Gross AM (ed). Handbook of Clinical Pediatrics. New York, Plenum, 1990, pp. 365-382.

66. Rapoff M, Barnard, MU: Compliance with pediatric medical regimens. In Cramer JA (ed). Patient Compliance in Medical Practice and Clinical Trials. New York, Raven Press, 1991, pp. 73-98.

67. Rapoff MA: Assessing and enhancing adherence to medical regimens for juvenile rheumatoid arthritis. Pediatr Ann 2002;31:373-379.

68. Fielding D, Duff A: Compliance with treatment protocols: interventions for children with chronic illness. Arch Dis Child 1999; 80:196-200.

69. Inge TH, Krebs NF, Garcia VF, et al: Bariatric surgery for severely overweight adolescents: concerns and recommendations. Pediatrics 2004;114:217-223.

70. Buchwald H: Overview of bariatric surgery. J Am Coll Surg 2002; 194:367-375.

71. Garcia VF, DeMaria EJ: Adolescent bariatric surgery: treatment delayed, treatment denied, a crisis invited. Obes Surg 2006;16:1-4.

72. Fernandez AZ Jr, Demaria EJ, Tichansky DS, et al: Multivariate analysis of risk factors for death following gastric bypass for treatment of morbid obesity. Ann Surg 2004;23:698-702.

73. Brolin RE, LaMarca LB, Kenler HA, Cody RP: Malabsorptive gastric bypass in patients with superobesity. J Gastrointest Surg 2002; 6:195-203.

74. American Society for Bariatric Surgery. Society of American Gastrointestinal Endoscopic Surgeons. Guidelines for laparoscopic and open surgical treatment of morbid obesity. Obes Surg 2000; 10:378-379.

75. Wang Y: Is obesity associated with early sexual maturation? A comparison of the association in American boys versus girls. Pediatrics 2002;110:903-910.

76. Eriksson J, Forsen T, Osmond C, Barker D: Obesity from cradle to grave. Int J Obes Relat Metab Disord 2003;27:722-727.

77. Eriksson J, Forsen T, Tuomilehto J, et al: Size at birth, childhood growth and obesity in adult life. Int J Obes Relat Metab Disord 2001; 25:735-740.

78. Forsen T, Eriksson J, Tuomilehto J, et al: The fetal and childhood growth of persons who develop type 2 diabetes. Ann Intern Med 2000;133:176-182.

79. Mi J, Law C, Zhang KL, et al: Effects of infant birthweight and maternal body mass index in pregnancy on components of the insulin resistance syndrome in China. Ann Intern Med 2000;132:253-260.

80. Ravelli AC, van der Meulen JH, Osmond C, et al: Obesity at the age of 50 y in men and women exposed to famine prenatally. Am J Clin Nutr 1999;70:811-816.

81. Roseboom TJ, van der Meulen JH, Ravelli AC, et al: Effects of prenatal exposure to the Dutch famine on adult disease in later life: an overview. Mol Cell Endocrinol 2001;185:93-98.

82. Birkmeyer JD, Dimick JB: Potential benefits of the new Leapfrog standards: effect of process and outcomes measures. Surgery 2004; 135:569-575.

83. Birkmeyer JD, Siewers AE, Marth NJ, Goodman DC: Regionalization of high-risk surgery and implications for patient travel times. JAMA 2003;290:2703-2708.

84. Kalkwarf HJ, Khoury JC, Lanphear BP: Milk intake during childhood and adolescence, adult bone density, and osteoporotic fractures in US women. 2003;77:257-265.

85. Daniels SR: Obesity in the pediatric patient: cardiovascular complications. Prog Pediatr Cardiol 2001;12:161-167.

86. Fujioka K: Follow-up of nutritional and metabolic problems after bariatric surgery. Diabetes Care 2005;28:481-484.

87. Hall JG, Solehdin F: Folate and its various ramifications. Adv Pediatr 1998;45:1-35.

88. Dixon JB, Dixon ME, O'Brien PE: Elevated homocysteine levels with weight loss after Lap-Band surgery: higher folate and vitamin B_{12} levels required to maintain homocysteine level. Int J Obes Relat Metab Disord 2001;25:219-227.

89. Ilich JZ, Badenhop NE, Matkovic V: Primary prevention of osteoporosis: pediatric approach to disease of the elderly. Womens Health Issues 1996;6:194-203.

90. Goulding A, Taylor RW, Jones IE, et al: Overweight and obese children have low bone mass and area for their weight. Int J Obes Relat Metab Disord 2000;24:627-632.

91. Consensus Development Conference Panel: Gastrointestinal surgery for severe obesity. Ann Intern Med 1991;115:956-961.

92. Anderson AE, Soper RT, Scott DH: Gastric bypass for morbid obesity in children and adolescents. J Pediatr Surg 1980;15:876-881.

93. Capella JF, Capella RF: Bariatric surgery in adolescence: is this the best age to operate? Obes Surg 2003;13:826-832.

94. Lawson ML, Kirk S, Mitchell T, et al: One-year outcomes of Roux-en-Y gastric bypass for morbidly obese adolescents: a multicenter study from the Pediatric Bariatric Study Group. J Pediatr Surg 2006; 41:137-143.

95. Strauss RS, Bradley LJ, Brolin RE: Gastric bypass surgery in adolescents with morbid obesity. J Pediatr 2001;138:499-504.

96. Abu-Abeid S, Gavert N, Klausner JM, Szold A: Bariatric surgery in adolescence. J Pediatr Surg 2003;38:1379-1382.

97. Dolan K, Creighton L, Hopkins G, Fielding G: Laparoscopic gastric banding in morbidly obese adolescents. 2003;13:101-104.

98. Inge TH, Garcia V, Daniels S, et al: A multidisciplinary approach to the adolescent bariatric surgical patient. J Pediatr Surg 2004;39:442-447.

38

Body Contouring After Massive Weight Loss

Marie-Claire Buckley, M.D.

With the number of bariatric surgery procedures being performed increasing each year, there has been a tremendous increase in the number of patients undergoing massive weight loss (MWL) who are seeking body-contouring procedures. According to the data of the American Society for Aesthetic Plastic Surgery (ASAPS) from 2004, the number of post-MWL procedures has increased from between 28% and 67% during 2003 and 2004 (Table 38-1).[1] For example, nearly 17,000 abdominoplasties were performed in 1994 compared with more than 34,000 in 1996 and 150,000 in 2003. Although these figures do not distinguish between MWL and cosmetics patients, the increase in numbers correlates with the rise in the number of bariatric procedures performed during that time, and the lower-body lift is directed almost exclusively toward the MWL population.

Plastic surgeons have been involved in removing excess tissue and in body contouring for decades in the cosmetic population, but the MWL patient presents unique challenges that require more than just the simple application of traditional techniques. Because of the distribution and quantity, as well as the quality, of inelastic skin and fat left behind, a straightforward tummy-tuck or liposuction would result in less than ideal body contouring. Although we have much to learn regarding patterns of fat distribution and loss, the development of new techniques to recontour the common areas of redundant ptotic tissue (i.e., the abdomen, thighs, buttocks, chest, arms, and face of the MWL patient) is the newest subspecialty in the field of plastic surgery.

In caring for the MWL patient, the goal of body contouring surgery is to relieve the functional disability associated with excess skin, to help remove the remaining physical stigmata of obesity, and to gain for the patient a healthier body image.

In this chapter, I provide an overview of the physical changes experienced by MWL patients and the current thoughts and practices that are developing to meet the needs of this new and growing population of MWL patients.

▶ HISTORY

The history of body contouring began nearly a century ago, before morbid obesity became an epidemic and before bariatric surgery was developed. As early as 1899, Kelly described the first abdominoplasty in the United States, performing a transverse excision of the pannus at the level of the umbilicus to facilitate a gynecologic procedure. Babcock used a vertical incision in 1916, and Galtier combined the two incisions in a *fleur de lis*-type pattern in 1955. This traditional approach, using direct excision of excess tissue from the anterior abdomen, is referred to as a panniculectomy.[2,3]

Despite the variations in incision placement, a formal anterior panniculectomy does not address the flank and back rolls so common in the MWL patient, and sometimes they become even more prominent. In 1940, Somalo described the concept of an extended panniculectomy, or circumferential torsoplasty, and Gonzalez-Ulloa developed the mid-trunk belt lipectomy in 1960.

A tummy tuck is not the same as a panniculectomy. Modern abdominoplasties differ from traditional anterior panniculectomies in a number of ways. Not only is the excess pannus removed, but also the remaining skin flaps

PROCEDURE	NO. CASES 2003-2004	% INCREASE 2003-2004	% INCREASE 1997-2004
Abdominoplasty	150,987	28	344
Breast lift	98,351	28	395
Upper-arm lift	17,052	61	578
Lower-body lift	15,094	38	610
Thigh lift	13,502	53	366
Buttocks lift	5,960	67	285

Table 38-1 **ASAPS 2004 COSMETIC SURGERY NATIONAL DATA**

ASAPS, American Society for Aesthetic Plastic Surgery. (From www.shaping-futures.com)

are undermined to allow the redraping of the tissues; the abdominal muscular fascia is plicated to tighten and flatten the profile as an "internal corset," and scars are minimized and camouflaged as much as possible in natural creases. Additional liposuction of remaining fat deposits for further thinning or contouring, introduced by Illouz in the 1980s,[2] can also be combined with abdominoplasty or "excisional body contouring."

Prior to the development of bariatric surgery, anterior panniculectomy was the only option for the morbidly obese patient with a symptomatic giant pannus, which carries its own significant risks and complications because of the multiple comorbidities associated with the obesity. As bariatric surgery procedures have become more accessible, more successful, and less risky, we are seeing more MWL patients with a different set of problems.

Despite the availability of the belt lipectomy and the abdominoplasty, many patients were dissatisfied with their appearance. The changes in skin elasticity and underlying connective tissue support did not go back to normal after MWL, leaving redundant ptotic skin involving not only the abdomen but also the buttocks, thighs, chest, arms, and face as well. A study by Young and Freiberg looked at the level of satisfaction in a small number of postbariatric surgery patients following panniculectomy and found them to be unhappy with their body images; they had expected to look better, in addition to obtaining relief from their symptoms.[4]

Perhaps the most significant development in the body contouring approach to the MWL patient is Lockwood's work. He described the anatomy of the superficial fascial system, a fibrous structural meshwork that encases fat beneath the skin, and used it to resuspend, or lift, the ptotic tissues of the thighs, buttocks, and abdomen of the MWL patient. His results were stunning.[5-8] He also proposed a shift in perspective from that of functional reconstruction to that of cosmetic contouring, looking at the body in terms of "aesthetic units" centered around the trunk.[9,10] Lockwood's high lateral tension abdominoplasty and lower-body lift techniques took body contouring for the MWL patient to a new level, treating the abdomen, flanks, back, buttocks, and thighs as an aesthetic whole.[8] His work laid the foundation for the continued evolution of body contouring.

▶ PREOPERATIVE CONSIDERATIONS

Before we look more closely at these new techniques, there are a number of preoperative criteria to consider. Although the MWL patient has worked hard to achieve his or her new weight and improved health, massive weight loss does not automatically make him or her a good candidate for further surgery.

Before considering body contouring surgery, the MWL patient must be committed to maintaining lifestyle changes, must have had bariatric surgery at least 1 year earlier, and must maintain a stable weight for a minimum of 3 to 6 months so as to avoid a false plateau. If there is any desire for or possibility of further significant weight loss, the patient is encouraged to reach that goal before taking the next step. If the patient still falls within the category of obesity, she or he should be reevaluated by the bariatric surgeon for a possible further revision procedure.

In addition to stable weight, medical comorbidities should also be stable or improved. They include any psychological issues, such as depression, personality disorders, or body dysmorphia. As part of the initial workup, a number of experts recommend using the Hopkins Symptom Checklist[11,12] or another standardized questionnaire to determine the patient's suitability as a surgical candidate. It is estimated that 50% of the MWL population suffer from Axis I disorders (depression, anxiety, or both; as compared to 17% in the general population); and that 30% suffer from Axis II disorders (personality disorders). Significant postoperative changes, including changing self-identity, new relationship demands, failure to achieve a normal body, and adjustments of body image, may have to be addressed prior to further surgery. Vineberg stresses the importance of matching patient expectations with potential outcomes and ruling out body dysmorphia.[13] Psychological illness does not preclude surgery, but it is recommended that a mental health provider evaluate the patient's stability and potential for compliance with a very stressful perioperative period and recovery phase.

Whether the new lifestyles of MWL patients include adequate nutrition, regular exercise, and generally healthful habits must be considered. MWL patients are often anemic and may also have other deficiencies requiring dietary supplementation to facilitate healing and postoperative recovery (e.g., Neferex Forte and vitamin K). They should have basic preoperative laboratory assessments, including prealbumin, hemoglobin, iron, calcium, magnesium, and phosphorus. Rubin even suggests preconditioning.[14] Patients who are smokers must quit at least 2 weeks prior to any surgery, if the surgeon agrees to operate at all.

If patients appear to have realistic goals and expectations of what body contouring surgery can achieve, attention then turns to which procedure or technique is most appropriate. This is based on the patients' priorities as well as on physical presentation. In addition to a thorough evaluation of the quantity and quality of skin, subcutaneous tissues, and the underlying musculature of individual areas, one must also consider the overall contour and proportions between regional aesthetic units.

Preoperative questions to be addressed include the following. Does the patient have an android ("apple," or centralized) body habitus or a gynoid ("pear-shaped") distribution of excess fat and skin? Are there adherent areas that result in "tiers," or festoons, of excess skin? Has the patient reached his or her near-ideal body weight, or is the patient still considered overweight or obese? What was the patient's highest body mass index (BMI) and his or her current BMI? What does the skin look like? (Are there gynecologic or open cholecystectomy scars, striae, evidence of sun damage?) What is the degree of ptosis and the degree of elasticity? Does the anterior abdominal pannus wrap around the flanks to the back rolls? Does the upper-arm excess continue onto the chest wall? Is the entire thigh circumference in need of tightening or just the medial aspect? How ptotic are the mons pubis, the breasts, the face, and the neck?

What about the underlying abdominal wall; is there diastasis, attenuation, true herniation? Is there good muscle tone or are the muscles patulous? Is there remaining intraabdominal fat that will determine the abdominal profile after the excess tissues are removed? Is the gluteal region atrophic?

All of these factors can affect the final outcome and must be discussed with the patient to ensure the best possible choice of procedures and techniques. If there is more than one area of concern for the patient, it must be decided whether the patient is a candidate for a combination of procedures or a staged approach.

▶ CONTRAINDICATIONS

Postbariatric body contouring is contraindicated in the following situations: unstable weight; noncompliance with lifestyle changes; unrealistic expectations of postoperative results (contour irregularities, scarring, revisions, possible complications, prolonged recovery, compression garments, and activity restrictions); smoking; malnutrition; unstable comorbidities; and psychological instability.

▶ POSTOPERATIVE CONSIDERATIONS

Because these procedures are essentially elective, it is important to discuss with patients what to expect and what is expected of them after surgery. Some of the operations can be done on an outpatient basis, but the more extensive belt lipectomies and body lifts require hospitalization, sometimes between 2 and 7 days. Immediate postsurgical pain management may include epidural, patient-controlled analgesia, or On-Q pumps, transitioning to oral medications prior to discharge. Most patients will have drains for at least a week and variable prophylactic antibiotic coverage. Binders or compression garments are also dependent on surgeon preference and procedure. The use of external compression has the potential to cause further tissue ischemia in undermined flaps, so some surgeons require patients to limit activity levels and dependent positioning for the first week or two to minimize postoperative edema. Activity levels and return to work can gradually increase over the second to fourth weeks. Throughout the recovery period, it is recommended that patients have adequate support systems.

It is very important to make sure that patients understand the outcomes and results they can expect on the basis of their current BMIs. Aly recommends showing before-and-after pictures of similar patients to provide realistic ideas about appearance. Ideally, bariatric patients should be educated before their bariatric procedures about "what they're going to look like after the weight is gone" so as to prepare them for the need for further surgery.[15]

After the early recovery phase, the healing process continues as scars remodel and settle down and edema resolves. By 3 months, patients can usually get a sense of their results, but final results should not be judged until about 1 year after surgery. It is important that patients know that they will probably experience recurrent skin laxity or rebound, perhaps even further weight loss, and widening scars and that they may indeed need additional revisions.[14]

▶ INFORMED CONSENT

Informed consent should include a description of the procedure, what is involved, any alternatives, and possible risks and complications. Because these procedures are essentially elective, patients must be fully aware of the possible risks and complications involved, particularly if they are undergoing a combination of procedures over a lengthy period under anesthesia. Most surgeons limit themselves to 6 to 8 hours at a time so as to minimize the risks of anesthesia, but there are some who have successfully done single-stage full-body lifts lasting up to 12 hours with no serious complications.[16]

The typical general surgical risks and complications include but are not limited to infection, bleeding, hematoma/seroma, bruising, swelling, pain, allergic reactions, deep venous thrombosis, and pulmonary embolus. Risks more specific to MWL procedures include skin and fat necrosis, including loss of umbilicus or nipples, delayed wound healing, scarring, asymmetries, altered sensation, lymphedema, contour irregularities and distortions, and the need for further revisions.

▶ COMPLICATIONS

Although comorbidities often improve, and complication rates are lower for MWL patients than for morbidly obese patients, there are still problems that can occur, no matter what procedure or perioperative precautions are taken.

Vastine and colleagues found that "obesity at the time of abdominoplasty has a profound influence on the wound complication rate following surgery, regardless of any previous weight reduction surgery." They compared nonobese (within 50 lbs), borderline (50-100 lb >ideal body weight), and obese (>100 lb >ideal body weight) patients undergoing abdominoplasty and noted a 42% overall complication rate. This was divided into major and minor categories, with 13% major and 29% minor complications. When stratified for weight, 80% of the complications occurred in the obese group compared to 33% in the borderline and nonobese groups. The most common complication was seroma formation. It is interesting to note that bariatric surgery itself did not decrease the complication rate if the patients were still considered obese; there was a 55% overall complication rate as opposed to a 33% complication rate in those with no previous bariatric surgery. It is not until patients lose the extra weight that they benefit from lower risks and complications.[17]

Complications are typically divided into early and late stages. Early complications include seroma, hematoma, infection, wound-healing problems, and skin necrosis. Late complications include dog-ears, asymmetries, residual laxity, contour irregularities, and widening or migrating scarring. The early complications are the more common and problematic, whereas the late complications are more of an aesthetic problem. Gmur and colleagues looked at the safety of abdominoplasty combined with other dermolipectomy procedures after MWL and had a total complication rate of 59% and no increased length in hospital stay.[18]

In the literature, early wound-healing complications range between 3% and 35% for abdominoplasties, with or without additional simultaneous procedures. Grazer and Goldwyn reviewed more than 10,000 abdominoplasties and found a 15% complication rate, with a predominance of wound infections and dehiscences.[19] Seromas may occur in up to 40%, despite postoperative drains, requiring repeated aspirations, ultrasound-guided percutaneous drain placement, or doxycycline sclerosis. On rare occasions, patients may need surgical revision of the seroma cavity to remove the lining. Although the literature shows a higher rate of wound infections in obese patients, the rate of postoperative infection in the MWL population is about 10% to 20%.[17] Perioperative prophylactic antibiotics are commonplace, but continued antibiotic coverage for drains is variable.

Postoperative bleeding and hematoma formation can occur in 3% to 10% of patients, possibly due to malabsorptive nutritional deficiencies; they may be prevented by preoperative vitamin K.[20] Although precautions are taken to decrease the incidence of deep vein thrombosis and pulmonary embolus by using sequential compression devices prior to the induction of anesthesia, early ambulation, and postoperative low-molecular-weight heparin therapy, there is still a rate of deep vein thrombosis as high as 10% and a rate of pulmonary embolism of 1%.[21]

The need for postoperative revisions ranges from 5% to 15%, even when multiple procedures are performed. "Additional dermolipectomies did not increase abdominoplasty-related morbidity, but revealed better long-term results."[18] The majority of revisions are small procedures for wound healing or residual deformities. But, as Vastine points out, "Complication rates are not equivalent to surgical failure rates."[17] Despite all of the possible risks and complications, post-MWL body contouring can provide these patients with long-awaited relief from years of physical and psychological suffering. Modolin noted, "Complications were not sufficient to contraindicate the procedures. Patients showed satisfaction with the surgical results: more social and professional integration, behavioral improvement, increment in walking capacity, and better performance in physical exercises, sexual life and recreational activities."[22]

▶ STAGING

A number of studies have already shown that combination surgeries can be performed without undue added risk,[3,7,23] so the decision to separate procedures by stages depends on patient priorities and finances as well as on the nature of the surgeon's practice. As in remodeling a house, if one cannot afford the massive payment or additional mortgage for a total-body "extreme makeover," one may start with the abdomen or the region that is most problematic and go from there, one project or area at a time.[20] Commonly, patients present with symptomatic panni, along with bothersome medial thighs, listing breasts, and arms as secondary concerns; a panniculectomy or perhaps a lower-body lift could be performed first, followed by an upper-body lift or surgery on individual areas. Rhomberg noted that patients undergoing single-stage operations had higher postoperative self-assessment scores, showing greater satisfaction than those undergoing multistage procedures.

They also had strong improvements in psyche, appearance, self-confidence, and vitality after surgery. By combining procedures, there were cost savings resulting from decreased lengths of hospital stay and periods of time off work.[24]

If the patient still has some residual regional fat deposits, it may be necessary to perform preliminary liposuction for debulking 6 months prior to thigh or arm plasty to achieve the best possible results.

It is a given that there will probably be future revisions, even after combined procedures, but these are usually minor alterations or touch-ups.

▶ SURGICAL OPTIONS

Massive weight loss can affect all areas of the body. Although we do not fully understand the physiologic or metabolic processes involved in the patterns of fat deposition and loss, which vary among people and even within the same person, there are certain areas that are commonly affected in MWL patients, including the abdomen, mons pubis, buttocks, thighs, chest/breast, arms, face, and neck. Each of these areas is addressed individually, looking at the residual deformities after MWL and the various surgical options available.

Abdomen

The most common request for post-MWL body contouring is the abdomen, where a majority of patients carry their excess weight. Even women with more gynoid distributions of fat seem to lose fat more easily from the central depots of the abdomen. Lockwood observed that the relaxation of abdominal tissues is closely associated with the general descent of the surrounding waist, groin, pubis, and upper thighs and should be considered the cornerstone for restoration of the truncal region.[9]

Following MWL, patients are commonly left with a symptomatic pannus, or apron of skin and fat, hanging from the lower abdomen. Because of the overlapping skin, patients often experience increased sweating with malodorous maceration, rashes, and skin breakdown in the intertriginous folds and umbilicus that usually persist despite conservative treatments. Maintaining personal hygiene and skin integrity can be a daily struggle, requiring frequent cleansing and application of creams and powders to prevent further breakdown. In some cases, the pannus is so excessive that it interferes with toileting. Even a moderately sized pannus can exacerbate lower back pain due to the translation of the forward pull and can interfere with daily activities and exercise. Uneven distribution of extra skin may make it difficult to find clothing that fits.

These patients have often accomplished considerable weight loss and improvement in overall health, but the loose skin is a physical reminder of their former selves that prevents them from developing new mental images of themselves, even in those patients reaching near ideal body weight. The appearance of their new bodies is almost more psychologically painful than it was when they were obese.

The redundant, inelastic, ptotic pannus rarely improves with exercise alone and ultimately requires excision.

The simplest method of removal of excess abdominal skin is the panniculectomy. This traditional approach to the anterior abdominal pannus was used in the past for morbidly obese patients, as well as to facilitate other general surgical procedures. It involves undermining only the extra tissue to be directly excised. This limited undermining decreases the risk for tissue necrosis of the skin flaps. Any protuberant abdominal profile, from either persistent intraabdominal fat or attenuated patulous abdominal muscles, remains unaddressed unless there is also a concomitant hernia that needs repair.

A transverse inguinal-crease incision is used for excess tissue along the horizontal plane, particularly if the patient is still considered obese. The incision usually stops around the flanks and leaves large dog-ear deformities. For the patient who has reached near ideal body weight, a vertical incision can be added to remove any additional excess tissue along the midline. This may result in an epigastric dog-ear deformity.[20,25]

This anterior "anchor" or "inverted-T" incision is considered old-fashioned by many of today's experts, and it may even accentuate the remaining flank and back rolls, but it is a useful and effective method for the removal of an often problematic pannus. An anterior panniculectomy does not preclude a completion circumferential abdominoplasty in the future,[20] and staging procedures allow the functional problems to be addressed early.

A formal abdominoplasty involves undermining the entire anterior skin flap up to the costal margins to allow redraping and removal of the excess skin along the horizontal plane, umbilicoplasty, and vertical plication of the anterior rectus sheath to tighten the "internal corset" and improve the abdominal profile. Variations, including external oblique fascial plication or combined vertical and horizontal plication, are possible but not common.[26,27] In the MWL patient, even tightening the anterior skin flap may still leave excess tissue behind. For this reason, the circumferential, or "belt," lipectomy, as developed by Somalo and Gonzalez-Ulloa, is now the favored approach to abdominal contouring.[26]

Aly's experience with the belt lipectomy elegantly demonstrates the distortions left by the traditional anterior panniculectomy, but he is careful to point out that even a belt lipectomy cannot correct for residual obesity after weight loss. He notes that it is not so much the total amount of weight lost, but rather the current BMI that dictates the final results.[28] This is illustrated by two nesting "balloons," representing the internal or intraabdominal fat and muscle envelope, and the external or skin envelope. Tightening the external skin envelope does not guarantee changing the profile of the internal abdominal balloon unless it can be tightened as well.[15] The goals of the belt lipectomy are to tighten the anterior abdomen and define the waist, but we must take into account the quality of the skin-fat envelope—its thickness, pliability, translation of pull and, ultimately, the underlying BMI. A superb series of photographs shows the possible results with belt lipectomy relative to remaining weight in individuals who are obese, 30 to 50 lb overweight, or near ideal body weight.[29,30]

Individual differences exist among surgeons with regard to preoperative markings, intraoperative positioning, and postoperative management, but most circumferential lipectomies or torsoplasties result in significant improvement in anterior abdomen, flank, and back rolls, as well as upper buttocks. The belt lipectomy has become the gold standard for optimal reconstructive outcomes.

As with most abdominoplasties, in an effort to remove and tighten skin as much as possible, the patient may be required to walk bent forward for a week or so and to avoid any excessive tension on the anterior closure that might result in dehiscence. Because of the undermining of the skin flaps, some surgeons prefer to forgo the use of compression garments or binders so as to avoid any risk for tissue ischemia. Drains are usually used for at least the first 2 weeks. The scars and redraped tissues may take up to a year to fully remodel and to relax.

Mons Pubis

The mons pubis is not usually an area of concern for most cosmetic patients, but in the MWL population, both female and male, there is often residual fat and redundant, ptotic skin that can interfere with personal hygiene and the aesthetically balanced appearance of the anterior abdomen.

The ptotic tissues can be lifted and reduced with the anterior abdominal excess, but the mons can appear distorted in the transverse dimension.[31,32] Several different techniques have been proposed to avoid this deformity, including wedge excisions in the inguinal creases or a vertical midline excision. Liposuction can also be used if there is considerable fatty tissue.

If direct excision is used, care must be taken to avoid disrupting the deeper lymphatics or overresection. Lymphedema of the mons can be extremely uncomfortable and distressing to the patient. Overzealous resection and lifting can also result in distortion of the labia and abnormal redirection of the external urethral opening. Procedures on the medial thighs may also affect the mons tissues and may require further revisions.

Buttocks

The buttocks in MWL patients often appear flat, having lost both fat and muscle mass as well as anatomic landmarks and natural folds. Pitanguy's[33] early attempts to camouflage incisions within the gluteal crease at the time of direct excision resulted in a distorted transition between gluteal mound and upper posterior thigh.[34-37] Other procedures (e.g., Ersek) have attempted to hide incisions in the medial gluteal crease.[38]

Although gluteal lift as part of the circumferential lipectomy or lower-body lift removes the redundant ptotic skin without violating the natural creases and redrapes the skin, there remains a lack of volume of the gluteal mounds. This lack of fullness or projection can be overcome by either synthetic or autologous means. Buried dermal flaps, as described by Isaacs,[37] give some fullness to the upper buttocks. Subgluteal solid silicone implants have been used to improve the contour of the buttocks, but they are subject to complications resulting from implant exposure, infection, and shifting implants.

Centeno[19] is developing a technique for autoaugmentation of the gluteal region that increases mass and projection without implants. Essentially, they preserve some of the tissue that would otherwise be removed during dermolipectomy as a deepithelialized tissue mound that adds volume under the redraped skin. They have found that the most aesthetically pleasing buttocks have the most projection at the level of the mons as seen from the side (lateral view).[40]

Thighs

In patients whose pattern of fat distribution is gynoid, MWL in the thighs and legs can leave a significant amount of redundant ptotic skin, particularly in the upper medial thighs. This often causes problems similar to those caused by the abdominal pannus, including excessive sweating, chafing, and skin irritation and breakdown that are very difficult to prevent. Excess tissue in the medial thigh region is also a problem during ambulatory activities and exercise and may limit the type of clothing patients can comfortably wear.

The traditional approach to post-MWL thigh deformities has been direct excision, pulling the excess skin medially and leaving a long scar along the inseam. This does not address any remaining fatty deformities in the lateral thigh and trochanteric region, nor does it consider the skin along the oblique inguinal-labial crease. In an effort to deal with the upper medial thigh skin, the medial thigh lift, with a transverse excision along the groin crease, has been tried,[41-43] but it is often plagued by migration of the scars and distortion of the labia due to the downward pull on the fascial suspension anchoring sutures. These deformities are even more difficult and unacceptable than the original problem, and for these reasons such an excision is not widely performed. The presence of varicosities can add to the risk of bleeding and hematoma formation. Dissection in the deeper planes can result in prolonged problems with lymphedema, adding to the risks for infection and poor wound healing. Postoperative compression is difficult because of the conical shape of the legs and should be done carefully to avoid ischemic injury to the skin.

If direct excision is attempted, great care should be taken to dissect in the superficial plane and minimize the undermining of the skin flaps. The surgeon should also be careful to avoid overresection, taking into account the thickness of the subcutaneous fat during closure. Some surgeons recommend the use of steroids to help minimize early edema and tension on the closure.

In looking at other areas of the thigh, Lockwood noted that many patients were left with abnormal circumferential fat deposits unresponsive to weight loss. He referred to this as "genetic fat" and felt that it was deep to the suspension tissues, preventing their mobilization and redraping. He proposed circumferential liposuction of the thigh to recontour the fatty deposits, as well as facilitate the lifting of the redundant ptotic thigh skin and the release of "zones of adherence."[5-7] Lockwood achieved remarkable improvement in the appearance of the thighs, allowing the underlying musculature to show as never before. Even with this circumferential treatment, an additional medial thigh excision may be necessary.

Lower-Body Lift

Lockwood is credited with the concept of the lower-body lift, combining the circumferential high lateral tension abdominoplasty with the transverse flank/thigh/buttock lift (including circumferential liposuction of thighs to the knees). His aesthetic approach to anatomic body "units" and the use of the superficial fascial system to support and maintain the lift resulted in the removal of excess tissue, rejuvenation and repositioning of the skin, and restoration of a more normal youthful contour.[6,7,9,10,34]

Considered to be the gold-standard procedure for lower-contouring in the MWL patient, the lower-body lift typically involves two surgeons and a trained team of assistants to help with intraoperative patient positioning. The procedure may last 6 to 8 hours and requires up to 1 week in hospital postoperatively.

In order to prevent the real possibility of posterior or anterior suture-line dehiscence, Aly does not allow patients to be repositioned postoperatively unless they are fully awake so it is possible to judge whether there is too much tension on the closure.[28] It is not surprising that in the lower-body lift, there are still more problems with wound healing and seroma formation than in some of the lesser procedures, despite careful planning and execution, advanced training, and experience in performing these surgeries.

Reverse Abdominoplasty

The upper-body areas are subject to the same forces of gravity and effects of morbid obesity on skin quality as is the lower body. An area of transition between the upper and lower trunk is just below the breasts, at the level of the lower thoracic cage. This is distinct from the lower abdomen and in some MWL patients this additional tier or roll of skin and fat can extend posteriorly to the spine, even interfering with respiratory efforts. Because the circumferential abdominoplasty does not extend this far superiorly, Grazer proposed a reverse abdominoplasty in which this lower costal roll could be undermined from above and removed along the inframammary crease, with an extension around to the back.[16] This operation was first described by Rebello in 1972, and Baroudi combined reverse abdominoplasty with breast reduction via a common incision (1979).[16] This procedure is distinct from the more oblique excision of lateral thoracic rolls that may be combined with the upper arms or upper-body lift, where it is more difficult to camouflage incisions.

Breast

Both male and female MWL patients experience changes in breast volume and shape. Women often have loss of volume due to glandular involution, with significant ptosis resulting from prolonged skin tension that leaves them with flat, elongated skin envelopes and displaced nipples. Men tend to have ptosis with varying degrees of excess fat or gynecomastia. In both cases, a breast lift is required to tighten the stretched skin envelope and to add volume to the female breast mound and reduce the male breast mound.

Traditionally, the ptotic female breast has been treated by mastopexy augmented by implants if more volume is needed. Rubin has developed an ingenious technique using excess lateral thoracic tissue to help autoaugment the breast mound at the time of mastopexy, with beautiful results. Essentially, he fashions a random flap of lateral wall skin to help reshape the parenchyma with dermal suspension suturing. Alloderm and synthetic mesh have been used to help resuspend the ptotic breast tissue, but autoaugmentation seems to be most practical, with additional improvement of the lateral chest wall contour where extra rolls of tissue are a problem, even in the non-MWL population. This maneuver also negates the need for staged implant augmentation and mastopexy; however, about 20% of patients will need implants because of insufficient tissue.[44]

Capella has analyzed the male breast deformity in MWL patients and developed a classification system of the nipple-areolar complex based on degree of ptosis and excess fat. The treatment of male gynecomastia involves removal of extra fatty tissue, either by liposuction or direct excision of more fibrous tissue in mild to moderate ptosis. For male breasts that are too ptotic, have a "lateral slide," or have skin quality that will not retract after reduction, formal mobilization of the upper skin flap and excision of excess skin is necessary, sometimes with replacement of the NAC as a free graft. As with females, the excision of extra breast skin can be extended laterally to include thoracic skin folds.[45] Rubin sometimes uses the inframammary fold to raise and suspend the abdominal tissues from the rib periosteum.[44]

Arms

The excess skin of the upper inner arms may vary among MWL patients. Although some toning can be done for the underlying musculature, there is usually the need for direct excision. To date, there are no arm lifts analogous to the thigh lifts that allow for avoidance of a long scar. Lockwood describes the stretching of anchoring septae, with the loosening of the interconnection between superficial fascial system of the arm and the axillary fascia.[6] Strauch describes "zones of treatment," including the forearm as well as the axilla.[46] Brachioplasty involves removal of excess skin and fat between the axilla and the elbow. If the skin is still too fat, preliminary liposuction can be done 6 months earlier. In patients whose deformities do not end at the axilla or elbow, a number of variations have been developed that extend beyond these areas, all of them avoiding straight-line incisions, which are prone to scar contracture. DiFrancesco presents an excellent review of the historical approaches to brachioplasty.[47] The two most favored incisions are linear and sinusoidal, placed in the bicipital groove or along the posterior axillary fold line so as to minimize scar visibility. Aly uses a close-as-you-go technique to avoid overresection and inability to close due to rapid onset of edema. Others undermine and advance the extra tissue to be excised, taking into account the thickness of the skin flaps. Axillary contractures are avoided with Z-plasty and T-incisions. Whichever technique is used, great care must be taken to avoid injury to the deeper neurovascular structures of the upper arm and axilla.

Like the thighs, the upper arms are also prone to difficulties with lymphedema and wound healing. Aly instructs his patients to keep their arms elevated as much as possible for at least 2 weeks.[48] Other surgeons use compression garments to try to prevent excessive edema, but they can run into problems with uneven or constricting pressure that result in ischemic skin or even nerve injury. Axillary contractures can occur if straight-line incisions cross the axillary crease. If the dissection plane is too deep, there is risk for cutaneous sensory nerve injury.

Upper-Body Lift

The upper-body lift "removes epigastric and midback rolls of skin, adjusts the inframammary fold, and reshapes the breast or corrects gynecomastia, leaving behind a near circumferential transverse scar partially hidden by the breasts."[16,23] Hurwitz is one of the few surgeons to include the upper arms, chest, and breast in one stage.[49,50] Vogt has also presented a combined approach to the arms, chest, and breast involving multiple areas of ellipse excisions and Z-plasty.[51,52] A flankoplasty, or "batwing" torsoplasty, is described by Freeman; it includes lateral truncal excision as well as excision in the axillae and upper arms.[26] Rubin estimates that 25% to 30% of female MWL patients will require an upper-body lift in addition to a breast lift to correct rolls on the lateral and posterior chest wall.[44]

Total-Body Lift

Many surgeons are performing separate lower- and upper-body lifts, but few have attempted them together in a total-body lift. With a specialized surgical team, Hurwitz and colleagues performed this complete torso correction (which requires 7 to 12 hours in the operating room, 0 to 4 transfusion units, and a 3- to 4-day hospital stay) in a small and select group of patients (n = 8). It is surprising to note that the only complications included three seromas, two wound infections resulting from fat and skin necrosis, and one small skin dehiscence. Overall, the results were impressive; seven of eight patients were satisfied, and only two revisions were planned.[16]

Face and Neck

When considering the distribution of excess skin in the MWL patient, we usually think of the abdomen, breast, thighs, and arms. For a fair number of patients, there is also significant weight loss from the face and neck area, leaving them with a noticeable wattle of excess skin on the anterior neck (the "turkey-gobbler deformity") and jowling. Traditional face and neck lift procedures can be applied with variations, and the results are good in most cases. Rarely, if there is an extreme amount of skin, direct excision by means of an anterior neck incision is considered. Only a small amount of published literature addresses facial rejuvenation specifically in the MWL population other than the modified application of traditional facelift techniques by Sclafani.[53]

▶ INSURANCE

Many MWL patients have the unfortunate expectation that insurance will cover their post-weight-loss surgeries because the initial bypass was covered. At present, insurance coverage for postbariatric body contouring has been limited to areas that result in functional problems. These include an abdominal pannus that causes intertriginous dermatitis, physical hindrance to personal hygiene, interference with activities of daily living, exacerbation of lower back pain, or the presence of an incisional hernia. Some insurance companies are now requiring up to 6 months of documentation of skin problems that persist despite conservative therapy, and they demand evidence of chiropractic or physical therapy treatment for lower back pain before they consider surgery "medically necessary." Some companies may even require that the pannus extend below the pubis to a certain distance. Coverage for surgery in areas other than the anterior abdomen, such as the upper arms, medial thighs, or breasts is even less likely because surgery in these areas is thought of as being purely cosmetic, despite the psychosocial impact on the patient. Presutti[54] recommends that we approach these surgeries as being "reconstructive," attempts to restore to normal that which has been rendered abnormal as the result of a disease process such as morbid obesity, rather than as being improvements on normal appearances through cosmetic procedures.[54] Even with a concomitant hernia repair, which is clearly reconstructive, the panniculectomy portion of the procedure must get prior authorization and can no longer be assumed to be covered.

"MWL achieved by bariatric surgery, while improving health... leaves a patient incompletely treated, analogous to a woman treated for breast cancer and left with an unreconstructed mastectomy defect."[55] Some centers offer "package deals" or combined insurance-self-pay "bargain packages" to lessen the financial burden on the MWL patient, but any efforts to challenge the insurance industry to change their policies will have to come from the bariatric community because support is unlikely to come from the plastic surgery establishment.

▶ CONCLUSION

In summary, body contouring procedures for the MWL patient have come a long way, from the traditional reconstructive approach of direct excision for localized functional problems to the recent cosmetic approach to entire anatomic regions through lifting and contouring. As more surgeons turn their efforts to serving this growing population of patients, new and improved techniques will continue to develop. It is to be hoped that efforts to make these procedures more readily available and more easily affordable by the majority of MWL patients will also progress.

▶ REFERENCES

1. American Society for Aesthetic Plastic Surgery (ASAPS): 2004 Cosmetic Surgery National Data Bank Statistics. www.shaping-futures.com. Accessed, 2004.
2. Shons AR: Plastic reconstruction after bypass surgery and massive weight loss. Surg Clin North Am 1979;59:1139-1152.
3. Fuente del Campo A, Rojas Allegretti E, Fernandez Filho JA, et al: Regional dermolipectomy as treatment for sequelae of massive weight loss. World J Surg 1998;22:974-980.
4. Young SC, Freiberg A: A critical look at abdominal lipectomy following morbid obesity surgery. Aesthetic Plast Surg 1991;15:81-84.
5. Lockwood TE: Fascial anchoring technique in medial thigh lifts. Plast Reconstr Surg 1988;82:299-304.
6. Lockwood TE: Superficial fascial system (SFS) of the trunk and extremities: a new Concept. Plast Reconstr Surg 1991;87:1009-1027.
7. Lockwood TE: Lower body lift with superficial fascial system suspension. Plast Reconstr Surg 1993;92:1112-1125.
8. Lockwood TE: High-lateral-tension abdominoplasty with superficial fascial system suspension. Plast Reconstr Surg 1995;96:603-615.
9. Lockwood TE: The role of excisional lifting in body contour surgery. Clin Plast Surg 1996;23:695-712.
10. Lockwood TE: Maximizing aesthetics in lateral-tension abdominoplasty and body lifts. Clin Plast Surg 2004;31:523-537.
11. Rubin JP: Body contouring after massive weight loss. American Society of Plastic Surgeons Symposia Series, panel discussion; April 2005:Dallas.
12. Rubin JP, Nguyen V, Schwentker A, et al: Perioperative management of the post-gastric-bypass patient presenting for body contouring surgery. Clin Plast Surg 2004;31:601-610.
13. Vineberg D: Mind and body: perspectives on the psychological presentation of massive weight loss patients. www.shaping-futures.com. Accessed, 2006.
14. Kenkel JM: Body contouring after massive weight loss: establishing realistic expectations....things to consider. American Society of Plastic Surgeons Symposia Series; April 2005:Dallas.
15. Aly AS: Body contouring after massive weight loss. American Society of Plastic Surgeons Symposia Series, panel discussion; April 2005: Dallas.
16. Hurwitz DJ: Single-staged total body lift after massive weight loss. Ann Plast Surg 2004;52:435-441.
17. Vastine VL, Morgan RF, Williams GS, et al: Wound complications of abdominoplasty in obese patients. Ann Plast Surg 1999;42:34-39.
18. Gmur RU, Banic A, Erni D, et al: Is it safe to combine abdominoplasty with other dermolipectomy procedures to correct skin excess after weight loss? Ann Plast Surg 2003;51:353-357.
19. Grazer FM, Goldwyn RM: Abdominoplasty assessed by survey with emphasis on complications. Plast Reconstr Surg 1977;59:513-517.
20. Downey S: A meter-long incision: special consideration for MWL patients and body contouring. www.shaping-futures.com. Accessed, 2006.
21. Fotopoulos L, Kehagias I, Kalfarentzos F, et al: Dermolipectomies following weight loss after surgery for morbid obesity. Obes Surg 2000;10:451-459.
22. Modolin M, Cintra W Jr, Gobbi CI, et al: Circumferential abdominoplasty for sequential treatment after morbid obesity. Obes Surg 2003;13:95-100.
23. Hurwitz JD, Zewert TE: Body contouring after bariatric surgery. Oper Tech Plast Reconstr Surg 2002;8:87-95.
24. Rhomberg M, Pulzl P, Piza-Katzer H, et al: Single-stage abdominoplasty and mastopexy after weight loss following gastric banding. Obes Surg 2003;3:418-423.
25. da Costa LF, Landecker A, Manta AM, et al: Optimizing body contour in massive weight loss patients: the modified vertical abdominoplasty. Plast Reconstr Surg 2004;114:1917-1923.
26. Freeman BG: Body contouring, flankoplasty and thigh lift. www.eMedicine.com/plastic. Accessed, 2005.
27. Carwell GR, Horton CE: Circumferential torsoplasty. Ann Plast Surg 1997;38:213-216.
28. Aly AS, Cram AE, Chao, M, et al: Belt lipectomy for circumferential truncal excess: the University of Iowa experience. Plast Reconstr Surg 2003;111:398-413.
29. Aly AS, Cram AE, Heddens C, et al: Truncal body contouring surgery in the massive weight loss patient. Clin Plast Surg 2004;31:611-624.
30. Aly AS: Balanced in the middle: truncal body contouring in massive weight loss patients. www.shaping-futures.com. Accessed, 2006.
31. Hurwitz DJ, Rubin PJ, Risin M, et al: Correcting the saddlebag deformity in the massive weight loss patient. Plast Reconstr Surg 2004;114:1313-1325.
32. Young L: Wrap your head around the body's circumference: innovative techniques in circumferential body lift and post-massive weight loss body contouring. www.shaping-futures.com. Accessed, 2006.
33. Pitanguy I: Trochanteric lipodystrophy. Plast Reconstr Surg 1964;34:280-286.
34. Lockwood TE: Body contouring after massive weight loss. Breast and Body Contouring Symposium, video #0246. Plastic Surgery

Educational Foundation/American Society of Aesthetic Plastic Surgery;2002.

35. Regnault P, Daniel R: Secondary thigh-buttock deformities after classical techniques: prevention and treatment. Clin Plast Surg 1984;11:505-516.
36. Guerrerosantos J: Secondary hip-buttock-thigh plasty. Clin Plast Surg 1984;11:491-503.
37. Isaacs G: Breast shaping procedures, abdominoplasty, and thigh-plasty in Australia. Clin Plast Surg 1984;11:525-548.
38. Ersek RA: The saddle lift for tight thighs. Aesthetic Plast Surg 1995;19:341-343.
39. Centeno R: Gluteal augmentation: an important component of lower body contouring in massive weight loss (MWL) patients. www.shaping-futures.com. Accessed, 2006.
40. Sozer SO, Agullo FJ, Wolf C, et al: Autoprosthesis buttock augmentation during lower body lift. Aesthetic Plast Surg 2005;29:133-137.
41. Capella FJ: Correcting the medial thighs: a whole-body approach to the medial thigh lift in massive weight loss patients. www.shaping-futures.com. Accessed, 2006.
42. Candiani P, Campiglio GL, Signorini M, et al: Fascio-fascial suspension technique in medial thigh lifts. Aesthetic Plast Surg 1995;19:137-140.
43. Le Louarn C, Pascal JF: The concentric medial thigh lift. Aesthetic Plast Surg 2004;28:20-23.
44. Rubin JP: Things are looking up: improving the results of mastopexy and upper-body lift in massive weight loss patients. www.shaping-futures.com. Accessed, 2006.
45. Capella FJ: Body contouring after massive weight loss. American Society of Plastic Surgeons Symposia Series; April 2005:Dallas.
46. Strauch B, Greenspun D, Levine J, et al: A technique of brachioplasty. Plast Reconstr Surg 2004;113:1044-1048.
47. diFrancesco L, Bruggeman B, Kennedy D, et al: Brachioplasty. Operative techniques in plastic and reconstructive surgery 2002;8:116-127.
48. Aly AS: Our traditional approach to arms doesn't fit everyone to a T: a new take on brachioplasty in massive weight loss patients. www.shaping-futures.com. Accessed, 2006.
49. Aly AS: One up: the unit principle applied to the upper body lift in massive weight loss patients. www.shaping-futures.com. Accessed, 2006.
50. Capella FJ: The sum is greater than the parts: upper body contouring in massive weight loss patients. www.shaping-futures.com. Accessed, 2006.
51. Vogt PA: A proposed algorithm for upper arms, back and chest laxity: body contouring after MWL. American Society of Plastic Surgeons Symposia Series; April 2005:Dallas.
52. Vogt PA: Body contouring: upper extremity. In Mathes SJ, Hentz V: Plastic Surgery, 2nd ed. Philadelphia, Saunders Elsevier, Vol. 6, 2006.
53. Sclafani AP: Restoration of the jawline and the neck after bariatric surgery. Facial Plast Surg 2005;21:28-32.
54. Presutti RJ, Gorman KS, Swain JM: Primary care perspective on bariatric surgery. Mayo Clin Proc 2004;79:1158-1166.
55. Taylor J, Shermak M: Body contouring following massive weight loss. Obes Surg 2004;14:1080-1085.

39

Ancillary Procedures in Bariatric Surgery

Thomas A. Stellato, M.D., M.B.A.

Although ancillary procedures are sporadically performed in conjunction with bariatric operations, the focus of the bariatric team and patient is on the weight-reduction effort.[1] Nonetheless, ancillary procedures are, and commonly should be, coordinated with the bariatric procedure. Any ancillary procedure has the potential to have a serious impact on patient outcome. It may increase or decrease the safety of the primary operation, treat an associated disease process, prolong the procedure, either increase or decrease the postoperative length of stay, and influence the liability associated with the bariatric operation. Consequently, the decision to supplement the primary indication for surgery (i.e., the correction of morbid obesity and its consequences) with any additional procedure must be made only after careful consideration by the surgeon and thorough discussion with the patient.[2]

This chapter critiques the numerous associated operations that have been performed in conjunction with the bariatric procedure. For convenience, these ancillary procedures have been grouped into the following four categories:

1. Procedures to make the bariatric operation safer
2. Procedures to treat other diseases
3. Procedures to prevent other diseases
4. Miscellaneous procedures.

These categories represent the overwhelming majority of indications for performing an ancillary procedure; the operations discussed in each category denote the more common procedures one might consider when executing a bariatric operation. The examples are, however, incomplete. No attempt has been made to be encyclopedic; the list of anecdotal individual ancillary procedures is endless.

▶ PROCEDURES TO MAKE THE BARIATRIC OPERATION SAFER

The morbidly obese patient presents with a variety of comorbid conditions that not only threaten the health and longevity of the patient, but also increase his or her risk when undergoing general anesthesia and a major operative procedure. Three procedures—tracheostomy, vena cava filters, and gastrostomy—have the potential to lower the risks involved in anesthesia and surgery. With the exception of gastrostomies, these procedures are utilized quite selectively; all three also have the potential to introduce additional complications.

Tracheostomy

Pulmonary decompensation represents one of the most common reasons for postoperative morbidity after major bariatric procedures. The spectrum of pulmonary compromise ranges from relatively innocuous atelectasis to life-threatening pulmonary embolization. Obesity as a disease can directly compromise hemodynamic and respiratory function; the obese patient is likely to have abnormal functional residual capacity and expiratory reserve volume with resultant depressed PaO_2,[3,4] as well as the associated problem of obstructive sleep apnea (OSA).[5] Tracheostomy was the first successful treatment for OSA[6] and represents the gold standard for OSA because it is successful essentially 100% of the time.[7]

Despite tracheostomy's eradication of sleep apnea, its application in the morbidly obese patient who is a candidate for bariatric surgery is quite limited. The dramatic improvement in OSA with successful weight reduction greatly limits the need for tracheostomy. Figure 39-1 illustrates the typical improvement in OSA in a patient whose body mass index (BMI) decreased from 44.6 kg per m^2 to 32.8 kg per m^2 6 months after Roux-en-Y gastric bypass.

Although the overwhelming majority of morbidly obese patients avoid preoperative tracheostomy, criteria do exist for those select few in whom this procedure may limit the operative risk of the bariatric surgery. Mickelson has suggested that tracheostomy is most commonly recommended in patients with severe oxygen desaturation or cardiac arrhythmias associated with severe sleep apnea when continuous positive airway pressure (CPAP) is refused, unsuccessful, or poorly tolerated.[7] Sugerman and colleagues concur with this recommendation and note that in their

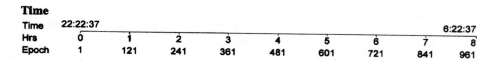

Time

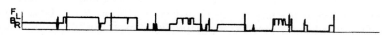

Body Position-Pre Operative

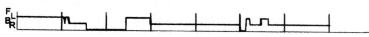

Body Position-Post Operative

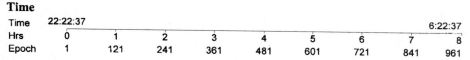

A

Figure 39-1. Polysomnography report (sleep study) of a morbidly obese patient comparing preoperative and postoperative results. The study is performed in a darkened room, with the patient sleeping in a comfortable bed. These charts are a portion of the entire study. **A.** Comparison of body position preoperatively and 6 months postoperatively. The body is significantly more still in the postoperative study. F, prone or front; L, left lateral decubitus; B, supine or back; R, right lateral decubitus. **B.** Respiratory events. The preoperative tracing demonstrates that the apneas that occur are obstructive in nature, not central. After weight loss, no obstructive apnea is seen, and only very rare hypopneas. Cn.A, central apnea; Ob.A, obstructive apnea; Mx.A, mixed central and obstructive apneas; Hyp, hypopnea; Uns, unscored. **C.** Hyponogram. MOV AWK, movement awake (basically, the patient is awake and moving for more than 30 seconds). This movement is shown in the bottom tracing to have been nearly eliminated.

Respiratory Events-Pre Operative

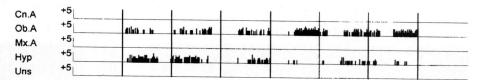

Respiratory Events-Post Operative

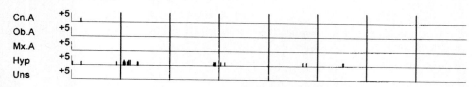

B

Time

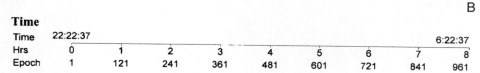

Hypnogram-Pre Operative

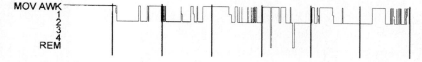

Hypnogram-Post Operative

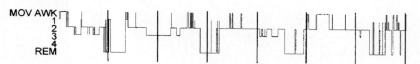

C

large series of bariatric patients, tracheostomy was performed only if the patient could not tolerate nasal CPAP.[4]

Mickelson further defines his recommendation as follows: "Sleep apnea is considered severe enough to consider tracheostomy if the respiratory disturbance index is above 50, the lowest oxygen saturation is below 60%, or there are significant cardiac arrhythmias (severe bradycardia, asystoles, frequent premature ventricular contractions, or runs of ventricular tachycardia) associated with respiratory events. Tracheostomy also should be considered when cardiac, pulmonary, or neurologic diseases are exacerbated or affected by the severity of the apnea (for example; a patient with coronary artery disease develops nocturnal angina, a patient with seizure disorder develops nocturnal seizures, a patient with emphysema develops worsening hypoxemia)."

It may seem that these examples describe patients who would be questionable candidates for a major bariatric procedure. That is exactly the situation when a tracheostomy is appropriate. If dramatic improvement in the OSA and its consequences occurs, the tracheostomy may improve the likelihood of tolerating the bariatric procedure. Figure 39-2 represents my personal experience with

a similar situation. This patient presented with severe morbid obesity with a BMI of 51.9 kg per m². His comorbid conditions included atrial fibrillation and left atrial thrombus with anticoagulation requirement, patent foramen ovale, type II diabetes, hypertension and severe, long-standing OSA. He described increasing exertional and resting dyspnea. The patient was unable to tolerate CPAP. It was felt that his OSA compounded his hypertension and contributed to his atrial arrhythmia. Because the use of CPAP was not a viable option, the patient underwent tracheostomy, and approximately 4 months later, an open Roux-en-Y gastric bypass. After 6 months, his weight had decreased by 102 lb (Fig. 39-3), and his BMI had improved from nearly 52 kg per m² preoperatively to 36.8 kg per m². His OSA had resolved, so the tracheostomy was removed. The patient's weight loss continued over the next 6 months.

Although tracheostomy can dramatically improve the health and the surgical and anesthesia risks for morbidly obese patients with severe OSA, it also imposes new risks, as does any ancillary procedure. Attention to the usual postoperative problems, such as infection and bleeding, are even more critical in the bariatric patient. Death attributed to

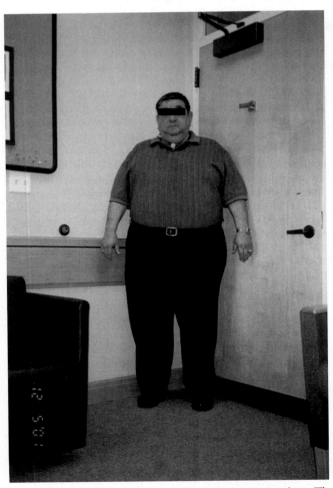

Figure 39-2. Preoperative patient with tracheostomy in place. The patient had a BMI of nearly 52 kg per m² and numerous comorbid problems, including severe obstructive sleep apnea. The patient was unable to tolerate continuous positive airway pressure.

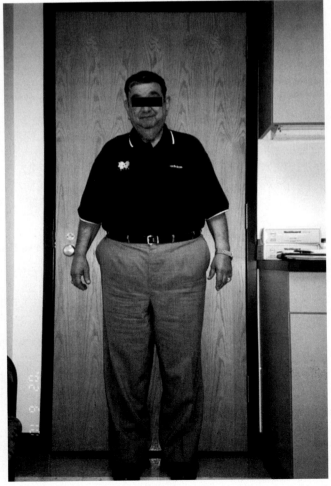

Figure 39-3. After successful open Roux-en-Y gastric bypass resulting in the loss of more than 100 lb, the patient's obstructive sleep apnea resolved and the tracheostomy was removed.

tracheostomy has been seen as the result of a mucous plug causing lethal respiratory obstruction.[4]

For patients who can tolerate CPAP and demonstrate improvement in OSA, CPAP is the treatment of choice, but it should be initiated prior to surgery. CPAP titration will be difficult or impossible in the early postoperative period. Concern about the use of CPAP in the immediate postoperative period is unwarranted; it has been shown to be safe and efficacious during this time without increasing the risk of anastomotic leak.[8]

Vena Cava Filters

Despite the recognition that pulmonary embolization is one of the most common causes of serious morbidity and mortality following bariatric surgery, a survey of the members of the American Society for Bariatric Surgery found little consensus regarding the method of prophylaxis of venous thromboembolism.[9] Although a large majority of surgeons (86%) acknowledge that bariatric patients are at high risk for developing venous thrombosis and pulmonary embolism (Fig. 39-4), and an even greater majority (95%) use routine prophylaxis in this high-risk population, only 50% of those who responded to the survey use low-dose heparin as their first choice for thromboembolism prophylaxis. Nearly half of the surgeons (48%)

responding to the survey had experienced at least one patient death due to a pulmonary embolism.

In addition to low-dose heparin, a number of other modalities have been utilized, singly or in combination, for venous thromboembolism prophylaxis. They include:

- Intermittent pneumatic compression stockings
- Low-molecular-weight heparin
- Antiplatelet agents
- Dextran
- Early ambulation
- Elastic stockings
- Leg elevation
- Inferior vena cava filter
- Oral anticoagulants

Of all these methods of prophylaxis, only inferior vena cava filters primarily address pulmonary emboli. Vena cava filters are ineffective in preventing or limiting thrombus generation; they work by interrupting the path of an established thrombus as it travels from the lower extremities or pelvis to the lungs.

Because of their inability to affect the production of thrombi, as well as their invasiveness and cost, vena cava filters are used only in very select subsets of the bariatric population. Recommendations for the prophylactic insertion of vena cava filters prior to bariatric surgery have been

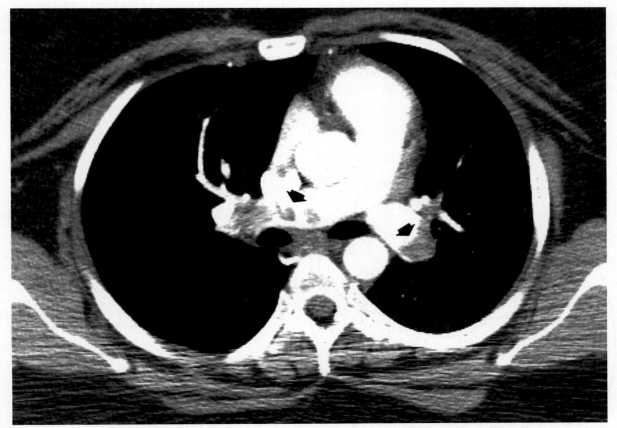

Figure 39-4. A spiral computed tomography scan demonstrates bilateral massive pulmonary emboli (arrows) that occurred in a young, morbidly obese female 9 days postoperatively, despite perioperative low-dose heparin, intermittent pneumatic compression stockings, and early mobilization. Survival required pulmonary embolectomy.

outlined by Sugerman and colleagues.[4,10] They suggest that specific high-risk groups that may benefit from preoperative vena cava filters include patients with severe venous stasis disease, patients with severe pulmonary hypertension (pulmonary artery pressure greater than or equal to 40 mmHg), and patients with obesity hypoventilation syndrome (PaO_2 less than or equal to 55 mmHg or $PaCO_2$ greater than or equal to 65 mmHg). In a retrospective study, they found that patients with severe venous stasis disease (examples included refractory pretibial venous stasis ulcers, recurrent lower extremity cellulitis secondary to venous disease, and pretibial bronze edema from extravasation of red blood cells) had a 4% incidence of fatal pulmonary embolism after gastric bypass compared to 0.2% for patients without severe venous stasis disease.[10] The authors note that patients with primary pulmonary hypertension and the pickwickian syndrome have a greater likelihood of fatality following pulmonary emboli. In addition to these indications, which reflect the morbidities associated with the bariatric patient, other potential indications for prophylactic vena cava filter placement include recurrent or prior deep venous thrombosis[11] and prior pulmonary emboli.

Vena cava filters can be placed intraoperatively under fluoroscopic control[12]; ultrasound guidance has been used for filter placement as an alternative to fluoroscopy in the superobese patient.[13] Although prophylactic vena cava filter placement is intended to avoid the serious and potentially fatal pulmonary embolus, vena cava filters carry their own intrinsic risks, including caval thrombosis and its consequences.[14]

Gastrostomy

Gastrostomies are constructed for a myriad of indications. The two most common reasons for gastrostomy placement are as a means for enteral nutrition and to provide gastric decompression.[15] Although no bariatric operation incorporates gastrostomy as a standard component of the procedure, gastrostomies, when used in bariatric surgery, most commonly complement the Roux-en-Y gastric bypass. As opposed to all other bariatric procedures, the Roux-en-Y gastric bypass has the potential to develop a closed-loop afferent (biliopancreatic) obstruction which may occur when obstruction secondary to adhesions or internal hernia develops anywhere along the biliopancreatic limb, up to and including the enteroenterostomy.

Although concomitant gastrostomy at the time of gastric bypass can circumvent serious and sometimes life-threatening postoperative complications, its benefits are seen in a relatively small percentage of patients. In a retrospective analysis of 1120 micropouch gastric bypass patients without gastrostomy, 33 patients (2.9%) developed a life-threatening postoperative complication requiring reoperation or prolonged hospitalization.[16] Analysis of this subset identified 19 patients (1.6% of the total cohort) in whom gastrostomy would have significantly affected the complication outcome. It was believed that gastrostomy would have prevented emergency reoperation in only four patients. Based on these data, the authors recommended gastrostomy only in select patients and voiced the opinion that routine gastrostomy could not be supported.

In my own experience, I have found gastrostomy to be extremely helpful in patients undergoing conversion of jejunoileal bypass to Roux-en-Y gastric bypass. The discrepancy in bowel lumen size of the enteroenterostomy and the delay in function of the small bowel put the biliopancreatic limb and bypassed stomach at an increased risk for both mechanical and functional obstruction. Other indications for gastrostomy placement, in my experience, include elective revisional gastric bypass and reoperative surgery for anastomotic complications (Fig. 39-5).

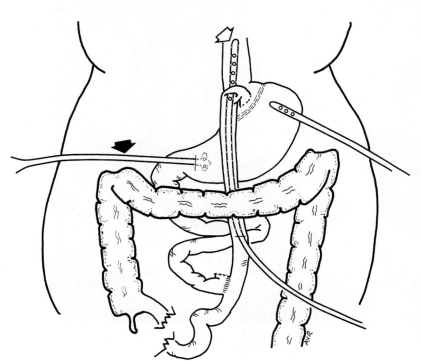

Figure 39-5. Surgical management of gastrojejunal anastomotic leak utilizing gastrostomy (closed arrow), transanastomotic stent (open arrow), and drainage catheter. The gastrostomy provides a means of supporting nutrition by the enteral route, thus avoiding total parenteral nutrition. The transanastomotic stent eliminates the need for long-term placement of a nasogastric tube.

Contrary to the selective application of gastrostomy, a minority of surgeons advocate routine gastrostomy placement. Among the most extensive experiences with this approach are those of Fobi and colleagues.[17] They note that gastrostomy allows mechanical, radiologic, and endoscopic evaluation and manipulation of the bypassed stomach. To maintain this benefit once the gastrostomy tube is removed, Fobi places a radiopaque marker around the gastrostomy site so that it can be identified by radiologic imaging and thus can be accessed percutaneously.

Schreiber and associates take an intermediate approach.[18] Rather than place a gastrostomy tube at the time of gastric bypass, these bariatric surgeons place a circular wire suture in the bypassed stomach and secure the area to the peritoneum of the anterior abdominal wall. Should gastric decompression become necessary postoperatively, this area can be identified and accessed as described earlier.

As noted previously, the most common indications for gastrostomy are decompression and feeding. However, in addition to the bypassed stomach, the common bile duct is also relatively inaccessible for direct evaluation or manipulation after Roux-en-Y gastric bypass. This has created a number of challenges for both the surgeon and the gastroenterologist when biliary disease, especially choledocholithiasis, develops after gastric bypass.[19] One approach to this dilemma has been the creation of a gastrostomy postoperatively as a means of endoscopic retrograde cholangeopancreatography access.[20]

▶ PROCEDURES TO TREAT OTHER DISEASES

Morbid obesity contributes to a variety of diseases and medical conditions that are routinely managed by surgical intervention. Nearly all of these patients have an abdominal panniculus. Umbilical, inguinal, and incisional hernias are commonplace, and symptomatic gastroesophageal reflux disease (GERD) is a common comorbid complaint elicited during the initial evaluation. The decision to address these and other presenting problems at the time of the bariatric procedure must be made with a careful understanding of the consequences of the additional operation and the changes that will take place postoperatively following substantial weight loss.

Panniculectomy

Excess skin, especially in the lower abdominal region, commonly occurs in association with morbid obesity and may be significantly increased following successful massive weight reduction. The obvious advantage of delaying panniculectomy until weight loss has been completed is the likelihood of achieving a more complete pannus removal, with an improved cosmetic result and greater patient satisfaction.

When abdominoplasty was compared in three groups of patients (obese, borderline, and nonobese), 80% of obese patients had complications as opposed to 33% of borderline and nonobese patients.[21] In my personal experience, plastic surgical procedures have been delayed until weight reduction is complete. At that time, the plastic surgery is coordinated with abdominal wall hernia repair, should the

latter be necessary. Thus, management of the redundant skin and repair of the abdominal hernia can be accomplished utilizing a single anesthetic in a patient who is optimally prepared, because the majority of any comorbid conditions have been eliminated or greatly improved with the achieved weight reduction. There is scant literature regarding concomitant panniculectomy at the time of the bariatric operation. Fobi and associates suggest that a select subgroup of patients may benefit from panniculectomy concurrent with gastric bypass.[22] These surgeons have formulated the following grading system to help quantitate the severity of the panniculus:

- Grade 1. Panniculus covers the pubic hairline but not the entire mons pubis.
- Grade 2. Panniculus extends to cover the entire mons pubis.
- Grade 3. Panniculus extends to cover the upper thigh.
- Grade 4. Panniculus extends to mid thigh.
- Grade 5. Panniculus extends to the knee and beyond.

They suggest that panniculectomy should be offered to patients with grades 2 to 5 panniculi. Concurrent panniculus removal adds 1.5 to 2.5 hours to the gastric bypass operating time, so Fobi and colleagues reserved this approach for patients without underlying cardiopulmonary disease. They suggest that panniculectomy at the time of bypass surgery can be physically, socially, and emotionally beneficial as well as cost-effective for patients with symptomatic panniculi. It has been theorized that the abdominal wall panniculus may actually contribute to the creation of incisional hernias by means of lateral traction on the abdominal incision.[23] If this theory is correct, the recommendation to address the panniculus at the time of the gastric bypass would have additional validity.

Hernia Repair

Hernias in obesity patients most commonly occur in the umbilicus, inguinal, and abdominal wall incisions. Hernia repair can be performed in advance of the bariatric procedure, concomitant with the bariatric operation, or postoperatively, when the benefits of the weight reduction have been realized. The advantages of using the last approach include an easier repair, less likelihood of recurrence, and less risk for mesh infection, should mesh be utilized. When morbidly obese patients present with significant symptoms attributed to the hernia or incarceration, correction of the hernia is appropriate, including delay of the bariatric procedure until recovery is achieved (mobility, properly healing wound, etc.).

Many obese patients have asymptomatic umbilical hernias. Not uncommonly, these can be identified at the time of open gastric bypass by identifying omentum adherent to an umbilical hernia defect. I make no attempt to repair these defects at the time of gastric bypass; the midline incision for gastric bypass is kept as short as possible (Fig. 39-6), and repair is delayed until weight loss has been maximized.[24] No adverse complication has been seen with this approach.

Delaying repair of ventral hernias is not universally recommended. The bariatric surgeons from the University

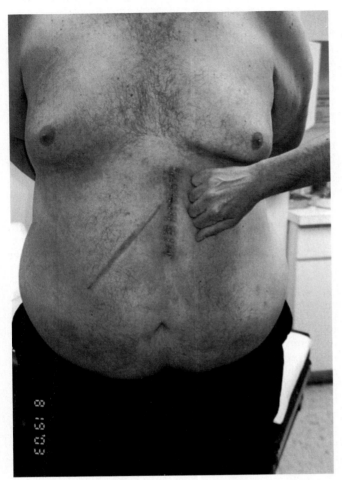

Figure 39-6. Early postoperative midline incision (staples still in place) following open Roux-en-Y gastric bypass. Incision is minimally larger than the surgeon's fist, which is shown for comparison. No attempt is made to extend the incision to the umbilicus, even if an umbilical hernia is identified. A remote right subcostal incision due to a prior cholecystectomy is seen. Note the comparative sizes of the respective incisions.

of Pittsburgh noted that more than one third (37%) of their patients whose ventral hernia repairs were deferred following laparoscopic gastric bypass developed incarceration.[25] In short-term follow-up, they noted no adverse sequelae when ventral hernias were repaired using biodegradable, small intestine submucosa mesh concomitant with laparoscopic gastric bypass.

Stringent recommendations for hernia repair in morbidly obese patients are not available. It is prudent to consider repair when hernia symptoms are present. Incarceration of omentum, especially in the umbilicus, may be asymptomatic and is unlikely to eventuate in a serious outcome. Incarceration of bowel mandates emergency correction, and its management takes precedence over the bariatric procedure.

When incisional hernias are present in the upper midline, they will, by necessity, be encountered during open surgery if the midline is utilized. Although the rate of recurrence with primary repair is high, the overwhelming majority remain intact, without the risk involved with mesh.[25] The use of synthetic mesh for hernia repair during

surgery involving bowel anastomosis must take into consideration the risks and benefits of the approach.

Surgery for Gastroesophageal Reflux Disease

GERD is a common comorbid problem in the morbidly obese patient. Significant advances in the management of GERD are now available, both medically (proton pump inhibitors, H_2 blockers) and surgically (laparoscopic antireflux procedures), but failure to address the underlying morbid obesity limits the success of these approaches. Successful Roux-en-Y gastric bypass provides correction of both the obesity and the reflux disease. This is probably the most suitable treatment for GERD associated with morbid obesity in appropriate patients.[26-28] The gastric pouch has been shown to contain negligible gastric acid and the long Roux limb prevents bile reflux. This benefit is generally not achieved with vertical banded gastroplasty.[29-31] Thus, an antireflux procedure in conjunction with gastric bypass is, arguably, unnecessary and can be technically challenging. An enlarged esophageal hiatus, however, does create concerns for some bariatric surgeons. Dr. Henry Buchwald, of the University of Minnesota, indicates that he reapproximates the diaphragmatic crura at the time of performing an open bariatric procedure when a hiatal hernia is present (personal communication). Other surgeons have performed hiatal hernia repair laparoscopically at the time of adjustable silicone gastric banding.[32]

There is scant literature available on management of paraesophageal hernias in conjunction with bariatric procedures. This anatomic defect would impart a much more serious risk than simple enlargement of the esophageal hiatus; repair in conjunction with whatever bariatric procedure is being undertaken would seem prudent. The necessity of performing an adjuvant antireflux procedure for GERD in association with procedures other than Roux-en-Y gastric bypass, such as biliopancreatic diversion and the duodenal switch procedure, remains unclear.

Miscellaneous

The potential for encountering numerous other conditions at the time of a bariatric procedure is great; they may be neoplastic (benign and malignant tumors), inflammatory, or congenital. Each requires an individual assessment of the risks and benefits of addressing the condition in concert with, or independent of, the bariatric procedure. If the weight loss, postoperative symptoms, and newly created anatomy will interfere with the subsequent evaluation and management of the associated nonbariatric problem (i.e., the follow-up of a malignant process or the management of inflammatory bowel disease), delay or exclusion of the bariatric procedure may be warranted. This may be especially challenging when one encounters an unexpected intraabdominal malignant process at the time of the bariatric procedure.

A patient in our bariatric program presented with a 1-cm nodule in the upper body of the stomach at the time of open Roux-en-Y gastric bypass. Full-thickness excisional biopsy was performed, and frozen section indicated that it probably represented a stromal cell tumor. All pathologic findings were favorable (size, clear margins, lack of mitosis).

After discussing the situation with the patient's wife, the decision was made to proceed with the bariatric procedure, which went without difficulty. The patient had an unremarkable recovery. Sound, basic surgical judgment must always prevail over the desire to perform the bariatric operation. When low-risk, early-stage malignancy, or benign neoplasms are encountered, management in concert with the weight-reduction surgery may be reasonable. Each situation, however, must be approached individually.

▶ PROCEDURES TO PREVENT OTHER DISEASES

Cholecystectomy

Patients undergoing bariatric procedures are at risk for biliary tract disease based on two related causes. First, obese patients have a greater likelihood of developing gallstones than do nonobese patients. With a normal bile-acid pool but greatly increased amounts of biliary cholesterol (which may occur following bariatric surgery), obese patients have cholesterol-supersaturated bile that predisposes to cholesterol gallstones.[32] Thus, morbidly obese patients have a greater probability of presenting with gallstones or having already undergone cholecystectomy at the time of the bariatric procedure than would nonobese patients undergoing any other surgical procedure. The second cause of biliary tract disease in obese patients is the correlation between weight loss and the development of gallstones.[33] Consequently, morbidly obese patients have a greater probability of developing gallstones postoperatively than other individuals who have undergone surgery without attendant weight loss.[34]

The likelihood of prior cholecystectomy in patients undergoing gastric bypass is approximately 20%. Pooled data (8097 patients) from the International Bariatric Surgery Registry revealed that 19% of the patients had had their gallbladders removed before surgical treatment of obesity.[1] Individual studies have suggested a slightly higher percentage of prior cholecystectomy, ranging from 19.4% to 26%.[35-38] Consequently, approximately 74% to 81% of morbidly obese patients have a gallbladder that is at risk prior to the bariatric operation. There is a wide variation in opinion among surgeons regarding the management of the gallbladder in these patients. A survey of the active contributors to the International Bariatric Surgery Registry indicates that 30% of surgeons performing standard Roux-en-Y gastric bypass remove normal-appearing gallbladders.[1] This same study, however, suggests that there is greater consensus when malabsorptive procedures, such as the biliopancreatic diversion, are performed; in this setting there appears to be fairly universal acceptance of concomitant cholecystectomy.

In our program, we screen all preoperative patients who have not undergone prior cholecystectomy by means of percutaneous ultrasound and we use this modality as the sole indicator for gallbladder removal at the time of Roux-en-Y gastric bypass. If the ultrasound examination demonstrates pathology, the gallbladder is removed at the time of either open or laparoscopic bypass. No attempt is made to evaluate the gallbladder intraoperatively if the ultrasound exam is normal.

Prophylactic postoperative administration of ursodiol has been shown to be effective in decreasing the incidence of gallstone formation following gastric bypass.[39] When begun 10 days after surgery and continued for 6 months, ursodiol (600 mg/day) reduced gallstone formation to 2%, compared to 32% in patients taking placebo.

Our program informs patients about the risk for gallstone formation and the availability and potential benefit of ursodiol; patients then decide whether they wish to embark on a program of ursodiol. In our region (northeast Ohio), a 6-month course of this medication costs approximately $600. Other bariatric programs routinely prescribe ursodiol after gastric bypass.[40] We have been reluctant to take this approach because of the difficulty some patients have with medications postoperatively, the side effects of ursodiol, and the cost.

▶ MISCELLANEOUS PROCEDURES

Liver Biopsy

The list of secondary miscellaneous procedures performed in conjunction with gastric bypass is lengthy. These procedures range from those familiar to most surgeons, such as appendectomy and removal of the Meckel diverticulum, to esoteric operations such as combining gastric bypass with partial ileal bypass for hypercholesterolemia.[41]

One of the more commonly performed procedures that falls outside of the categories of making the operation safer, treating other diseases, or preventing other diseases, is liver biopsy. It has been suggested that liver biopsy during bariatric surgery may be helpful to screen for the presence of steatohepatitis and fibrosis.[42] Obesity may be the most common cause of nonalcoholic steatohepatitis (NASH). When a group of consecutive, morbidly obese patients undergoing gastric bypass was evaluated by liver biopsy, 90% had abnormal liver histology, and 56% qualified for the diagnosis of NASH.[43] In the same study, unsuspected cirrhosis was found in 2%. Others have found up to 91% of morbidly obese patients manifesting liver biopsies consistent with NASH.[44] Because the diagnosis of NASH can only be made histologically, and because the liver pathology seen in this entity may progress, possibly, to cryptogenic cirrhosis,[45] liver biopsy may be reasonable to consider.

▶ CONCLUSION

As noted in the introduction, no attempt has been made to be encyclopedic in the presentation of ancillary procedures. Rather, an attempt has been put forward to provide the bariatric surgeon with some information that can justify the additional time, effort, and possible risk intrinsic to the addition of any procedure or intervention at the time of the bariatric operation. Whenever possible, this decision should be discussed with the patient so that valid informed consent can be obtained. The decision to perform prophylactic procedures that may have little benefit should be discouraged. This caveat, however, mandates an individual appraisal of every patient and every ancillary procedure.

▶ REFERENCES

1. Mason EE, Renquist KE, IBSR Data Contributors, et al: Gallbladder management in obesity surgery. Obes Surg 2002;12:222-229.

2. Mason EE, Hesson WW: Informed consent for obesity surgery. Obes Surg 1998;8:419-428.

3. Jenkins SC, Moxham J: The effects of mild obesity on lung function. Respir Med 1991;85:309-311.

4. Sugerman HJ, Baron PL, Fairman RP, et al: Hemodynamic dysfunction in obesity hypoventilation syndrome and the effects of treatment with surgically induced weight loss. Ann Surg 1988;207:604-613.

5. Kyzer S, Charuzi I: Obstructive sleep apnea in the obese. World J Surg 1998;22:998-1001.

6. Fee WE, Ward PH: Permanent tracheostomy. Ann Otol, Rhinol Laryngol 1977;86.635-638.

7. Mickelson SA: Upper airway bypass surgery for obstructive sleep apnea syndrome. Otolaryngol Clin North Am 1998;31:1013-1023.

8. Huerta S, DeShields S, Shipner R, et al: Safety and efficacy of postoperative continuous positive airway pressure to prevent pulmonary complications after Roux-en-Y gastric bypass. J Gastrointest Surg 2002;6:354-358.

9. Wu EC, Barba CA: Current practices in the prophylaxis of venous thromboembolism in bariatric surgery. Obes Surg 2000;10:7-13.

10. Sugerman HJ, Sugerman EL, Wolfe L: Risks and benefits of gastric bypass in morbidly obese patients with severe venous stasis disease. Ann Surg 2001;234:41-46.

11. Gargiulo NJ, Goodman E, Veith FJ, et al: Experience with prophylactic inferior vena cava filter placement during Roux-en-Y gastric bypass surgery in the super-obese. Obes Surg 2002;12:213.

12. Kazmers A, Ramnauth S, Williams M: Intraoperative insertion of Greenfield filters: lessons learned in a personal series of 152 cases. Am Surg 2002;68:877-882.

13. Snyder JM, Arita A, Inampudi C, et al: Intra-operative ultrasound guidance of vena caval umbrella placement in a super obese patient. Obes Surg 2002;12:679-681.

14. Chopra AK, Gorecki P, D'Ayala M, et al: Prophylactic vena cava filter placement in the morbidly obese: a case report of caval thrombosis. Obes Surg 2003;13:21-29.

15. Gauderer MWL, Stellato TA: Gastrostomies: evolution, techniques, indications and complications. Curr Probl Surg 1986;23:657-719.

16. Wood MF, Sapak JA, Schuhknecht MP, et al: Micropouch gastric bypass: indications for gastrostomy tube placement in the bypass stomach. Obes Surg 2000;10:413-419.

17. Fobi MA, Chicola K, Lee H: Access to the bypassed stomach after gastric bypass. Obes Surg 1998;8:289-285.

18. Schreiber H, Sonpal I, Patterson L: The routine use of a gastropexy with a radiologic marker without gastrostomy after Roux-en-Y gastric bypass. Obes Surg 2002;12:217.

19. Stellato TA, Crouse C, Hallowell PT: Bariatric surgery: creating new challenges for the endoscopist. Gastrointest Endosc 2003;57:86-94.

20. Baron TH, Vickers SM: Surgical gastrostomy placement as access for diagnostic and therapeutic ERCP. Gastrointest Endosc 1998; 48:640-641.

21. Vastine VL, Morgan RF, Williams GS, et al: Wound complications of abdominoplasty in obese patients. Ann Plast Surg 1999;42:34-39.

22. Igwe D Jr, Stanczyk M, Lee H, et al: Panniculectomy adjuvant to obesity surgery. Obes Surg 2000;10:530-539.

23. Byrne TK: Complications of surgery for obesity. Surg Clin North Am 2001;81:1181-1193.

24. Stellato TA, Hallowell PT, Crouse C, et al: Two-day length of stay following open Roux-en-Y gastric bypass: is it feasible, safe and reasonable? Obes Surg 2004;14:27-34.

25. Eid GM, Mattar SG, Hamad G, et al: Repair of ventral hernias in morbidly obese patients undergoing laparoscopic gastric bypass should not be deferred. Surg Endosc 2004;18:207-210.

26. Frezza EE, Ikramuddin S, Gourash W, et al: Symptomatic improvement in gastroesophageal reflux disease (GERD) following laparoscopic Roux-en-Y gastric bypass. Surg Endosc 2002;16:1027-1031.

27. Smith SC, Edwards CB, Goodman GN: Symptomatic and clinical improvement in morbidly obese patients with gastroesophageal reflux disease following Roux-en-Y gastric bypass. Obes Surg 1997;67:479-484.

28. Jones KB: Roux-en-Y gastric bypass: an effective antireflux procedure in the less than morbidly obese. Obes Surg 1991;1:295-298.

29. Ovrebo K, Hatlebakk J, Viste A, et al: Gastroesophageal reflux in morbidly obese patients treated with gastric banding or vertical banded gastroplasty. Ann Surg 1998;228:51-58.

30. Kim CH, Sarr MG: Severe reflux esophagitis after vertical banded gastroplasty for treatment of morbid obesity. Mayo Clin Proc 1992;67:33-35.

31. Balsiger BM, Murr MM, Mai J, et al: Gastroesophageal reflux after intact vertical banded gastroplasty: correction by conversion to Roux-en-Y gastric bypass. J Gastrointest Surg 2000;4:276-281.

32. Szold A, Abu-Abeid S: Laparoscopic adjustable silicone gastric banding for morbid obesity: results and complications in 715 patients. Surg Endosc 2002;16:230-233.

33. Mabee TM, Meyer P, DenBesten L, et al: The mechanism of increased gallstone formation in obese human subjects. Surgery 1976;79:460-468.

34. Syngal S, Coakley EH, Willett WC, et al: Long-term weight patterns and risk for cholecystectomy in women. Ann Int Med 1999;130:471-477.

35. Hamad GG, Ikramuddin S, Gourash WF, et al: Elective cholecystectomy during laparoscopic Roux-en-Y gastric bypass: is it worth the wait? Obes Surg 2003;13:76-81.

36. Villegas L, Schneider B, Chang C, et al: Is routine cholecystectomy required during laparoscopic gastric bypass? Obes Surg 2004;14:60-66.

37. Fobi, MA, Lee H, Igwe D Jr, et al: Prophylactic cholecystectomy with gastric bypass operation: incidence of gallbladder disease. Obes Surg 2002;12:350-353.

38. Czerniach DR, Novitsky YW, Perugini RA, et al: Avoidance of simultaneous cholecystectomy in laparoscopic bariatric surgery patients: a case for conservative management. Obes Surg 2002;12:211.

39. Sugerman HJ, Brewer WH, Shiffman ML, et al: A multicenter, placebo-controlled, randomized, double-blind, prospective trial of prophylactic ursodiol for the prevention of gallstone formation following gastric-bypass-induced rapid weight loss. Am J Surg 1995;169:91-96.

40. Higa KD, Boone KB, Ho T: Complications of the laparoscopic Roux-en-Y gastric bypass: 1,040 patients: what have we learned? Obes Surg 2000;10:509-513.

41. Buchwald H, Schone JL: Gastric obesity surgery combined with partial ileal bypass for hypercholesterolemia. Obes Surg 1997;7:313-316.

42. Gholam PM, Kotler DP, Flancbaum LJ: Liver pathology in morbidly obese patients undergoing Roux-en-Y gastric bypass surgery. Obes Surg 2002;12:49-51.

43. Spaulding L, Trainer T, Janiec D: Prevalence of non-alcoholic steatohepatitis in morbidly obese subjects undergoing gastric bypass. Obes Surg 2003;13:347-349.

44. Crespo J, Fernandez-Gil P, Hernandez-Guerra M, et al: Are there predictive factors of severe liver fibrosis in morbidly obese patients with non-alcoholic steatohepatitis? Obes Surg 2001;11:254-257.

45. Garcia-Monzon C, Martin-Perez E, Lo Iacono O, et al: Characterization of pathogenic and prognostic factors of nonalcoholic steatohepatitis associated with obesity. J Hepatol 2000;33:716-724.

section VIII

OUTCOMES

40

Long-Term Follow-Up and Evaluation of Results in Bariatric Surgery

Horacio E. Oria, M.D., F.A.C.S.

The assessment of outcomes of the surgical treatment of morbid obesity is complicated by, among other factors, the scarcity of data in large series with adequate long-term surveillance, the high percentage of patients lost to follow-up, the lack of standards for comparison of results, poor statistical reporting, and the urgent need for clear definitions of success and failure.

This chapter first reviews the methods for assessing quality of care and the types of outcome measures and data sources that can be used. Then it discusses the follow-up of bariatric surgery patients and the evaluation of outcomes, which should include weight loss parameters, analysis of improvement in comorbidities, and changes in quality of life after the treatment. The next two sections cover the need to compare results among different operations and patient subgroups, and the presentation of data according to clinical, quality-of-life, and economic outcomes. The last part reviews the international experience using the Bariatric Analysis and Reporting Outcome System (BAROS), a unique and simple method of classifying outcome groups and defining success or failure based on a scoring key that takes into account weight loss, changes in comorbidities and quality of life, complications, and reoperations.

▶ ASSESSING QUALITY OF CARE

History's earliest standard of care based on outcomes dates back nearly 4000 years. It was written in Babylon during the reign of Hammurabi: "If a physician shall make a severe wound with the bronze operating knife and kill him [the patient] or shall open a growth with a bronze knife and destroy his eye, [the surgeon's] hands shall be cut off."[1] Perhaps today, surgeons should meditate on this extreme form of punishment when we are confronted by liability crises, the public, insurers, managed care companies, government agencies, and private organizations, all clamoring for accountability.

It was a surgeon at the Massachusetts General Hospital in Boston, Dr. Ernest Codman, who pioneered modern outcomes research in the early 1900s.[2] He proposed that surgeons' performance should be evaluated by measuring how their patients progressed after leaving the hospital. This was to be done by using a card that included the symptoms, initial diagnosis, treatment, complications during the hospital stay, diagnosis at discharge, and the result each year afterwards for each patient treated. Codman suggested that to improve the processes of care, all problems in outcomes be noted and investigated. He also developed a charting system that used cost and the patient's functional status as key variables to measure surgeons' performance, and he recommended that hospitals appoint efficiency committees to analyze results before allocating funds for new buildings and equipment. Unfortunately, his novel ideas were not implemented, possibly because he was opinionated and had a difficult personality, which created conflicts with the hospital authorities. Codman's concepts, however, were not totally forgotten.

Another leading figure in outcomes research, Dr. John Wennberg of Darmouth Medical School, introduced in the early 1970s a simple technique: small-area analysis. This method measures variations in surgical-use rates in neighboring communities and compares the results within similar geographic areas. Wennberg's research during the past few decades has discovered striking differences in the use of common surgical operations within areas that have comparable patient populations. A significant drop in utilization was observed after he presented his results to the medical societies and published his observations. Another critical concept that Wennberg introduced was the importance of providing better information to patients prior to any intervention and allowing them to participate actively in decisions regarding their medical care. In 1989, he founded the Foundation for Informed Medical Decision Making, which develops interactive video disks to help patients understand the risks and benefits of various treatments.

The Rand Corporation (Santa Monica, California) has used similar techniques since the early 1980s to analyze the appropriateness of treatment of large numbers of Medicare patients. Dr. Robert Brook, professor at the UCLA School of Medicine, directed the investigations. Rand teams conduct literature reviews, analyze patient records, and consult experts to assess quality of care. The Medical Outcomes Study is one of the corporation's major efforts. The Medical Outcomes Study Short Form Survey (SF-36),[3] the most widely used generic instrument to measure health-related quality of life, was developed by researcher John Ware while he worked for Rand during the 1980s.

In 1988, Dr. Paul Ellwood, who also coined the term *health maintenance organization*, introduced the concept of outcomes management.[4] "Outcomes measurement would draw on four already rapidly maturing technologies." Ellwood elaborated, "First, it would place greater reliance on standards and guidelines that physicians can use in selecting appropriate interventions. Second, it would routinely and systematically measure the functioning and well-being of patients, along with disease-specific clinical outcomes at appropriate time intervals. Third, it would pool clinical and outcomes data on a massive scale. Fourth, it would analyze and disseminate results from the segment of the database most appropriate to the concerns of each decision-maker. This should allow the entire outcomes-management system to be modified continuously and improved with advances in medical science, changes in people's expectations, and alterations in the availability of resources." Some of these concepts are based on the industrial-management theory pioneered by W. Edwards Deming and others.

Ellwood believed that the government, through the U.S. Health Care Financing Administration, should play an important role in this initiative. The Agency for Health Care Policy and Research, an entity entirely separate from the Health Care Financing Administration, was created in 1989. Among other missions, the agency was to conduct long-term outcomes research through Patient Outcomes Research Teams, and develop practice guidelines, beginning with high-volume conditions affecting Medicare patients. *Guidelines* are defined by the Institute of Medicine as "systematically developed statements to assist practitioner and patient decisions about appropriate health care for specific clinical circumstances." The first federal clinical practice guideline, on postoperative pain management, was issued in March of 1992. However, private groups had already begun to do so in 1976, when the Blue Cross and Blue Shield Association asked the American College of Physicians to review the appropriateness of certain questionable tests and procedures submitted for payment. This initiative evolved into the Clinical Efficacy Assessment Project, created in 1981. The guidelines are peer-reviewed and then published in the *Annals of Internal Medicine*.

The American College of Physicians considers cost to be a criterion in the evaluation of appropriateness of care, a position that divides it from other institutions, such as the American Medical Association, which insists that cost considerations should not be included. Moreover, the American Medical Association prefers the term *parameter* instead of *guideline*. Its *Directory of Practice Parameters* includes thousands of parameters developed by more than 45 physician organizations. The problem with this approach, say some experts such as Brook and Dr. David Eddy of Duke University, is that the parameters are developed by consensus panels of specialists, based on these experts' opinions, without following a methodology structured on metaanalysis and statistical modeling. Eddy, an influential decision-maker on the Clinical Efficacy Assessment Project, strongly believes that costs should be addressed while developing a practice policy.

The National Academy of Science's Institute of Medicine lists some conditions that should characterize a guideline: validity based on the strength of the evidence and estimated outcomes, reliability and reproducibility, clinical applicability, flexibility, and clarity. After a guideline is implemented, review criteria need to be used for evaluation. The Institute of Medicine also defines attributes for these criteria: sensitivity, specificity, patient responsiveness, readability, minimal intrusiveness, feasibility, and computer compatibility.

In addition to the difficulties in developing appropriate and useful guidelines, another dilemma the outcome researchers face is how to disseminate and facilitate physicians' implementation of the parameters. Some experts, such as Wennberg, believe that doctors can change practice patterns if they are aware of comparative performance data. Others think that strong peer and institutional pressures, supported by medical organizations and external review entities, including the government, are necessary to lead practitioners to adopt the guidelines and improve performance. To further complicate these issues, in the past decade several states, led by New York, began releasing to the general public individual surgeons' and hospitals' data on surgical volumes and outcomes.

As a result, the Leapfrog Group, a consortium of health care purchasers with 33 million customers, is directing their customers to hospitals and other institutions that meet the group's volume criteria for several surgical procedures. The most contentious issue in the current debate over surgical quality is whether higher volume means better outcomes. Even though no study has confirmed an absolute relationship between quality of care and number of cases performed, there seems to be a consensus that volume has a significant impact on outcomes of many surgical procedures, especially when evaluating complication rates and length of hospital stay, as compared with mortality data. One of the best examples of a performance-improvement project is the Veteran Affairs Administration's National Surgical Quality Improvement Program, which has led to a 27% decrease in mortality and 45% reduction in perioperative morbidity since 1991. This was the first national, validated, outcome-based, risk-adjusted, and peer-controlled program for measuring and improving surgical care.

Structure, Process, and Outcome

The decade of the 1980s was enlightened by the contributions of Dr. Avedis Donabedian, Professor Emeritus of Public Health at the University of Michigan. In numerous publications he defined quality and suggested approaches and methods of its assessment; he also established criteria and standards of quality.[5] The classic triad for the evaluation of quality of care is based on structure, process, and outcome. In bariatric surgery, structural data can include, among many other elements, the experience of the surgeon, surgical technique, office and hospital facilities, equipment and personnel, and more. For example, surgeons can improve outcomes by increasing their training, gaining more experience, changing their technique, or switching to another type of operation. Hospitals can do the same by updating equipment or educating the staff.[6] The events that occur before, during, and after the encounter between the medical care provider and the patient constitute part of the process information. Diagnosis, assessment, and management of obesity comorbidities; preoperative testing; treatment of surgical complications; and development of clinical pathways are some examples of the data to be studied. *Analysis of outcomes* refers to the patient's health status after the medical intervention.

According to Brook, process data are usually more sensitive than outcome information, because a poor outcome does not occur every time there is an error in the provision of care.[7] In the surgical treatment of obesity, this issue is further complicated by the long time required in between the key process (surgery) and important outcomes such as reduction in mortality or increase in life expectancy. Brook defines five methods of assessing quality. Three of them are *implicit*, meaning that a professional who reviews data sources does not follow prior standards to render an opinion about the quality of care. The fourth method assesses the provision of care using *explicit* process criteria; the fifth analyzes the results of care by using explicit a priori criteria and comparing the data with the outcome predicted by a validated model. The last two methods are more strict.

Types of Outcome Measures

Bariatric surgeons are familiar with *clinical* outcomes data, such as early and late complications, mortality, reoperation rates, and weight loss. In the late 1980s, Brolin and colleagues introduced another important parameter, the resolution or improvement in obesity comorbidities.[8] These authors considered medical disorders "resolved" when controlled without medication and "improved" when fewer medications were required after surgery.

Functional outcomes evaluate the effect of the treatment on the patient's ability to do something. This is important, for example, in orthopedic surgery, rehabilitation medicine, and certain types of cancer, but it can also be applied to general surgery procedures, including bariatrics. The analysis of *economic* outcomes has significant importance not only at the individual (patient), institutional (hospital), and payer (insurance companies, government) levels but also as an overall social responsibility. The concept of value is defined as the ratio of the quality of medical care divided by the cost of such care. As mentioned before, it is a contentious issue, but one that physicians need to recognize, accept, and include in the evaluation of medical care. In these days of escalating health care costs, dwindling resources, climbing numbers of uninsured people, and increasing demands by the aging population, assessment of the cost-effectiveness of treatments, especially surgery, should be a priority. In other words, any medical intervention should aim to be effective and efficacious (producing the desired effect), but also efficient, that is, productive of the desired effects without waste.

Another type of outcome measure is patient perception and satisfaction with the medical intervention. It is the most difficult outcome to analyze by strict scientific standards, but its importance in the evaluation of quality of care continues to grow.[9] Closely related to this topic is the analysis of quality of life (QOL), the subjective value that an individual places upon satisfaction with his or her life. More specifically, the term *health-related QOL (HRQL)* refers to the physical, psychological, and social domains of health, seen as distinct areas influenced by a person's experience, beliefs, expectations, and perceptions.[10] This measure, for some researchers the final health outcome, focuses on the person and not on the disease. However, the concept is intrinsically subjective and difficult to quantitate. Essential features of a QOL instrument are validity, reliability, responsiveness (sensitivity to change), appropriateness, and practicality.[11] Typical domains included in a HRQL assessment are physical function, mental or psychological status, social and role function, general health perception, and symptom perception.

Instruments to measure QOL can be generic or disease-specific. Examples of sophisticated and validated generic questionnaires are the Sickness Impact Profile, the Quality of Well-Being Scale, the Nottingham Health Profile, and the Gothenburg Quality of Life Scale.[12] However, these surveys are long and comprehensive, and some require an interviewer, which renders them less practical. Probably the most widely used generic QOL instrument is the SF-36.[3] This questionnaire contains 36 questions to measure eight domains. It is self-administered and can be completed in less than 10 minutes. The SF-36 has been used in numerous studies of obese patients.[13,14] Other generic inventories developed for special populations such as pediatrics were applied to study QOL in obesity.[15] Some surgeons use disease-specific instruments that were created to analyze life quality in many disorders, such as gastrointestinal diseases (Gastrointestinal Quality of Life Index) or reflux (Gastroesophageal Reflux Disease-Health-Related Quality-of-Life).[16,17]

Two disease-specific questionnaires were developed in the past decade to evaluate QOL in the obese population. Kolotkin and colleagues originally included 74 items in their Impact of Weight on Quality of Life (IWQOL) survey, which was later shortened to a 31-item self-reporting instrument (IWQOL-Lite), following a format and domains similar to those of the SF-36.[18] This scale has been used with bariatric surgery patients along with the SF-36 and has also been applied to compare prospective surgical patients with obese controls.[19] Another obesity-specific instrument is the Moorehead-Ardelt Quality of Life Questionnaire (M-A QOLQ), created in response to my request for a simple, one-page survey that could be included in the Bariatric Analysis and Reporting Outcome System (BAROS) that I was developing in the 1990s.[20] This outcome-evaluating system is amply discussed in a later section of the chapter.

Data Sources for Outcomes Evaluation

The appropriate source of information for quality evaluation depends on the objective of the study. The selection of data sources is the following step after deciding what method of quality assessment (implicit or explicit) will be used. Information can be collected before and after treatment. The medical record is the most common source of data for clinical outcomes, whereas patient questionnaires and other validated instruments can be used to analyze health status, functional outcomes, and QOL. Patient self-assessment should be applied before and after treatment, and at periodic intervals thereafter because of the continuous changes expected in patients' perceptions as time passes, particularly in view of the weight regain commonly observed years after surgery for obesity and the possibility that older patients will develop other medical conditions or a recurrence of those successfully treated before.

On the other hand, to study economic outcomes, it would be more appropriate to use hospitals' financial records, which should include the real hospital costs and the charges submitted to the health care payer. State and national billing records, from both private and governmental entities, can be utilized to compare individual physicians' and hospitals' cost-effectiveness and the appropriateness of tests, treatments, and other interventions, especially those that require high technology and invasiveness. Examples that apply to bariatric surgery are the costs of preoperative tests, drugs, and supplies; laparoscopic instruments; anesthesia; operative and recovery room times; and length of hospital stay, as well as the costs of readmissions, complications, and other necessary interventions such as adjustable band adjustments. More difficult to quantitate are other economic measures, such as lost wages or unearned income incurred by patients during the recovery period and the costs of medicines, vitamins, supplements, and medical care needed after the operation, especially if the bariatric procedure was a malabsorptive operation. This type of information is very important for comparing the long-term results of various techniques and for assessing the outcomes of patients who had surgery with those of controls.

▶ FOLLOW-UP OF BARIATRIC SURGICAL PATIENTS

Length and Type of Follow-up

The 1991 National Institutes of Health (NIH) Consensus Development Conference on Gastrointestinal Surgery for Severe Obesity recommended: "Postoperative care, nutritional counseling, and surveillance should continue for an indefinitely long period. The surveillance should include the monitoring of indices of inadequate nutrition and of amelioration of any preoperative disorders such as diabetes, hypertension, and dyslipidemia. The monitoring should include not only indices of macronutrients but also of mineral and vitamin nutrition."[21] The NIH statement, understandably, did not advise specific intervals for the postoperative visits nor the tests required to assess clinical changes.

In an attempt to clarify these issues, the Standards Committee of the American Society for Bariatric Surgery (ASBS) developed two sets of guidelines that were approved by the membership in plenary sessions at the annual meetings. The first included guidelines for postoperative follow-up care.[22] It recommended visits during the immediate postoperative period, then within 3 months of the operation, at 6 months, yearly for 3 years, at 5 years, then at 5-year intervals for life, with additional visits as indicated by the patient's condition. The visits had to include a history and physical examination followed by laboratory tests; radiographic, endoscopic, or other studies; and consultations as indicated. The second ASBS statement is related to the length of follow-up necessary for a classification of results.[23] It defined results as preliminary (less than 2 years of follow-up); intermediate (2 to 5 years); long-term (5 to 10 years); and very-long-term (more than 10 years). This statement also discouraged the presentation of preliminary results. Statistical data must include the mean and median lengths of follow-up, in months. Unfortunately, the bariatric surgery literature is plagued by case series with inadequate lengths of surveillance.

The importance of long-term follow-up in surgery for morbid obesity cannot be overemphasized. The history of this particular field is abundant in techniques that showed promise in the short term, only to be abandoned years later because of poor results, or serious side effects or complications. Typical examples are the jejunoileal bypass, horizontal gastroplasties, gastric partition, and wrapping. In the United States, the decade of the 1980s was dominated by the vertical gastroplasties, which were later replaced in preference by the Roux-en-Y gastric bypass. However, in many other countries, laparoscopic adjustable banding is currently the technique most used because of its low level of invasiveness and low morbidity and mortality rates, in spite of poorer weight loss. On the other side of the surgical spectrum, the biliopancreatic diversion and its variants are preferred by a relatively sizable percentage of surgeons because of the excellent weight loss it produces over time, even though the technical challenges, complications, and long-term sequelae are much higher than in other procedures.

These considerations, better discussed elsewhere in this book, bring up another issue related to our subject: the intensity of the follow-up. Clearly, the necessary frequency and thoroughness of the surveillance of a patient after a pure gastric restrictive operation are different from those in surveillance of one who had a mostly malabsorptive operation. For this reason, the ASBS Standards Committee decided against setting specific guidelines, not only for the required preoperative assessment but also for the postoperative testing during follow-up, opting to leave it at the surgeon's discretion, according to the individual needs of the patient. However, the committee advised, if indicated, obtaining a complete blood count, and albumin and electrolyte levels if the patient is vomiting or eating improperly, as well as vitamin B_{12}, iron, iron-binding capacity, calcium, and alkaline phosphatase if the duodenum has been bypassed.

Weight and Follow-up Calculations

The ASBS published in 1994 a review of factors to be considered when evaluating and reporting results of the surgical treatment of morbid obesity.[24] These recommendations were followed in 1997 by another statement from the Standards Committee.[25] The latter included more guidelines for reporting results and a classification of obesity based on body mass index (BMI). The ASBS

Table 40-1	FORMULAS TO CALCULATE RELATIVE WEIGHT PARAMETERS	

Percent ideal weight (%IW) $= \dfrac{\text{weight}}{\text{ideal weight}} \times 100$

Percent excess weight (%EW) $= \dfrac{\text{weight} - \text{ideal weight}}{\text{ideal weight}} \times 100$

Percent weight loss (%WL) $= \dfrac{\text{operative weight} - \text{follow-up weight}}{\text{operative weight}} \times 100$

Percent excess weight loss (%EWL) $= \dfrac{\text{operative weight} - \text{follow-up weight}}{\text{ideal weight}} \times 100$

Percent BMI loss (%BMIL) $= \dfrac{\text{operative BMI} - \text{follow-up BMI}}{\text{operative BMI}} \times 100$

Percent excess BMI loss (%EBMIL) $= \dfrac{\text{operative BMI} - \text{follow-up BMI}}{\text{operative BMI} - 25} \times 100$

%BMIL, percent body mass index loss; %EBMIL, percent excess body mass index loss; %EW, percent excess weight; %EWL, percent excess weight loss; %IW, percent ideal weight; %WL, percent weight loss.

recommended, among other topics, the use of the metric system, BMI, measures of fat distribution, and the analysis of subgroups of patients. It also discouraged the presentation of weight loss in series with fewer than 2 years of follow-up.

To report results, various measures and weight calculations are necessary. These can be absolute, such as the patient's weight in pounds or, preferably, in kilograms, and the patient's excess weight, that is, the difference between the patient's weight and the "ideal weight," usually taken from the 1983 Metropolitan Life Insurance Company's tables. Another absolute parameter is the weight loss, expressed in units, comparing the pre- and postoperative weights. This is not advisable as a measure for presenting results. Commonly used relative weight calculations, shown in Table 40-1, include percent ideal weight, percent excess weight, percent weight loss and percent excess weight loss (%EWL). More recently, the postoperative changes in BMI are also being utilized. A BMI of 25 is recognized as the lowest limit of overweight. This allows for the calculation of percent BMI loss and percent excess BMI loss. The ASBS recommends using %EWL and reduction of BMI as measures of weight loss following bariatric surgery.[25]

Standardized Follow-up Calculations

The 1994 ASBS guidelines stipulated that follow-up data should be provided for each analysis presented: "The numerator should indicate the number of patients whose data are included in the group analyzed and the denominator is recommended to be the number of patients eligible for follow-up."[24] Adequate postoperative surveillance remains the most important means of identifying the completeness of the data reported. More than 60% follow-up is accepted by statisticians as being satisfactory for significance.[26] The percentage of patients followed has to be determined at periodic intervals during the first 6 postoperative months and at 12-month intervals thereafter.

According to the International Bariatric Surgery Registry (IBSR), these time intervals are also used for presenting weight loss, but all other data collected after the primary operation is considered follow-up, with the following order of dominance: mortality, reoperation, readmission, subsequent procedure, and office visits or questionnaire responses. Only one visit per patient is selected within each time interval, choosing the one that is most conservative and closest to the midpoint of the interval if more visits are recorded. Weight-loss parameters should reflect the midpoint value for the interval examined.

Difficulties in Obtaining Adequate Follow-up

Severe obesity is a complex, life-long, chronic, epidemic and, at this time, incurable disease. Hence, gathering long-term data on patients, either treated or not, is of crucial relevance for the study of this metabolic disorder. Unfortunately, it has proven very difficult to obtain appropriate information about the morbidly obese population after surgery. Very few centers have the resources to obtain adequate follow-up data on significant numbers of patients years after the operation. The IBSR, for example, records a pale 10.9% follow-up among 1781 patients eligible 8 years after surgery.

However, some anecdotal presentations have pointed out that patients lost to follow-up do not necessarily constitute failure of the treatment. This impression was confirmed by the majority of respondents to a survey that I conducted among experienced bariatric surgeons in 1996.[27] It appears that an approximately equal number of patients do not respond to surveillance inquiries either because they have not lost enough weight and consider themselves failures, or because they have progressed so well after the operation that they think it is unnecessary to report to the surgeon's office. In any event, it is important to report the number and percentage of patients lost to follow-up for each time period and to specify how those patients are accounted for in the outcome analysis.[25]

▶ EVALUATION OF OUTCOMES IN BARIATRIC SURGERY

Parameters to Present Weight Loss

Weight loss has been used, erroneously, as the main outcome parameter of surgery for morbid obesity for many decades. In the 1960s and 1970s, results were presented as mean weight loss over time, without strict criteria for defining success or failure. Many surgeons developed their own criteria for a successful operation during the following decade, creating numerous definitions that often differed significantly. Pories and colleagues defined success as a loss of 25% or more of the operative weight,[28] similar to the criterion used by MacLean and associates in 1981[29] but more strict than the loss of more than 15% of initial weight utilized by Freeman.[30] Other investigators used %EWL as the main outcome measure. Mason defined success as more than 25%EWL,[31] whereas Halverson opted for a threshold of 50%EWL, 100% higher than the former.[32] Many bariatric surgeons currently use Halverson's definition, but neither the ASBS nor the International Federation for the Surgery of Obesity (IFSO) has adopted standards to define success or failure.

Reinhold proposed, in 1982, a weight-loss classification based on another parameter: postoperative weight as percentage within the ideal. He used quartiles of the percentage within ideal weight to classify his results as excellent, good, fair, or poor. A final weight more than 100% of the ideal was considered a failure, certainly a very low threshold for defining an unsuccessful operation.[33] A year later, Lechner and Elliott published different criteria, considering more than 80%EWL to be an excellent result, 50% to 80%EWL to be a good result, and less than 50% EWL was deemed a poor result.[34] The respondents to the survey previously mentioned did not select any of these definitions as a possible standard.[27]

Analysis of Comorbidity Improvements

Weight loss is clearly insufficient as a single outcome criterion in bariatric treatments. The ultimate goal of weight reduction is improving patients' health, reducing mortality, and enhancing their psychological and socioeconomic well-being. As indicated earlier, Brolin and colleagues introduced the concept of accounting for the improvement in obesity-related diseases in the evaluation of results.[7] They established three outcome groups, according to weight loss in comparison to ideal weight and changes in comorbidities. Brolin and his colleagues, however, failed to define which medical conditions should be analyzed, their degree of severity, and the criteria needed for diagnosis; those are the reasons, among others, that their method was not accepted.

Several problems are encountered in the analysis of this topic. First, morbid obesity can affect almost any organ system in various degrees of severity. Not even an exhaustive list of comorbidities could cover all possibilities. Therefore, it is necessary to develop a concise list of the most common and serious obesity-related diseases. Second, we need to define strict diagnostic criteria so as to avoid observer's bias in the preoperative assessment and in the evaluation after the surgery. Third, we should establish a classification of severity according to health risks (a severity stratification). Finally, we need to clarify the terms *resolution* and *improvement* on the basis of concrete parameters.

Some answers to these dilemmas were provided by the development-committee members convened in 1996 at the request of the Shape Up America! Foundation and the American Obesity Association.[35] They defined a comorbid condition as "any condition associated with obesity that (1) usually worsens as the degree of obesity increases and (2) often improves as the obesity is successfully treated." Seven major comorbidities were listed: hypertension, cardiovascular disease, dyslipidemia, type 2 diabetes, sleep apnea/obesity hypoventilation syndrome, osteoarthritis, and infertility. The panelists also set diagnostic criteria for these comorbidities. They also listed four other medical problems that "become comorbid conditions when they impair or diminish QOL or require chronic treatment." These diseases are idiopathic intracranial hypertension, lower-extremity venous stasis disease, gastroesophageal reflux, and urinary stress incontinence. The statement recommended identifying other risk factors, especially fat distribution, by using anthropomorphic measures such as waist-to-hip ratio and waist circumference.

Assessment of Quality of Life After Surgery

The 1991 NIH statement also recommended that "quality of life considerations in patients undergoing surgical treatment of obesity must be considered...."[21] In addition, the experts urged "the development of standardized, reliable, and valid questionnaires with which to evaluate patients' expectations about changes and the psychological changes actually experienced during weight loss and maintenance." These instruments must be validated by appropriate psychometric techniques for reliability, consistency, robustness, and reproducibility. They should be reliable (yield consistent value); valid (target what they claim to measure); responsive (detect changes over time); and sensitive (reflect true changes in individual patients). As discussed before, numerous lengthy and comprehensive generic questionnaires are available. It is difficult, however, to obtain a balance between practicality and thoroughness of evaluation when selecting a survey to assess the elusive concept of QOL. One dilemma in evaluating life quality after obesity surgery is the choice of the appropriate instrument. Do we select an elaborate, long survey and risk a poor response rate, or do we rather choose a short and simple questionnaire that is more likely to be completed and returned? Outcome-management researchers advise the use of a well-validated generic instrument, such as the SF-36, complemented by an additional specific questionnaire focusing on the condition being examined.

How to Account for Reoperations and Complications in the Evaluation of Results

Complicating further the issues presented before, it is not clear how to account for reoperations caused by complications or side effects of the surgery or by failure to lose enough weight. Half of the respondents to my questionnaire considered a reoperation to be a failure, whereas the other half did not.[27] These experienced surgeons agreed that the number and percentage of reoperations should be included in the analysis, but few supported using the reoperation rate per year, as proposed by Mason.[36] However, considering that morbid obesity is a chronic, complex and, at this time, incurable condition, even after surgery, I agree with Dr. Mason. Too many surgical techniques were thought to be successful for a while, only to be abandoned later because of their poor results or long-term complications.

Similarly, the assessment of surgical complications presents another problem. Early postoperative events are usually well documented in the literature, but late complications and side effects are more difficult to evaluate and report, principally because of the poor long-term surveillance characteristic in bariatric surgery. Once again, we lack clear definitions of what constitutes a major or a minor morbidity, as well as a list of complications, including varying degrees of severity, that can be taken into account in the outcome analysis. The IBSR defines a major complication as one that results in a hospital stay of 7 days or longer, and a minor complication as one that does not.[36] It should be noted, however, that in many countries outside the United States, the hospital stay is sometimes longer than 7 days because of socioeconomic factors, not because of complications. Appendix 1 in the 1998 BAROS publication lists surgical and medical complications, dividing them into major and minor, as well as early and late.[20] This list was used to develop the list included in the ASBS booklet of information for patients.[37]

▶ COMPARISON AND PRESENTATION OF RESULTS

An important difficulty encountered by the 1991 NIH panelists was summarized in a simple sentence: "One of the key problems in evaluating the current reports of case series in surgical therapy is the lack of standards for comparison."[21] They recommended that various surgical procedures be compared for complications rates, weight loss, long-term maintenance, and improvement in secondary complications of obesity. Furthermore, the consensus panel found a critical need for clear definitions of terms related to obesity, especially terms defining outcomes, and for better statistical reporting of surgical results, which are necessary for clearer assessments of outcomes.

The NIH statement also advised that the effects of surgical therapy be defined in various subgroups stratified for gender, age, ethnicity, socioeconomic status, comorbidity, and fat distribution. These recommendations were included in the 1997 ASBS Standards Committee guidelines.[25] Other suggestions listed in these guidelines were: analyze separately patients who had had previous surgery for obesity and those requiring reoperations; and state clearly that percentage of the total series and the reasons for reintervention. The details of the surgical technique, as well as modifications implemented during the course of the study, must be included. It would also be useful to assess the results in superobese patients separately from results in the cohort who have BMIs of 40 to 50 kg per m² because of the significant differences in comorbidities, surgical risk, and weight loss between the two groups. Unfortunately, very few case series in the literature publish results according to these subgroups.

Another important consideration is the geographic, social, and economic differences, not to mention the genetic differences, when trying to compare outcomes in various countries. This is paramount in the selection of a QOL instrument, which should be simple for the patient to complete, regardless of educational level or cultural background. In addition, an appropriate questionnaire has to be easily translated into other languages so as to eliminate the cross-cultural and linguistic factors that influence its reliability.

In summary, an adequate presentation of results of the surgical treatment of morbid obesity must include clinical, QOL, and economic outcomes. Table 40-2 summarizes

Table 40-2	OUTCOME MEASURES AND DATA SOURCES	
PARAMETERS	**DATA SOURCES**
Preoperative	
Demographics: age, sex, height, weight	Patient information form
Ideal and excess weight, %EW, BMI	Tables, nomograms, formulas
History, clinical factors, comorbidities, medications, physical examination, measures of fat distribution, presurgical testing, consultations, final diagnoses	Office medical record
Health status, generic quality-of-life instrument	SF-36
Disease-specific questionnaire	Obesity-specific QOL survey
Perioperative	
Surgical technique, intraoperative events, anesthesia	Operative report
Anesthesia/operative/recovery unit time, ICU, LOS	Hospital records
Early (<30 days) morbidity/mortality, reoperations	Hospital chart
Financial data: costs, charges to payer	Billing records
Recovery/return to work time, income loss	Office and work records
Postoperative	
Late complications, readmissions, reoperations	Office and hospital records
Weight loss, improvements in comorbidities, % patients followed/lost, mean time of F/U	Office records, database
Changes in quality of life/health status % success, failures, outcome groups	QOL questionnaires Outcome system (BAROS)
Patient satisfaction	Patient surveys

BAROS, Bariatric Analysis and Reporting Outcome System; BMI, body mass index; F/U, follow-up; ICU, intensive care unit; LOS, length of hospital stay; %EW, percent of excess weight; QOL, quality of life; SF-36 Short Form 36. (Modified from the Recommended American College of Surgeons Core Data Collection Set, developed by the American College of Surgeons Advisory Council Task Force on Outcomes, 1997.)

the principal measures and data sources that can be used for the assessment and reporting of surgical outcomes.

THE BARIATRIC ANALYSIS AND REPORTING OUTCOME SYSTEM

The BAROS instrument allows for the analysis, evaluation, and classification of the results of bariatric surgery in a single page, shown in Figure 40-1.[20] The groundwork of this project was the survey cited before. In addition to weight loss, the majority of the surgeons agreed with the concept of including the changes in obesity-related diseases and QOL in the assessment of outcomes, but there was no consensus of how this should be accomplished. Likewise, clear definitions of success and failure were not obtained.[27]

The idea of creating a scoring system to standardize the reporting of outcomes was then developed further by selecting three principal domains: weight loss, improvements in comorbidities, and changes in quality of life.

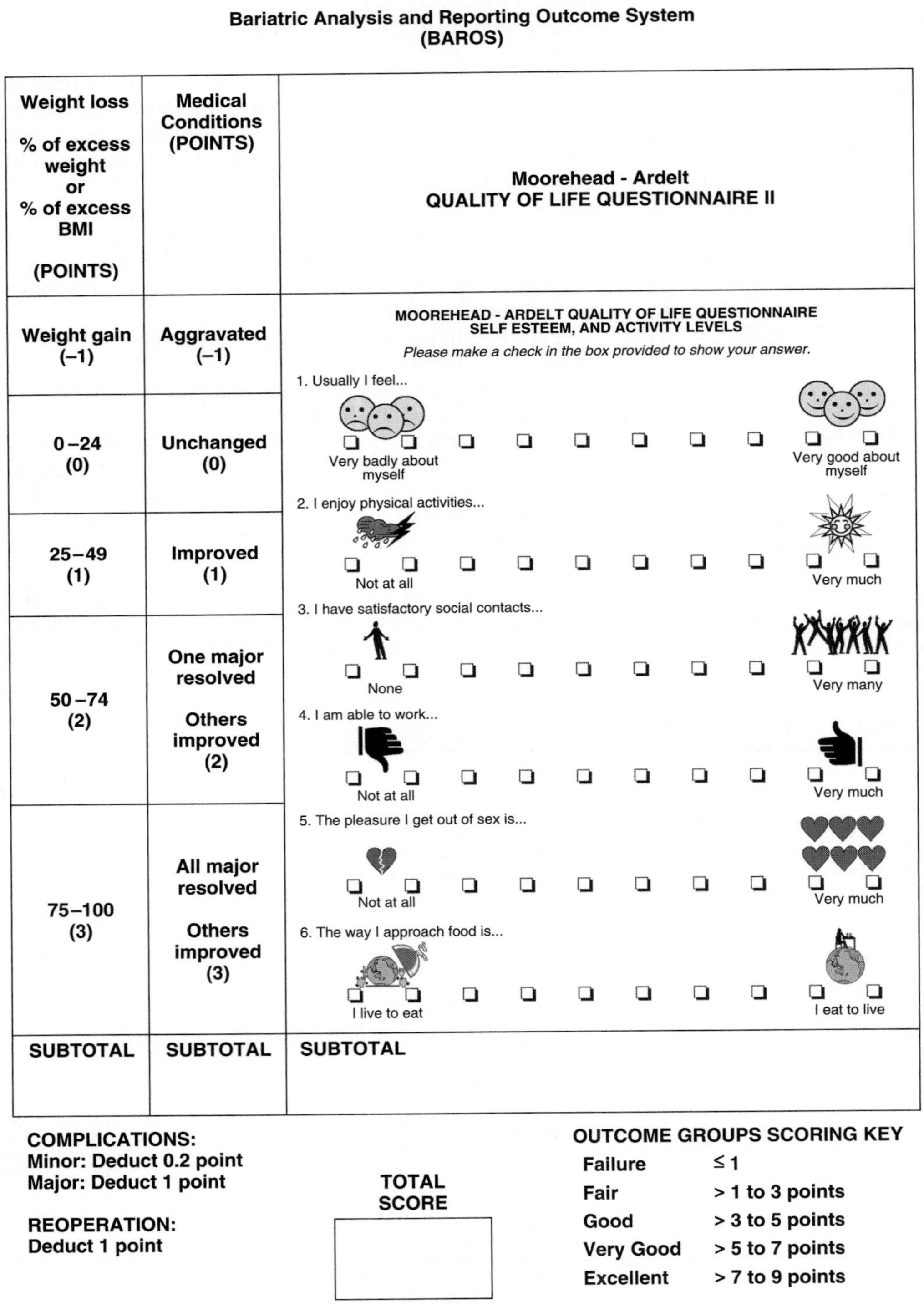

**Bariatric Analysis and Reporting Outcome System
(BAROS)**

Weight loss % of excess weight or % of excess BMI (POINTS)	Medical Conditions (POINTS)	Moorehead - Ardelt QUALITY OF LIFE QUESTIONNAIRE II
Weight gain (−1)	Aggravated (−1)	**MOOREHEAD - ARDELT QUALITY OF LIFE QUESTIONNAIRE SELF ESTEEM, AND ACTIVITY LEVELS** *Please make a check in the box provided to show your answer.* 1. Usually I feel...
0−24 (0)	Unchanged (0)	Very badly about myself ... Very good about myself 2. I enjoy physical activities...
25−49 (1)	Improved (1)	Not at all ... Very much 3. I have satisfactory social contacts...
50−74 (2)	One major resolved Others improved (2)	None ... Very many 4. I am able to work... Not at all ... Very much
75−100 (3)	All major resolved Others improved (3)	5. The pleasure I get out of sex is... Not at all ... Very much 6. The way I approach food is... I live to eat ... I eat to live
SUBTOTAL	SUBTOTAL	SUBTOTAL

COMPLICATIONS:
Minor: Deduct 0.2 point
Major: Deduct 1 point

REOPERATION:
Deduct 1 point

TOTAL SCORE

OUTCOME GROUPS SCORING KEY

Failure	≤ 1
Fair	> 1 to 3 points
Good	> 3 to 5 points
Very Good	> 5 to 7 points
Excellent	> 7 to 9 points

Figure 40-1. The Bariatric Analysis and Reporting Outcome System (BAROS). *(Copyright 2002, H.E. Orio, M.D., and M.K. Moorehead, Ph.D.)*

Points are added or deducted according to the postoperative results. A maximum of three points is given for each domain. The %EWL was originally selected because it is the parameter most widely used, and it is easy to calculate and represent in graphic form. The division into quartiles follows the classification proposed by Reinhold.[33] The assessment of medical conditions was modified from Brolin and colleagues;[8] the comorbidities list and diagnostic criteria were selected on the basis of the recommendations by the American Obesity Association and the Shape Up America! Foundation.[35] A list of possible early and late complications, classified as major and minor, was created according to the IBSR protocols. Points are deducted for complications and reoperations, without classifying them as failures.

Another difficulty encountered was to find a simple, short, and reliable obesity-specific QOL instrument, which prompted my request for contributions from several psychologists active in the ASBS. Self-esteem and four domains of daily activities were to be included in the questionnaire, following the work of Wyss and colleagues[38] and Delin and coworkers.[39] The M-A QOLQ was thus developed and incorporated into the BAROS. This instrument is designed on a single page, using colored drawings as a visual aid. Originally, the questions addressed five main areas: self-esteem, physical activity, social life, work conditions,

MOOREHEAD - ARDELT QUALITY OF LIFE QUESTIONNAIRE
SELF ESTEEM, AND ACTIVITY LEVELS

Please make a check in the box provided to show your answer.

1. Usually I feel... Very badly about myself ❑ ❑ ❑ ❑ ❑ ❑ ❑ ❑ ❑ ❑ Very good about myself
2. I enjoy physical activities... Not at all ❑ ❑ ❑ ❑ ❑ ❑ ❑ ❑ ❑ ❑ Very much
3. I have satisfactory social contacts... None ❑ ❑ ❑ ❑ ❑ ❑ ❑ ❑ ❑ ❑ Very many
4. I am able to work... Not at all ❑ ❑ ❑ ❑ ❑ ❑ ❑ ❑ ❑ ❑ Very much
5. The pleasure I get out of sex is... Not at all ❑ ❑ ❑ ❑ ❑ ❑ ❑ ❑ ❑ ❑ Very much
6. The way I approach food is... I live to eat ❑ ❑ ❑ ❑ ❑ ❑ ❑ ❑ ❑ ❑ I eat to live

Melodie K. Moorehead, Ph. D., Bariatric Surgery Clinical Psychologist, 1201 E. Broward Blvd., Ft. Lauderdale, FL 33301.
Elizabeth Ardelt, Ph. D., Institute für Psychologic, Universität Salzburg.
MOOREHEAD - ARDELT QUALITY OF LIFE QUESTIONNAIRE
SELF ESTEEM, AND ACTIVITY LEVELS
Copyright 1997 M.K. MOOREHEAD, Ph. D. (954) 524-5244

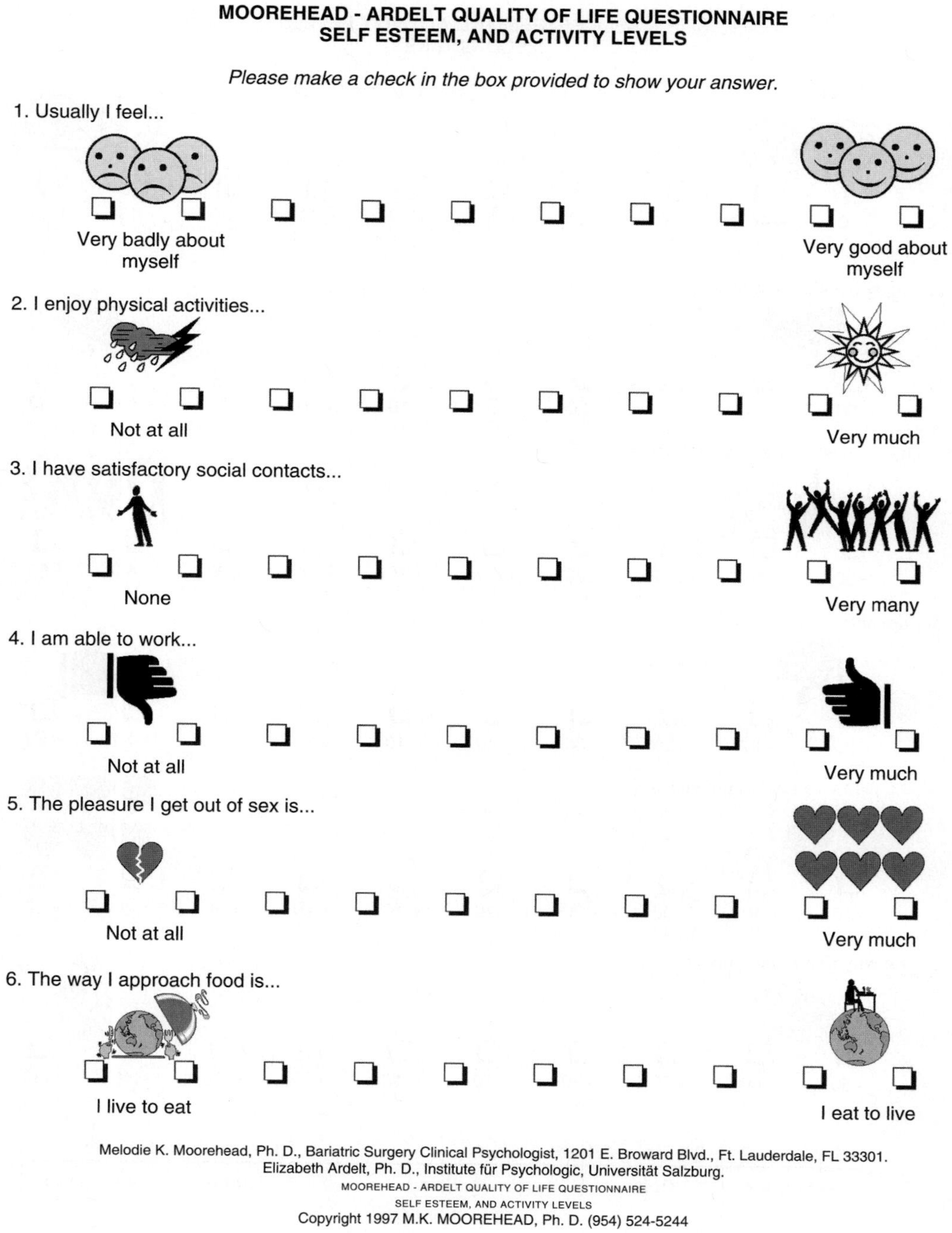

Figure 40-2. The Moorehead-Ardelt Quality of Life Questionnaire II. *(Copyright 1997, M.K. Moorehead, PhD.)*

and sexual activity. The simple vocabulary allows for easy translation into other languages, overcoming cultural, educational-level, and linguistic barriers. The inventory does not require an interviewer and can be completed by the patient in less than a minute, a fact important in reducing costs and increasing the response rate.

While the questionnaire was being developed, we considered that patients' self-esteem was a priority compared to the other four items. However, after trying the instrument in clinical settings, we realized that this assumption was inaccurate. We also found it appropriate to include a sixth question regarding patients' approach to food. In addition, the drawings were slightly modified, and a 10-point visual analogue scale was adopted, which required changes in the scoring key. The new M-A QOLQ II, shown in Figure 40-2, has recently been validated in clinical trials in the United States and Austria.[40] Figure 40-3 depicts the scoring key for the new questionnaire.

The final BAROS point score is used to classify results in five outcome groups: failure, fair, good, very good, and excellent, hence establishing a clear definition of success and failure. This allows for an objective assessment of

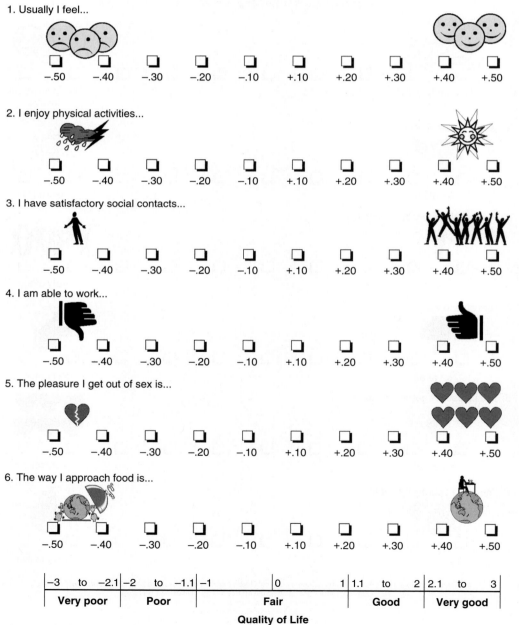

Figure 40-3. The Moorehead-Ardelt Quality of Life Questionnaire II scoring key. *(Copyright 1997, M.K. Moorehead, PhD.)*

Table 40-3	APPLICATION OF THE BAROS SCORE	
PREOPERATIVE	POSTOPERATIVE	POINTS
150% excess weight	Lost 45%	1
Sleep apnea/OHS	Resolved	2
Hypertension	Improved	
Dyslipidemia	Improved	
Self-esteem	Better	2
Activities	Improved	
Total		5
BAROS outcome score	GOOD	

Example of a male patient, 45 years old; height: 183 cm (6 ft); weight: 185 kg (410 lb); BMI: 55; ideal weight: 74 kg (164 lb); excess weight: 111 kg (246 lb); no complications or reoperations.

BAROS, Bariatric Analysis and Reporting Outcome System; OHS, obesity hypoventilation syndrome.

outcomes and facilitates a comparison of results among various surgical techniques, subgroups of patients, and surgeons. Table 40-3 demonstrates the usefulness of the system in impartially evaluating criteria other than weight loss. This hypothetical superobese male lost only 45% of his excess weight. According to some definitions of success, this would be a poor result or even a failure. However, this patient had significant improvement in comorbidities and QOL. The BAROS final score of five points classifies him as having a "good result," an outcome more objective than having "a failure." This innovative scoring system can be applied to healthy patients with no obesity-related conditions and also can be used if the postoperative QOL has not been studied (Table 40-4).

The BAROS has been extensively utilized internationally for many years in presenting results of individual series studying one or more operations and in comparing outcomes from various authors and countries, even if different operative techniques have been performed.[41-47] This method has been accepted as the standard for reporting results in Austria and all German-speaking countries, and in Brazil and Spain. Prestigious surgeons have recommended that the BAROS be adopted as a standard by the ASBS and IFSO.[48-50]

CONCLUSIONS

The evaluation of postoperative outcomes is of significant relevance to surgical investigators. It is clear now that the assessment and presentation of surgical results should include other end-points besides mortality, complication, and reoperation rates. The risks and side effects of the

Table 40-4	THE BAROS MODIFIED SCORING KEY
Failure	0 points or less
Fair	>0 to 1.5 points
Good	>1.5 to 3 points
Very good	>3 to 4.5 points
Excellent	>4.5 to 6 points

Classifies outcome groups in patients without comorbidities; it can also be used if quality of life is not included in the analysis.

BAROS, Bariatric Analysis and Reporting Outcome System.

operation may diminish the benefits of the treatment, especially in quality of life. In the particular field of surgery for morbid obesity, weight loss is clearly an insufficient criterion of overall success.

A satisfactory presentation of results after bariatric surgery should include long-term weight loss, details of the surgical technique, mortality, early and late morbidity, and reoperations caused by either complications or failure to lose weight. The rate of reoperation per year is another valuable parameter. The report would state the percentage of patients followed, the mean and median follow-up time, and how patients lost to follow-up are accounted for in the final analysis. The study of subgroups of patients is also desirable. As this chapter extensively discussed, a good-quality outcome report should include an objective assessment of the postoperative changes in obesity comorbidities and modifications in QOL that the patients experienced.

Outcomes evaluation in bariatric surgery is complicated by the lack of standards for comparison and the multiple and arbitrary definitions of success and failure encountered in the literature. Organizations such as the ASBS and IFSO should establish appropriate criteria to define a successful operation and should adopt uniform standards for outcome assessment and reporting of results. Such standards also could be helpful in comparing the effects of surgery against nonsurgical methods for the control of obesity. The BAROS fulfills all the requirements of a valuable instrument in international research. This method provides an evidence-based evaluation in a simple, unbiased, patient-friendly, and objective way. It analyzes weight loss, changes in obesity comorbidities, and QOL, and it defines diagnostic criteria and severity stratification of medical conditions. The instrument also takes into account early and late morbidity and reoperations. The final point-scoring key provides the much-needed classification of success and failure by dividing the patients into five groups.

The BAROS is a unique evaluation method for helping in the development of standards for the assessment and reporting of results in bariatric surgery.

REFERENCES

1. Rutkow IM: Surgery: An Illustrated History, p. 7. St. Louis, Mosby-Year Book, 1993.
2. Vibbert S: What Works: How Outcomes Research Will Change Medical Practice. Knoxville, Tenn., The Grand Rounds Press, Whittle Communications, 1993.
3. Ware JE, Sherbourne CD: The MOS Short-Form Survey (SF-36). I: Conceptual framework and item selection. Med Care 1992;30: 473-483.
4. Ellwood PM: Outcomes management: a technology of patient experience. N Engl J Med 1988;318:1549-1556.
5. Donabedian A: The quality of care: how can it be assessed? JAMA 1988;260:1743-1748.
6. Oria HE, Brolin RE: Performance standards in bariatric surgery. Eur J Gastroenterol Hepatol 1999;11:77-84; and in Deitel M, Cowan G (eds): Update: Surgery for the Morbidly Obese Patient, pp. 85-93. Toronto, FD-Communications, 2000.
7. Brook RH, McGlynn EA: Quality of health care. 2: Measuring quality of care. N Engl J Med 1996;335:966-969.
8. Brolin RE, Kasnetz KA, Greenfield DP, et al: A new classification system for weight loss analysis after bariatric operations. Clin Nutr 1986;5:5-8.
9. Fischer D, Stewart AL, Bloch DA, et al: Capturing the patient's view of change as a clinical outcome measure. JAMA 1999;282:1157-1162.

10. Testa MA, Simonson DC: Assessment of quality-of-life outcomes. N Engl J Med 1996;334:835-840.

11. Velanovich V: The quality of life studies in general surgical journals. J Am Coll Surg 2001;193:288-296.

12. Sullivan MBE, Sullivan LGM, Kral KG: Quality of life assessment in obesity: physical, psychological, and social function. Gastroenterol Clin North Am 1987;16:33-42.

13. Choban PS, Onyejekwe J, Burge JC, et al: A health status assessment of the impact of weight loss following Roux-en-Y gastric bypass for clinically severe obesity. J Am Coll Surg 1999;188:491-497.

14. Dixon JB, Dixon ME, O'Brien PE: Quality of life after Lap-Band placement: influence of time, weight loss, and comorbidities. Obes Res 2001;9:713-721.

15. Schwimmer JB, Burwinkle TM, Varni JW: Health-related quality of life of severely obese children and adolescents. JAMA 2003;289: 1813-1819.

16. Freys SM, Tigges H, Heimbucher J, et al: Quality of life following laparoscopic gastric banding in patients with morbid obesity. J Gastrointest Surg 2001;5:401-407.

17. Velanovich V: Comparison of generic (SF-36) vs. disease-specific (GERD-HRQL) quality-of-life scales for gastroesophageal reflux disease. J Gastrointest Surg 1998;2:141-145.

18. Kolotkin RL, Crosby RD, Kosloski KD, et al: Development of a brief measure to assess quality of life in obesity. Obes Res 2001;9: 102-111.

19. Kolotkin RL, Crosby RD, Pendleton R, et al: Health-related quality of life in patients seeking gastric bypass surgery vs. non-treatment-seeking controls. Obes Surg 2003;13:371-377.

20. Oria HE, Moorehead MK: Bariatric Analysis and Reporting Outcome System (BAROS). Obes Surg 1998;8:487-499.

21. National Institutes of Health Consensus Development Panel: National Institutes of Health Consensus Development Conference Statement, Gastrointestinal surgery for severe obesity. Ann Intern Med 1991;115:956-961.

22. Mason EE, Amaral JF, Cowan GSM, et al: Guidelines for selection of patients for surgical treatment of obesity. Obes Surg 1993;3:429.

23. American Society for Bariatric Surgery: Standards Committee Statement on length and percentage of follow-up. Obes Surg 2000;10:1.

24. Mason EE, Amaral JF, Cowan GSM, et al: Standards for reporting results. Obes Surg 1994;4:56-65.

25. Oria HE, Standards Committee, American Society for Bariatric Surgery: Guidelines for reporting results in bariatric surgery. Obes Surg 1997;7:521-522.

26. Renquist KE, Cullen JJ, Barnes D, et al: The effect of follow-up on reporting success for obesity surgery. Obes Surg 1995;5:285-292.

27. Oria HE: Reporting results in obesity surgery: evaluation of a limited survey. Obes Surg 1996;6:361-368.

28. Pories WJ, Flickinger EC, Meelheim D, et al: The effectiveness of gastric bypass over gastric partition in morbid obesity. Ann Surg 1982;196:389-399.

29. MacLean LD, Rhode BM, Shizgal HM: Gastroplasty for obesity. Surg Gynecol Obstet 1981;253:200-207.

30. Freeman JB, Burchett H: Failure rate with gastric partitioning for morbid obesity. Am J Surg 1983;145:113-119.

31. Mason EE, Maher JW, Scott DH, et al: Ten years of vertical banded gastroplasty for severe obesity. Probl Gen Surg 1992;9:280-289.

32. Halverson JD, Zuckerman GR, Koehler RE, et al: Gastric bypass for morbid obesity: a medical-surgical assessment. Ann Surg 1981;194: 152-160.

33. Reinhold RB: Critical analysis of long-term weight loss following gastric bypass. Surg Gynecol Obstet 1982;155:385-394.

34. Lechner GW, Elliott DW: Comparison of weight loss after gastric exclusion and partitioning. Arch Surg 1983;118:685-692.

35. Shape Up America! Organization and the American Obesity Association. Guidance for treatment of adult obesity. Bethesda, Maryland, 1996.

36. Mason EE, Tang T, Renquist KE, et al: A decade of change in obesity surgery. Obes Surg 1997;7:189-197.

37. Oria HE, American Society for Bariatric Surgery. Surgery for Morbid Obesity: What Patients Should Know. Toronto, FD-Communications, 2000. (Spanish translation, 2002.)

38. Wyss C, Laurent-Jaccard A, Burckhardt P, et al: Long-term results on quality of life of surgical treatment of obesity with vertical banded gastroplasty. Obes Surg 1995;5:387-392.

39. Delin CR, Watts JM, Bassett DL, et al: An exploration of the outcomes of gastric bypass surgery for morbid obesity: patient characteristics and indices of success. Obes Surg 1995;5:159-170.

40. Moorehead MK, Ardelt-Gattinger E, Lechner H, et al: The validation of the Moorehead-Ardelt Quality of Life Questionnaire II. Obes Surg 2003;13:684-692.

41. Favretti F, Cadiere GB, Segato G, et al: Bariatric Analysis and Reporting Outcome System (BAROS). Obes Surg 1998;8:500-504.

42. Hell E, Miller KA, Moorehead MK, et al: Evaluation of health status and quality of life after bariatric surgery: comparison of standard Roux-en-Y gastric bypass, vertical banded gastroplasty and laparoscopic adjustable silicone gastric banding. Obes Surg 2000;10: 214-219.

43. Wolf AM, Falcone AR, Kortner B, et al: BAROS: an effective system to evaluate the results of patients after bariatric surgery. Obes Surg 2000;10:445-450.

44. Nguyen NT, Goldman C, Rosenquist CT, et al: Laparoscopic versus open gastric bypass: a randomized study of outcomes, quality of life, and costs. Ann Surg 2001;11:265-270.

45. Victorzon M, Tolonen P: Bariatric Analysis and Reporting Outcome System (BAROS) following laparoscopic adjustable gastric banding in Finland. Obes Surg 2001;11:740-743.

46. Kalfarentzos F, Kechagias MD, Soulikia K, et al: Weight loss following vertical banded gastroplasty: intermediate results of a prospective study. Obes Surg 2001;11:265-270.

47. Nini E, Slim K, Scesa JL, et al: Evaluation of laparoscopic bariatric surgery using the BAROS score. Ann Chir 2002;127:107-114.

48. Hell E: IFSO and the future of surgery. Fifth Congress of the International Federation for the Surgery of Obesity, Genoa, September 22, 2000. Obes Surg 2000;10:495-497.

49. Cowan Jr GSM: Obligations of the bariatric surgeon. Fourth Congress of the International Federation for the Surgery of Obesity, Salzburg, September 24, 1999. Obes Surg 2000;10:498-501.

50. Scopinaro N: Outcome evaluation after bariatric surgery. Obes Surg 2002;12:253.

41

Nutritional Outcomes of Bariatric Surgery

John B. Dixon, M.B.B.S., Ph.D., F.R.A.C.G.P. and Paul E. O'Brien, M.D., F.R.A.C.S.

For the obese, the benefits of weight loss are overwhelming. The comorbidities of obesity improve or are resolved completely, the quality of life improves, and there are major psychosocial benefits.[1] However, in achieving these benefits, we must remember the first dictum of health care: *primum non nocere*—first do no harm. There may be a nutritional price to be paid for the weight loss. We must be committed to minimizing or deleting this cost in order that the full nutritional benefits of weight loss, especially secondary to bariatric surgery, can also be achieved. In this chapter, we review the range of nutritional problems that have been identified in association with bariatric surgery, characterize the mechanisms of their occurrence, and define strategies to minimize the problems.

The nutritional problems of bariatric procedures reflect the mechanisms of effect of each procedure. Weight loss is achieved by reducing the intake or the absorption of nutrients. There are two fundamental mechanisms for reducing the intake. First, it may be reduced by creating a sense of satiety, of reducing the almost constant background sense of hunger, so that food is not sought. It is probable that this is a component of most bariatric procedures but, in general, this mechanism has been poorly studied and documented. We have demonstrated this to be an important effect after laparoscopic adjustable gastric banding surgery (LAGB). Second, bariatric procedures may create a sense of fullness early after commencing eating, thereby inducing early satiety. This is the so-called restrictive effect, most prominent as a mechanism in gastroplasty but also important in LAGB and Roux-en-Y gastric bypass (RYGB). The role of malabsorption of nutrients as a mechanism of current bariatric procedures varies greatly with the procedure used. It is most prominent after biliopancreatic diversion (BPD) and its duodenal switch variant, but is undoubtedly significant after all forms of RYGB. A profile of possible malnutrition can be established for each current bariatric procedure and an awareness of this profile is mandatory if adequate follow-up care of the patient is to occur.

The following nutritional criteria have been enunciated by Dr. Luc Van Gaal for dietary weight-loss programs.[2]

We believe that these criteria are equally appropriate for bariatric surgical procedures:

1. The diet should be safe and include adequate vitamins, minerals, and protein. It should be low in energy but not in essential nutrients. The diet should provide adequate dietary fiber.
2. Weight-loss programs should be directed toward a slow, steady weight loss unless the health condition of the patient requires more rapid weight loss.
3. The diet must be palatable and acceptable to the patient to achieve high patient compliance.
4. Strategies for weight maintenance should be implemented.

Thus dietary strategies have to be complemented by behavioral change and increased physical activity. In addition, there are specific considerations related to each of the surgical techniques used to achieve weight loss. Procedures with a diversionary or malabsorptive component are more likely to produce specific deficiencies or metabolic risks, and procedures that are too restrictive may lead to maladaptive eating patterns, producing significant changes in nutrient intake.

Jejunoileal bypass (JIB), a procedure no longer performed, provided the paradigm for a malabsorptive procedure that produced a plethora of major metabolic problems and nutritional deficiencies. It perhaps provides a model of the potential nutritional problems that may follow less intrusive surgery. The long-term complications of JIB included arthralgia or arthritis, oxalate urolithiasis, metabolic bone disease,[3] multiple vitamin and mineral deficiencies,[4-6] and liver failure.[7] These effects resulted not only from malabsorption but also from the additional toxic effects of gastrointestinal bacterial overgrowth.

▶ MACRONUTRIENT DEFICIENCY

Protein deficiency, or malnutrition, has until recently been the only focus of investigation into macronutrient deficiency following bariatric surgery. Deficiency of carbohydrate has not been an issue, but concern has recently been raised regarding deficiency in essential fatty acids in association with fat malabsorption.

Protein Malnutrition

A major reduction in energy intake or absorption following bariatric surgery leads to rapid weight loss. Mobilization of free fatty acids from adipose tissue and amino acids from muscle are needed to provide essential oxidative substrates for metabolic and brain function. As amino acids are diverted to gluconeogenesis, protein synthesis and metabolic rate are reduced. There is a concomitant reduction in both fat and lean body mass. Protein intake may be disproportionately reduced as a result of intolerance to high protein foods, increasing loss of lean body mass.[8] Mobilization of amino acids from muscle supports some albumin synthesis; low albumin levels postoperatively reflect significant protein depletion.

The degree of protein malnutrition following bariatric surgery is uncertain because diagnostic criteria vary from study to study. However, protein malnutrition is a serious complication and may occur with continued rapid weight loss or excessive weight loss after any form of bariatric surgery. Protein malnutrition is likely to be accompanied by a range of nutritional deficiencies. Several case reports discuss the results of gastroplasty,[9,10] but the risk appears to be greater with procedures that have a significant component of malabsorption such as RYGB, especially distal gastric bypass,[11,12] and BPD.[13,14] The duodenal switch variant of BPD may produce a lower risk than the original operation.[15]

The management of protein malnutrition requires an assessment of the underlying problem, assisted enteral feeding or parenteral nutrition, and correction of any associated nutritional deficiency. Revisional surgery may be necessary to improve intestinal absorption. Recovery may be quite slow and must be carefully monitored.

Essential Fatty Acids

Procedures producing significant fat malabsorption also impair the absorption of fat-soluble vitamins and essential fatty acids. The essential fatty acids linoleic and α-linolenic acid are the precursors for prostaglandin and leukotriene production. Deficiency can lead to alopecia, dermatitis, thrombocytopenia, and anemia. Unfortunately, very few studies have looked at the potential problems associated with essential fatty acids following bariatric surgery. Obese subjects have low levels of essential fatty acids and vitamin E in their plasma during dietary restriction, and fat malabsorption is very likely to be associated with fatty-acid deficiency.[16,17] One study has reported deficiency of essential fatty acids 1 year following biliopancreatic diversion/duodenal switch (BPD/DS).[18] The quality of dietary fat may be very important after bariatric surgery, especially surgery causing fat malabsorption.

▶ MICRONUTRIENT DEFICIENCY

Iron

Iron is absorbed as the ferrous form, and gastric acid aids in conversion from the ferric ion in food to its ferrous form.

Iron is best absorbed in the duodenum and upper jejunum. Iron deficiency anemia is a common complication of gastric bypass surgery.[19] This may result from several surgically induced factors: gastric bypass limits the exposure of food to gastric acid; the region of optimal iron absorption is bypassed by the surgery; and meat intake is often reduced after gastric bypass.[20,21] Brolin and colleagues reported iron deficiency in 32% of patients at a mean follow-up of 2 years after bypass and of these, 67% developed anemia.[22] By 42 months after surgery, 47% were iron deficient and almost one third had microcytic anemia.[23] Iron deficiency does not appear to be more common in subjects having long-limb gastric bypass (150-cm defunctionalized jejunum) when compared with the standard (75-cm defunctionalized jejunum). Low iron levels continue to be a significant problem years after gastric bypass surgery when weight is stable and therefore energy intake and expenditure are balanced.[24] Routine micronutrient supplementation did not prevent iron deficiency or anemia, but significant oral iron supplementation of 350 mg twice daily was able to prevent the development of iron deficiency in the majority of menstruating women.[25] It is important to have adequate stores before the last trimester of pregnancy because refractory iron deficiency anemia may occur when fetal iron demands are very high. Thus, significant iron supplementation, for an indefinite period, is required to prevent iron deficiency, especially in menstruating women.[26] It is relevant to note that low iron levels are expected after both partial and total gastrectomy. Late follow-up, 25 to 30 years after subtotal gastrectomy, found iron deficiency and B_{12} deficiency in 90% of women and 70% of men, indicating the need for indefinite long-term biochemical monitoring and supplementation.[27] The gastric bypass should be expected to cause no less a problem.

Iron deficiency may occur after gastroplasty or LAGB as a result of reduced dietary intake, related principally to a reduction in meat intake, but it is not a common or predictable event.[27] BPD may also reduce the opportunity for iron absorption within the gut, and iron deficiency anemia has been reported as a common event if careful supplementation is not provided.[28,29] Limiting gastric resection and retaining the continuity of the antrum, pylorus, and cuff of the duodenum may help to minimize the effect. Indeed, one study has reported ferritin levels are better maintained after the BPD/DS variant of the operation.[15] The duodenal switch procedure may also reduce the risk for iron loss associated with gastrointestinal bleeding resulting from stomal ulcers.

Regular adequate iron supplementation is needed to prevent iron deficiency after any surgery with a diversionary component. Hemoglobin, serum iron status, and ferritin should be monitored after all bariatric surgery. Iron deficiency should be treated with oral iron. Ferrous sulfate, 200 mg three times a day, is a simple and cheap choice.[30] Iron tablets can cause local irritation and erosion of the gastric mucosa. Consequently, if significant gastric restriction or delayed emptying is suspected, a liquid preparation may be more appropriate.[31] Iron tablets are often coated and gastric acid is required to allow full bioavailability. Thus, a liquid preparation may also be appropriate after gastric bypass. The addition of ascorbic acid may enhance absorption. Once iron stores have been replenished, the daily iron dose can usually be reduced to improve compliance; lower doses reduce the incidence of the common gastrointestinal side effects. Compliance is important. If supplementation is inadequate, iron deficiency anemia returns.[32] Parenteral iron should be used only if there is intolerance to at least two iron preparations or if there is noncompliance.[30]

Vitamin B₁₂

The only dietary sources of vitamin B_{12} are animal products—meat and dairy. Vitamin B_{12} deficiency leads to megaloblastic anemia and, via demyelination, to potentially irreversible neurologic changes, including peripheral neuropathy, subacute combined degeneration of the spinal chord, optic atrophy, and dementia. Inadequacy or deficiency of vitamin B_{12} raises homocysteine concentrations, leading to greater endothelial dysfunction and increasing the risk for both arteriosclerotic and venous thromboembolic diseases. It is also likely to increase the risk for birth defects, including neural tube defects.

Gastric acid facilitates vitamin B_{12} release from food and its attachment to gastric R binder. Digestion of this complex in the duodenum allows the release of vitamin B_{12}, which then binds to intrinsic factor (IF), a product of the gastric parietal cells. The vitamin B_{12}-IF complex is then absorbed with the assistance of specific receptors in the distal ileum. Body stores of vitamin B_{12} are usually considerable and if absorption were to cease abruptly it may take more than a year for deficiency to present. Vitamin B_{12} absorption is not likely to be an issue in gastric restrictive procedures.

Vitamin B_{12} deficiency is common following RYGB,[33,34] and the deficiency may not be prevented by a standard multivitamin preparation.[23,35] The Schillings test may be normal or abnormal. An abnormal Schillings test is generally associated with reduced or absent IF in the gastric juice.[36,37] Deficiency in the presence of a normal Schillings test possibly results from reduced acid-pepsin activity, which may fail to release protein-bound vitamin B_{12}, or from inadequate intestinal vitamin B_{12}-IF mixing, which may not allow therapeutic reliability.[38] Vitamin B_{12} deficiency is seen in up to 30% of patients who receive the recommended daily intake of vitamin B_{12}, indicating that routine supplementation is often inadequate.[35] Specific vitamin B_{12} supplementation following gastric bypass is required, and 350 µg of oral crystalline B_{12} has been shown to provide adequate replacement of vitamin B_{12} in 95% of patients.[38] Low vitamin B_{12} is seen in a high percentage of patients (36%) 22 months following gastric bypass surgery. Vitamin B_{12} deficiency in nursing mothers is associated with low breast milk vitamin B_{12}, and vitamin B_{12} deficiency has been reported in breast-fed infants.[39,40] Vitamin B_{12} deficiency does not appear to be more common in patients having long-limb gastric bypass than in those undergoing the standard technique.[23]

Reports of significant vitamin B_{12} deficiency following BPD are few but are similar to those seen following RYGB.[41] Theoretically, the duodenal switch variant of this operation should provide less risk for vitamin B_{12} deficiency. No data on this comparison are available.

Folate

Folate is a water-soluble vitamin that functions as a one-carbon-unit transfer coenzyme for the synthesis of purines and pyramidines and for amino acid conversions. Folate is absorbed principally in the proximal third of the small intestine and is partly pH dependent. Gastric atrophy, achlorhydria, and gastrectomy have all been associated with some malabsorption of folate.[42] However, increased bacterial presence in the small bowel may allow for increased bacterial folate production, countering this effect.[43] Low folate levels were found in 30% of patients following total or subtotal gastrectomy. Deficiency can be attributed to inadequate intake; to increased demand, for example during pregnancy; or to malabsorption. Stores last no more than a few months after intake ceases.

It has been established that folic acid supplements can prevent neural tube defects.[44] Mills and colleagues have shown increased homocysteine levels in women carrying fetuses with neural tube defects.[45,46] They hypothesize that the folate- and vitamin B_{12}-dependent enzyme methionine synthetase is likely to be the critical pathway, and that adequate methionine is needed for neural tube closure. Cuskelly and colleagues[47] showed that increasing dietary folic acid in food was inadequate, so folate supplementation of 400 µg per day is recommended for women who could become pregnant so as to prevent neural tube defects.[44,48] Folate deficiency is also associated with megaloblastic anemia and increased cardiovascular risk.

Folate deficiency has been reported to be common after RYGB surgery.[9,49] However, the incidence varies greatly, and with adequate oral intake of supplements, deficiency is readily prevented.[50,51] A folate supplement of 400 µg per day will minimize homocysteine levels in most people,[52] and this is the minimum recommended dosage for all patients after bariatric surgery. We have demonstrated that this dosage is sufficient to maintain both adequate folate and optimal low homocysteine concentrations following LAGB surgery. There are no data to indicate an appropriate dosage of folate to maintain optimal homocysteine levels following RYGB or BPD.

Vitamin B₆

The coenzyme form of vitamin B_6 is pyridoxal phosphate, an essential cofactor and stabilizer for many enzymes involved in amino acid metabolism. Vitamin B_6 is available in many foods and is readily absorbed; deficiency is rare. Requirements are increased by pregnancy and by estrogens. Deficiency may be seen in those taking drugs that have a pyridoxal-antagonist effect, for example, isoniazid and penicillamine. Supplementation may be required during pregnancy and for those taking oral contraceptives. Specific deficiencies have not been reported following bariatric surgery.

Homocysteine: Weight Loss and Raised Plasma Homocysteine Levels

There is now consistent evidence that fasting plasma homocysteine levels rise with weight loss.[53-55] A raised level of homocysteine, an amino acid, is associated with a broad range of cardiovascular events, including myocardial infarction, stroke, and thromboembolic disease,[56] and is a recognized independent risk factor for cardiovascular disease,[57] along with overweight, smoking, high blood pressure, hypercholesterolemia, and type 2 diabetes. It has a direct toxic effect on vascular endothelium, leading to dysfunction, a key early step in the atherogenic process.[58] Three micronutrients are important cofactors in homocysteine metabolism. Folate and vitamin B_{12} are cofactors for the methylation of homocysteine into the essential amino acid methionine, and vitamin B_6 is involved in its catabolism. The rise in homocysteine levels with weight loss occurs independently of the plasma levels of folate and vitamin B_{12}, but responds to supplementary folate and vitamin B_{12}. With weight loss, higher levels of plasma micronutrients are required to maintain optimal low homocysteine levels.[55] It is, therefore, recommended that all bariatric surgical patients take adequate supplements of folate, vitamin B_{12}, and vitamin B_6, and that fasting plasma homocysteine levels be monitored.[59] Homocysteine levels greater than 15 µmol/l are abnormally high. The American Heart Association recommends that levels of homocysteine be maintained below 10 µmol/l. Supplementation should be provided to achieve levels below 10 µmol/l.

Thiamine (Vitamin B_1)

Thiamine pyrophosphate is required for branched amino acid and carbohydrate metabolism. It is readily absorbed by both passive and active mechanisms, with the greatest deficiency resulting from poor dietary intake. Total body storage is approximately 30 mg, and biological half-life ranges from 9 to 18 days.

Deficiency induces anorexia, irritability, apathy, and generalized weakness. More prolonged deficiency produces wet or dry beriberi syndromes. In both forms, patients complain of pain and paraesthesia. Wet beriberi presents with high-output congestive cardiac failure and peripheral neuritis. Dry beriberi presents with a symmetrical mixed motor and sensory peripheral neuropathy. The central nervous system can also be affected by Wernicke encephalopathy, which is characterized by nystagmus, ophthalmoplegia, cerebellar ataxia, and mental impairment. The addition of loss of memory and confabulation is known as Wernicke-Korsakoff syndrome, a condition usually described in alcoholics.

Wernicke-Korsakoff syndrome is a serious nutritional complication that can follow rapid weight loss after bariatric surgery. Most case reports cite persistent or severe vomiting in conjunction with rapid weight loss soon after the surgery as the usual precipitating conditions. Thiamine-related neurologic disorders should be prevented by appropriately managing any complication leading to vomiting and by instituting parenteral vitamin B_1 supplementation early, should persistent vomiting occur.[60-64] Neurologic conditions occurring soon after surgery should be viewed with a high degree of suspicion, and urgent vitamin B_1 therapy should be commenced.[65] Routine multivitamin supplementation after all forms of bariatric surgery should include vitamin B_1.

Of interest is a recent report describing a fall in vitamin B_1 levels following distal or total gastrectomy for cancer. The problem usually occurred in the first 6 months following surgery,[66] and this further emphasizes the need for early supplementation. The laboratory diagnosis of thiamine deficiency is usually made by measuring transketolase activity. Thiamine is a coenzyme for the transketolase reaction. Acute deficiency should be treated with 100 mg per day of thiamine parenterally for 7 days. followed by adequate oral supplementation.

Calcium, Vitamin D, and Metabolic Bone Disease

Vitamin D is functionally a hormone rather than a vitamin and, with adequate sunlight exposure, no dietary intake is necessary. Production of the active form, $1,25(OH)_2D_3$, appears to be regulated physiologically by extracellular calcium and parathyroid hormone concentrations. Oral vitamin D absorption occurs via chylomicrons and is impaired by conditions causing steatorrhea. Skin production of vitamin D may be inadequate if ultraviolet exposure is poor, as is during limited sun exposure, in higher latitudes in winter, in cases of increased melanin pigmentation, and because of atmospheric factors such as smog. Calcium is absorbed principally by active transport in the duodenum and upper jejunum, a process closely linked to that of the active form of vitamin D.

Metabolic bone disease is a well-documented long-term complication of bariatric surgery. Symptoms of metabolic bone disease in adults are often nonspecific, and the diagnosis is commonly delayed. Generalized skeletal pain, muscle weakness, and bony tenderness are usual symptoms, and pathologic fractures may occur. The diagnosis of metabolic bone disease is often difficult because symptoms can mimic other diseases. Those who care for patients after bariatric surgery should have a low threshold for the exclusion of metabolic bone disease when vague but suspicious symptoms occur.

Gastric restrictive procedures do not impair calcium or vitamin D absorption and, if intake remains adequate, metabolic bone disease is unlikely. A study of 18 patients followed for up to 2 years after vertical banded gastroplasty (VBG) found a small but significant fall in upper femoral but not in lumbar bone density. There was an increase in urinary hydroxyproline excretion but no evidence of hyperparathyroidism or vitamin D deficiency.[67] These findings have been confirmed following LAGB surgery.[68] In a small study of 17 patients after LAGB, we found no reduction in total body bone mineral density at a median of 30 months after surgery.[69]

Gastric bypass with duodenal exclusion is likely to reduce the absorption of calcium, which is absorbed principally in the duodenum and upper jejunum; insufficient intake of calcium or vitamin D leads to secondary hyperparathyroidism and metabolic bone disease.[70,71] There is detailed knowledge about the bone changes following gastrectomy for ulcer or cancer,[72,73] but less is known about the effects of gastric and duodenal exclusion following bariatric surgery.[74] Metabolic bone disease following gastrectomy may not present for many years; it is characterized by low urinary calcium, raised alkaline phosphatase, high parathyroid hormone, and in some cases low $25(OH)D_3$. Bone histology may show a mixed picture of osteoporosis and osteomalacia.[75] Metabolic bone disease has been reported following RYGB. Shaker and colleagues describe two women with metabolic bone disease associated with secondary hyperparathyroidism. Another six were also examined. Seven of the eight had raised parathyroid hormone, and six had low urinary calcium excretion; both mean lumbar spine and hip mineral density were below predicted levels in the group.[76] It is of concern that Crowley and colleagues found that after RYGB surgery, 90% of patients were taking inadequate vitamin D and 54% inadequate calcium.[70] A case report of severe metabolic bone disease 17 years after gastric bypass has been published.[77] Hypocalcemia has been reported to occur in 13% and low vitamin A and D in 23% of patients after distal RYGB.[12]

A study in the United States of 17 consecutive adults with vitamin D-deficient osteomalacia indicated that all had gastrointestinal disorders, and 12 had histories of gastrointestinal surgery producing malabsorption. The procedures included six bariatric surgeries, four gastrectomies, one intestinal resection for Crohn disease, and one Whipple procedure. Patients almost always had significant symptoms of osteomalacia, but only in the minority had the diagnosis been considered prior to referral. There was a long period between the gastrointestinal surgery and the development of osteomalacia, and there was a long delay between the development of symptoms and the diagnosis. The best noninvasive clues to diagnosis were the patients' histories and raised levels of serum alkaline phosphatase and parathyroid hormone. In all persons in whom vitamin D deficiency is a possibility, yearly examination of $25(OH)D_3$ and parathyroid hormone levels is recommended.[78]

Metabolic bone disease commonly follows BPD surgery. Compston and colleagues described it as being characterized in the majority of patients by defective mineralization, decreased bone formation rate, and increased bone resorption. Of the group, 22% were hypocalcemic, but serum $25(OH)D_3$ concentrations were normal in all patients.[79] A high oral intake of calcium and supplementary vitamin D is advised in order to prevent the problem.[28] The duodenal switch variant may provide the advantages of higher mean calcium concentrations, lower parathyroid levels, and a significantly smaller proportion of patients complaining of bone pain than is found after the BPD with distal gastrectomy procedure.[15] A recent report concerning nutritional markers following the duodenal switch procedure found mean parathyroid hormone levels to be abnormal 2 years after surgery, indicating a high risk for metabolic bone disease in the majority of patients.[80] It is of interest that peak bone demineralization appears to occur at around 4 years after surgery but has not been found to be an increasing problem thereafter.[13,28] Some late spontaneous improvement in metabolic bone disease has also been reported following JIB, suggesting long-term adaptation.[81]

Vitamin D and calcium intake should be assessed in all patients after they have undergone bariatric surgery, and all patients should receive 1200 to 1500 mg calcium and 800 IU vitamin D per day. After procedures in which malabsorption of calcium or vitamin D is likely, yearly screening of calcium, alkaline phosphatase, $25(OH)D_3$, and parathyroid hormone levels is recommended.[77] A rise in alkaline phosphatase or parathyroid hormone would be the first biochemical sign of metabolic bone disease and would indicate the need to increase calcium and vitamin D therapy. Metabolic bone disease is treated with calcium and vitamin D supplementation; often, high doses are required, and the adequacy of treatment should be monitored by biochemical assessment.

Micronutrients

ZINC

Low zinc intake has been reported in obese subjects, and intake falls with reduced caloric consumption.[82] It has been proposed that hair loss following VBG may be caused by zinc deficiency because zinc supplementation arrested hair loss and promoted hair growth.[83] Malabsorptive procedures, too, are likely to reduce zinc levels; one report indicates that 69% of patients had low zinc levels 1 year after BPD/DS surgery.[18] Zinc should be included in the multivitamin supplementation after all forms of bariatric surgery.

VITAMINS A, E, AND K

Procedures producing significant fat malabsorption also impair the absorption of fat-soluble vitamins and essential fatty acids. Symptomatic deficiency has been reported. Night blindness and prolonged prothrombin time have responded to vitamin A and D supplementation following JIB. A case report of maternal night blindness and fetal retinal damage has been reported following BPD.[84] Few studies have looked at the potential problems associated with fat-soluble vitamins and essential fatty acids following bariatric surgery. A single study has reported deficiencies in essential fatty acids 1 year after BPD/DS, and the same study found that one third of subjects had low vitamin A levels.[18] The quality of dietary fat may be very important after bariatric surgery, especially surgery causing fat malabsorption.

MAGNESIUM

Very low magnesium levels have been reported after JIB, and normal levels have been reported after gastric restrictive procedures, but the effect on magnesium levels of the currently performed malabsorptive procedures, such as BPD and BPD/DS, is unknown.

▶ SUMMARY OF THE NUTRITIONAL CONSEQUENCES OF CURRENT BARIATRIC PROCEDURES

This summary of nutritional consequences must consider the surgeries in the following sequence: LAGB, VBG, RYBG, and finally BPD or BPD/DS. The challenges associated with the less intrusive procedures increase greatly in the more intrusive diversionary and malabsorptive procedures (Table 41-1).

Laparoscopic Adjustable Gastric Band

Weight loss following LAGB is usually well controlled, and the risk for persistent vomiting and maladaptive eating behavior is very low as a result of adjustability. This reduces the risk for nutritional deficit. However, adequate folate, vitamin B_{12}, and vitamin B_6 are needed to maintain low homocysteine levels. Foods high in iron content such as red meats are often avoided, putting premenopausal women at risk for iron deficiency. Appropriate dietary advice must be provided and iron status should be monitored and supplements provided if necessary. Optimal maternal weight gain and fetal nutrition during pregnancy can be achieved by

Table 41-1	ESTIMATED RISK FOR SPECIFIC DEFICIENCIES OR INCREASED REQUIREMENTS BASED ON THE TYPE OF SURGERY PERFORMED

	LAGB	VBG	RYGB	BPD	BPD/DS
Iron	+	+	+++	+++	++
Thiamine	+	++	+	+	+
Vitamin B_{12}	+	+	+++	++	++
Folate	++	++	++	++	++
Calcium	+	+	++	+++	+++
Vitamin D	+	+	+	+++	+++
Protein	+	+	+	++	++
Fat-soluble vitamins and essential fatty acids	+	+	+	+++	+++

+, Recommended dietary allowance or standard multivitamin preparation is likely to be sufficient.

++, Significant risk for deficiency or increased requirements; specific supplementation is appropriate, especially in higher risk groups.

+++, High risk for deficiency; additional specific supplementation is necessary to prevent deficiency. Careful monitoring is recommended. Supplementation well in excess of daily requirements may be necessary.

LAGB, laparoscopic adjustable gastric banding; VBG, vertical banded gastroplasty; RYGB, Roux-en-Y gastric bypass; BPD, biliopancreatic diversion; BPD/DS, biliopancreatic diversion/duodenal switch.

judicious band adjustment, a facility that should be used.[85] Complications involved with the band should be recognized early, and if they are compromising nutritional status, they should be treated promptly. Parenteral thiamine should be administered if there are any persistent obstructive symptoms or vomiting.

A simple daily multivitamin preparation containing vitamin B_{12}, vitamin B_6, and at least 400 μg of folic acid is recommended for all patients. These vitamins can readily be obtained in preparations containing a range of other vitamins and minerals, including vitamin B_1 and zinc. The addition of a small quantity of iron to this preparation is appropriate for premenopausal women.

Vertical Banded Gastroplasty

After VBG, nutritional issues are similar to those that occur after the performance of LAGB. However, the fact that in this procedure the gastric stoma cannot be readily adjusted is likely to lead to an increased risk for food intolerance and maladaptive eating and therefore to nutritional imbalance. Multivitamin supplementation is recommended and additional nutritional support may be required during pregnancy. Persistent food intolerance may occur and additional thiamine may be necessary.

Roux-en-Y Gastric Bypass

In addition to the nutritional considerations after a VBG, which forms an essential element of RYGB, the partial gastric and duodenal exclusion involved in a RYGB add additional considerations; there is a major risk for iron and vitamin B_{12} deficiency and significant risk for inadequate folate and calcium intake. Careful, permanent nutritional

follow-up is essential. Vitamin B_{12}, folate, fasting homocysteine, and iron studies must be performed annually to assess the adequacy of supplementation. Metabolic bone disease is a possibility and should be monitored by measuring alkaline phosphatase and parathyroid hormone levels. Osteoporosis should be assessed by bone density measurement. The risk that nutritional deficiencies will present is high, even after many years.

Biliopancreatic Diversion and Biliopancreatic Diversion/Duodenal Switch

BPD has been proven to provide excellent weight loss over a prolonged period.[13] BPD and BPD/DS are the only commonly used bariatric surgical procedures that provide a major change in energy balance through the malabsorption of macronutrients. The balance of malabsorption and reduced caloric intake in BDP and BPD/DS is problematic and needs to be very finely balanced. If the patient continues to consume all foods at the presurgery rate, it is likely to lead to frequent bulky stools and significant diarrhea. The risk for broad-range nutritional problems is very high. In addition to all the concerns described previously in VBG and RYGB, there is also a greater likelihood of calcium and vitamin D deficiency, which increases the risk for metabolic bone disease. Alkaline phosphatase, $25(OH)D_3$, and parathyroid hormone levels must be regularly monitored, and there should be a low threshold for investigating any symptoms that may indicate bone pain. The risk for deficiencies in other fat-soluble vitamins or essential fatty acids must be further investigated. Protein levels need to be monitored closely, especially during the phase of rapid weight loss. Patients electing to have this form of bariatric surgery should be counseled that they will require a broad range of vitamin, mineral, and possibly macronutrient supplementation regularly, along with careful nutritional monitoring indefinitely.

There are theoretical reasons and some limited data to suggest that with the BPD/DS there is a lower risk for nutritional deficiency.[15] At the present time, however, there is insufficient evidence that a less intense or varied program of supplementation and monitoring could be followed.

▶ REFERENCES

1. Dixon JB, O'Brien PE: Changes in comorbidities and improvements in quality of life after LAP-BAND placement. Am J Surg 2002; 184:S51-S54.
2. Van Gaal L: Dietary treatment of obesity. In Bray GA, James WPT (eds): Handbook of Obesity, pp. 875-890. New York, Marcel Dekker, 1998.
3. Parfitt AM, Podenphant J, Villanueva AR, et al: Metabolic bone disease with and without osteomalacia after intestinal bypass surgery: a bone histomorphometric study. Bone 1985;6:211-220.
4. Atkinson RL, Dahms WT, Bray GA, et al: Plasma zinc and copper in obesity and after intestinal bypass. Ann Intern Med 1978;89:491-493.
5. Lavery JP: Magnesium deficiency in a pregnancy six years after jejunoileal bypass. J Am Coll Nutr 1984;3:187-191.
6. Enat R, Nagler A, Bassan L, et al: Night blindness and liver cirrhosis as late complications of jejunoileal bypass surgery for morbid obesity. Isr J Med Sci 1984;20:543-546.
7. Rucker RD Jr, Horstmann J, Schneider PD, et al: Comparisons between jejunoileal and gastric bypass operations for morbid obesity. Surgery 1982;92:241-249.

8. Moize V, Geliebter A, Gluck ME, et al: Obese patients have inadequate protein intake related to protein intolerance up to 1 year following Roux-en-Y gastric bypass. Obes Surg 2003;13:23-28.

9. MacLean LD, Rhode BM, Shizgal HM: Nutrition following gastric operations for morbid obesity. Ann Surg 1983;198:347-355.

10. Schneider SB, Erikson N, Gebel HM, et al: Cutaneous anergy and marrow suppression as complications of gastroplasty for morbid obesity. Surgery 1983;94:109-111.

11. Fobi MA, Lee H, Igwe D Jr, et al: Revision of failed gastric bypass to distal Roux-en-Y gastric bypass: a review of 65 cases. Obes Surg 2001;11:190-195.

12. Fox SR, Oh KH, Fox K: Vertical banded gastroplasty and distal gastric bypass as primary procedures: a comparison. Obes Surg 1996;6:421-425.

13. Scopinaro N, Gianetta E, Adami GF, et al: Biliopancreatic diversion for obesity at eighteen years. Surgery 1996;119:261-268.

14. Antal S: Treatment of protein malnutrition and uncontrollable diarrhea following biliopancreatic diversion with pancreas extract viokase. Obes Surg 1993;3:279-283.

15. Marceau P, Hould FS, Simard S, et al: Biliopancreatic diversion with duodenal switch. World J Surg 1998;22:947-954.

16. Reitman A, Friedrich I, Ben-Amotz A, et al: Low plasma antioxidants and normal plasma B vitamins and homocysteine in patients with severe obesity. Isr Med Assoc J 2002;4:590-593.

17. Rossner S, Walldius G, Bjorvell H: Fatty acid composition in serum lipids and adipose tissue in severe obesity before and after six weeks of weight loss. Int J Obes 1989;13:603-612.

18. Siegel N, Dugay G, Wolfe B, et al: Fat-soluable nutrient deficiency after malabsorptive operations for morbid obesity. Obes Surg 2003;13:204(abstr).

19. Blake M, Fazio V, O'Brien P: Assessment of nutrient intake in association with weight loss after gastric restrictive procedures for morbid obesity. Aust N Z J Surg 1991;61:195-199.

20. Amaral JF, Thompson WR, Caldwell MD, et al: Prospective hematologic evaluation of gastric exclusion surgery for morbid obesity. Ann Surg 1985;201:186-193.

21. Avinoah E, Ovnat A, Charuzi I: Nutritional status seven years after Roux-en-Y gastric bypass surgery. Surgery 1992;111:137-142.

22. Brolin RE, Gorman RC, Milgrim LM, et al: Multivitamin prophylaxis in prevention of post-gastric bypass vitamin and mineral deficiencies. Int J Obes 1991;15:661-667.

23. Brolin RE, Gorman JH, Gorman RC, et al: Are vitamin B12 and folate deficiency clinically important after Roux- en-Y gastric bypass? J Gastrointest Surg 1998;2:436-442.

24. Brolin RE, Kenler HA, Gorman JH, et al: Long-limb gastric bypass in the superobese: a prospective randomized study. Ann Surg 1992;215:387-395.

25. Brolin RE, Gorman JH, Gorman RC, et al: Prophylactic iron supplementation after Roux-en-Y gastric bypass: a prospective, double-blind, randomized study. Arch Surg 1998;133:740-744.

26. Gurewitsch ED, Smith-Levitin M, Mack J: Pregnancy following gastric bypass surgery for morbid obesity. Obstet Gynecol 1996;88:658-661.

27. Tovey FI, Godfrey JE, Lewin MR: A gastrectomy population: 25-30 years on. Postgrad Med J 1990;66:450-456.

28. Scopinaro N, Adami GF, Marinari GM, et al: Biliopancreatic diversion. World J Surg 1998;22:936-946.

29. Sileo F, Bonassi U, Bolognini C, et al: Biliopancreatic bypass in the treatment of severe obesity: long-term clinical, nutritional and metabolic evaluation. Minerva Gastroenterol Dietol 1995;41:149-155.

30. Goddard AF, McIntyre AS, Scott BB: Guidelines for the management of iron deficiency anaemia. Gut 2000;46(suppl 3-4):IV1-IV5.

31. Eckstein RP, Symons P: Iron tablets cause histopathologically distinctive lesions in mucosal biopsies of the stomach and esophagus. Pathology 1996;28:142-145.

32. Rhode BM, Shustik C, Christou NV, et al: Iron absorption and therapy after gastric bypass. Obes Surg 1999;9:17-21.

33. Yale CE, Gohdes PN, Schilling RF: Cobalamin absorption and hematologic status after two types of gastric surgery for obesity. Am J Hematol 1993;42:63-66.

34. Sugerman HJ, Starkey JV, Birkenhauer R: A randomized prospective trial of gastric bypass versus vertical banded gastroplasty for morbid obesity and their effects on sweets versus non-sweets eaters. Ann Surg 1987;205:613-624.

35. Provenzale D, Reinhold RB, Golner B, et al: Evidence for diminished B12 absorption after gastric bypass: oral supplementation does not prevent low plasma B12 levels in bypass patients. J Am Coll Nutr 1992;11:29-35.

36. Marcuard SP, Sinar DR, Swanson MS, et al: Absence of luminal intrinsic factor after gastric bypass surgery for morbid obesity. Dig Dis Sci 1989;34:1238-1242.

37. Crowley LV, Olson RW: Megaloblastic anemia after gastric bypass for obesity. Am J Gastroenterol 1983;78:406-410.

38. Rhode BM, Tamin H, Gilfix BM, et al: Treatment of vitamin B12 deficiency after gastric surgery for severe obesity. Obes Surg 1995;5:154-158.

39. Grange DK, Finlay JL: Nutritional vitamin B12 deficiency in a breastfed infant following maternal gastric bypass. Pediatr Hematol Oncol 1994;11:311-318.

40. Wardinski T, Montes R, Friederich R, et-al: Vitamin B12 deficiency associated with low breast milk vitamin B12 concentration in an infant following maternal gastric bypass. Arch Pediatr Adolesc Med 1995;149:1281-1284.

41. Skroubis G, Sakellaropoulos G, Pouggouras K, et al: Comparison of nutritional deficiencies after Roux-en-Y gastric bypass and after biliopancreatic diversion with Roux-en-Y gastric bypass. Obes Surg 2002;12:551-558.

42. Halsted CH: The intestinal absorption of dietary folates in health and disease. J Am Coll Nutr 1989;8:650-658.

43. Krasinski SD, Russell RM, Samloff IM, et al: Fundic atrophic gastritis in an elderly population: effect on hemoglobin and several serum nutritional indicators. J Am Geriatr Soc 1986;34:800-806.

44. Medical Research Council Vitamin Research Group: Prevention of neural tube defects: results of vitamin study. Lancet 1991;338:131-137.

45. Mills J, McPartlin J, Kirke P, et al: Homocysteine metabolism in pregnancy complicated by neural-tube defects. Lancet 1995;345:149-151.

46. Mills J, Scott J, Kirke P, et al: Homocysteine and neural tube defects. J Nutr 1996;126:756-760.

47. Cuskelly G, McNulty H, Scott J: Effect on increasing dietary folate on red-cell folate: implications for prevention of neural tube defects. Lancet 1996;347:657-659.

48. Medical Research Council Vitamin Research Group: Recommendation for the use of folic acid to reduce the number of cases of spina bifida and other neural tube defects. MMWR Morb Mortal Wkly Rep 1992;41:1-7.

49. Halverson J: Micronutrient deficiencies after gastric bypass for morbid obesity. Am J Surg 1986;52:594-598.

50. Mallory GN, Macgregor AM: Folate status following gastric bypass surgery (the great folate mystery). Obes Surg 1991;1:69-72.

51. Boylan LM, Sugerman HJ, Driskell JA: Vitamin E, vitamin B6, vitamin B12, and folate status of gastric bypass surgery patients. J Am Diet Assoc 1988;88:579-585.

52. Oakley GJ: Eat right and take a multivitamin. N Engl J Med 1998;338:1060-1061.

53. Henning B, Tepel M, Riezler R, et al: Vitamin supplementation during weight reduction: favourable effect on homocysteine metabolism. Res Exp Med 1998;198:37-42.

54. Borson-Chazot F, Harthe C, Teboul F, et al: Occurrence of hyperhomocysteinemia 1 year after gastroplasty for severe obesity. J Clin Endocrinol Metab 1999;84:541-545.

55. Dixon JB, Dixon ME, O'Brien PE: Elevated homocysteine levels with weight loss after Lap-Band surgery: higher folate and vitamin B12 levels required to maintain homocysteine level. Int J Obes Relat Metab Disord 2001;25:219-227.

56. Welsh G, Loscalzo J: Mechanisms of disease: homocysteine and atherothrombosis. N Engl J Med 1998;338:1042-1050.

57. Hankey GJ, Eikelboom JW: Homocysteine and vascular disease. Indian Heart J 2000;52:S18-S26.

58. Bellamy MF, McDowell IF, Ramsey MW, et al: Hyperhomocysteinemia after an oral methionine load acutely impairs endothelial function in healthy adults. Circulation 1998;98:1848-1852.

59. Dixon JB: Elevated homocysteine with weight loss. Obes Surg 2001;11:537-538.

60. Chaves LC, Faintuch J, Kahwage S, et al: A cluster of polyneuropathy and Wernicke-Korsakoff syndrome in a bariatric unit. Obes Surg 2002;12:328-334.

61. Bozbora A, Coskun H, Ozarmagan S, et al: A rare complication of adjustable gastric banding: Wernicke's encephalopathy. Obes Surg 2000;10:274-275.

62. Salas-Salvado J, Garcia-Lorda P, Cuatrecasas G, et al: Wernicke's syndrome after bariatric surgery. Clin Nutr 2000;19:371-373.

63. Toth C, Voll C: Wernicke's encephalopathy following gastroplasty for morbid obesity. Can J Neurol Sci 2001;28:89-92.

64. Seehra H, MacDermott N, Lascelles R, et al: Lesson of the week: Wernicke's encephalopathy after vertical banded gastroplasty for morbid obesity. BMJ 1996;312:43.

65. Maryniak O: Severe peripheral neuropathy following gastric bypass surgery for morbid obesity. CMAJ 1984;131:119-120.

66. Iwase K, Higaki J, Yoon HE, et al: Reduced thiamine (vitamin B_1) levels following gastrectomy for gastric cancer. Gastric Cancer 2002;5:77-82.

67. Cundy T, Evans MC, Kay RG, et al: Effects of vertical-banded gastroplasty on bone and mineral metabolism in obese patients. Br J Surg 1996;83:1468-1472.

68. Pugnale N, Giusti V, Suter M, et al: Bone metabolism and risk of secondary hyperparathyroidism 12 months after gastric banding in obese pre-menopausal women. Int J Obes Relat Metabol Disord 2003;27:110-116.

69. Strauss BJG, Marks SJ, Growcott JP, et al: Body composition changes following laparoscopic gastric banding for morbid obesity. Act a Diabetologica 2003;40(suppl. 1):S266-S269.

70. Crowley LV, Seay J, Mullin G: Late effects of gastric bypass for obesity. Am J Gastroenterol 1984;79:850-860.

71. Parfitt AM, Miller MJ, Frame B, et al: Metabolic bone disease after intestinal bypass for treatment of obesity. Ann Intern Med 1978;89:193-199.

72. Zittel TT, Zeeb B, Maier GW, et al: High prevalence of bone disorders after gastrectomy. Am J Surg 1997;174:431-438.

73. Tovey FI, Hall ML, Ell PJ, et al: A review of postgastrectomy bone disease. J Gastroenterol Hepatol 1992;7:639-645.

74. Mason EE: Bone disease from duodenal exclusion. Obes Surg 2000;10:585-586.

75. Fitzpatrick LA: Secondary causes of osteoporosis. Mayo Clin Proc 2002;77:453-468.

76. Shaker JL, Norton AJ, Woods MF, et al: Secondary hyperparathyroidism and asteopenia in women following gastric exclusion surgery for obesity. Osteoporosis International 1991;1:177-181.

77. Goldner WS, O'Dorisio TM, Dillon JS, et al: Severe metabolic bone disease as a long-term complication of obesity surgery. Obes Surg 2002;12:685-692.

78. Basha B, Rao DS, Han ZH, et al: Osteomalacia due to vitamin D depletion: a neglected consequence of intestinal malabsorption. Am J Med 2000;108:296-300.

79. Compston JE, Vedi S, Gianetta E, et al: Bone histomorphometry and vitamin D status after biliopancreatic bypass for obesity. Gastroenterology 1984;87:350-356.

80. Rabkin RA, Rabkin JM: Nutritional markers following the duodenal switch procedure. Obes Surg 2003;13:197(abstr).

81. Halverson JD, Haddad JG, Bergfeld M: Spontaneous healing of jejunoileal bypass-induced osteomalacia. Int J Obes 1989;13:497-504.

82. Cooper PL, Brearley LK, Jamieson AC, et al: Nutritional consequences of modified vertical gastroplasty in obese subjects. Int J Obes Relat Metabol Disord 1999;23:382-388.

83. Neve HJ, Bhatti WA, Soulsby C, et al: Reversal of hair loss following vertical gastroplasty when treated with zinc sulphate. Obes Surg 1996;6:63-65.

84. Huerta S, Rogers LM, Li Z, et al: Vitamin A deficiency in a newborn resulting from maternal hypovitaminosis A after biliopancreatic diversion for the treatment of morbid obesity. Am J Clin Nutr 2002;76:426-429.

85. Dixon JB, Dixon ME, O'Brien PE: Pregnancy after Lap-Band surgery: management of the band to achieve healthy weight outcomes. Obes Surg 2001;11:59-65.

42

Resolution of Bariatric Comorbidities: Diabetes

Walter J. Pories, M.D., F.A.C.S. and Stewart E. Rendon, M.D.

We were not prepared for the observation that the gastric bypass could make diabetes go away. It's not the way discoveries are made. Usually laboratories get the good news first from test tubes, sometimes from animal experiments. Further, totally new findings on the big diseases, like diabetes or cancer, just don't come along very often.

It happened during the early days of bariatric surgery when our group at East Carolina University, after testing several variations of the gastric bypass, found that the version shown in Figure 42-1 produced durable weight loss with an acceptable rate of complications. Initially, we did not

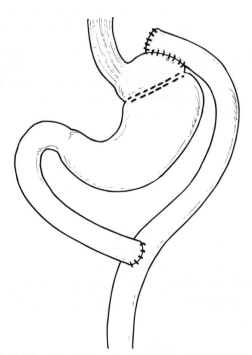

Figure 42-1. The Greenville version of the gastric bypass. The critical elements of the bypass included a small proximal gastric pouch between 15 and 30 ml, a gastrojejunostomy of 8 to 10 mm, and an alimentary Roux-en-Y loop of 60 cm.

accept diabetic patients. Morbid obesity offered enough challenges without adding the higher rates of infection and the difficulties of glucose control. In addition, the diabetic morbidly obese had higher rates of serious cardiopulmonary comorbidities. However, when it became apparent that at least one third of our patients were diabetic or glucose impaired we reconsidered our decision.

We had to deal with the issue of performing elective surgery on a morbidly obese diabetic patient. From our experience with other major operations in diabetics, we were aware that diabetes control could be difficult during the stress of postoperative recovery, especially if there were infectious complications. Therefore, we made elaborate preparations and instructed the patients and their families about the increased risk. Approaches to giving continuous intravenous insulin with sliding-scale protocols were elaborately devised. To our surprise, the need for increased insulin supplements failed to materialize; in fact, after a few days of sharply reduced doses of 4 to 8 units per day, the patients no longer needed the insulin at all. This observation was not expected.

Medical investigators are just like everyone else: we tend to see only the familiar, the expected. When the blood glucose levels came back to being within normal limits, we challenged these results and were initially convinced that the samples had been drawn incorrectly or that the hospital's laboratory was at fault. By the fourth patient, we actually accused the laboratory of sloppy work with the comment: "How can we take care of these sick folks if we can't trust tests as simple as blood sugar levels?" But those technicians were correct, and later, embarrassingly much later, we formally apologized for our unwarranted accusations.

The fifth patient's course is shown in Table 42-1. This woman, a same-day admission known for her poor compliance, reported to the hospital in November 1982 with a blood glucose level of 490, in spite of a morning dose of 90μ of insulin. She looked well otherwise, so we brought her to more reasonable levels with additional intravenous insulin doses and, after considerable discussion with her and among ourselves, we proceeded with surgery. By the next morning, on her first postoperative day, her daily

Table 42-1	EFFECT OF GASTRIC BYPASS ON PLASMA GLUCOSE AND SLIDING-SCALE INSULIN REQUIREMENTS	
DATE	GLUCOSE	INSULIN BY SLIDING SCALE
16 Nov., 1982 (preoperative)	495	90
17 Nov.	281	8
18 Nov.	308	16
19 Nov.	240	8
20 Nov.	210	4
21 Nov.	230	8
22 Nov.	216	4
28 Nov.	193	0
30 Nov.	153	0
14 Dec.	155	0

requirement had dropped to 8μ and within 6 days she no longer required insulin. She returned to fully normal glucose values within 3 months and has remained euglycemic, even with resumption of a diet that includes an unlimited choice of food but, of course, a limitation in volume because of the small gastric pouch.

▶ CONFIRMATION: GASTRIC BYPASS CAN CONTROL TYPE 2 DIABETES

Our experience with subsequent diabetic patients supported the initial observation and produced the surprising thesis that the gastric bypass operation can control type 2 diabetes. We continued to use the Greenville version of the gastric bypass, an operation that was developed through observations in about 200 patients between 1978 and 1980. The operation, shown in Figure 42-1, provides a gastric pouch of less than 30 ml, a gastrojejunostomy of 8 to 10 mm, and a Roux-en-Y conformation with a 60-cm limb. We carried out the identical, rigorously controlled operation for 16 years from 1980 to 1996.[1,2] In 1997, we altered our surgical approaches with the introduction of laparoscopy and, based on the work of Brolin and colleagues,[3] we lengthened our alimentary limbs to 100 cm for the morbidly obese and 150 cm for the superobese.

Figure 42-2 demonstrates our findings after we performed the gastric bypass operations on 608 patients. Of these individuals, 165 had type 2 diabetes and another 165 proved to have impaired glucose tolerance. Patients were allowed 6 months for equilibration, leaving for study 146 diabetics and 152 patients with impaired glucose tolerance. Over the 16 years during which we observed this group, with a 97.3% follow-up, we found that 121 of the 146 diabetics (83%) were returned to euglycemia, and of the 152 patients with impaired glucose tolerance, 150 (99%) were restored to euglycemia.[4]

The resolution of the hyperglycemia is also associated with a rapid correction of the hyperinsulinemia of diabetes. Levels drop sharply within a matter of days and reach normal values long before normal weight is attained.

In fact, the gastric bypass can overcorrect the problems of hyperglycemia and hyperinsulinemia. We recently reported our experience with 47 patients who suffered documented attacks of severe hypoglycemia following the operation. Fortunately, the problem was self-limited in all patients, usually clearing within a year and controllable by hard candy during the prodrome of the attacks.[5]

Why Did Some Fail?

The 27 patients who did not return to full euglycemia are of special interest. The situations in the 10 patients who had disruptions of their staple lines were easy to explain. The flow of their intake was not diverted; food continued to flow into the distal stomach. The remaining 17 patients, however, had intact operations documented by gastrointestinal series. They lost weight and although their diabetes was under better control, some hyperglycemia still persisted. What differentiated these individuals from the group was that they were older and had been burdened with diabetes longer than those who had had successful procedures.[6-8]

We concluded that durable control of diabetes was more likely to be attained in those who are young and have had diabetes for a shorter time. Or, to put it another way, morbidly obese patients who are diabetic should be considered for early bariatric surgery to obtain optimal results.

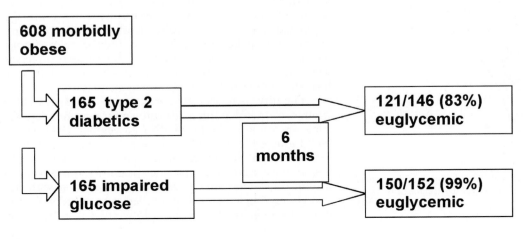

Figure 42-2. Durable control of type 2 diabetes following the gastric bypass operation.

Reduction in Mortality Rates

The question remained whether the gastric bypass merely corrected glucose levels or whether the operation also mitigated the effects of diabetes. We explored this question by comparing our surgical group with a matched cohort who did not undergo the procedure.

During the same period during which we performed gastric bypasses in the 154 patients noted previously, another 78 patients were evaluated and scheduled for surgery but, just prior to the planned surgery, cancelled the procedures for personal reasons or, more commonly, because insurance approval was refused. The two groups did not differ significantly in terms of gender, age, body mass index, or comorbidities. All mortalities were included, whether they were due to perioperative complications, automobile accidents, return to substance abuse, suicide, or other causes. In the surgical group, 14 of 154 (9%) died during 9 years of follow-up; in those who did not undergo the gastric bypass, 22 of 78 (28%) died during 6.2 years ($P < 0.0003$).[6] Although these are remarkable observations and are the first indication that mortality due to diabetes can be reduced by any measure, there are limitations to this study: the two groups are not tightly matched, the study is retrospective, and the numbers are small.

The effect of the operation on long-term mortality needs to be explored further, especially in light of Fobi's presentation, which stated that his series of patients over 70, primarily nondiabetic, who underwent the gastric bypass had a mean survival of only 36 months.[7] This figure is difficult to interpret because the patients varied significantly in their comorbidities and because we do not have mortality data for a group of matched older morbidly obese patients.

When the Gastric Bypass Fails, the Diabetes Returns

If the gastric bypass is the real reason for the remission of diabetes, the disease should return when the operation fails. This is indeed true. Our experience with staple-line failures taught us that hyperglycemia and the rise of hemoglobin A_{1c} levels are reliable indicators that the staple line is no longer intact.

Confirmation of our Findings

Although there have been a number of reports corroborating our finding that the gastric bypass can induce full remission of type 2 diabetes, the most rigorous of these is the paper by Schauer's group at the University of Pittsburgh.[8] After their initial studies demonstrated full clinical remission of diabetes in 82% of patients and significant improvement in 18% following the gastric bypass, they initiated a much larger 5-year study involving 1160 patients. Of these, 240 demonstrated either glucose impairment or diabetes. Follow-up was possible in 119 of these patients (80%). No patient experienced worsening of diabetes. Fasting blood glucose and hemoglobin A_{1c} levels were markedly improved or returned to normal levels in all patients and most dramatically, in the patients with less severe or shorter duration of diabetes. A significant reduction in the use of oral antidiabetic agents (80%) and insulin (79%) followed surgical treatment in all patients who required pharmacologic management. The authors concluded that "laparoscopic gastric bypass results in significant weight loss (60% excess body weight) and resolution (83%) or improvement (17%) of type 2 diabetes mellitus." They also confirmed that the gastric bypass resolved or ameliorated the major comorbidities of diabetes (Table 42-2).

Questioning a Concept: Is Type 2 Diabetes Really Due to Insulin Resistance and Failure of the Islets?

The traditional explanation of type 2 diabetes contends that the basic cause of the disease is insulin resistance, that the islets are unable to maintain adequate production of the hormone, and that eventually hyperglycemia becomes uncontrollable, even with the external administration of insulin, therefore explaining the increase in both insulin and glucose. The disease is considered inexorable and incurable, although rigorous maintenance of euglycemic protocols can produce symptomatic benefits.

The observation that the gastric bypass induces rapid, durable, and complete remission of the disease and the amelioration of the comorbidities forces us to reexamine the traditional explanations. The operation has shown that diabetes is reversible, that it is not incurable, and that its effects can be mitigated.

How Does the Gastric Bypass Control Diabetes?

Accordingly, the question is no longer whether the gastric bypass can induce full and durable control of diabetes. The puzzle is how. Let's examine the possible causes for the remission. The gastric bypass produces three known effects on energy intake and the physiology of the gut: reduction in caloric intake; change in the composition of the diet; and exclusion of food from the stomach, the entire duodenum, and a major portion of the jejunum, with flow of the food from the stomach directly into the distal jejunum.

Table 42-2	EFFECT OF GASTRIC BYPASS ON THE MAJOR COMORBIDITIES OF TYPE 2 DIABETES					
COMORBIDITIES	TOTAL POPULATION	RESOLVED	IMPROVED	UNCHANGED	WORSE	UNKNOWN
Hypertension	134 (70%)	36%	53%	2%	2%	0
Hyper-cholesterolemia	107 (56%)	37%	41%	3%	1%	18%
Hyper-triglyceridemia	86 (45%)	31%	44%	5%	1%	19%
Sleep apnea	109 (57%)	33%	47%	10%	1%	9%

(Reproduced from Schauer PR, Burguera B, Ikramuddin S, et al: Effect of laparoscopic Roux-en-Y gastric bypass on type 2 diabetes mellitus. Ann Surg 2003;238:467-484.)

REDUCTION IN CALORIC INTAKE

The small gastric pouch, with its ½- to 1-ounce volume, and the gastrojejunostomy, with an opening barely larger than a pencil, reduce caloric intake by limiting intake and delaying emptying. The magnitude of the reduction in caloric intake varies after the gastric bypass. Bobbioni-Harsch and colleagues concluded that "gastric bypass-induced body weight loss is mainly due to the reduction of energy intake, whereas the qualitative modifications of the diet do not play a role. Younger subjects have a greater capacity to reduce energy intake and, therefore, lose more weight. A preoperative high degree of obesity leads to a larger weight reduction, probably because of a greater energy deficit."[9] Similar reductions of caloric intake in nonoperated diabetic patients can also return these individuals to euglycemia. However, perhaps due to noncompliance with such rigorous quality-of-life changes, these measures have not been successful in the long-term control of diabetics.

The inclusion of a single-patient anecdote is always questionable, but our experience with one individual bears inclusion. This 47-year-old man was a morbidly obese diabetic who was found, at surgery, to have a stomach distended with recently eaten food. He had apparently dined very late at night. Fortunately, he did not aspirate during induction. We backed out because we did not feel that we could achieve competent stapling of the stomach in the presence of undigested corn and collards. When he awoke, confronted with the disappointing findings, he agreed to follow the same postoperative dietary regimen prescribed for gastric bypass patients. He complied for about 2 weeks: clear liquids for 2 days, 2 ounces of Ensure Plus three times a day, and water ad libitum for an additional week, with a slow progression to a soft diet. His glucose levels also returned to normal, similar to the levels in those who had undergone the full gastric bypass surgery. Based on these observations, as well as on the experience of decades of diabetes therapy, it is safe to conclude that the amount of food plays a role in the control of glucose metabolism.

CHANGE IN THE COMPOSITION OF THE DIET

The changes in diets after the gastric bypass vary considerably from patient to patient. Most patients learn to avoid sweets because their ingestion produces dumping in about two thirds of patients who undergo the surgery. Some have difficulty managing beef, preferring poultry and pork. Others state that they enjoy salads and vegetables far more than they had in the past. Almost all fail to ingest adequate vitamins and minerals and require supplementation with multivitamin and mineral preparations, as well as calcium, iron (for menstruating females), B_{12}, and the other B vitamins. Although there is a paucity of studies evaluating diet composition after gastric bypass, it is our opinion that the diets tend to be more balanced and to include fewer candies and a diminished intake of glucose.

Additional data are available from the studies of Moize and associates, who concluded that: "daily energy intake (kcal/day) increased from 849 ± 329 (SD) at 3 months to 1101 ± 400 at 12 months ($P = .009$). Protein intake also increased (g/day) from 45.6 ± 14.2 at 3 months to 58.5 ± 17.1 at 12 months ($P = .04$), and as a percentage of goal protein intake from $55.1\% \pm 23.0$ at 3 months to $73.5\% \pm 38.0$ at

12 months ($P = .02$).[10] Although energy and protein intake increased significantly over the 12-month period, protein intake at 12 months remained significantly lower ($P = 0.01$) than the daily recommended guidelines (1.5 g/kg initial body weight) for a low-energy restrictive diet.

The gastric bypass is clearly followed by sharp changes in diet, including a reduction in calories and changes in diet composition. Many of the patients probably develop deficiencies in protein, vitamins, and minerals, especially during the first 2 years after the surgery. These dietary changes probably have a favorable effect on diabetes but, do not explain *full* remission, especially for the long term, when many of the dietary changes have disappeared. Patients who comply with dietary recommendations often improve their diabetes control but certainly do not lose their disease.

There has to be at least one other reason for the full remission.

EXCLUSION OF FOOD FROM ITS NORMAL PATHWAYS

The gastric bypass operation, in addition to limiting intake and slowing emptying time, changes the flow of food drastically so that the stomach, the entire duodenum, and a major portion of the jejunum are excluded from contact with nutrients. Or, to put it another way, the undigested food is emptied directly into the distal gut. We believe that this is the critical change responsible for the remission of diabetes.

▶ COMPLEXITY OF GLUCOSE METABOLISM

The control of carbohydrate metabolism and the conservation of energy must be one of our most primitive and complex metabolic processes. It is controlled by a variety of mechanisms that have developed during our evolution. The production and use of insulin by an organism requires delivery of insulin at a moment's notice, despite limited facilities for insulin storage and the maintenance of glucose levels within a narrow range of normal values. To regulate production and distribution, early notice that food is being consumed is necessary. Once food is consumed, the modulation of insulin distribution requires information about where the food is within the gut, the speed of transit, and when it is likely that the food will have been digested. If appropriate signals are not received, overproduction or underproduction of insulin ensues. Simultaneously, signals from adipose tissues provide measures of insulin storage, while those from muscle indicate utilization. The insulin regulatory system must also monitor the rates of insulin and glucose clearance as a measure of energy production and utilization. In short, it is likely that insulin production and the control of glucose use require highly complex interactions between the gut and the islets. It is likely that the antidiabetic effects of gastric bypass are achieved through alteration of these interactions.

Hyperinsulinemia of Type 2 Diabetes Mellitus

Let us examine a theoretical model in which managing insulin supply is the immediate concern, and insulin production has to be adequate to meet metabolic needs. In type 1 diabetes, the islets are destroyed and production is certainly inadequate. In type 2 diabetes, however, insulin shortage is only relative. Even though the traditional explanations indicate that "the islets wear out in diabetics," hyperinsulinemia is a characteristic of the disease even into its late stages. In fact, even in the late stages of type 2 diabetes, oral glucose tolerance tests provoke insulin levels that are twice as high as those seen in normal patients. No, the islets are not the problem. The capacity to manufacture and store insulin is probably not the primary cause of type 2 disease.

Insulin Resistance: Cause or a Protective Mechanism?

Type 2 diabetics display a resistance to insulin; that is, it takes ever greater amounts of the hormone to initiate its functions. Because this resistance continues to increase over the course of the disease and because it can be overcome by increasing the dosages of insulin, insulin resistance has become recognized as the cause of the disease. In accord with that concept, diabetics today are treated with drugs that increase insulin production, medications that decrease insulin resistance and, when these measure fail, with injections of insulin that increase with time.

The observations that the gastric bypass abolishes insulin resistance, reduces insulin levels to normal in a matter of days, and allows insulin to remain at these normal levels even after resumption of a full diet, are not consistent with the theory that insulin resistance is the cause of the disease. Merely bypassing a segment of the gut is not likely to be capable of changing insulin resistance on a body-wide cellular level in a matter of a few days.

The more likely explanation is that insulin resistance is, indeed, resistance—that is, a protective mechanism of the cells working against the excess production of insulin by the β cells. According to that concept, diabetes is due to hyperactivity of the islets as they produce large excesses of insulin, just as other glands can become overactive (e.g., hyperthyroidism or Cushing syndrome).

Is the Overactivity of the Islets Primary or Secondary?

The overactivity of endocrine organs is usually classified as intrinsic, as in primary hyperthyroidism, or extrinsic, due to stimulation by other endocrine organs such as in the hyperadrenalism of a pituitary tumor in Cushing disease. If hyperinsulinism were caused by an intrinsic disease of the islets, it would disappear only with the removal of some or all of the β cells. The excessive production clears within days after a gastric bypass, so the likely conclusion is that the islets were overactive because of an external stimulus. Further, because euglycemia follows a rearrangement of the gut, it seems reasonable to conclude that the stimulus for the hyperinsulinism comes from the gut.

Regulation of Insulin Production by the Gut

The participation of intestinal hormones in insulin production has been known about since the 1930s, when investigators called these factors incretins. Since then, a number of hormones have been shown to be insulinogogues, including glucose-dependent insulinotropic polypeptide (GIP), glucagonlike peptide-1 (GLP-1), cholecystokinin, peptide YY and, most recently, ghrelin. Exactly how they interact with each other and with other hormones involved in glucose metabolism, such as leptin and adiponectin from the adipose tissues, remains to be shown.

If we return to the idea that management by the islets resides in their monitoring of the location of food within the gut, it seems likely that the various hormonal signals interact to reveal transit time and probably composition of the chyme. Reinforcing this concept is the finding that the gut hormones are not secreted uniformly throughout the gut but, instead, tend to increase or decrease as food proceeds. Thus ghrelin is at its highest concentration in the stomach when there is a gradual diminution of its concentration in the small bowel; in contrast, GLP-1 is lowest in the proximal gut and highest near the cecum. The islets could, therefore, be signaled regarding the level of food in the intestine either via changes in the concentration of the hormones or, perhaps, by comparison of ratios of one hormone to another, such as GLP-1 versus ghrelin. The sensing of ratios is not a radical new suggestion; organisms use that process commonly, as in the sensing of the concentrations of phosphorus-carbon; potassium-sodium; zinc-calcium; iron-copper; and oxygen-carbon dioxide.

Effect of the Gastric Bypass on the Gut Hormones

The effects of the gastric bypass on the gut hormones are not well known, but there are indications that they can be profound. For example, prior to surgery the levels of ghrelin, sometimes called the hunger hormone, rise in sharp spikes just before breakfast, lunch, and supper and somewhat more modestly at bedtime. The gastric bypass abolishes these responses, reducing ghrelin secretion to minimal levels without any periodic spikes. Studies have shown similar changes in the concentration of other gut hormones. Of particular interest are the observations that the gastric bypass produces more significant changes (because of its alteration of gut sequence) than does the purely restrictive procedures such as gastric banding.

A full discussion of these interactions is beyond the scope of this chapter. Additional information, however, can be found in several excellent reports about ghrelin by Leonetti,[11] Tritos,[12] Holdstock,[13] and Cummings[14] and their colleagues. Discussions of incretin signaling are to be found in the publications of Perfetti[15] and Vahl and their colleagues.[16] In addition, the articles by Mortensen,[17] Vilsboll,[18] and Gault[19] and their colleagues provide a good overview of GLP-1 and GIP, two powerful gut-signal hormones.

▶ CONCLUSION

The gastric bypass provides, for the first time, a therapy that induces full and durable remission of type 2 diabetes mellitus, with a rapid reduction of hyperglycemia and a significant reduction in the morbidity and mortality rates of this disease. The effect of the bypass suggests that our current concepts about the pathophysiology of type 2 diabetes should be reexamined. The recognition that the hyperinsulinemia and hyperglycemia clear within days after surgery suggests that the cause of diabetes is not insulin resistance but is more likely overstimulation of the islets by hyperactive intestinal hormones.

Future areas of research should compare the effects of the common bariatric operations (gastric bypass, duodenal switch, and gastric banding) on diabetes, with its hyperinsulinemia and hyperglycemia, with the effects of diet and exercise in diabetics and in euglycemic individuals. Profiles of hormones from the gut, adipose tissues, muscles, and hypothalamus should be measured in rapidly timed sequences after food intake. Similar studies also should be conducted in patients with gestational diabetes before and after delivery. The mechanism of relief of the diabetes may well be the same in the pregnant and the morbidly obese female. The hope is that these studies will reveal one or several diabetogenic hormones that can be controlled by molecular biologic approaches, including metabolic surgery.

▶ REFERENCES

1. Flickinger EG, Pories WJ, Meelheim HD, et al: The Greenville gastric bypass: progress report at three years. Ann Surg 1984;199:555-562.
2. Pories WJ, Swanson MS, MacDonald KG, et al: Who would have thought it: an operation proves to be the most effective therapy for adult-onset diabetes mellitus. Ann Surg 1995;222:339-352.
3. Brolin RE, LaMarca LB, Kenler HA, et al: Malabsorptive gastric bypass in patients with superobesity. J Gastrointest Surg 2002;6:195-203.
4. Hickey MS, Pories WJ, MacDonald KG, et al: A new paradigm for type 2 diabetes mellitus: could it be a disease of the foregut? Ann Surg 1998;227:637-644.
5. Pories WJ, Stearns JD, Swanson MS, et al: Episodic severe hypoglycemia following gastric bypass. Ann Surg 2006(accepted for publication).
6. MacDonald KG, Long SD, Swanson MS, et al: The gastric bypass operation reduces the progression and mortality of non-insulin dependent diabetes mellitus. J Gastrointest Surg 1997;1:213-220.
7. Fobi M: Gastric bypass operations in elderly patients. International Federation for Surgery of Obesity 2003; Salamanca, Spain.
8. Schauer PR, Burguera B, Ikramuddin S, et al: Effect of laparoscopic Roux-en-Y gastric bypass on type 2 diabetes mellitus. Ann Surg 2003;(in press).
9. Bobbioni-Harsch E, Huber O, Morel P, et al: Factors influencing energy intake and body weight loss after gastric bypass. Eur J Clin Nutr 2002;56:551-556.
10. Moize V, Geliebter A, Gluck ME, et al: Obese patients have inadequate protein intake related to protein intolerance up to 1 year following Roux-en-Y gastric bypass. Obes Surg 2003;13:23-28.
11. Leonetti F, Silecchia G, Iacobellis G, et al: Different plasma ghrelin levels after laparoscopic gastric bypass and adjustable gastric banding in morbid obese subjects. J Clin Endocrinol Metab 2003;88:4227-4231.
12. Tritos NA, Mun E, Bertkau A, et al: Serum ghrelin levels in response to glucose load in obese subjects post-gastric bypass surgery. Obes Res 2003;11:919-924.
13. Holdstock C, Engstrom BE, Ohrvall M, et al: Ghrelin and adipose tissue regulatory peptides: effect of gastric bypass surgery in obese humans. J Clin Endocrinol Metab 2003;88:3177-3183.
14. Cummings DE, Shannon MH: Ghrelin and gastric bypass: is there a hormonal contribution to surgical weight loss? J Clin Endocrinol Metab 2003;88:2999-3002.
15. Perfetti R, Brown TA, Velikina R, et al: Control of glucose homeostasis by incretin hormones. Diabetes Technol Ther 1999;1:297-305.
16. Vahl T, D'Alessio D: Enteroinsular signaling: perspectives on the role of the gastrointestinal hormones glucagon-like peptide 1 and glucose-dependent insulinotropic polypeptide in normal and abnormal glucose metabolism. Curr Opin Clin Nutr Metab Care 2003;6:461-468
17. Mortensen K, Christensen LL, Holst JJ, et al: GLP-1 and GIP are colocalized in a subset of endocrine cells in the small intestine. Regul Pept 2003;15:114,189-196.
18. Vilsboll T, Krarup T, Madsbad S, et al: Both GLP-1 and GIP are insulinotropic at basal and postprandial glucose levels and contribute nearly equally to the incretin effect of a meal in healthy subjects. Regul Pept 2003;114:115-121.
19. Gault VA, Flatt PR, O'Harte FP: Glucose-dependent insulinotropic polypeptide analogues and their therapeutic potential for the treatment of obesity-diabetes. Biochem Biophys Res Commun 2003;308:207-213.

43

Resolution of Bariatric Comorbidities: Hypertension

Kenneth G. MacDonald, Jr., M.D. and John R. Pender, IV, M.D.

Hypertension is a risk factor for coronary artery disease, renal disease, peripheral vascular disease, stroke, and congestive heart failure. One 18-year observational study of 8690 patients whose hypertension was medically managed showed that cardiovascular events continue to be the principal cause of morbidity and mortality in this population.[1] The causes of hypertension are multifactorial, and in 95% of cases of primary, or essential, hypertension, a specific cause cannot be defined. There is a strong genetic component in hypertension, as evidenced by its greater prevalence in certain ethnic groups. The overall prevalence of hypertension has increased over the past decade, with almost 29% of the population meeting the criteria for diagnosis of hypertension.[2] The number of Americans with hypertension is estimated to be in the range of 50 million, with 2 million new cases diagnosed yearly.[3,4]

There is an established relationship between obesity and hypertension, and obesity is recognized as an independent risk factor for hypertension. Excess adiposity accounts for 70% of hypertension in men and 60% in women,[5] and it has been claimed that the strongest predictor of hypertension is excess body weight.[6] A relationship between degree of obesity and severity of hypertension has been demonstrated. A report from the Framingham Heart Study showed that for every 10% increase in weight, the systolic blood pressure increased by 6.5 mm Hg.[7] A Swedish study of a large number of that country's homogeneous population showed a 3-mm Hg increase in systolic and a 2-mm Hg increase in diastolic pressures for each 10-kg increase in weight.[8] The longer an individual is obese, the greater his or her chance of developing hypertension.

Central fat distribution, or truncal obesity, correlates more closely with the incidence of hypertension than does overall fat mass. Increased systolic and diastolic blood pressures have been positively correlated with measures showing increased visceral fat, such as waist -to-hip ratios,[9] abdominal computed tomography,[10] and waist circumference measurements.[11]

A prospective study of more than a million men and women found obesity to be the most strongly predictive factor for death from cardiovascular disease.[12] Data from the National Health and Nutrition Evaluation Survey III (NHANES III) demonstrated that obese individuals are at risk for other causes of coronary heart disease in addition to their obesity, such as hypertension. In an analysis of 662,443 records from the National Health Interview Survey database, Livingston and Ko found that the presence of diabetes or hypertension substantially increased age-adjusted mortality rates, independent of body weight.[13] It is interesting that in this analysis, mortality rates decreased with increasing body mass index in patients with either diabetes or hypertension, suggesting some benefit of adiposity with these diseases. Others have confirmed higher mortality rates in lean hypertensive patients than in obese patients.[14] This observed protective effect of increased obesity is not understood, but it could be explained by a variety of causes or by the differing cardiovascular effects of hypertension in lean and obese patients.

▶ METABOLIC SYNDROME

Individuals have been identified with a clustering of cardiovascular risk factors, including central obesity, insulin resistance with hyperinsulinemia, dyslipidemia, and hypertension.[15] The association of these conditions has been termed metabolic syndrome, or syndrome X (Table 43-1), and individuals with this syndrome are well documented to be at higher risk for coronary heart disease.[16] Abdominal, central, or visceral fat distribution has long been shown to correlate with elevated glucose and insulin levels,[17] hypertension, and hyperlipidemia. There is even evidence that subcutaneous or peripheral fat has a beneficial effect on lipid profiles, compared with the decreased high-density lipoprotein and increased low-density lipoprotein seen with visceral fat deposition.[18] The pathophysiology of

Table 43-1	NATIONAL CHOLESTEROL EDUCATION PROGRAM ADULT TREATMENT PANEL III: THE METABOLIC SYNDROME
RISK FACTOR	DEFINING LEVEL
Abdominal obesity (waist circumference)	
Men	>102 cm (>40 in)
Women	>88 cm (>35 in)
Triglycerides	>150 mg/dl
HDL C	
Men	<40 mg/dl
Women	<50 mg/dl
Blood pressure	>130/80 mm Hg
Fasting glucose	>110 mg/dl

Diagnosis is established when more than three of these risk factors are present.
HDL C, high-density lipoprotein cholesterol.
(Haffner S, Taegtmyer H: Epidemic obesity and the metabolic syndrome. Circulation 2003;108:1541-1545. Copyright © Lippincott, Williams & Wilkins.)

the role of central adiposity is probably multifactorial, with evidence for genetic, mechanical, and biochemical mechanisms.

▶ PATHOPHYSIOLOGY OF HYPERTENSION IN OBESITY

There is no single unifying explanation for the cause of hypertension with obesity. There is evidence to support genetic predisposition, hyperinsulinemia, overactivity of the sympathetic nervous system, the renin-angiotensin-aldosterone system (RAAS), salt retention, and leptin, among others (Table 43-2). There are close ties between two of the most common obesity comorbidities, diabetes and hypertension. Hypertension is present in 70% of obese type 2 diabetics, and 50% of patients with hypertension have insulin resistance. Hyperglycemia has been linked to increases in plasma renin levels, renal vascular resistance, and mean arterial pressure.[19]

Genetics

Obesity is a risk factor for hypertension, but not all obese people have hypertension and not all hypertensive people are obese. The incidence of hypertension actually declined between the times of NHANES II and NHANES III, whereas the prevalence of obesity was increasing.[20] There is evidence that there may a genetic link to the development of obesity and hypertension. Studies have demonstrated

Table 43-2	PATHOPHYSIOLOGY OF HYPERTENSION IN OBESITY

Genetic
Increased intraabdominal pressure
Insulin resistance/hyperinsulinemia
Sympathetic nervous system stimulation
Vascular resistance/Na-K-ATPase
Renin-angiotensin-aldosterone system
Leptin

Na-K-ATPase, sodium-potassium-adenosinetriphosphatase.

that a family history of hypertension may be linked to an increased propensity to develop insulin resistance. The relationship among central obesity, insulin resistance, hypertension, and hyperlipidemia discussed previously in terms of metabolic syndrome suggests a possible genetic basis for this association of conditions, although other mechanisms are likely to be involved.[21,22]

Increased Intraabdominal Pressure

Sugerman and colleagues have postulated that the increased intraabdominal pressure documented in the obese is one of the causes of systemic hypertension, particularly in cases of central obesity.[23] Possible mechanisms suggested include stimulation of the RAAS due to increased venous pressure; direct renal compression; and increased intrathoracic pressure with decreased venous return to the heart and a resultant fall in cardiac output. Activation of the RAAS would then result in sodium and water retention and increased blood pressure. The Medical College of Virginia group has provided experimental data with animal models to support each of these three possible mechanisms leading to RAAS activation.[24-26]

Insulin Resistance and Hyperinsulinemia

Insulin resistance and the resultant hyperinsulinemia have long been suggested as the pathologic link between obesity, glucose intolerance, and hypertension.[27] Excess free fatty acids found in the obese are thought to lead to an increase in triglyceride accumulation in muscle and liver. Insulin resistance then results from the inhibition of insulin action by these triglycerides.[28]

Insulin is a potent stimulant of renal sodium absorption, leading to hypervolemia. Thus, increased insulin levels can result in increased sodium retention, hypervolemia, and increased peripheral vascular resistance (Fig. 43-1).[29] The underlying mechanism may be explained by an insulin-related increase in sensitivity to angiotensin II and catecholamines, as well as activation of angiotensinogen secretion by adipocytes.[30]

Sympathetic Nervous System Stimulation

Several studies support the association of increased sympathetic stimulation in obesity with the higher incidence of hypertension in this population.[31,32] A collaborative study with the Normative Aging Study provided data from 24-hour urinary norepinephrine levels and postprandial insulin levels, relating both to hypertension.[33] The levels of norepinephrine in urinary samples of the cohort demonstrated significantly higher levels in obese individuals than in lean individuals. Those individuals in the lowest third for both norepinephrine excretion and insulin levels had a 10% incidence of hypertension, whereas those in the highest third had a 35% incidence of hypertension.

Proposed mechanisms of sympathetic nervous system activation with obesity include stimulation by both insulin (Fig. 43-2) and leptin directly, stimulation by angiotensin II, and arterial baroreflex and hypothalamic-pituitary axis dysfunction.[2] As with many other possible mechanisms causing obesity-related hypertension, there is a positive

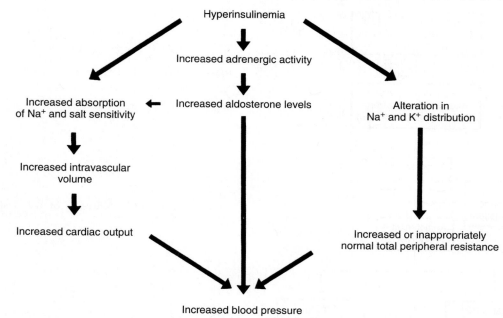

Figure 43-1. Role of hyperinsulinemia in obesity-related hypertension. K, potassium; Na, sodium. (Maxwell M, Herber D, Waks AV, et al: Role of insulin and norepinephrine in the hypertension of obesity. Am J Hypertens 1995;7:402-408. Copyright © Elsevier Science Inc.)

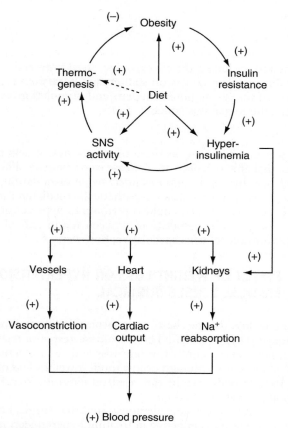

Figure 43-2. Insulin-stimulated sympathetic nervous system activity and hypertension with obesity. (Landsberg L: Insulin-mediated sympathetic stimulation: role in the pathogenesis of obesity-related hypertension (or, how insulin affects blood pressure, and why). J Hypertens 2001; 19:523-528. Copyright © Lippincott Williams & Wilkins.)

correlation with the degree of visceral or central adiposity and increased muscle sympathetic neural activity.[34]

Intracellular Calcium and Sodium-Potassium-Adenosinetriphosphatase: Vascular Resistance

In lean individuals, blood volume is inversely related to blood pressure; the higher the blood pressure, the lower the blood volume. However, obese individuals have higher blood volume, which results in a higher cardiac output due to increased stroke volume. A significant percentage of this increased blood volume is used to perfuse the excess adipose tissue. In addition, the compensatory decrease in peripheral vascular resistance in response to the increased blood volume seen in lean individuals is inhibited in the obese.[29] Generally, insulin is a direct vasodilator, and an acute increase in plasma insulin in the nonobese does not increase blood pressure despite the concurrent stimulation of the sympathetic nervous system.[35]

The absence of the normal vasodilatory response to increased blood volume and to hyperinsulinemia in obesity may in part be the result of increased intracellular calcium due to the decrease in sodium-potassium-adenosinetriphosphatase (ATPase) seen in obese persons.[36] This increase in intracellular calcium leads to increased tone in vascular smooth muscle, with a corresponding increase in peripheral vascular resistance. Other possible explanations for the lack of vasodilation include the chronic opposing sympathetic nervous system stimulation discussed earlier and the autonomic dysfunction with parasympathetic withdrawal related to insulin resistance.[37]

Renin-Angiotensin-Aldosterone System

The RAAS is an important regulator of blood pressure and electrolyte homeostasis. The juxtaglomerular cells of the

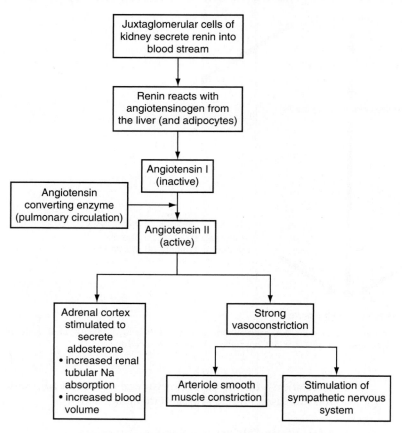

Figure 43-3. Schematic of renin-angiotensin-aldosterone system.

afferent arterioles of the kidneys release renin, which cleaves amino acids from angiotensinogen, a precursor produced by the liver, to form angiotensin I. Angiotensin converting enzyme then converts the inactive angiotensin I into angiotensin II, primarily in the pulmonary circulation. Angiotensin II is a potent vasoconstrictor, both by direct effect on arteriolar smooth muscle and by stimulation of the sympathetic nervous system. It also stimulates aldosterone release from the adrenal cortex, which promotes reabsorption of sodium by the renal tubules. These actions increase blood pressure by increasing plasma volume and by causing vasoconstriction (Fig. 43-3).

Angiotensinogen is formed primarily in the liver, but it has also been found in adipose tissue in the obese, suggesting a possible role for tissue angiotensinogen in the development of obesity-related hypertension.[38] Of interest is the discovery that angiotensinogen is secreted more from visceral than from subcutaneous adipocytes,[39] which suggests one explanation for the association of central obesity with metabolic syndrome and increased risk for cardiovascular mortality.

The role of the RAAS in obesity-related hypertension is supported by evidence of increased activity of several components with obesity[40] and decreased activity with weight loss, accompanied by reduction in blood pressure. There is conflicting data, however, as some have reported renin levels to be no different in obese compared to lean patients, with a progressive decrease as weight increases.[41] There are likely multiple pathways leading to involvement of the RAAS with obesity, some of which have been reviewed, including the effects of increased intra-abdominal pressure, insulin effects on sodium and potassium regulation, adipocyte angiotensinogen, and stimulation of the sympathetic nervous system.

LEPTIN

Leptin is a hormone secreted by adipocytes; it acts upon hypothalamic receptors to decrease caloric intake. There is evidence that leptin opposes nitric oxide vasodilation, acts as a pressor, and also has sympathetically mediated cardiac and renal actions that could contribute to hypertension in the obese.[42] The association between leptin and obesity hypertension remains speculative, however.

▶ EFFECT OF WEIGHT LOSS ON HYPERTENSION: MEDICAL VERSUS SURGICAL

Weight loss is the best nonpharmacologic method of managing hypertension. There is a dose-response relationship between amount of weight loss and the reduction in blood pressure, although even a modest weight loss of 5% to 10% of body weight can result in clinically significant blood pressure reduction.[43,44]

Several studies have demonstrated that surgical treatment of obesity is effective in treating hypertension in the obese hypertensive patient.[45-47] Sugerman and colleagues reported that hypertension resolved in 69% of their patients following gastric bypass, and that those patients had greater weight loss than those in whom hypertension did not resolve.[47] Resolution of hypertension was less likely in black than in white patients (60% versus 73%), although blacks also had significantly less excess weight loss. Schauer and others reported resolution of hypertension in 70% and improvement in another 18% of their patients after gastric bypass.[48] Despite less mean weight loss with the purely restrictive procedures, resolution of hypertension has been reported in 65.5% of patients after vertical banded gastroplasty[49] and in 55% after adjustable gastric banding.[50]

The metaanalysis of Buchwald and colleagues showed significant improvement in hypertension in the total surgical population reviewed and with all types of surgical procedures.[51] Hypertension resolved in 38.4% of patients after gastric banding, in 72.5% after gastroplasty, in 75.4% after gastric bypass, and in 81.3% after biliopancreatic diversion or duodenal switch. The percentage of patients with either resolution or improvement in hypertension ranged from 71.5% with gastric banding to 91.8% with the malabsorptive procedures. Although it was stated in this review that reduction in blood pressure seemed less dependent on the operative procedure performed than did the effects on diabetes and hyperlipidemia, there did appear to be higher rates of resolution or improvement of hypertension with the procedures that resulted in greater average weight loss.

There are few long-term analyses to assess the durability of the improvements in comorbidities after surgical weight loss, but data from the Swedish Obesity Study have shown that initial improvements in blood pressure after surgical weight loss dissipate over time.[52] Another report from the Swedish Obesity Study, however, showed that patients who had gastric bypass maintained significant reductions in blood pressure at 5 years after surgery.[53]

Apart from type of procedure and amount of weight loss, it has been postulated that duration of exposure to any risk factor, such as obesity-related hypertension or diabetes, increases the likelihood of irreversibility of these comorbid states due to permanent end-organ damage, both functional and structural.[9,54] Various studies have demonstrated increased rates of diabetes and hypertension in the obese with increasing age, as well as decreased rates of resolution of both after surgical weight loss.[9,55] The obvious implication is that earlier treatment of obesity by surgery either prevents the development or increases the rate of resolution of the comorbidity.

CONCLUSION

There is a clear association between obesity and hypertension. The pathophysiology is complex because of the many interrelated mechanisms. Although the cause of obesity-related hypertension is clearly multifactorial, visceral or central adiposity, insulin resistance with resultant hyperinsulinemia, RAAS effects, and sympathetic nervous system stimulation appear to be the most important contributors. Weight loss results in improvement in hypertension, with increased benefit seen with greater weight loss. Nevertheless, modest weight loss is associated with clinically significant improvement in blood pressure. Long-term benefits in health and longevity may seem intuitive but have not yet been well demonstrated in clinical trials. As with diabetes,

there is clinical evidence that increased duration of hypertension with obesity results in end-organ damage that lessens the effects of weight loss in overall health benefits and improvement in blood pressure. Earlier intervention is therefore recommended.

REFERENCES

1. Alderman MH, Cohen H, Madhavan S: Epidemiology of risk in hypertensives: experience in treated patients. Am J Hypertens 1998; 11:874-876.
2. Davy KP, Hall JE: Obesity and hypertension: two epidemics or one? Am J Physiol Regul Integr Comp Physiol 2004;286: R803-R813.
3. The fifth report of the Joint National Committee on Detection, Evaluation, and Treatment of High Blood Pressure. Arch Int Med 1993;153:154-183.
4. National High Blood Pressure Education Program Working Group report on primary prevention of hypertension. Arch Intern Med 1993;153:186-208.
5. Kannel WB, Garrison RJ, Dannenberg AL: Secular blood pressure trends in normotensive persons: the Framingham Study. Am Heart J 1993;125:1154-1158.
6. Eckle RH: Obesity and heart disease: a statement for health care professionals from the nutrition committee, American Heart Association. Circulation 1997;96:3248-3250.
7. Kannel WB, Gordon T, et al: Left ventricular hypertrophy by electrocardiogram: prevalence, incidence and mortality in the Framingham study. Ann Intern Med 1969;71:89-105.
8. Bjerkedal T: Overweight and hypertension. Acta Med Scand 1957; 13-26.
9. Lapidus L, Bengtsson C, Larsson B, et al: Distribution of adipose tissue and risk of cardiovascular death: a 12-year follow up of participants in the population study of women in Gothenburg, Sweden. BMJ 1984;289:1257-1261.
10. Kanai H, Tokunaga K, Fujioka S, et al: Decrease in intra-abdominal visceral fat may reduce blood pressure in obese hypertensive women. Hypertension 1996;27:125-129.
11. Han TS, van Leer EM, Seidell JC, et al: Waist circumference action levels in the identification of cardiovascular risk factors: prevalence study in a random sample. BMJ 1995;311:1401-1405.
12. Calle E, Thun MJ, Petrelli JM, et al: Body-mass index and mortality in a prospective cohort of U.S. adults. N Engl J Med 1999;341: 1097-1105.
13. Livingston EH, Ko CY: Effect of diabetes and hypertension on obesity-related mortality. Surgery 2005;137:16-25.
14. Stamler R, Ford CE, Stamler J: Why do lean hypertensives have higher mortality rates than other hypertensives: findings of the Hypertension Detection and Follow-Up Program. Hypertension 1991;17:553-564.
15. Gillum RF: The association of body fat distribution with hypertension, hypertensive heart disease, coronary heart disease, diabetes and cardiovascular risk factors in men and women aged 18-79 years. J Chron Dis 1987;40:421-428.
16. Kissebah AH, Vydelingum N, Murray R, et al: Relation of body fat distribution to metabolic complications of obesity. J Clin Endocrinol Metab 1982;54:254-257.
17. Despres JP: Visceral obesity: a component of the insulin resistance-dyslipidemic syndrome. Can J Cardiol 1991;10:17B-22B.
18. Terry RB, Stefanick ML, Haskell WL, et al: Contributions of regional adipose tissue depots to plasma lipoprotein concentrations in overweight men and women: possible protective effects of thigh fat. Metabolism 1991;40:733-740.
19. Lim HS, MacFadyen RJ, Lip GY: Diabetes mellitus, the renin-angiotensin-aldosterone system, and the heart. Arch Intern Med 2004;164:1737-1748.
20. Burt VL, Cutler JA, Higgins M, et al: Trends in the prevalence, awareness, treatment and control of hypertension in the adult US population: data from the Health Examination surveys, 1960-1991. Hypertension 1995;26:60-69.
21. Allemann Y, Horber FF, Colombo M, et al: Insulin sensitivity and body fat distribution in normotensive offspring of hypertensive patients. Lancet 1993;341;327-331.

22. Pausova Z, Gossard F, Gaudet D, et al: Heritability estimates of obesity measures in siblings with and without hypertension. Hypertension 2001;38:41-47.

23. Sugerman HJ: Effects of increased intra-abdominal pressure in severe obesity. Surg Clin North Am 2001;81:1063-1075.

24. Bloomfield GL, Blocher CR, Fakhry IF, et al: Elevated intra-abdominal pressure increases plasma renin activity and aldosterone levels. J Trauma 1997;42:997-1005.

25. Doty JM, Saggi BH, Blocher CR, et al: The effect of increased renal venous pressure on renal function. J Trauma 1999;47:1000-1003.

26. Bloomfield GL, Sugerman HJ, Blocher CR, et al: Chronically increased intra-abdominal pressure produces systemic hypertension in dogs. Int J Obes Relat Metabol Disord 2000;24:819-824.

27. Ferannini E, Seghieri G, Muscelli E: Insulin and the renin-angiotensin-aldosterone system: influence of ACE inhibition. J Cardiovasc Pharmacol 1994;24(suppl 3):S61-S69.

28. Krotkiewski M, Bjorntorp P, Sjostrom L, et al: Impact of obesity on metabolism in men and women: importance of regional adipose tissue distribution. J Clin Invest 1983;72:1150-1162.

29. Thakur V, Richards R, Reisin E: Obesity, hypertension and the heart. Am J Med Sci 2001;321:242-248.

30. Ruano M, Silvestre V, Dominguez Y, et al: Morbid obesity, hypertensive disease and the renin-angiotensin-aldosterone axis. Obes Surg 2005;15:670-676.

31. Grassi G, Seravalle G, Dell'Oro R, et al: Adrenergic and reflex abnormalities in obesity-related hypertension. Hypertension 2000;36:538-542.

32. Landsberg L: Insulin-mediated sympathetic stimulation: role in the pathogenesis of obesity-related hypertension. J Hypertension 2001;19:523-528.

33. Ward KD, Sparrow D, Landsberg L, et al: Influence of obesity, insulin, and sympathetic nervous system activity on blood pressure: the Normative Aging Study. J Hypertens 1996;14:301-308.

34. Alvarez GE, Beske SD, Ballard TP, et al: Sympathetic neural activation in visceral obesity. Circulation 2002;106;2533-2536.

35. Anderson EA, Hoffman RP, Balon TW, et al: Hyperinsulinemia produces both sympathetic neural activation and vasodilation in normal humans. J Clin Invest 1991;87:2246-2252.

36. Avenel A, Leeds AR: Sodium intake, inhibition of Na-K-ATPase, and obesity. Lancet 1981;1:836.

37. Perin PC, Maule S, Quadri R: Sympathetic nervous system, diabetes, and hypertension. Clin Exper Hypertens 2001;23:45-55.

38. Engeli S, Negrel R, Sharma A: Physiology and pathophysiology of the adipose tissue renin-angiotensin system. Hypertension 2000;35:1270-1277.

39. Van Harmelen V, Elizalde M, Ariapart P, et al: The association of human adipose angiotensinogen gene expression with abdominal fat distribution in obesity. Int J Obes Relat Metab Disord 2000;24:673-678.

40. Umemura S, Nyui N, Tamura K, et al: Plasma angiotensinogen concentrations in obese patients. Am J Hypertens 1997;10:629-633.

41. Messerli F, Christie B, DeCarvalho G, et al: Obesity and essential hypertension, intravascular volume, sodium excretion and plasma renin activity. Arch Intern Med 1981;141:81-85.

42. Coatmellec-Taglioni G, Ribiere C: Factors that influence the risk of hypertension in obese individuals. Curr Opin Nephrol Hypertens 2003;12:305-308.

43. Stevens VJ, Obarzanek E, Cook NR, et al: Long-term weight loss and changes in blood pressure: results of the Trials of Hypertension Prevention, phase II. Ann Intern Med 2001;134:1-11.

44. National Heart, Lung, and Blood Institute: Clinical guidelines on the identification, evaluation, and treatment of overweight and obesity in adults: The Evidence Report. Obes Res 1998;6:51S-209S.

45. Carson JL, Ruddy ME, Duff AE, et al: The effect of gastric bypass surgery on hypertension in morbidly obese patients. Arch Intern Med 1994;154:193-200.

46. Foley EF, Benotti PN, Borlase BC: Impact of gastric restrictive surgery on hypertension in the morbidly obese. Am J Surg 1992;163:294-297.

47. Sugerman HJ, Wolfe LG, Sica DA, et al: Diabetes and hypertension in severe obesity and effects of gastric bypass induced weight loss. Ann Surg 2003;237:751-758.

48. Schauer PR, Ikramuddin S, Gourash W, et al: Outcomes after laparoscopic Roux-en-Y gastric bypass for morbid obesity. Ann Surg 2000;232:515-529.

49. del Amo A: Effect of vertical banded gastroplasty on hypertension, diabetes and dyslipidemia. Obes Surg 2002;12:319-323.

50. Dixon JB, O'Brien PE: Changes in comorbidities and improvements in quality of life after LAP-BAND placement. Am J Surg 2002;184(supple 2):S51-S54.

51. Buchwald H, Avidor Y, Braunwald E, et al: Bariatric surgery: a systematic review and meta-analysis. JAMA 2004;292:1724-1737.

52. Sjostrom CD, Peltonen M, Wedel H, et al: Differentiated long-term effects of intentional weight loss on diabetes and hypertension. Hypertension 2000;36:20-25.

53. Sjostrom CD, Peltonen M, Sjostrom L: Blood pressure and pulse pressure during long-term weight loss in the obese: the Swedish Obese Subjects (SOS) intervention study. Obes Res 2001;9:188-195.

54. Kral JG: Morbidity of severe obesity. Surg Clin North Am 2001;81:1039-1061.

55. Pories WJ, MacDonald KG, Flickinger EG, et al: Is type 2 diabetes mellitus (NIDDM) a surgical disease? Ann Surg 1992;215:633-642.

44

Resolution of Bariatric Comorbidities: Sleep Apnea

Ido Nachmany, M.D., Amir Szold, M.D., Joseph Klausner, M.D., and Subhi Abu-Abeid, M.D.

Obstructive sleep apnea was clinically recognized more than 30 years ago, but awareness of this phenomenon and its occurrence in the obese was known long before that. In his book *The Posthumous Papers of the Pickwick Club*, Charles Dickens describes a young patient who is undoubtedly morbidly obese and suffers from a severe sleep apnea syndrome. The boy, Joe is described as follows: "... and on the box sat a fat and red-faced boy, in a state of somnolency." And he writes, "Joe snores as he waits at the table...the snoring of the fat boy penetrated in a low and monotonous sound from the distant kitchen." There are several other precise clinical observations in Dickens' book that led Osler and later Burwell to apply the term *pickwickian syndrome* to the combination of obesity, hypersomnolence, and the signs of chronic alveolar hypoventilation.

Gastaut and coworkers are responsible for defining sleep apnea in 1965.[1] They simultaneously recorded sleep and breathing electrophysiologically in a patient with the pickwickian syndrome. They also described all three types of apnea (central, obstructive, and mixed), and postulated that the daytime sleepiness was due to the repetitive arousals and impairment of normal sleep pattern associated with the resumption of breathing.

Sleep apnea is a temporary cessation of breathing during sleep. Breathing cessation must be long enough to be considered an apnea. It is arbitrarily defined as a 10-second stop in the breathing cycle. Sleep apnea syndromes are divided, according to mechanism, into three groups. In central apnea, there is a pathologic reduction in respiratory drive and no effort to breathe is made. In obstructive sleep apnea (OSA), there is a ventilatory effort but no airflow because the upper airway is closed. This form of sleep apnea is far more prevalent than the central one. A mixed apnea represents a combination of low respiratory effort and obstruction to airflow.

The definition of hypopneas is more problematic. A hypopnea is a temporary decrease in inspiratory airflow that is out of proportion to the individual's effort or to metabolic demand. Practically speaking, it means a marked reduction in tidal volume. Because measuring airflow, respiratory effort, and alveolar or arterial carbon dioxide tension is difficult under usual clinical conditions, the most common indicator in use for the assessment of respiratory function in sleep is the oxygen saturation, measured by pulse oximetry.

The total number of apneas in a given sleep time yields the apnea index—the average number of apneas per hour of sleep. The apnea/hypopnea index (AHI) is the number of apneas plus hypopneas per hour of sleep. Obstructive apneas and hypopneas are terminated by an arousal, a transient partial or complete return to awake physiology. Arousals resulting in sleep fragmentation appear to be the primary cause of daytime hypersomnolence. Central apneas or hypopneas that do not lead to arousals may be clinically trivial.

The spectrum of sleep-related obstructed breathing is considered by many researchers to include increased upper airway resistance, which is manifested as snoring without frank apnea or hypopnea events, and episodic flow limitation, which terminates in central nervous system arousals and is often called upper airway resistance syndrome. These conditions may represent the earliest stages of OSA and may be important in investigating disease progression.

▶ EPIDEMIOLOGY

OSA is a highly common disorder that is seen not only in the morbidly obese and that is recognized as a major public health problem. An AHI of at least 5 is found to occur in 24% of men and 9% of women. An AHI of 5 or higher, in association with excessive daytime somnolence, occurs in 4% of men and 2% of women who are 30 to 60 years of age.[2]

In the United States, it is estimated that more than 3 million men and 1.5 million women meet at least one definition of OSA (an AHI of 5 or more plus a complaint of daytime sleepiness). In most population-based studies that have estimated sex-specific prevalence, the risk for men has been found to be two- to threefold greater than the risk for women, but little progress has been made in understanding the reasons for this risk difference. OSA prevalence appears to increase steadily with age in midlife, but age trends in childhood, adolescence, and older age do not indicate a simple positive correlation of OSA with age. Several studies have found OSA to be highly prevalent in people older than age 65 years. Although there are many studies regarding the prevalence of the disease, little is known about incidence (i.e., the occurrence of new cases over a given time interval) or progression (i.e., worsening over time) of OSA.

Only preliminary findings of OSA progression are currently available from population studies. Data from baseline and 8-year follow-up studies of 282 participants in the Wisconsin Sleep Cohort show a significant increase in OSA severity over this interval. The overall mean AHI increased by 2.6 events per hour, from 2.5 at baseline to 5.1 at follow-up. Progression was significantly greater in obese compared with nonobese, older compared with younger, and habitually snoring compared with nonhabitually snoring subjects.[3,4]

However, the most significant risk factor for OSA is obesity. The incidence of OSA in morbidly obese patients is 12- to 30-fold higher than in the general population. Clinical and laboratory investigations in obese patients have showed that the incidence of OSA is 42% to 48% among males and 8% to 38% among females.

At least 70% of patients with OSA are morbidly obese; in particular, some have special occupations such as truck driver, and some have various syndromes associated with obesity, including the night eating syndrome, the Prader-Willi syndrome, Cushing disease, and hypothyroidism.

▶ PATHOPHYSIOLOGY

The pathophysiology of OSA is incompletely understood, although many factors are known to serve as predisposing factors for its occurrence. Upper-airway narrowing or closure in sleep occurs as a result of a combination of anatomic and functional abnormalities of upper-airway regulation. Anatomic susceptibility to sleep apnea is determined by the relationship between the fixed dimensions of the craniofacial skeleton and the distribution of soft-tissue structures and adipose tissues that reside in the skeletal compartment. It is important to note that in the majority of patients, the structural "defect" predisposing the patient to the development of sleep apnea is simply a subtle reduction in airway size that can often be appreciated clinically as "pharyngeal crowding."

Superimposed on this anatomic substrate are complex neurophysiologic mechanisms that regulate the patency of the upper airway during sleep.[5] The relative contribution of anatomic and functional factors is likely to vary greatly among individuals and may vary considerably among groups of apneic patients defined on the basis of age, sex, body habitus, race, or ethnicity, although there are no data that address this.[3]

Normally, airway size is dynamic and depends upon a balance between factors exerting an outward force, thereby maintaining luminal diameter and patency (e.g., contraction of the dilator muscles of the upper airway), and factors exerting an inward force, decreasing luminal diameter (and most important, reduced intraluminal pressure). It appears that during sleep, a reduction in drive to the dilator muscles of the upper airway is the primary cause of airway narrowing and obstructive events. This change may be a direct result of a decrease in medullary respiratory activity. It may translate into a reduction in activity of those respiratory muscles with both respiratory and postural functions, such as the muscles of the upper airway.[6]

The activity of the upper airway dilator muscles can be divided into two components: phasic and tonic. The phasic activity is inspiratory, and its onset precedes diaphragmatic activity, thus preparing the pharyngeal airway for the development of negative pressure during inspiration. Tonic activity, on the other hand, refers to the activity during expiration, or the level of activation in muscles without any phasic activity, and may be looked upon as a baseline function of muscle tension.

In wakeful patients with OSA, there is an augmented tonic activity of the genioglossus muscle as well as of other pharyngeal dilators (such as the tensor palatini), when compared with healthy subjects. This activity is thought to represent a neuromuscular compensatory mechanism for an anatomically small and more collapsible pharyngeal airway. This augmented dilator muscle activity is lost at sleep onset and is associated with pharyngeal collapse. Numerous variables, including blood oxygen and carbon dioxide levels, sleep-wake state, gender-specific hormones, blood pressure, temperature, lung inflation, pharyngeal airflow, and intrapharyngeal negative pressure, influence the activity of the pharyngeal dilator muscles. However, most data suggest that intrapharyngeal pressure is the primary stimulus for phasic pharyngeal dilator muscle activation. It is well known that the application of negative pressure to the pharyngeal airway in animals and in humans leads to a substantial increase in the activity of the genioglossus as well as other upper airway muscles. It has also been found that the responsiveness of the genioglossus to different negative pressures is remarkably constant in a given individual. The increased dilator muscle activity in a patient with sleep apnea is not due to an increased responsiveness of the genioglossus to changes in pharyngeal pressure during inspiration. In fact, under all conditions, there is no difference in the response of the muscle between patients with OSA and control subjects. This was found to be true over a substantial range of pharyngeal negative pressures. It thus appears that the higher peak phasic genioglossus activity seen in apneic patients is caused by a combination of two factors. First, under all conditions, tonic activity is higher in apneic patients. Second, as intrinsic upper airway resistance is higher in these patients, they generate more negative intrapharyngeal pressures under all conditions which, in the face of an identical response to negative pressure, yields increased phasic activity.[7]

Some other factors in the genesis of upper airway obstruction merit discussion. Although not a primary mechanism for upper airway obstruction, body position may play an important role in the obstructive events. Some individuals with position-dependent sleep apnea obstruct exclusively in the supine position. When an individual is in the supine position, soft structures such as the tongue and soft palate can be drawn into the pharyngeal airway by the effects of gravity. As a result, the area behind the tongue and soft palate becomes a site of airway narrowing which can lead to upper-airway obstruction. Alcohol, benzodiazepines, and other similar agents have been shown to cause or worsen sleep-disordered breathing in nonsnorers, snorers, and patients with OSA. These substances may increase sleep-disordered breathing by depressing respiration or by preferentially inhibiting upper airway muscle activity.[5]

▶ PATHOPYSIOLOGY OF OBSTRUCTIVE SLEEP APNEA IN THE OBESE PATIENT

Overweight and obesity are highly prevalent and are increasing in Western societies, and they have long been known to be associated with OSA. Many studies have found significant associations between OSA and measures of excess body weight. There seems to be little controversy that the associations seen in observational studies represent a causal role of excess weight in OSA.[3]

As mentioned earlier, the anatomic prerequisite to the development of OSA is the narrowing of the upper airways (i.e., "pharyngeal crowding"). It is common for obesity to contribute to the reduction in size of the upper airway because of fat deposition in the soft tissues of the pharynx or because of compression of the pharynx by superficial fat masses in the neck.[8] Metabolic and hormonal changes associated with obesity could increase airway collapsibility[6] and also disturb the relationship between respiratory drive and load; the reduction in functional residual capacity and increased whole-body oxygen demand may exacerbate OSA events in the obese patient. Specific anatomic locations of excess fat deposition may be important. A variety of body habitus measures, including neck morphology, general obesity, and central obesity, have been associated with OSA. At present, there is no consensus that a particular habitus phenotype is causatively important in the pathophysiology of OSA.

The effect of weight change on OSA has been most commonly examined in clinical weight-loss studies of morbidly obese patients. Typically, these studies assessed indexes of OSA before and after either surgical or dietary weight loss. Only two studies included an appropriate control group. In the only randomized study, the therapeutic effects of weight loss were evaluated in 15 hypersomnolent patients with moderately severe OSA. As patients decreased their body weight from an average of 106 kg to 97 kg, apnea frequency fell from 55 to 29 episodes per hour. Sleep patterns also improved, with a reduction in stage I sleep and a rise in stage II sleep. In the 9 patients with the most marked fall in apnea frequency, the tendency to experience daytime hypersomnolence decreased ($P < 0.05$). No significant changes in sleep patterns occurred in 8 age- and weight-matched control patients who did not lose weight.[9]

In the other controlled study, the effect of dietary weight loss on apnea severity was examined in 13 obese patients and 13 age- and weight-matched obese control subjects. The upper airway critical closing pressure before and after a $17.4\% \pm 3.4\%$ reduction in body mass index was

tested in order to estimate the influence of diet on airway collapsibility. Also included in the study were 13 controls—weight-stable male subjects matched for age, body mass index, and disordered breathing rate during the non-rapid-eye-movement stage of sleep. In the weight-loss group, there was a significant decrease in the number of obstructive events from 83 to 32 episodes per hour, and a decrease in critical pressure from 3 cm to −2.5 cm H_2O was demonstrated. Moreover, the decreases in critical pressures were associated with nearly complete elimination of apnea in each patient with critical pressure below −4 cm H_2O. In contrast, no significant change was observed in the usual-care group. Therefore, it seems that weight loss is associated with decreases in upper airway collapsibility in obstructive sleep apnea, and that the resolution of sleep apnea depends on the absolute level to which the negative pressure falls.[10]

These results were mirrored in several uncontrolled dietary and surgical weight-loss studies. The relationship between mean weight change and mean AHI reduction among the weight-change studies is depicted in Figure 44-1. Generally, there was greater relative weight loss (i.e., mean percent reduction from baseline weight) in the studies of surgical weight loss than in those of dietary loss. Overall, across the several studies, there is a clear and consistent trend in the relationship of mean weight loss and mean reduction in AHI.

There are probably multiple mechanisms by which obesity predisposes to airway collapse during sleep. (1) Increased fat deposits in tissues surrounding the upper airway in obese patients with OSA (in comparison to weight-matched controls) may directly impinge on the airway lumen. (2) These fat deposits may also increase airway collapsibility by altering tissue compliance, producing an elastic "loading" effect. (3) Fat deposits may interfere with

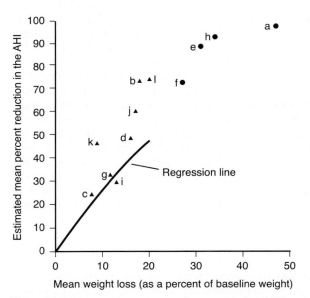

Figure 44-1. Estimated mean apnea-hypopnea index (AHI) reduction, as a percentage of baseline AHI, associated with mean weight loss, as a percentage of baseline weight, from clinical studies of dietary weight loss (*triangles*) and surgical weight loss (*circles*). From Young T, Peppard PE, Gottlieb DJ: Epidemiology of obstructive sleep apnea: a population health perspective. Am J Respir Crit Care Med 2002;165:1217-1239.

the function of inspiratory and expiratory muscles that normally maintain upper airway caliber. (4) Metabolic and hormonal changes associated with obesity could increase airway collapsibility via several mechanisms. Regardless of the mechanism, upper airway collapsibility has been shown to decrease after weight loss in obese patients with OSA.[6]

▶ CLINICAL PRESENTATION AND COMPLICATIONS OF OSA

The cardinal manifestations of the OSA syndrome are stentorian snoring and severe daytime sleepiness. In most patients, snoring antedates the development of obstructive events by many years. It is important to stress that the majority of snoring individuals do not have OSA. The recurrent episodes of nocturnal asphyxia and arousal from sleep that characterize OSA lead to a series of secondary physiologic events, which in turn give rise in some patients to the clinical complications of the syndrome.

The most common manifestations are neuropsychiatric and behavioral disturbances that are thought to arise from the fragmentation of sleep and the loss of slow-wave sleep induced by the recurrent arousal responses. Nocturnal cerebral hypoxia may also play an important role in the well-known manifestation of daytime sleepiness. Initially, daytime sleepiness manifests under passive conditions, such as reading or watching television. As the disorder progresses, sleepiness encroaches onto all daily activities and can become disabling and dangerous.[8] Both snoring and sleepiness may be denied or minimized by the patient. Snorers may be unaware of the sounds of their nightly battles to breathe unless there are listeners to tell them. There are at least two problems with sleepiness as a symptom. One is that patients may develop sleepiness so slowly over years that they forget what normal alertness is like. The other is that sleep deprivation is so common in our society that sleepiness is ubiquitous and thus nonspecific. The observations of people who have seen the patients' sleep behaviors can be very helpful to clinicians.

Other reported manifestations of OSA include physically restless sleep, night sweats, morning dry mouth or sore throat, personality change, morning confusion, intellectual impairment, impotence, and morning headaches.

It is well known that OSA is associated with some of the leading causes of mortality in adults: hypertension and cardiovascular and cerebrovascular diseases. In addition, several neurobehavioral morbidities that are of potentially great public health and economic importance are linked with OSA, including daytime sleepiness and impaired cognitive function that may, in turn, contribute to motor vehicle crashes and job-related accidents.[3]

Hypertension

Apnea and hypopnea episodes during sleep cause acute, transient blood pressure perturbations, inducing elevations of 30 mm Hg or more in mean arterial pressure. Nightly episodes of hypoxia, arousals, and swings in intrathoracic pressure due to OSA may lead to sustained elevation of blood pressure via pathophysiologic mechanisms that include chronically elevated sympathetic tone, alterations in baroreceptor function, and cardiovascular remodeling.

Several epidemiologic studies have consistently found positive associations between OSA and hypertension.[11-16]

There is, therefore, a growing consensus that OSA is an important risk factor for hypertension, independent of excess weight and other potentially confounding factors. An association appears to be present even at the mild end of the OSA severity spectrum. Despite the generally modest magnitude of the association, the high prevalence of OSA implies that it may be responsible for a substantial portion of the population burden of hypertension.

In a prospective study over a 4-year period, and after adjustment for habitus, age, sex, and cigarette and alcohol use, persons with few episodes of apnea or hypopnea (up to 4.9 events per hour) at baseline had 42% greater odds of having hypertension at follow-up than did persons with no episodes.[15] Persons with mild sleep-disordered breathing (as defined by an AHI of 5.0 to 14.9 events per hour) and those with more severe sleep-disordered breathing (as defined by an AHI of 15.0 or more events per hour) had approximately two and three times, respectively, the odds of having hypertension at follow-up than those with no episodes of apnea or hypopnea.

The fact that the association was tested prospectively lends support to the evidence of a causal role of sleep-disordered breathing in hypertension. The presence of sleep-disordered breathing was predictive of the presence of hypertension 4 years later. This finding may indicate that sleep-disordered breathing accelerates the progression of blood-pressure levels. Because sleep-disordered breathing is highly prevalent, a causal association could be responsible for a substantial number of cases of hypertension and its sequelae, such as cardiovascular and cerebrovascular morbidity and mortality.[15]

Cardiovascular and Cerebrovascular Morbidity and Mortality

Many studies of sleep and breathing suggest an independent association between coronary artery disease and obstructive sleep apnea. There are several suggested mechanisms, including the high prevalence of hypertension, chronic sympathetic stimulation, hypoxemia, and others. Most of the studies regarding the question of whether OSA is a risk factor for coronary artery disease test the prevalence of sleep apnea in patients who have had an acute coronary event. These studies, therefore, cannot determine a direct and independent causality between OSA and ischemic heart disease. This question will have to await resolution for the incidence data from several ongoing population-based cohort studies of objectively assessed OSA.

If OSA does cause hypertension, then OSA should also contribute to cardiovascular and cerebrovascular morbidity and mortality, given their incontrovertible link to hypertension. In addition to chronically elevated blood pressure, a number of possible mechanisms by which OSA might affect cardiovascular function have been hypothesized, including vascular injury and acceleration of atherosclerosis due to episodic hypoxemia, chronic sympathetic hyperactivity, elevated fibrinogen and homocysteine levels, elevated pulmonary blood pressure, and the consequent risk for right heart hypertrophy and heart failure and an increased risk for plaque ruptures and subsequent cardiovascular or cerebrovascular events.

▶ DIAGNOSIS

Diagnosis of OSA requires that the patient be examined during sleep. The extent and location of the examination is the subject of considerable debate, but it is likely that full laboratory polysomnography is not necessary in most cases. Advances in technology now allow patients to be examined while sleeping (or presumed to be sleeping) in their own homes. The diagnosis of OSA is determined when there are 5 or more episodes of apnea per hour or 30 episodes during an average night's sleep.

▶ TREATMENT

There are no controlled trials that compare medically induced and surgically induced weight loss as a treatment for sleep apnea. In an observational study, an average weight loss of 10 kg reduced the mean AHI from 55 to 29, and a 10% weight-loss was associated with a 26% decrease in the AHI in patients with OSA syndrome.[9]

Nonsurgical Treatment

Nonsurgical therapy can be classified as behavioral, pharmacologic, or mechanical. Behavioral treatments include dietary modification for weight loss, restriction of body position during sleep, avoidance of alcohol and other substances known to make apnea worse, avoidance of upper airway mucosal irritants and, possibly, avoidance of altitude.

A variety of drugs have been used for treatment of obstructive sleep apnea, most with only limited success. Supplemental oxygen may be helpful in a small subset of patients, especially those who sleep in high-altitude environments. The categories of drug therapy that have been tried are drugs that increase upper-airway patency (e.g., nasal decongestants and steroids); drugs that cause respiratory stimulation (e.g., progesterone and acetazolamide); and more generalized neuroactive drugs (e.g., protriptyline). Despite much interest in the past in pharmacologic therapy of OSA, most agents have fallen out of favor.

Mechanical devices aimed at altering the configuration or compliance of the upper airway may be useful in selected patients, especially those with mild or positional apnea. The major advance in mechanical treatment, however, is nasal continuous positive airway pressure (nasal CPAP). It has largely replaced tracheostomy as the immediate, demonstrably effective therapy for OSA. However, compliance with CPAP treatment remains a major problem.

Surgical Treatment

Tracheostomy was the first treatment used in obstructive sleep apnea.[17] It was uniformly successful because it established a continuously patent airway. However, tracheostomy is associated with medical and psychosocial morbidity. For this reason, as well as because of the successful use of CPAP therapy, the frequency of using tracheostomy has decreased significantly.[18] Nevertheless, this procedure remains an option in patients who have severe disease and are unable to use other forms of treatment.[17]

Surgery to reconfigure the upper airway so that it remains patent during sleep is a valid treatment option.[19] Tonsillectomy, with or without adenoidectomy; nasal surgery; and uvulopalatopharyngoplasty are the most common procedures performed.[19]

In the past decade, anterior sagittal osteotomy of the mandible with hyoid myotomy and suspension, and mandibular advancement (Le Fort type 1 osteotomy) have been employed in the treatment of OSA. Most recently, maxillomandibular and hyoid advancement has been performed by Riley and Powell,[20] and laser midline glossectomy has been performed by Fujita and colleagues.[21]

It is obviously desirable to have a clear definition of the specific location within the upper airway at which the obstruction is occurring during sleep. With this information, the surgical procedure can be tailored to the pathophysiology operative in the particular patient, and the chance of a successful surgical outcome is improved. The reported rates of improvement in the AHI with uvulopalatopharyngoplasty vary. The rate of long-term effectiveness (a reduction in the AHI of at least 50% and a postoperative AHI below 10) is less than 50%.[19] Also, the procedure has been associated with complications, including postoperative pain, bleeding, nasopharyngeal stenosis, changes in the voice and, in rare cases, death.

BARIATRIC SURGERY

In morbidly obese subjects, weight loss remains the ideal treatment. Low-calorie diet together with dramatic changes in lifestyle may succeed, but the long-term results are disappointing. Surgical treatment remains the most effective treatment for morbid obesity.[22,23]

Charuzi and colleagues have reported results of short- and long-term follow-up (42 ± 30 weeks and 6.3 years, respectively) in morbidly obese OSA patients undergoing bariatric surgery. In the short term, a significant decrease in the number of apneic episodes and a significant improvement in all measures related to sleep quality were found. Long-term follow-up revealed that regaining weight was associated with recurrence of OSA.[24]

Pillar and colleagues demonstrated the results of 7.5 years of follow-up in morbidly obese patients undergoing obesity surgery; a significant increase in the AHI was shown, along with a slight, nonsignificant decrease in the body mass index of the patient. They concluded that morbid obesity is probably not the only cause of OSA in these patients, and that weight reduction alone does not cure OSA. In other words, obese patients who lose weight following obesity surgery are still at risk for the recurrence of OSA.[25]

Longstanding significant improvement in the AHI and in arterial blood gases, pulmonary hypertension, left ventricular dysfunction, and lung volumes was, however, demonstrated by Sugerman and colleagues in patients following bariatric surgery.[26]

Profound improvement in OSA in morbidly obese patients was also demonstrated, by Rasheid and colleagues, in 100 patients following gastric bypass with accompanying reductions in body mass index.[27] We saw similar results when reporting on the effects of gastric banding on weight reduction; there were marked improvements in respiratory parameters.[28]

We believe that the preponderance of the evidence favors improvement in OSA after bariatric surgery.

This was dramatically confirmed in the metaanalysis published by Buchwald and colleagues, wherein OSA was resolved in 85.7% of patients and was resolved or improved in 83.6%.[29]

PERIOPERATIVE MANAGEMENT

OSA patients should be diagnosed and evaluated preoperatively in order to improve the immediate postoperative course and prevent postoperative respiratory complications, including apnea and long-term mechanical ventilation. It is well known that OSA patients may suffer exacerbation of the disease after general anesthesia. Clinical symptoms of OSA include a history of snoring, daytime somnolence, short sleep, latency, and reported history of observed apnea. Physical examination may show a crowded oropharynx, enlarged uvula, redundant pharyngeal folds, relative macroglossia, and excessive neck circumference.

In subjects suspected of having OSA, additional preoperative evaluations should be made, including flexible laryngoscopy and polysomnography. Special efforts should be made to bring patients with moderate and severe OSA to surgery in optimal respiratory function and ready for possible flexible fiberoptic intubation or even tracheostomy.

The use of postoperative narcotics and sedatives should be minimized. Patients should be monitored using pulse oximetry. Patients with severe OSA should be in an intensive care unit for optimal monitoring. Patients who were using CPAP before surgery should be encouraged to continue using the device postoperatively.

▶ CONCLUSION

OSA is a highly common disorder, not only in the morbidly obese; it is recognized as a major health problem that may lead to various medical disturbances, including hypertension, left and right ventricular hypertrophy, pulmonary hypertension, and increased risk for sudden death.

Obesity plays an important role in the pathogenesis of OSA. A special effort should be made to identify those with OSA prior to surgery. Patients suspected of having OSA should undergo preoperative evaluation and management so they arrive at surgery in optimal respiratory status.

Weight loss leads to a significant improvement in all OSA patients. Medical and conservative treatment in morbid obesity is generally ineffective; bariatric surgery seems to be the treatment of choice. Weight loss in these patients results in OSA resolution or improvement.

▶ REFERENCES

1. Gastaut H, Tassarini CA, Duron B: Polygraphic study of the episodic diurnal and nocturnal manifestations of the Pickwick syndrome. Brain Res 1965;2:167.
2. Flemons WW: Obstructive sleep apnea. N Engl J Med 2002;347:498-504.
3. Young T, Peppard PE, Gottlieb DJ: Epidemiology of obstructive sleep apnea: a population health perspective. Am J Respir Crit Care Med 2002;165:1217-1239.
4. Young T, Palta M, Dempsey J, et al: The occurrence of sleep-disordered breathing among middle-aged adults. N Engl J Med 1993;328:1230-1235.
5. Dempsey JA, Skatrud JB, Jacques AJ, et al: Anatomic determinants of sleep-disordered breathing across the spectrum of clinical and nonclinical male subjects. Chest 2002;122:840-851.
6. Westbrook PR: An overview of obstructive sleep apnea: epidemiology, pathophysiology, clinical presentation, and treatment. UpToDate, version 10.2, April 2002.
7. Fogel RB, Malhotra A, Pillar G, et al: White genioglossal activation in patients with obstructive sleep apnea versus control subjects. Am J Respir Crit Care Med 2001;164:2025-2030.
8. Phillipson EA: Sleep apnea. In Isselbacher KJ, Braunwald E, Wilson JD, et al (eds): Harrison's Principles of Internal Medicine, ed 14, pp. 1483-1998. New York, McGraw-Hill, 1998.
9. Smith PL, Gold AR, Meyers DA, et al: Weight loss in mildly to moderately obese patients with obstructive sleep apnea. Ann Intern Med 1985;103:850-855.
10. Schwartz AR, Gold AR, Schubert N, et al: Effect of weight loss on upper airway collapsibility in obstructive sleep apnea. Am Rev Respir Dis 1991;144:494-498.
11. Durán J, Esnaola S, Rubio R, et al: Obstructive sleep apnea-hypopnea and related clinical features in a population-based sample of subjects aged 30 to 70 years. Am J Respir Crit Care Med 2001;163:685-689.
12. Nieto FJ, Young TB, Lind BK, et al: Association of sleep-disordered breathing, sleep apnea, and hypertension in a large community-based study. JAMA 2000;283:1829-1836.
13. Bixler EO, Vgontzas AN, Lin HM, et al: Association of hypertension and sleep-disordered breathing. Arch Intern Med 2000;160:2289-2295.
14. Young T, Peppard P, Palta M, et al: Population-based study of sleep-disordered breathing as a risk factor for hypertension. Arch Intern Med 1997;157:1746-1752.
15. Peppard PE, Young T, Palta M, et al: Prospective study of the association between sleep-disordered breathing and hypertension. N Engl J Med 2000;342:1378-1384.
16. Peppard PE, Young T: Sleep-disordered breathing and hypertension: reply. N Engl J Med 2000;343:967.
17. White D, Douglas N, Pickett C, et al: Sleep deprivation and control of ventilation. Am Rev Respir Dis 1983;128:984-986.
18. Lin C: Effect of nasal CPAP on ventilatory drive in sleep apnea syndrome. Eur Respir J 1994;7:2005-2010.
19. Loube D, Loube A, Milter M: Weight loss for obstructive sleep apnea: the optimal therapy for obese patients. J Am Diet Assoc 1994;94:1291-1295.
20. Riley RW, Powell NB, Guilleminault C: Maxillary, mandibular and hyoid advancement for treatment of obstructive sleep apnea: a review of 40 patients. J Oral Maxillofac Surg 1990;48:20-26.
21. Fujita S, Woodson BT, Clark JL, et al: Laser midline glossectomy as a treatment for obstructive sleep apnea. Laryngoscope 1991;101:805-809.
22. Abu-Abeid S, Szold A: Results and complications of laparoscopic adjustable gastric banding: an early and intermediate experience. Obes Surg 1999;9:188-190.
23. Abu-Abeid S, Keidar A, Szold A: Resolution of chronic medical conditions after laparoscopic adjustable silicon gastric banding for the treatment of morbid obesity in the elderly. Surg Endosc 2001;15:132-1324.
24. Charuzi I, Lavie P, Peiser J: Bariatric surgery in morbidly obese sleep apnea patients: short- and long-term follow-up. Am J Clin Nutr 1992;55(suppl):S945-S946.
25. Pillar G, Peled N, Lavie P: Recurrence of sleep apnea without concomitant weight increase 7.5 years after weight reduction surgery. Chest 1994;106:1702-1704.
26. Sugerman H, Faiman R, Sood R, et al: Long-term effect of gastric surgery for treating respiratory insufficiency of obesity. Am J Clin Nutr 1992;55(suppl):S597-S601.
27. Rasheid S, Banasiak M, Gallagher S, et al: Gastric bypass is an effective treatment for obstructive sleep apnea in patients with clinically significant obesity. Obes Surg 2003;13:58-61.
28. Szold A, Abu-Abeid S: Laparoscopic adjustable silicone gastric banding for morbid obesity: results and complications in 715 patients. Surg Endosc 2002;16:230-233.
29. Buchwald H, Avidor Y, Braunwald E, et al: Bariatric surgery: a systematic review and meta-analysis. JAMA 2004;292:1724-1737. (Erratum), JAMA 2005;293:1728.

45

Orthopedic Conditions and Obesity: Changes with Weight Loss

John B. Dixon, M.B.B.S., F.R.A.C.G.P. and Paul E. O'Brien, M.D., F.R.A.C.S.

Although most severely obese patients suffer from joint or musculoskeletal discomfort, many aspects of the relationship between orthopedic conditions and obesity have a low level of evidence-based support. In this chapter, the limited data regarding this important relationship are explored. Understanding the interaction among weight, weight loss, and arthritis, especially osteoarthritis, may prove crucial to the optimal management and prevention of some very common orthopedic conditions.

▶ OBESITY AND ORTHOPEDIC PATHOLOGY

Impaired Mobility

Obesity is associated with major mobility problems and a range of musculoskeletal pains that reduce quality of life.[1,2] Shortness of breath can make everyday tasks such as walking to the shop or up a flight of stairs difficult and exercise impossible. Physical constraints can make personal hygiene and cleanliness difficult, with simple tasks such as drying oneself after a shower, cutting toenails, or tying shoelaces becoming major challenges. Seats are often too small to sit in comfortably, making travel, especially air travel, difficult.

Mobility problems associated with obesity appear to be most common in women, and they increase with age.[3] Elderly obese women have been found to suffer significantly greater functional limitations than those of normal weight.[4] Women report that their main mobility disabilities are with strain and pain at work, sports, walking outdoors and up stairs, getting off the sofa, and housework that requires squatting, stooping, or lifting.[5] Obesity has also been associated with a rapid decline in mobility, independent of baseline mobility.[6]

It is not surprising that the degree of disability suffered by obese subjects appears most strongly related to lower-body pain. Common examples include pain in the feet[7] and knees following periods of standing and walking, along with persistent heel pain[8] and nagging lower-back pain.[9] Neck and shoulder pain is also common among women with large breasts.[10] Such joint and musculoskeletal complaints have now been clearly shown to have a major negative impact on quality-of-life (QOL) measures among obese persons.[2,11]

Osteoarthritis

The association between obesity and osteoarthritis is strongest in the knee joint in women.[12-15] The relative risk for developing knee osteoarthritis is two- to sevenfold for women in the upper third of the body mass index (BMI) and is 18-fold for bilateral disease. The proportion of osteoarthritis attributable to obesity in middle-aged women is estimated to be 63%.[16] The Framingham Heart Study demonstrated, 1948 to 1951, a strong association between obesity and the subsequent development of osteoarthritis in women 36 years later. The relationship was not as strong for men.[12,15] Twin studies confirmed the importance of BMI as a risk factor for knee arthritis in women with an estimate that the risk for knee osteoarthritis increases by 35% for every 5 kg of weight gain.[17,18]

Current evidence suggests that the increased risk is probably due to direct mechanical stress on the joint rather than to metabolic factors.[14,16,19] Sharma and colleagues found that obesity was related to knee arthritis more strongly in those individuals with a varus malalignment and hypothesized that this local effect may render the knee more susceptible to arthritis in obese subjects.[20] Biomechanical factors associated with the gait in obese individuals may also predispose to knee arthritis.[21] It is important to recognize that obesity contributes not only to the progression of knee arthritis but also to the disability associated with it.[22]

There is no clear relationship between obesity and osteoarthritis in joints other than the knee. Some studies have suggested an increase in risk for hand[23,24] and hip arthritis,[25,26] but these findings have not been consistent.[27,28] Many studies have shown an increased prevalence of back pain in patients with severe obesity,[29-31] but the nature and mechanisms of pain have not been well studied.

A study of the 1958 British birth cohort found an interesting interaction between back pain and obesity in women. Women with chronic back pain gained more weight between ages 23 and 33 than those without pain. Women who were obese at age 23 years had an elevated risk for subsequent onset of back pain over the next 10 years (adjusted relative risk = 1.78). There were no similar relationships found for men.[32] It has been hypothesized that loss of lower limb muscle in association with central obesity with aging is associated with lower back pain.[33] In our consecutive series of 1000 severely obese patients presenting for laparoscopic adjustable banding surgery, 56% complained of recent lower-back pain. Obesity is a risk factor for transition from acute to chronic occupational back pain.[34] A systematic review of the literature found that two thirds of studies showed a positive relationship between back pain and obesity, but that the relative risk was generally less than 2.0.[35]

Gout

Cross-sectional and longitudinal studies have consistently shown an association between obesity, hyperuricemia, and gout in both men and women. Hyperuricemia is associated with central weight distribution and insulin resistance. Hyperuricemia develops as a result of both increased production and reduced renal clearance.[16] In addition to obesity, excessive weight gain in young adulthood and hypertension are risk factors for the development of gout.[36] Weight reduction has been associated with a modest lowering of serum uric acid concentration.[37]

▶ EFFECT OF WEIGHT LOSS

Quality of Life

Almost all subjects losing significant weight report improvements in their levels of energy, physical mobility, general mood, self-confidence, and physical health.[38]

Studies of QOL following bariatric surgery consistently demonstrate sustained improvements in physical function and reduction in pain.[11,39,40]

We have performed a large prospective study of health-related QOL in severely obese subjects before and following weight loss induced by laparoscopic adjustable gastric banding.[11] We used the validated Medical Outcomes Trust Short Form-36 (SF-36). Subjects with preoperative lower-limb arthritis or a history of lower-limb joint pain reported significantly poorer QOL scores preoperatively and had significantly greater improvement than other patients in seven of the eight SF-36 domains at 1 year. SF-36 scores at 1 year for patients with arthritis and joint pain were not different from those of nonobese community norms (Fig. 45-1).[11] The major improvement in QOL in subjects with knee, ankle, and foot pain supports the hypothesis that obesity causes or aggravates conditions that produce these symptoms.

Osteoarthritis

There is a paucity of data on weight loss as a treatment for osteoarthritis, but the limited information suggests that it is effective, especially in patients with knee disease, and that even small amounts of weight reduction may have favorable effects.[41] A reduction in weight has been shown at least to slow the progression of knee osteoarthritis.[16]

Weight loss and exercise lead to improvements in pain levels, disability, and performance in obese elderly subjects with established knee osteoarthritis.[42] A 6-week intervention program found that increased exercise and reduced fat mass were correlated with greater symptomatic relief in overweight subjects with osteoarthritis.[43] Overweight and obese women participating in the Framingham Knee Osteoarthritis study who had lost weight in the preceding 10 years had a reduced risk for developing symptomatic knee osteoarthritis.[44]

Bariatric surgery has been shown to reduce medication requirements by those with osteoarthritis.[45] Several series

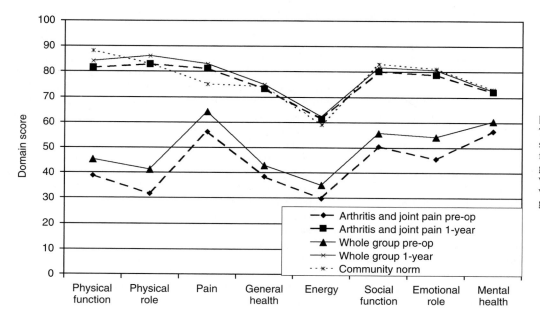

Figure 45-1. Medical Outcomes Trust Short Form-36 (SF-36) scores preoperatively and at 1 year following laparoscopic adjustable gastric bypass surgery. Patients with arthritis or joint pain (n = 158) were compared with the whole goup (n = 218).

reporting the outcomes of obesity surgery indicate improvement or resolution of symptoms related to arthritis but have not provided specific details.[46-48] There is a need for greater specificity in reporting the musculoskeletal outcomes of bariatric surgery.

▶ ORTHOPEDIC SURGERY IN THE OBESE SUBJECT

Risks of Surgery

Problems associated with joint replacement surgery have a positive relationship with BMI. Obese patients have greater preoperative comorbidities, such as type 2 diabetes, obstructive sleep apnea, and heart disease. Obese patients, especially those with BMIs greater than 35 kg per m^2, require longer hospitalization and more intensive rehabilitation and have an increased incidence of postoperative complications following knee arthroplasty.[49] There is consistent evidence that obesity is a risk factor for venous thromboembolism, greater operative blood loss, delayed wound healing, and deep joint infection following both hip and knee replacement surgery.[50-58]

Surgical Outcomes in Obese Subjects

There is a broadly held attitude in the orthopedic community that severe obesity will compromise the long-term outcome of joint replacement to such an extent that surgery should be deferred until substantial weight loss has been achieved. The available published data do not provide strong or consistent support for this view. Obesity is associated with increased perioperative risk in joint replacement, but long-term outcomes are generally favorable and are comparable to those in nonobese subjects. In a study performed 10 years after total knee arthroplasty, Griffin and colleagues found obese subjects to have greater improvement in functional scores than nonobese subjects.[59] Scores at 10 years were comparable, but the obese subjects had lower baseline functional scores. A community-based, cross-sectional survey showed that age and obesity do not have negative impacts on health-related QOL following knee replacement.[60] Stickles and colleagues found that obese patients enjoy the same improvement and satisfaction after hip and knee arthroplasty as other patients.[61] In a consecutive series of 180 knee arthroplasties, BMI did not adversely influence the outcome at 1 year.[62] Spicer and colleagues confirmed the improvement in functional knee scores following surgery appears to be similar in obese and nonobese groups.[63]

Obesity, however, has been demonstrated to be a risk factor for some late complications that require revisional surgery after knee arthroplasty.[64] Spicer and colleagues reported an increase in focal osteolysis on radiograph in subjects with BMIs greater than 40 kg per m^2 and a trend toward increased need for revisional surgery.[63] Obesity appears also to be one of a number of important risk factors for late deep-joint infection following knee replacement.[65] The possibility that obesity increases stress and wear on the implanted prosthesis remains possible, although one study examining this did not find polyethylene wear in hip and knee prostheses to be weight dependent.[66]

Thus, although functional outcomes are good, there is not only an increased risk for perioperative complications, but there continues to be the later risk for infection and revision in obese subjects.

Weight Loss Following Joint Replacement

The physical restriction and reduced mobility associated with osteoarthritis have often been blamed for leading to weight gain in obese patients who suffer from significant joint pain; this hypothesis is supported by some epidemiologic evidence.[32] Could improvements following joint replacement lead to weight loss? Two small observational studies have indirectly addressed this issue. Neither found that functional improvement following hip or knee surgery facilitated weight loss.[67,68] The relationships between pain and weight gain and between pain resolution and weight loss clearly require further careful exploration.

Effect of Weight Loss Prior to Arthroplasty

Given the increased risk for both early and late complications following joint replacement surgery in obese people, it would seem appropriate to test the effect of weight loss prior to surgery. There are limited data, but a single observational study has reported favorable outcomes for joint replacement following bariatric surgery.[69] It is perhaps surprising that there are so few data in this important area. Obese patients who require joint replacement are almost certainly advised to lose weight. Some surgeons advise delaying the joint replacement until weight is lost. Important questions remain unanswered. How much weight should be lost? How to lose it? And, will weight loss lead to better outcomes?

The risks in joint replacement surgery are greatest in those with BMIs greater than 35 kg per m^2. The only reliable way to achieve and sustain significant weight loss in this weight range is with bariatric surgery. Bariatric surgery is now safer, minimally invasive, and more broadly acceptable. Given that conditions caused by or aggravated by obesity are often best treated by substantial sustained weight loss, and that exercise is especially difficult for obese people with arthritis, it would therefore appear important to test formally the place of modern bariatric surgery prior to joint replacement surgery.

There is no doubt that severe obesity is associated with grossly impaired physical quality of life. This provides an important challenge for both bariatric and orthopedic specialists. Trials that carefully assess various management options are urgently needed.

▶ REFERENCES

1. Han TS, Tijhuis MA, Lean ME, et al: Quality of life in relation to overweight and body fat distribution. Am J Public Health 1998;88:1814-1820.
2. Barofsky I, Fontaine KR, Cheskin LJ: Pain in the obese: impact on health-related quality-of-life. Ann Behav Med 1998;19:408-410.
3. Himes CL: Obesity, disease, and functional limitation in later life. Demography 2000;37:73-82.
4. Davison KK, Ford ES, Cogswell ME, et al: Percentage of body fat and body mass index are associated with mobility limitations in people

aged 70 and older from NHANES III. J Am Geriatr Soc 2002;50:1802-1809.

5. Larsson UE, Mattsson E: Perceived disability and observed functional limitations in obese women. Int J Obes Relat Metab Disord 2001;25:1705-1712.

6. Damush TM, Stump TE, Clark DO: Body-mass index and 4-year change in health-related quality of life. J Aging Health 2002;14:195-210.

7. Chan MK, Chong LY: A prospective epidemiologic survey on the prevalence of foot disease in Hong Kong. J Am Podiatr Med Assoc 2002;92:450-456.

8. Wolgin M, Cook C, Graham C, et al: Conservative treatment of plantar heel pain: long-term follow-up. Foot Ankle Int 1994;15:97-102.

9. Brown WJ, Mishra G, Kenardy J, et al: Relationships between body mass index and well-being in young Australian women. Int J Obes Relat Metab Disord 2000;24:1360-1368.

10. Netscher DT, Meade RA, Goodman CM, et al: Physical and psychosocial symptoms among 88 volunteer subjects compared with patients seeking plastic surgery procedures to the breast. Plast Reconstr Surg 2000;105:2366-2373.

11. Dixon JB, Dixon ME, O'Brien PE: Quality of life after lap-band placement: influence of time, weight loss, and comorbidities. Obes Res 2001;9:713-721.

12. Sandmark H, Hogstedt C, Lewold S, et al: Osteoarthrosis of the knee in men and women in association with overweight, smoking, and hormone therapy. Ann Rheum Dis 1999;58:151-155.

13. Coggon D, Reading I, Croft P, et al: Knee osteoarthritis and obesity. Int J Obes Relat Metab Disord 2001;25:622-627.

14. Davis MA, Ettinger WH, Neuhaus JM: Obesity and osteoarthritis of the knee: evidence from the National Health and Nutrition Examination Survey (NHANES I). Semin Arthritis Rheum 1990;20:34-41.

15. Felson DT, Anderson JJ, Naimark A, et al: Obesity and knee osteoarthritis: The Framingham Study. Ann Intern Med 1988;109:18-24.

16. Cicuttini FM, Spector TD: Obesity Osteoarthritis and Gout. In George A, Bray CB, James WPT (eds): Handbook of Obesity, pp. 741-752. New York, Marcel Dekker, 1998.

17. Spector T, Cicuttini F, Baker J, et al: Genetic influences on osteoarthritis in women: a twin study. BMJ 1996;312:940-943.

18. Cicuttini FM, Baker JR, Spector TD: The association of obesity with osteoarthritis of the hand and knee in women: a twin study. J Rheumatol 1996;23:1221-1226.

19. Martin K, Lethbridge-Cejku M, Muller DC, et al: Metabolic correlates of obesity and radiographic features of knee osteoarthritis: data from the Baltimore Longitudinal Study of Aging. J Rheumatol 1997;24:702-707.

20. Sharma L, Lou C, Cahue S, Dunlop DD: The mechanism of the effect of obesity in knee osteoarthritis: the mediating role of malalignment. Arthritis Rheum 2000;43:568-575.

21. Messier SP: Osteoarthritis of the knee and associated factors of age and obesity: effects on gait. Med Sci Sports Exerc 1994;26:1446-1452.

22. Lamb SE, Guralnik JM, Buchner DM, et al: Factors that modify the association between knee pain and mobility limitation in older women: the Women's Health and Aging Study. Ann Rheum Dis 2000;59:331-337.

23. Carman WJ, Sowers M, Hawthorne VM, et al: Obesity as a risk factor for osteoarthritis of the hand and wrist: a prospective study. Am J Epidemiol 1994;139:119-129.

24. Hart DJ, Spector TD: The relationship of obesity, fat distribution and osteoarthritis in women in the general population: the Chingford Study. J Rheumatol 1993;20:331-335.

25. Hartz AJ, Fischer ME, Bril G, et al: The association of obesity with joint pain and osteoarthritis in the HANES data. J Chronic Dis 1986;39:311-319.

26. Cooper C, Inskip H, Croft P, et al: Individual risk factors for hip osteoarthritis: obesity, hip injury, and physical activity. Am J Epidemiol 1998;147:516-522.

27. Sturmer T, Gunther KP, Brenner H: Obesity, overweight and patterns of osteoarthritis: the Ulm Osteoarthritis Study. J Clin Epidemiol 2000;53:307-313.

28. Hochberg MC, Lethbridge-Cejku M, Scott WW Jr: Obesity and osteoarthritis of the hands in women. Osteoarthritis Cartilage 1993;1:129-135.

29. Garzillo MJ, Garzillo TA: Does obesity cause low back pain? J Manipulative Physiol Ther 1994;17:601-604.

30. Deyo RA, Bass JE: Lifestyle and low-back pain: the influence of smoking and obesity. Spine 1989;14:501-506.

31. Leboeuf-Yde C, Kyvik KO, Bruun NH: Low back pain and lifestyle. II: Obesity. Information from a population-based sample of 29,424 twin subjects. Spine 1999;24:779-783.

32. Lake JK, Power C, Cole TJ: Back pain and obesity in the 1958 British birth cohort: cause or effect? J Clin Epidemiol 2000;53:245-250.

33. Toda Y, Segal N, Toda T, et al: Lean body mass and body fat distribution in participants with chronic low back pain. Arch Intern Med 2000;160:3265-3269.

34. Fransen M, Woodward M, Norton R, et al: Risk factors associated with the transition from acute to chronic occupational back pain. Spine 2002;27:92-98.

35. Leboeuf-Yde C: Body weight and low back pain: a systematic literature review of 56 journal articles reporting on 65 epidemiologic studies. Spine 2000;25:226-237.

36. Roubenoff R, Klag MJ, Mead LA, et al: Incidence and risk factors for gout in white men. JAMA 1991;266:3004-3007.

37. Scott JT: Obesity and uricaemia. Clin Rheum Dis 1977;3:25-35.

38. Klem ML, Wing RR, McGuire MT, et al: A descriptive study of individuals successful at long-term maintenance of substantial weight loss. Am J Clin Nutr 1997;66:239-246.

39. Kral JG, Sjostrom LV, Sullivan MB: Assessment of quality of life before and after surgery for severe obesity. Am J Clin Nutr 1992;55:611S-614S.

40. van Gemert WG, Adang EM, Greve JW, et al: Quality of life assessment of morbidly obese patients: effect of weight-reducing surgery. Am J Clin Nutr 1998;67:197-201.

41. Felson DT, Chaisson CE: Understanding the relationship between body weight and osteoarthritis. Baillieres Clin Rheumatol 1997;11:671-681.

42. Messier SP, Loeser RF, Mitchell MN, et al: Exercise and weight loss in obese older adults with knee osteoarthritis: a preliminary study. J Am Geriatr Soc 2000;48:1062-1072.

43. Toda Y, Toda T, Takemura S, et al: Change in body fat, but not body weight or metabolic correlates of obesity, is related to symptomatic relief of obese patients with knee osteoarthritis after a weight control program. J Rheumatol 1998;25:2181-2186.

44. Felson DT, Zhang Y, Anthony JM, et al: Weight loss reduces the risk for symptomatic knee osteoarthritis in women: The Framingham Study. Ann Intern Med 1992;116:535-539.

45. Murr MM, Siadati MR, Sarr MG: Results of bariatric surgery for morbid obesity in patients older than 50 years. Obes Surg 1995;5:399-402.

46. Pories WJ, Swanson MS, MacDonald KG, et al: Who would have thought it? An operation proves to be the most effective therapy for adult-onset diabetes mellitus. Ann Surg 1995;222:339-350.

47. Buchwald H, Rucker RD, Schwartz MZ, et al: Positive results of jejunoileal bypass surgery: emphasis on lipids with comparison to gastric bypass. Int J Obes 1981;5:399-404.

48. Melissas J, Christodoulakis M, Schoretsanitis G, et al: Obesity-associated disorders before and after weight reduction by vertical banded gastroplasty in morbidly vs super obese individuals. Obes Surg 2001;11:475-481.

49. Miric A, Lim M, Kahn B, et al: Perioperative morbidity following total knee arthroplasty among obese patients. J Knee Surg 2002;15:77-83.

50. White RH, Henderson MC: Risk factors for venous thromboembolism after total hip and knee replacement surgery. Curr Opin Pulm Med 2002;8:365-371.

51. Winiarsky R, Barth P, Lotke P: Total knee arthroplasty in morbidly obese patients. J Bone Joint Surg Am 1998;80:1770-1774.

52. Wilson MG, Kelley K, Thornhill TS: Infection as a complication of total knee-replacement arthroplasty: risk factors and treatment in sixty-seven cases. J Bone Joint Surg Am 1990;72:878-883.

53. Soballe K, Christensen F, Luxhoj T: Hip replacement in obese patients. Acta Orthop Scand 1987;58:223-225.

54. Lowe GD, Haverkate F, Thompson SG, et al: Prediction of deep vein thrombosis after elective hip replacement surgery by preoperative clinical and haemostatic variables: the ECAT DVT Study: European Concerted Action on Thrombosis. Thromb Haemost 1999;81:879-886.

55. Yong KS, Kareem BA, Ruslan GN, et al: Risk factors for infection in total hip replacement surgery at Hospital Kuala Lumpur. Med J Malaysia 2001;56(supplC):57-60.

56. Eveillard M, Mertl P, Canarelli, B et al: Risk of deep infection in first-intention total hip replacement: evaluation concerning a continuous series of 790 cases. Presse Med 2001;30:1868-1875 (in French).

57. Kim YH, Choi IY, Park MR, et al: Deep vein thrombosis after uncemented total hip replacement. Bull Hosp Jt Dis 1997;56:133-139.

58. Grosflam JM, Wright EA, Cleary PD, et al: Predictors of blood loss during total hip replacement surgery. Arthritis Care Res 1995;8:167-173.

59. Griffin FM, Scuderi GR, Insall JN, et al: Total knee arthroplasty in patients who were obese with 10 years follow-up. Clin Orthoped Rel Res 1998:28-33.

60. Hawker G, Wright J, Coyte P, et al. Health-related quality of life after knee replacement. J Bone Joint Surg 1998;80:163-173.

61. Stickles B, Phillips L, Brox WT, et al: Defining the relationship between obesity and total joint arthroplasty. Obes Res 2001;9:219-223.

62. Deshmukh RG, Hayes JH, Pinder IM: Does body weight influence outcome after total knee arthroplasty? A 1-year analysis. J Arthroplasty 2002;17:315-319.

63. Spicer DD, Pomeroy DL, Badenhausen WE, et al: Body mass index as a predictor of outcome in total knee replacement. Int Orthop 2001;25:246-249.

64. Ahlberg A, Lunden A: Secondary operations after knee joint replacement. Clin Orthop 1981;156:170-174.

65. Peersman G, Laskin R, Davis J, et al: Infection in total knee replacement: a retrospective review of 6489 total knee replacements. Clin Orthop Rel Res 2001;392:15-23.

66. McClung CD, Zahiri CA, Higa JK, et al: Relationship between body mass index and activity in hip or knee arthroplasty patients. J Orthop Res 2000;18:35-39.

67. Woolf VJ, Charnley GJ, Goddard NJ: Weight changes after total hip arthroplasty. J Arthroplasty 1994;9:389-391.

68. Pritchett JW, Bortel DT: Knee replacement in morbidly obese women. Surg Gynecol Obstet 1991;173:119-122.

69. Parvizi J, Trousdale RT, Sarr MG: Total joint arthroplasty in patients surgically treated for morbid obesity. J Arthroplasty 2000;15:1003-1008.

46

Metabolic Outcomes of Bariatric Surgery

Athanassios Petrotos, M.D. and Louis Flancbaum, M.D., F.A.C.S., F.C.C.M., F.C.C.P.

Obesity causes numerous metabolic and physiologic perturbations, most of which are positively affected by surgically induced weight loss. In addition, bariatric surgical procedures themselves, by virtue of the changes in anatomy and gastrointestinal physiology inherent in them, lead to significant changes in body composition and energy metabolism. This chapter discusses both of these subjects.

▶ METABOLIC ABNORMALITIES ASSOCIATED WITH OBESITY

Metabolic Syndrome

The ominous association between upper-body obesity, glucose intolerance, hypertriglyceridemia, and hypertension was termed the deadly quartet and was elaborated upon by Kaplan in 1989.[1] This constellation was later called metabolic syndrome, syndrome X, or the insulin-resistance metabolic syndrome of obesity.

Metabolic syndrome is defined as the presence of three or more of the following criteria[2]:

1. Abdominal obesity: waist circumference larger than 102 cm in men and larger than 88 cm in women;
2. Hypertriglyceridemia, above 150 mg per dl (1.69 mmol/l);
3. Low high-density lipoprotein (HDL) cholesterol, below 40 mg per dl (1.04 mmol/l) in men and below 50 mg per dl (1.29 mmol/l) in women;
4. High blood pressure, above 130/85 mm Hg;
5. High fasting glucose, above 110 mg per dl (6.1 mmol/l).

In one study, the unadjusted and age-adjusted prevalences of the metabolic syndrome were 21.8% and 23.7%, respectively.[2] The prevalence increased from 6.7% in participants aged 20 through 29 years, to 43.5% in those 60 through 69 years, and to 42% in those at least 70 years of age. Mexican-Americans had the highest age-adjusted prevalence of the metabolic syndrome (31.9%). The age-adjusted prevalence was similar for men (24%) and women (23.4%). However, among African-Americans, women had a 57% higher prevalence than men, and among Mexican-Americans, women had a 26% higher prevalence than men. Using census data from 2000, it is estimated that about 47 million U.S. residents have the metabolic syndrome. People with the metabolic syndrome are at increased risk for developing diabetes mellitus and cardiovascular disease, as well as being at increased risk for death from cardiovascular disease and all other causes.

Insulin Resistance

A reduction in sensitivity to insulin can occur as a result of a genetic defect or it can be acquired as a metabolic consequence of obesity. In both the fasting and postprandial states, obese individuals require insulin levels that are several times higher than those of nonobese individuals to maintain euglycemia.[3] On a cellular level, insulin binds to its receptors on the surfaces of target cells, triggering tyrosine autophosphorylation and consequent intracellular signaling. These events culminate in cellular responses, such as the translocation of glucose transporters to the cell surface to allow glucose uptake for use in glycogen storage. In obesity, insulin signaling is defective. Insulin-stimulated protein kinase activity of the insulin receptor, which mediates tyrosine autophosphorylation, is lower in obese subjects than in nonobese individuals, and it is even lower in people with obesity-engendered type 2 diabetes. Obesity is associated with other defects in insulin action, including impaired generation of second messengers, reduced glucose transport in skeletal muscle, and abnormalities in some critical enzymatic steps involved in glucose use.[4] Obese individuals with depressed insulin-mediated glucose transport can reverse this defect after weight loss.[4]

The increased levels of free fatty acids (FFAs) found in obese individuals also contribute to the defects in glucose use and storage. As body fat increases, the rate of lipolysis rises, leading to increased FFA mobilization and, consequently, to increased FFA oxidation in muscle and liver. In turn, glucose use by muscle declines as FFAs are used as an alternative energy source, and hepatic glucose production increases in response to the higher FFA oxidation. These actions result in hyperglycemia and impaired glucose tolerance. This mechanism is particularly important among individuals with upper-body or central obesity. The liver is also less responsive to insulin. As the insulin resistance becomes more profound, glucose uptake in peripheral tissues is impaired and hepatic glucose output increases.[3]

Type 2 Diabetes Mellitus

The risk for developing type 2 diabetes increases significantly with increasing body mass index (BMI). This relationship was demonstrated by the Nurses' Health study, which prospectively followed a cohort of more than 114,000 registered nurses for 14 years.[5] Relative to women with BMIs below 22 kg/m², age-adjusted risk for developing type 2 diabetes rose steadily with increasing BMI. Women with BMIs of 35 kg/m² or greater had a 93 times higher risk for developing diabetes than those with BMIs of less than 22 kg/m². Even women who were overweight had higher risk; those with BMIs of 25.0 to 26.9 kg/m² and 27.0 to 28.9 kg/m² had relative risks of 8.1 and 15.8, respectively. These findings emphasize the importance of maintaining a constant body weight throughout life. In the United States, about 85% of patients with type 2 diabetes mellitus are obese.

The exact mechanism by which the constellation of obesity and insulin resistance transform obesity into type 2 diabetes is unclear. Also, by an unknown mechanism, β-cell failure occurs after years of chronic hyperinsulinemia.[6]

Dyslipidemia

Dyslipidemias are common metabolic abnormalities associated with obesity. The pattern of plasma lipoproteins in obese individuals is altered. Hypertriglyceridemia is common, possibly because the insulin resistance and hyperinsulinemia of obesity lead to increased hepatic production of triglycerides. Two basic mechanisms exist for the hypertriglyceridemia of obesity: overproduction of very-low-density lipoprotein (VLDL) triglycerides and defective lipolysis of triglyceride-rich lipoproteins.[7] High caloric intake in obese individuals induces an overproduction of VLDL triglycerides, but because many of these individuals respond by increasing their clearance capacity for VLDLs, overt hypertriglyceridemia is often avoided.

Hypercholesterolemia is also common in obesity. Hypercholesterolemia usually consists of elevated serum low-density lipoprotein (LDL) concentrations and can result from defects in either the input or the clearance of LDL.[7]

Nonalcoholic Fatty Liver Disease

The term *nonalcoholic steatohepatitis* refers to a condition characterized by two main diagnostic criteria: (1) evidence of fatty changes, with lobular hepatitis; and (2) absence of alcoholism.[8] Other terms used to describe this condition include *fatty-liver hepatitis*, *nonalcoholic Laennec disease*, *diabetes hepatitis*, *alcohol-like liver disease*, and *nonalcoholic steatohepatitis*. Nonalcoholic fatty liver disease (NAFLD) is becoming the preferred term. The spectrum of NAFLD ranges from benign steatosis to cirrhosis. Obesity, type 2 diabetes mellitus, and hyperlipidemia are associated with NAFLD.

NAFLD is the most common cause of abnormal liver tests (most commonly a mild to moderate elevation of liver function enzymes (AST/ALT) in adults in the United States. The diagnosis of NAFLD is best made with liver biopsy. On the basis of the U.S. population in the year 2000, an estimated 30.1 million obese adults may have steatosis, and about 8.6 million may have steatohepatitis.[9] Among 92 consecutive morbidly obese patients undergoing bariatric surgery, routine liver biopsy demonstrated steatosis in 84%, moderate to severe inflammation in 20%, and, bridging fibrosis or cirrhosis in 8%.[10] There was no correlation with age, sex, BMI, or the presence or absence of liver function abnormality.

Body Composition and Energy Metabolism in Obesity

Obesity and weight loss result in significant alterations in body composition and energy expenditure. Energy expenditure is composed of three parts: basal metabolic rate (BMR) or resting energy expenditure (REE); thermic effect of food (TEF), also known as dietary-induced thermogenesis; and the thermic effect of exercise or activity (TEE). BMR is the minimal energy expenditure of an organism necessary for life, normally constituting about two thirds of daily energy expenditure, with the heart, liver, kidney, and brain accounting for approximately 60% of REE. In practice, because of the difficulty in measuring BMR, the REE, which is the energy expenditure of an organism measured at rest in a postabsorptive state, is used. If not measured by calorimetry or double-labeled water, BMR is usually estimated using the Harris-Benedict equation and is a function of height, weight, gender, and age. BMR and REE are predictably lower in women and the aged because these two populations have a greater percentage of body fat than lean body mass (e.g., skeletal muscle, bone, visceral protein).

Obese individuals have higher metabolic rates than lean individuals primarily because obese individuals, in addition to having significantly more fat mass, have more fat-free mass (FFM), or lean body tissue, which is more metabolically active. FFM is responsible for about 75% of REE.[11] The TEF, which is the amount of energy consumed as a result of eating and digestion, is responsible for approximately 5% to 10% of energy expenditure. For this reason, it is more energy-efficient to eat several smaller meals over the course of a day than one or two large meals. Whether TEF in obese patients is lower or the same as it is in lean counterparts is controversial. However, it is clear that TEF represents the smallest component contributing to daily energy expenditure.

TEE is the most variable component of 24-hour energy expenditure. Obese and lean subjects are equally efficient and expend equivalent amounts of energy for the same activity.[12] For any given activity, however, in which obese individuals need to support their own weight, such as walking or running, they expend more energy than lean counterparts because of the increased work requirements. For activities such as swimming or biking, where carrying their own weight is not necessary, obese and lean subjects are equally efficient. Thus, the common perception that severely obese individuals are hypometabolic is incorrect.[13]

▶ **METABOLIC EFFECTS OF BARIATRIC SURGICAL PROCEDURES**

Insulin Resistance and Type 2 Diabetes Mellitus

Glucose levels normalize in approximately 56% of patients with preoperative type 2 diabetes after vertical banded gastroplasty (VBG).[14] Fasting insulin is lowered significantly soon after VBG in hyperinsulinemic and diabetic patients.[15]

Roux-en-Y gastric bypass (RYGB) provides long-term control of non-insulin-dependent diabetes mellitus. With 14-year follow-up, 82% of obese patients with type 2 diabetes and 98% with impaired glucose tolerance maintained normal levels of plasma glucose, glycosylated hemoglobin, and insulin.[16] These effects of RYGB on glucose-insulin are observed even when individuals have relatively high proportions of body fat. The exact mechanism by which RYGB ameliorates or even treats the obesity-associated diabetes is not known. Proposed mechanisms include reduced caloric intake and synchronous reversal of insulin resistance in muscle. Pories and colleagues have documented dramatic improvement in type 2 diabetes mellitus within days of surgery, with reduction in fasting blood glucose, serum insulin, and serum leptin, as well as a lower rate of progression to and mortality from type 2 diabetes.[16,17] The Swedish Obese Subjects Intervention Study reported significant reductions in the incidence of type 2 diabetes, hyperinsulinemia, hypertension, and dyslipidemia at 2 years in their surgery cohort, which consisted of patients with BMIs above 34 kg/m².[18]

Malabsorptive procedures cause alterations in the hormonal milieu of the gastrointestinal tract. After biliopancreatic diversion (BPD), a rise in enteroglucagon levels is observed.[19] Enteroglucagon reduces the rate of glucose production by the liver, thus improving insulin metabolism. Scopinaro and colleagues observed a 100% resolution of hyperglycemia, diabetes mellitus, and diabetes mellitus requiring insulin in patients who underwent BPD.[20] Marceau and colleagues have found that blood glucose levels decreased after BPD, even when diabetes was not present preoperatively.[21]

Dyslipidemia

Obesity is associated with increased risk for cardiovascular disease due to elevated lipid levels. Serum triglyceride levels decrease early after VBG and hypertriglyceridemia normalizes in approximately 78% of the hypertriglyceridemic obese. Triglyceride levels remain low at 5 and 10 years of follow-up. Both triglyceride and glucose levels remain low, even after weight is regained.[14]

The beneficial effects of RYGB in lowering triglycerides and LDL, with synchronous increase in high-density lipoprotein (HDL), have been cited.[22] The mechanism by which these changes take place remains unclear. Brolin and colleagues prospectively studied obese patients who were hyperlipidemic in the preoperative period and subsequently underwent RYGB.[23] By the sixth postoperative month, they found a greater than 20% mean reduction in total cholesterol and a greater than 50% mean reduction in triglycerides.[23] Lipid profiles became normal in 84% of

the patients. There was a correlation between magnitude of weight loss and improvement in the lipid profile. Better results were observed in patients with satisfactory weight loss; in patients who did not lose more than 50% of their excess weight, hyperlipidemia regressed after 12 months.

As a result of decreased fat absorption after BPD, a decrease in LDL, total cholesterol, and triglycerides and an increase in HDL cholesterol were observed up to 10 years after the surgery.[21] In a study by Scopinaro and colleagues, more than 50% of patients undergoing BPD were hypercholesterolemic.[20] Normalization of cholesterol levels was observed as early as 1 month postoperatively, and the levels remained normal in subsequent measurements. Because of the interruption of the enterohepatic circulation in patients who undergo BPD, there is an increased de novo synthesis of bile acids, which accounts for the greater than expected reduction in cholesterol.

Nonalcoholic Fatty Liver Disease

Evidence is slowly beginning to appear that weight loss may result in histopathologic improvement in patients with NAFLD. Improvement in grade, stage, degree of fibrosis, and inflammation have been noted after weight loss in two small cohorts of patients with NAFLD that was identified at the time of RYGB.[24,25] The correction of metabolic abnormalities after BPD can lead to an improvement in liver function and morphology. Reversible NAFLD, even in advanced cases, was documented in one series over a period of 10 years.[21] The effects of VBG on NAFLD have not been studied.

▶ **MECHANISMS OF SURGICALLY INDUCED WEIGHT LOSS**

Prior to discussing the mechanisms by which various bariatric surgical procedures induce weight loss, a brief review of the physiology of weight homeostasis is in order. Caloric restriction produces changes in body composition and energy expenditure that lead to weight loss, as well as to compensatory changes designed to prevent it. It is these adaptive responses that make it so difficult to lose weight on diets and to maintain the weight that is lost.

Both low-calorie (800 to 1500 kcal per day) and very-low-calorie (less than 800 kcal per day) diets result in semi-starvation, a condition in which the individual experiences sustained negative nitrogen balance.[26] These dietary weight-loss regimens generally consist of an active weight-loss period of 3 to 4 months, followed by a prolonged maintenance phase. During the active phase, patients on low-calorie diets typically lose 9 to 18 kg, or 20 to 40 lb (10% to 15% of body weight) and those on very-low-calorie diets lose 14 to 27 kg, or 30 to 60 lb (15% to 20% of body weight).[26] The weight loss tends to be more rapid at first, then tapers off over time, reaching a plateau.

During this energy-deficient period, the body adapts by decreasing energy consumption commensurate with the decline in intake and by utilizing stored endogenous energy to meet its metabolic demands.[27] Initially, carbohydrates, in the form of hepatic glycogen, are broken down. However, these stores are usually depleted within 24 hours.

Following this, endogenous protein, predominantly from skeletal muscle, is degraded, producing carbon skeletons that are shunted to the liver for gluconeogenesis and resulting in negative nitrogen balance. The resultant decrease in lean body mass leads to a fall in measured resting energy expenditure (MREE) because, as noted earlier, FFM is the greatest contributor to REE. However, to prevent a reduction in lean body mass to critically low levels that would endanger health, an additional adaptive mechanism, the metabolism of fat stores into ketone bodies, is utilized. By day 7 of semistarvation, ketone bodies constitute the predominant metabolic fuel, although an obligatory nitrogen loss persists.

With the provision of adequate hydration, human beings can subsist in such a condition for several months. Although fat and FFM are lost during semistarvation, their relative contributions change over time as physiologic adaptation occurs. Because of the obligatory loss of protein that occurs, it is essential to supply adequate amounts of dietary protein to prevent compromise of essential bodily functions and processes such as immune function and wound healing and to avoid skeletal muscle atrophy. In the presence of adequate protein intake (approximately 1.2 to 1.5 g per kg ideal body weight per day), most patients on caloric restriction diets eventually lose about 75% fat and 25% lean body mass.[13,28] Energy metabolism concurrently declines during semistarvation, with most patients on low- and very-low-calorie diets manifesting a decrease in MREE of 15% to 30%, which returns toward normal during refeeding and maintenance.[29] Several factors contribute to this fall: a decrease in the amount of external work and activity; changes in thyroid hormone and sympathetic nervous system activity; and, most important, the decrease in body mass associated with weight loss, which is the factor responsible for the majority of REE.[13,29,30] However, the decline in MREE tends to be greater than can be accounted for by the loss of FFM alone, suggesting that there may also be a depression in MREE resulting from caloric restriction.[30] The efficiency of these adaptive mechanisms in semistarvation are partly responsible for the high failure rate of most dieters.

Weight regain remains a formidable problem, with most patients returning to their baseline weight by 3 years, and many exceeding it by 5 years.[26] Furthermore, in nonobese subjects experiencing increases and decreases in body weight, total, resting, and nonresting energy expenditure are significantly lower following a 10% and 20% reduction in body weight after an 800 kcal per day diet,[31] suggesting that changes in energy expenditure tend to oppose the weight change. These results have led to the implementation of additional modalities such as exercise to overcome the physiologic obstacles to weight loss.

Exercise is commonly promoted as an important component of a weight-loss regimen. In this regard, it is important to be aware that moderate exercise, per se, is ineffective as a means of achieving weight loss. Exercise alone, in the absence of dietary restriction, produces little, if any, weight loss.[32] Although there are a number of studies showing that exercise increases MREE, others have shown no effect or even a decrease in energy expenditure.[33] It does appear clear that exercise is an excellent way to promote the preservation of lean body mass during dieting.[34]

If exercise is combined with caloric restriction, it is probably better that it be done early in the day, so that any increase in metabolic rate that does occur can be combined with the increased TEE due to exercise and sustained throughout the day. Thus, exercise appears to be more important in maintaining weight loss than in achieving it.[34]

Surgical treatment for obesity is offered to patients who have clinically severe obesity or are considered morbidly obese (BMI >40 kg/m^2 or >35 kg/m^2 in the presence of associated obesity-related comorbid conditions). The role of surgery in the treatment of clinically severe obesity was evaluated in depth at a National Institutes of Health-sponsored Consensus Conference in 1991. The panel concluded that "the surgical procedures currently in use (gastric bypass and vertical banded gastroplasty) are capable of inducing significant weight loss (in severely obese patients), and in turn, have been associated with amelioration of most of the comorbid conditions that have been studied."[35]

Historically, operations for weight loss have been classified as restrictive, malabsorptive, or both, based on the proposed mechanism used for the induction of weight loss. The gastroplasties (horizontal banded gastroplasty, VBG, and laparoscopic adjustable gastric banding [LAGB]) are restrictive procedures, inducing weight loss by limiting caloric intake. The jejunoileal bypass (JIB) and its more recent modifications, BPD and BPD with duodenal switch (DS), are classified as primarily malabsorptive procedures. The most widely used procedure, the RYGB, represents a combination of these two mechanisms, although most categorize it primarily as a restrictive procedure.[36]

Caloric restriction is a major component of all bariatric surgical procedures. Weight loss following VBG appears to be similar to that in other forms of caloric restriction, although the weight loss tends to be more pronounced and persists over a longer period. The rate of weight loss after VBG ranges from 7% the first month postoperatively to 35% the twelfth month, when it stabilizes.[36] Although somewhat counterintuitive, caloric restriction played a significant role in weight loss after JIB, where it was documented that patients reduced their caloric intake by 50%.[37] Caloric intake after BPD and BPD-DS has not been published, but it stands to reason that it should fall substantially because gastric volume is reduced.[20,21] RYGB causes a profound decrease in protein and calorie intake. In the early postoperative period, up to 3 months, caloric intake ranges between 400 and 600 kcal per day. The caloric intake increases to 800 to 1000 kcal per day by 6 months, and reaches a plateau of 1200 to 1400 kcal per day.[38] Of greater concern is the inadequate protein intake up to 1 year after surgery.[39]

JIB, the prototypical malabsorptive operation, is no longer in use. Although highly effective in producing weight loss, it was associated with major long-term metabolic side effects, including diarrhea, malnutrition, gallstones, kidney stones, and liver failure, causing it to be abandoned after 1980. It has been suggested that the enhanced weight loss after BPD is related to the combination of a short common channel (approximately 50 to 100 cm), which limits fat absorption, and a long biliopancreatic limb (usually >250 cm), which is not in direct contact with food, therefore limiting the length of the alimentary (Roux) limb where protein and carbohydrates are absorbed.[40]

Limb length also affects weight loss after RYGB. Success after RYGB has varied with the degree of overweight, with so-called superobese patients (BMIs >50 kg/m², or approximately 200 lb overweight) achieving greater absolute, but smaller percent excess weight loss than less obese patients. Several studies have now demonstrated improved percentage of excess weight loss in superobese patients undergoing RYGB with longer Roux limbs of up to 250 cm[41,42] and with distal RYGB, in which gastrointestinal continuity is reestablished 75 cm proximal to the ileocecal valve.[43] For patients with BMIs below 50 kg/m², Roux limb length does not appear to affect absolute or percentage of excess weight loss.

VBG is associated with a fall in REE[44] which, in the early postoperative period, has been shown to parallel the marked decrease in caloric intake, similar to a very-low-calorie diet, rather than weight loss. For this reason, VBG is also plagued by the same difficulty in maintaining weight loss as diets, and weight regain as high as 40% has been reported. Mean body mass, fat free mass, and fat mass are significantly reduced after VBG,[45] but malnutrition is seen only rarely. Body composition studies have shown that the majority of weight loss (75%) is loss of fat, similar to that with diets. Although studies of energy expenditure and body composition after LAGB have not been reported, one would anticipate that they would be similar to those after VBG, because their mechanisms of action are identical.

Early after BPD (during the first 6 months), a rapid loss of weight is observed; it is characterized by loss of both adipose tissue (73%) and lean body mass (27%). Adipose tissue is lost mainly from arms, legs, and trunk; meanwhile, lean body mass is decreased in the trunk. The subsequent weight loss is then primarily at the expense of adipose tissue and leads to normalization of body weight and body composition after 2 years.[20,46] Scopinaro and colleagues found no differences in REE between post-BPD and control subjects.[20] However, in the same study, subjects who had decreased their weights by dieting had lower REE values.

RYGB is associated with significant changes in MREE over time.[38] A group of 70 patients undergoing RYGB were studied preoperatively and for 2 years postoperatively. Although patients manifested a decline in MREE levels over time, the values fell within the normal range of predicted values according to the Harris-Benedict equation. When stratified according to baseline MREE, patients who were initially hypometabolic (MREE <85% of the Harris-Benedict predicted value) experienced an increase in MREE to normal, beginning immediately after operation, and it remained normal over time. These changes in MREE occurred despite a marked reduction in energy intake to levels comparable with those that are present in a very-low-calorie diet (<800 kcal/day); this may contribute to the enhanced weight loss noted with RYGB compared to VBG. Furthermore, these changes in MREE are not related to the length of the Roux or alimentary limb of the bypass.[47] Similar findings of MREE in patients at their plateau weight following RYGB have recently been reported[48] and are consistent with the findings of Scopinaro.[20] In terms of body composition, preliminary data from our laboratory in patients before and 8 weeks after RYGB demonstrated an increased loss of lean body mass (30% to 36% as opposed to the recommended 25%), which normalized at 2 years with weight stabilization. These long-term results, as well as those from our laboratory concerning changes in MREE after RYGB,[49] have recently been corroborated,[48] providing valuable data about the long-term safety of RYGB.

Postsurgical subclinical malabsorption, satiety and, occasionally, dumping syndrome have also been hypothesized to play roles in weight reduction. The mechanisms, however, that govern these changes have not yet been elucidated. Ghrelin is a gastric hormone produced mainly in the cardia and fundus. Fasting causes ghrelin elevation, which induces appetite. RYGB is thought to induce anorexia by bypassing the ghrelin-producing areas of the stomach.[50]

▶ CONCLUSION

In conclusion, bariatric surgical procedures induce weight loss and profound changes in body composition and energy expenditure. The mechanisms by which these changes are produced are largely unknown or poorly defined. Some of these changes are similar to those found with diets, but some appear to be distinct, even independent of weight loss. Further studies are needed to better clarify the changes produced by these powerful operations in order to optimize outcomes and minimize complications.

▶ REFERENCES

1. Kaplan MN: The deadly quartet: upper-body obesity, glucose intolerance, hypertriglyceridemia, and hypertension. Arch Intern Med 1989;149:1514-1520.
2. Ford SE, Giles HW, Dietz HW: Prevalence of the metabolic syndrome among US adults. JAMA 2002;287:356-359.
3. Pi-Sunyer FX: The obesity epidemic: pathophysiology and consequences of obesity. Obes Res 2002;10:97S-104S.
4. Friedman JE, Dohm GL, Leggett-Frazier N, et al: Restoration of insulin responsiveness in skeletal muscle of morbidly obese patients after weight loss: effect on muscle glucose transport and glucose transporter GLUT4. J Clin Invest 1992;89:701-705.
5. Colditz GA, Willett WC, Rotnitzky A, et al: Weight gain as a risk factor for clinical diabetes mellitus in women. Ann Intern Med 1995;122:481-486.
6. Smith RS: The endocrinology of obesity: endocrinology and metabolism. Clin North Am 1996;25:921-942.
7. Grundy MS, Barnett PJ: Metabolic and health complications of obesity. Dis Mon 1990;23:643-731.
8. Ludwig J, Viggiano TR, McGill DB, et al: Nonalcoholic steatohepatitis: Mayo Clinic experiences with a hitherto unnamed disease. Mayo Clin Proc 1980;55:434-438.
9. Angulo P: Nonalcoholic fatty liver disease. N Engl J Med 2002; 346:1221-1231.
10. Gholam PM, Kotler DP, Flancbaum LJ: Liver pathology in morbidly obese patients undergoing Roux-en-Y gastric bypass surgery. Obes Surg 2002;12:49-51.
11. Segal KR, Edano A, Thomas MB: Thermic effect of a meal over 3 and 6 hours in lean obese men. Metabolism 1990;38:985-992.
12. Welle S, Forbes GB, Statt M, et al: Energy expenditure under free-living conditions in normal weight and overweight women. Am J Clin Nutr 1992;55:14-21.
13. Stallone DD, Stunkard AJ: The regulation of body weight: evidence and clinical implications. Ann Behav Med 1991;13:220-230.

14. Arribas del Amo D, Guedea EM, Diago A, et al: Effect of vertical banded gastroplasty on hypertension, diabetes and dyslipidemia. Obes Surg 2002;12:319-323.

15. Yashkov YI, Vinnitsky LI, Poroykova MV, et al: Obes Surg 2000;10:48-53.

16. Pories WJ, Swanson MS, MacDonald KG Jr, et al: Who would have thought it? An operation proves to be the most effective therapy for adult-onset diabetes mellitus. Ann Surg 1995;222:339-352.

17. MacDonald KG Jr, Long SD, Swanson MS, et al: The gastric bypass operation reduces the progression and mortality of non-insulin dependent diabetes mellitus. J Gastrointest Surg 1997;1:213-220.

18. Sjostrom CD, Lissner L, Wedel H, et al: Reduction in incidence of diabetes, hypertension and lipid disturbances after intentional weight loss induced by bariatric surgery: the SOS Intervention Study. Obes Res 1999;7:477-484.

19. Sarson DL, Scopinaro N, Bloom SR: Gut hormone changes after jejunoileal bypass or biliopancreatic bypass surgery for morbid obesity. Int J Obes 1981;5:471-480.

20. Scopinaro N, Gianetta E, Friedman D, et al: Biliopancreatic Diversion for Obesity. Problems in General Surgery. 1992;9:362-379.

21. Marceau P, Hould SF, Lebel S, et al: Malabsorptive obesity surgery. Surg Clin North Am 2001;81:1113-1127.

22. Gleysteen JJ, Barboriak JJ: Improvement in heart disease risk factors after gastric bypass. Arch Surg 1983;118:681-684.

23. Brolin ER, Kenler AH, Wilson CA, et al: Serum lipids after gastric bypass surgery for morbid obesity. Int J Obes 1990;14:939-950.

24. Clark JM, Alkhuraishi AR, Solga SF, et al: Roux-en-Y gastric bypass improves liver histology in patients with non-alcoholic fatty liver disease. Obes Res 2005;13:1180-1186.

25. Clark JM, Alkhuraishi AR, Solga SF, et al: Roux-en-Y gastric bypass improves liver histology in patients with non-alcoholic fatty liver disease. Gastroenterology 2003;124(suppl 1):A746.

26. National Taskforce on the Prevention and Treatment of Obesity: Very-low-calorie diets. JAMA 1993;270:967-974.

27. Gelfand RA, Hendler R: Effect of nutrient composition on the metabolic response to very low calorie diets: learning more and more about less and less. Diabetes Metab Res 1989;5:17-30.

28. Burgess NS: Effect of a very low-calorie diet on body composition and resting metabolic rate in obese men and women. J Am Diet Assoc 1991;91:430-434.

29. Wadden TA, Foster GD, Letizia KA, et al: Long-term effects of dieting on resting metabolic rate in obese outpatients. JAMA 1990;264:707-711.

30. Heshka S, Yang MU, Wang J, et al: Weight loss and change in resting metabolic rate. Am J Clin Nutr 1990;52:981-986.

31. Leibel RL, Rosenbaum M, Hirsh J: Changes in energy expenditure resulting from altered body weight. N Engl J Med 1995;332:621-628.

32. Meredith CN, Frontera WR, Fisher EC, et al: Peripheral effects of endurance training in young and old subjects. J Appl Physiol 1989;66:2844-2849.

33. Phinney SD, LaGrange BM, O'Conell M, et al: Effects of aerobic exercise on energy expenditure and nitrogen balance during very low-calorie dieting. Metabolism 1988;37:758-765.

34. Pavlou KN, Krey S, Stefee WP: Exercise as an adjunct to weight loss and maintenance in moderately obese subjects. Am J Clin Nutr 1989;49:1115-1123.

35. National Institutes of Health Consensus Development Conference: Gastrointestinal surgery for severe obesity: proceedings of the NIH conference. Am J Clin Nutr 1992;55(suppl 2):487S-699S.

36. Doherty C: Vertical banded gastroplasty. Surg Clin North Am 2001;81:1097-1112.

37. Condon SC, Janes NJ, Wise L, et al: Role of caloric intake in the weight loss after jejunoileal bypass for obesity. Gastroenterology 1978;74:34-37.

38. Flancbaum L, Choban PS, Bradley L, et al: Changes in measured resting energy expenditure after Roux-en-Y gastric bypass for clinically severe obesity. Surgery 1997;122:943-949.

39. Moize N, Geliebter A, Gluck EM, et al: Obese patients have inadequate protein intake related to protein intolerance up to 1 year following Roux-en-Y gastric bypass. Obes Surg 2003;13:23-28

40. Scopinaro N, Gianetta E, Adami GF, et al: Biliopancreatic diversion for obesity at eighteen years. Surgery 1996;119:261-268.

41. Brolin RE, Kenler HA, Gorman JH, et al: Long-limb gastric bypass in the superobese: a prospective, randomized trial. Ann Surg 1992;215:387-397.

42. Choban PS, Flancbaum L: The impact of limb length on weight loss following Roux-en-Y gastric bypass: a randomized prospective trial. Obes Surg 1999;9:124-125.

43. Brolin RE, LaMarca LB, Kenler HA, et al: Malabsorptive gastrointestinal bypass for patients with superobesity. J Gastrointest Surg 2002;6:195-205.

44. Van Gemert WG, Westerterp KR, Greve JWM, et al: Reduction of sleeping metabolic rate after vertical banded gastroplasty. Int J Obes Relat Metab Disord 1998;22:343-348.

45. Westerterp RK, Saris HMW, Soeters BP, et al: Determinants of weight loss after vertical banded gastroplasty. Int J Obes 1991;15:529-534.

46. Buscemi S, Caimi G, Verga S: Resting metabolic rate and postabsorptive substrate oxidation in morbidly obese subjects before and after massive weight loss. Int J Obes 1996;20:41-46.

47. Flancbaum LJ, Verducci SJ, Choban PS: Changes in measured resting energy expenditure after Roux-en-Y gastric bypass for clinically severe obesity are not related to bypass limb-length. Obes Surg 1998;8:437-443.

48. Das KS, Roberts BS, McCrory AM, et al: Long-term changes in energy expenditure and body composition after massive weight loss induced by gastric bypass surgery. Am J Clin Nutr 2003;78:22-30.

49. Geliebter A, Gluck M, Lorence M, et al: Early changes in body composition following Roux-en-Y gastric bypass for obesity. Gastroenterology 2003;124(suppl 1):A813.

50. Tritos AN, Mun E, Bertkau A, et al: Serum ghrelin levels in response to glucose load in obese patients post-gastric bypass surgery. Obes Res 2003;11:919-924.

section IX

EDUCATION, PRACTICE, AND REPORTING

47

Academic Training of Bariatric Surgeons

Daniel Kaufman, M.D. and John G. Kral, M.D., Ph.D.

As quoted from Sir William Osler (1849-1919): A man cannot become a competent surgeon without the full knowledge of human anatomy and physiology, and the physician without physiology and chemistry flounders along in aimless fashion....

The exponential rise in the number of bariatric procedures performed in the past decade (Fig. 47-1)[1] is the result of increased awareness of the major beneficial effects of surgical weight loss and of substantial advances in laparoscopic technology, but other factors may contribute to the rise. Increased demand for surgical weight-loss treatment parallels the increased prevalence of obesity in adults and adolescents, but it also reflects the publicity by obese celebrities who have undergone bariatric surgery. On the supply side, surgeons have realized that bariatric surgery is lucrative and are using their laparoscopic skills to profit from it.

Obesity is a disease with multiple causes and numerous serious comorbidities, often difficult to detect and to treat, that in turn affect both the performance and the outcome of surgery. Bariatric surgery is different from other gastrointestinal surgeries, especially with respect to the behavioral effects related to mechanism of action, and to patient selection and the evaluation of outcomes. In contrast to extirpative and reconstructive operations, bariatric surgery is "behavioral" surgery. Results are more dependent on the nutritional and lifestyle adaptations by the patient and the patient's adherence to treatment and monitoring plans than they are on the technical performance of the operation alone. For this reason, bariatric surgeons must provide for their patients thorough preoperative education and diligent long-term postoperative care. Recent findings demonstrate the appropriateness of a holistic approach, often disparaged by surgeons. Bariatric surgery, more than any other kind of surgery, requires a holistic view, and if performed by educated and committed surgeons, it can serve as an important arm in the treatment of this chronic disease.

As bariatric surgery is increasingly recognized for the role it can play in the treatment of obesity, the discipline must define itself as other surgical subspecialties have.

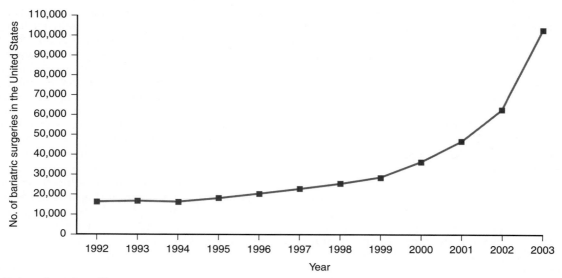

Figure 47-1. Estimated number of bariatric operations performed in the United States between 1992 and 2003. (From Steinbrook RA: Surgery for severe obesity. N Engl J Med 2004;350:1075-1079. By permission.)

This entails facing important challenges, such as establishing a consensus regarding practice standards and the qualifications and training of prospective surgeons.

▶ PROBLEMS

It is our opinion that traditional surgical residency and fellowship training, with its emphasis on technical proficiency, although unquestionably important does not provide sufficient knowledge about or skill in bariatric surgery. Careful study of the American College of Surgeons (ACS) Statement on Principles Underlying Perioperative Responsibility demonstrates the way in which applying these principles in bariatric surgery is difficult.[2]

The ACS states that "...proper preoperative preparation...requires full appreciation...of the patient's condition." Today's crash courses in bariatric surgery, while attempting to compensate for the neglect of nutrition and metabolism by most medical school curricula, are simply not sufficient to prepare the hordes of wannabe bariatric surgeons to take on the scope of responsibility to achieve "optimal... preparation," as the ACS defines it. The ACS statement continues: "The surgeon is responsible for presenting...the range of options...including...rationale for...approach to treatment." In the case of bariatric surgery, it is inadequate merely to state that diet, exercise, and drugs are ineffective treatments for severe obesity. Furthermore, because the majority of surgeons recently recruited to bariatric surgery offer only one surgical option, it is not likely that such surgeons are able to describe objectively the chronic effects of procedures with which they do not have hands-on experience. Indeed, this represents a conflict between the financial interests of the surgeon and the legitimate informational needs of the patient that potentially invalidates the consent process. Ultimately, this leaves the patient without the requisite range of options.

Regarding postoperative care, the ACS states that "even when...care may best be delegated...the surgeon must maintain an essential coordinating role...until the residual effects...are minimal, and the risk of complications... predictably small." Given the manifest and covert complexity of the comorbidities of obesity, it is unacceptable simply to refer the patient to a consultant, because many medical consultants themselves do not have specific knowledge about obesity. In addition, a surgeon must ensure "...appropriate long-term follow-up for continuing problems..." yet most surgeons have not elected a surgical career based on their dedication to long-term care of chronic conditions. Here also, a conflict may develop between surgeons' financial interests and patients' medical needs, because the number and severity of postoperative complications of bariatric surgery can limit a surgeon's lifetime case load.[3]

The evolution of a medical specialty is a notoriously messy process, generating anxiety in the parent field as well as in the new specialty, and often resulting in "turf battles."[4] Recognizing the growing expertise in various surgical fields, in 1998 the American Board of Surgery (ABS) created Specialty Boards and Advisory Councils in order to meet the needs of new surgical subspecialties with regard to education, training, examination, and certification.[5] Although only pediatric and vascular surgery currently offer independent Specialty Board certifications within the ABS structure, with the maturation of other subspecialty areas, additional boards will be needed.[6] Indeed, the omission of bariatric surgery education from the ABS document Specialty of Surgery Defined[7] demonstrates the lack of understanding of the special needs of the obese surgical patient, a fact that in itself might support the creation of separate Specialty Boards in bariatric surgery.

Bariatric surgery is currently practiced by a diverse group of general and laparoscopic surgeons, few of whom are specifically trained in the management of severely obese patients. So who should be doing bariatric surgery?[8] Although general guidelines for privileging and credentialing have been proposed by the American Society for Bariatric Surgery (ASBS)[9] and the Society of American Gastrointestinal Endoscopic Surgeons,[10] no consensus has been reached on the training requirements for prospective bariatric surgeons.

▶ SOLUTIONS

Patient Selection

The side effects and complications of bariatric surgery can be burdensome, taxing, and discouraging. These factors, which may have tremendous influence on the outcome of surgery, must be balanced in the preoperative risk-benefit analysis. Although no general outcome predictors are currently available, a surgeon must be very selective when evaluating a patient's ability to meet successfully the physiologic and psychological demands of bariatric operations. This involves careful evaluation of the patient's motivations to undergo the surgery and his or her expectations of it, as well as any possible investment the patient may have in remaining obese.[11]

Staged Approach to Bariatric Surgery

As bariatric surgery indications evolve, with trends downward in the body mass index (BMI) and minimum age of the patient, a staged algorithm or step-care approach to weight loss can assist surgeons in individualizing treatment (Fig. 47-2). The staged approach allows for selection of operation type based on disease severity and for its use as a rescue strategy for failed operations. Although a patient's BMI can be used as a rough guide for determining an appropriate bariatric operation, more comprehensive physiologic scales, such as the Obesity Severity Index[12] or the Bariatric Analysis and Reporting Outcome System[13] may yield a more appropriate determination.

Bariatric surgery today is undertaken as a treatment of last resort, often after years of unsuccessful noninvasive methods, including dietary modifications, exercise, and pharmacologic intervention. Laparoscopic gastric restriction is a relatively simple and effective operation, provided the patient understands and adheres to the prescribed rules for eating.[14] Adjustable gastric banding allows for continued education and assessment of the patient and can serve as a behavioral test for subsequent operations, possibly improving the selection process. If these operations fail, they can be revised by pouch banding or converted to

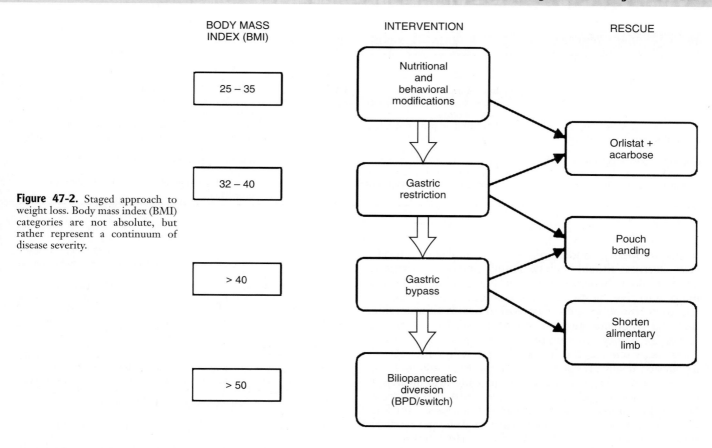

BODY MASS INDEX (BMI)

INTERVENTION

RESCUE

Figure 47-2. Staged approach to weight loss. Body mass index (BMI) categories are not absolute, but rather represent a continuum of disease severity.

combined restrictive-diversionary procedures (such as the Roux-en-Y gastric bypass) that can effect greater weight loss. Gastric bypass, in turn, could be rescued with pouch revision or shortening of the alimentary limb. Biliopancreatic diversion with duodenal switch may be reserved for the heaviest patients because this operation can yield the greatest amount of weight loss. This algorithm implies the need for advanced competency in bariatric surgery.

▶ TWO-TRACK MODEL FOR TRAINING BARIATRIC SURGEONS

Evidence of lower mortality rates and improved outcomes after major surgical procedures that are performed at high-volume compared to low-volume hospitals has been recognized for decades[15,16] and has prompted several initiatives aimed at regionalizing surgical care.[17-20] Underlying these strong volume-outcome associations are multiple factors, including patient characteristics, experience of the surgical team, care of various perioperative comorbidities, and substantial differences in the analytic techniques used in numerous studies.[21] Recently, the ASBS established a peer-review organization for identifying bariatric surgery "centers of excellence" that have high volume and comprehensive surgical-care programs. These centers, where surgical expertise has developed, can provide optimal training grounds for prospective bariatric surgeons. However, with the recognition that not all obese patients present complicated cases, nor are all bariatric procedures complex, we have designed a training program that addresses a continuum of

motives, from the altruistic to the avaricious, for seeking training in bariatric surgery. We suggest two curricula: Track A, for the basic bariatric surgeon, and Track B, for the complete bariatric surgeon (Table 47-1).

Track A prepares surgeons for simple bariatric procedures such as laparoscopic gastric banding in moderately obese, young patients. The premedical curriculum for Track A may include undergraduate courses in business, human resource management, and economics. In medical school, the 2-month break between years 1 and 2 can be used for an internship in a private surgical practice. During the clinical years, electives in this track may include anesthesia, orthopedics, and laparoscopic or bariatric surgery to quickly familiarize the student with the practical aspects of an operating lifestyle. The basic surgeon will benefit from a surgical residency with a high-volume laparoscopic bariatric surgery program with clinical rotations at least during years 1 and 2. This experience will introduce the resident to some bariatric procedures and to pre- and postoperative ancillary care. Finally, a fellowship for Track A will involve 1 year in a high-volume laparoscopic bariatric surgery program, allowing the surgeon to become technically proficient, yet with limited exposure to follow-up care.

Track B prepares surgeons for the performance of all the bariatric operations, including restrictive and diversionary procedures as well as reoperations, that are available for the management of all degrees of obesity. In this track, undergraduate courses may include epidemiology, psychology, sociology, and behavioral neuroscience, and the break between the first 2 years of medical school can be used for basic science or clinical research experience, preferably

Table 47-1	TWO-TRACK MODEL FOR TRAINING BARIATRIC SURGEONS	
EDUCATION LEVEL	**TRACK A**	**TRACK B**
	Basic bariatric surgeon	**Complete bariatric surgeon**
Premedical	Business, management, economics, accounting	Epidemiology, psychology, sociology, behavioral neuroscience
Medical school years 1 and 2	Internship in private surgical practice	Basic science or clinical research experience
Medical school years 3 and 4	Electives in anesthesia, orthopedics, cardiothoracic surgery	Electives in family practice, nutrition, endocrinology, critical care
General surgery residency	Program with high-volume laparoscopic bariatric surgery	Academic program with 2-year research fellowship
Bariatric surgery fellowship	1-year fellowship in high-volume laparoscopic program	2-year fellowship in bariatric surgery "center of excellence"

related to obesity, endocrinology, or metabolism. Clinical-year electives should include family practice, nutrition, endocrinology, hypertension, neurology, and critical care, in order to give the student a more comprehensive medical approach to obesity and its comorbidities. It is preferable that the complete surgeon attend an academic general surgery residency program that provides opportunity for a 2-year basic science and clinical research fellowship related to obesity, insulin resistance, endocrinology, metabolism, and bariatric surgery. This will provide the in-depth knowledge of the pathophysiology of obesity that is necessary for becoming a competent bariatric surgeon. Track B concludes with a 2-year fellowship in a laparoscopic bariatric surgery center of excellence, with the fellow acting in a capacity of ever-increasing responsibility and acquiring a knowledge base appropriate to the management of all morbidly obese patients, with proficiency in the full range of bariatric procedures and reoperative surgery.

◗ CONCLUSION

Training in bariatric surgery is not standardized. Because bariatric surgery is complex, we suggest two fellowship training pathways for surgeons who wish to perform bariatric procedures. Only holistic training in centers of excellence, emphasizing both scholarship and technical proficiency, will produce complete bariatric surgeons.

◗ REFERENCES

1. Steinbrook RA: Surgery for severe obesity. N Engl J Med 2004;350:1075-1079.
2. American College of Surgeons: ACS statement on principles underlying perioperative responsibility. Bull Am Coll Surg 1996;81:39. http://www.facs.org/fellows_info/statements/st-25.html. Accessed March 17, 2004.
3. McFarland RJ, Gazet JC, Pilkington TR: A 13-year review of jejunoileal bypass. Br J Surg 1985;72:81-87.
4. Lewis FR Jr: Surgical fellowships and specialization. Surgery 2002; 132:529-530.
5. American Board of Surgery: Component Boards and Advisory Councils. http://www.absurgery.org/default.asp?aboutcompboards. Accessed March 17, 2004.
6. Ritchie WP Jr: Basic certification in surgery by the American Board of Surgery (ABS): What does it mean? Does it have value? Is it relevant? A personal opinion. Ann Surg 2004;239:133-139.
7. American Board of Surgery: Component Boards and Advisory Councils. http://www.absurgery.org/default.asp?aboutsurgerydefined. Accessed March 17, 2004.
8. Al-Saif O, Gallagher SF, Banasiak M, et al: Who should be doing laparoscopic bariatric surgery? Obes Surg 2003;13:82-87.
9. American Society for Bariatric Surgery: Guidelines for laparoscopic and open surgical treatment of morbid obesity. Obes Surg 2000; 10:378-379. http://www.asbs.org/html/guidelines. Accessed March 17, 2004.
10. Society of American Gastrointestinal Endoscopic Surgeons: Guidelines for institutions granting bariatric privileges utilizing laparoscopic techniques. Surg Endosc 2003;17:2037-2040. http://www.sages.org/sg_pub31.html. Accessed March 17, 2004.
11. Kral JG: Selection of patients for anti-obesity surgery. Int J Obes Relat Metab Disord 2001;25(suppl 1):S107-S112.
12. Kral JG: Side effects, complications and problems in antiobesity surgery: introduction of the obesity severity index. In Angel A, Anderson H, Bouchard C, et al (eds): Progress in Obesity Research 7, pp. 655-661. London, John Libbey, 1999.
13. Oria HE, Moorehead MK: Bariatric analysis and reporting outcome system (BAROS). Obes Surg 1998;8:487-499.
14. Kral JG: Surgical treatment of obesity. Med Clin North Am 1989; 73:251-264.
15. Lee JA, Morrison SL, Morris JN: Fatality from three common surgical conditions in teaching and non-teaching hospitals. Lancet 1957; 273:785-790.
16. Birkmeyer JD, Stukel TA, Siewers AE, et al: Surgeon volume and operative mortality in the United States. N Engl J Med 2003; 349:2117-2127.
17. Luft HS, Bunker JP, Enthoven AC: Should operations be regionalized? The empirical relation between surgical volume and mortality. N Engl J Med 1979;301:1364-1369.
18. Birkmeyer JD: Should we regionalize major surgery? Potential benefits and policy considerations. J Am Coll Surg 2000;190:341-349.
19. Select Quality Care. http://www.selectqualitycare.com/p-pro.htm. Accessed March 17, 2004.
20. The Leapfrog Group. http://www.leapfroggroup.org/FactSheets/EHR_FactSheet. Accessed March 17, 2004.
21. Halm EA, Lee C, Chassin MR: Is volume related to outcome in health care? A systematic review and methodologic critique of the literature. Ann Intern Med 2002;137:511-520.

48

Practical Training
of the Bariatric Surgeon

Latham Flanagan, Jr., M.D.

The practical training of the bariatric surgeon pertains to the experienced, board-certified, general surgeon who wishes to be a bariatric surgeon. This chapter addresses the cross-training of the experienced general surgeon who wishes to make a commitment to bariatric surgery as a significant, if not principal, part of his or her practice. The complexities of patient selection, pre- and postoperative care, prolonged teaching and training of the patient, and long-term follow-up make it very difficult to perform bariatric surgery as a casual part of a general surgeon's practice (i.e., fewer than 20 to 30 cases per year). A number equal to or greater than that is required to create and maintain the skills of a support team of medical office assistants, nurses, consulting physicians, dietitians, and psychologists, as well as hospital facilities and personnel, all of which comprise the bariatric surgical team necessary to provide high-quality care. Even an effective support group requires a certain level of membership in order to create and maintain a dynamic, positive, and productive organization.

The purpose of this cross-training is to flatten and shorten the learning curve of beginning a bariatric surgical practice. We often refer flippantly to the learning curve. We are all very aware that there is an increased morbidity and mortality rate associated with an inexperienced surgeon in any area of surgery; the more complex and challenging the area of surgery, the more likely it is to see an increase in morbidity and mortality rates. It behooves us, occasionally, to jolt our sensibilities with the realization that the terms *morbidity* and *mortality* refer to very real damage to those people, our patients, who come to us confident of obtaining relief from their present and future suffering.

▶ THE RISKS OF BARIATRIC SURGERY

What are the risks for mortality and morbidity in bariatric surgery? Until October 2002, our profession had no reliable and unbiased description of the mortality and morbidity rates in bariatric surgery in a large geographic community.

The University of South Florida published data arising from a state mandate that all hospitals report to the Florida Board of Health all hospital admissions, discharges, diagnoses, deaths, complications, and certain financial issues. The office selected for review 34 surgeons who were performing fewer than two bariatric surgical procedures per month, but limited their evaluation to 10 bariatric surgeons (4 in academia and 6 in private practice) who performed more than two bariatric procedures per month. There was no significant difference in the mortality and morbidity rates between surgeons in academia and those in private practice, as one would expect. The development of the data, based on the proprietary Yale Scale, demonstrated that in the 612 patients who were considered low risk, there were no deaths and less than a 5% complication rate. However, in the 152 patients who were considered high risk, there were three deaths and a 42% complication rate.[1]

With Florida's long tradition of excellent practitioners and teachers of bariatric surgery, this alarming level of complications in the high-risk patients, nearly 20% of the total number, very likely reflected the outcomes of most, if not all, of the other states. Our previous impression of complication rates came from papers published by individual surgeons or individual institutions that are, by human nature, more likely to present better-than-average data or not publish at all. This bias toward better-than-average results even occurs to some degree in surgery registries such as the International Bariatric Surgery Registry, to which most of the contributing surgeons have proven their commitment to their profession not only by laboriously providing data to the registry, but also by being members of the American Society for Bariatric Surgery (ASBS). Thus, these data from the state of Florida have greater importance for those of us in private practice—on the firing line, at risk for losing hospital privileges, and at risk for malpractice actions.

It should be emphasized that the data from Florida come from 1999, the beginning of a dramatic increase of interest in bariatric surgery in this country and a responsive rise in the number of bariatric surgeons and the number of procedures being performed. The learning-curve effect on the very large number of these surgeons doing bariatric surgery, with the resultant increase in morbidity and mortality rates, certainly claimed the attention of the trial lawyers and augmented the number of malpractice actions. The rate of malpractice actions seems to be increasing relative to the number of deaths and complications, and with the increasing dollar amount of the awards sought, the cost of malpractice protection is escalating. Therefore, the premiums demanded by the few insurance companies still offering coverage to bariatric surgeons have risen dramatically. The malpractice insurance industry has also become more sophisticated and is stratifying bariatric surgeons in several ways. Most obvious is the number of claims brought against surgeons. But increasingly, insurance companies are looking at the surgeons' educational backgrounds in bariatric surgery and the surgeons' participation in appropriate surgical societies, such as the ASBS and The Society of American Gastrointestinal Endoscopic Surgeons (SAGES). One might predict that the state of readiness of the hospital facility will also have an effect on malpractice coverage stratification in the future. Indeed, there are many good reasons for an experienced general surgeon *not* to go into bariatric surgery, unless he or she is willing to make a significant commitment of time and energy to the field.

Should this in any way be interpreted as an effort to discourage general surgeons from becoming bariatric surgeons? In my personal view, as a general/thoracic/vascular/endocrine surgeon with 30 years of experience, and a bariatric surgeon with 27 years of experience, there is no phase of general surgery that even approaches the challenges and rewards of bariatric surgery. Experienced bariatric surgeons are and should be actively recruiting appropriate general surgeons to bariatric surgery. The need for more good bariatric surgeons is immense. In the past few years, the ASBS estimated that the number of bariatric procedures performed per year in the United States was increasing exponentially. For 2003, it was estimated that the number of bariatric procedures would approach or exceed 100,000, and for 2004, that it would exceed 140,000. However, these large numbers hardly scratch the surface of the need for bariatric surgery to be available to the 10 to 15 million Americans who *currently* meet the established indications for a bariatric surgical procedure.

There is and should be no external competition for bariatric surgery patients, at least in this decade. There is no need for extensive advertising when almost any established bariatric surgeon has a waiting list many months long. This lack of external competition is particularly important to those surgeons who are trying to decide whether to perform open bariatric procedures or to become involved in the acknowledged challenge and longer learning curve of laparoscopic bariatric surgery. For bariatric surgeons today, the competition should be an internal one—to be the best bariatric surgeon one can be.

▶ THE LEARNING CURVES

Much has been written about the learning curve in bariatric surgery. It is curious that in the era of exclusively open bariatric surgical procedures, this term was seldom heard, although the concept of improvement of performance in surgery has been the credo of surgeons for many decades, if not centuries. With the advent of laparoscopic surgery, the concept of the learning curve has been and remains a significant issue. There is not just one learning curve; there are actually three. First, the development of skills for patient selection, preoperative preparation, perioperative management, and long-term follow-up; second, the development of the skills of open bariatric surgical procedures; and third, based on the previous two skill sets, the learning curve of laparoscopic bariatric surgery.

The first learning curve is that of perioperative management in a larger sense. To become a good bariatric surgeon, a surgeon must also have a basic knowledge of morbidly obese persons. Psychologically, they are not different from any other patients, except for the defense mechanisms and feelings they have developed as the result of being extremely obese persons in a society that does not tolerate extreme obesity.[2] Many of our patients, if not most, have at one time or another been verbally abused by physicians who do not understand or accept the nature of this organic disease of metabolism based in the hypothalamus, or who have responded negatively due to their frustration with inadequate tools with which to achieve for their patients significant, lasting weight loss. Indeed, morbid obesity is the "last bastion of prejudice."[3] Along this same line, a surgeon is more likely to become a successful, effective, and contented bariatric surgeon if he or she is also a "people person." The surgeon who has a significant bias against the morbidly obese is not likely to be either successful or contented in bariatric surgical practice. Indeed, that surgeon is likely to have a higher malpractice risk in this field of surgery in which significant complications are unavoidable.

In addition to his or her own training, the bariatric surgeon is responsible for accomplishing the preparation of the hospital facility. The basic criteria for facility preparation were published in the Bulletin of the American College of Surgeons in September 2000.[4] Ordinarily, to obtain the skills necessary, in-service teaching of both operating room and hospital staff nurses is part of the surgeon's responsibility. There are available proprietary organizations that, for a significant fee, are prepared to prepare facilities appropriately.

Bariatric surgeons should have available skilled consultation, particularly in the cardiology, pulmonology, and nephrology specialties, because serious complications involving these specialized fields are, unfortunately, not uncommon in these sick patients. Perhaps the physicians whose education is most important are the emergency department physicians, who must handle the special needs of postoperative bariatric surgery patients. An evaluation of abdominal pain with obstructive symptoms can be dangerously different from the norm in a patient with a biliopancreatic limb.

The postoperative follow-up requires a great deal of time on the part of the surgeon's staff, as well as the surgeon. Some of the issues are procedure specific. Although medical community-wide experience is changing as the number of bariatric surgical procedures increase, there is still a vast lack of information in the general medical community about the specific needs and problems of the postoperative bariatric surgical patient. This includes not only under-diagnosis of a patient's problems but also overdiagnosis, as in attributing difficult-to-diagnose situations inappropriately to bariatric surgery. It is, therefore, particularly important for bariatric surgeons to follow their own patients in the posthospital setting, particularly those who have rapidly changing metabolic situations involving potentially dangerous medications (e.g., anticoagulant, diabetic, and hypertensive agents).

Our final charge to new and experienced bariatric surgeons is the development of well-run support groups that offer assistance to these patients that, in many ways, simply cannot be given by medical professionals. These support groups are also very useful in reducing preoperative patient anxiety over the anticipated procedure and, in many cases, in turning fear into eager anticipation of the procedure.

The second learning curve, that of learning the open procedure, has its own set of challenges. Surgeons who came to the field two decades ago were familiar with the problems of gastric surgery because of their experience in gastric operations for ulcers and cancer. It was not unusual for surgeons starting out with open bariatric surgery to perform several hundred operations without a mortality, especially in morbidly obese as opposed to superobese patients.[5] Surgeons trained in the most recent era face a greater challenge because of the relative paucity of gastric procedures, excluding bariatric surgery, that are performed today, even in our teaching institutions. As a matter of fact, one of the more attractive parts of a bariatric surgical program in a general surgeon residency is that the bariatric surgical program gives residents and fellows experience in dealing with stomach surgery. In any event, the general surgeon wishing to become an open-bariatric surgeon requires a distinct training period, which is described subsequently.

The third learning curve, laparoscopic bariatric surgery, is significantly more challenging and complex than the second. Indeed, the learning curve for laparoscopic bariatric surgery can be long and arduous for the surgeon and harmful to the morbidly obese patient.[6-12] In my own state, I am aware of three bariatric surgeons who have recently lost their privileges at their hospitals because of excessive complications. Two of the three had received no bariatric surgery orientation sessions and were not members of the ASBS. Even when done well, within an established bariatric surgery program, the mortality and morbidity rates during early experience can be severe.[13-15] Indeed, even in the experience of those who are leaders in the field of laparoscopic surgery, the initial learning curve resulted in more significant complications, particularly leaks, and even in more deaths.[6-9] Recently, there have been reports of very carefully and painstakingly prepared laparoscopic programs that have minimized this learning curve, flattened it, if you will, quite effectively because of their longstanding open-bariatric surgical experience.[16]

For the experienced general surgeon who is not versed in advanced laparoscopic skills, the question must be asked if there is a need to perform the surgery laparoscopically. Two recent publications ask this question directly.[13,17] In the 1990s, it was necessary to learn basic laparoscopic skills to remain financially competitive in private practice. As mentioned previously, that is hardly the case in bariatric surgery in this decade, when there is such a very great need for more operations to be done. There are few, if any, advantages to performing bariatric surgery laparoscopically that extend beyond the first 3 to 6 months postoperatively. Even the cosmetic effect of smaller scars often disappears in the face of the patients' commonly desired abdominal panniculectomy and abdominoplasty. It is rather uncommon to find candidates for bariatric surgery in a job situation that requires heavy lifting and straining, and most open-surgery patients return to their usual work within 3 weeks, depending more on their motivation to return to work than on any physical disability. In elite programs, laparoscopic bariatric surgery is performed with a complication rate equal, or nearly equal, to that of open surgery. However, no data currently available tell us how to translate the data from elite programs to community surgeons. Our own local experience in the state of Oregon suggests that there is, indeed, a higher morbidity and mortality rate with the laparoscopic approach. There is reason to remember the time-hallowed credo of physicians: *primum non nocere*.

▶ SUGGESTED GUIDELINES FOR CREDENTIALING BODIES

It is a relatively new concept for professional organizations to publish guidelines for credentialing bodies. The first guidelines to be published by the ASBS were published in the journal *Obesity Surgery* in 2000; they were the result of efforts by the leadership of the ASBS and SAGES.[18] Both organizations submitted these guidelines to their respective boards of governors. It is important to note that neither one of these organizations is a credentialing organization; credentialing organizations are the local hospitals or state boards of medical examiners. Professional organizations only propose guidelines for the use of those credentialing organizations. These guidelines are not only new, they are proposed for a dynamic, changing field of surgery. It is anticipated that there will be further changes to these guidelines, even in the next 5 years, to reflect the improvements in the understanding of the pitfalls of previous practices and innovations in training methodology. The initial guidelines, published in 2000, were general and nonspecific. The more current ASBS guidelines are more specific and are divided into three parts: global credentialing requirements, open bariatric surgery requirements, and laparoscopic bariatric surgery requirements.

The ASBS global credentialing requirements for both open and laparoscopic surgery are as follows. A candidate for privileges to perform bariatric surgery should

1. Have credentials at an accredited facility to perform gastrointestinal and biliary surgery;
2. Be able to state that he or she is working with an integrated program for the care of the morbidly obese patient that provides ancillary services, such as specialized nursing care, dietary instruction, counseling, support groups, exercise instruction and training, and psychological assistance as needed;
3. Know that there is a program in place to prevent, monitor, and manage short-term and long-term complications;

4. Know that there is a system in place that would ensure at least 50% patient follow-up at 2 years postoperatively for restrictive surgical patients and 75% for malabsorptive surgical patients;

5. Demonstrate that there is a follow-up system in place to provide for follow-up of all patients, including those who live outside of the customary driving distance;

6. Be a member of the American Society for Bariatric Surgery.

To obtain open-bariatric surgical privileges, the surgeon should meet the ASBS global credentialing requirements and (1) document three proctored cases in which the assistant is a fully trained bariatric surgeon and (2) document the successful outcomes (with acceptable perioperative complication rates) of 10 open bariatric surgical cases performed by the applicant.

To obtain laparoscopic bariatric surgical credentialing, the surgeon must meet the ASBS global credentialing requirements and (1) have privileges to perform open bariatric surgery at an approved facility; (2) have privileges at the given facility to perform advanced laparoscopic surgery; (3) document three proctored cases in which the assistant is a fully trained laparoscopic bariatric surgery; and (4) document the outcomes of 15 laparoscopic bariatric surgical procedures performed as the primary surgeon demonstrating an acceptable perioperative complication rate.

The pace for updating guidelines has accelerated and is now complemented by a credentialing body. Under the sponsorship of the ASBS, a Consensus Conference was held in May 2004 in Washington, D.C., to update the 1991 National Institutes of Health bariatric surgery guidelines and recommendations.[19] In 2004, also under the auspices of the ASBS, the Surgical Review Corporation was founded to serve as a credentialing body and to designate Bariatric Surgery Centers of Excellence. The Surgical Review Corporation is the first credentialing organization in the field of bariatric surgery.

▶ OPPORTUNITIES FOR CROSS-TRAINING IN BARIATRIC SURGERY

As a method of achieving these goals and becoming a full, active member in the ASBS, a general surgeon has several options. He or she can be working within an established bariatric surgical program with an experienced bariatric surgeon who will act as his or her mentor. If mentoring is not available, or even in addition to mentoring, a surgeon may choose to take a week-long preceptor course sponsored by and available through the ASBS.[20] The preceptors are experienced bariatric surgeons, and the preceptorships are available in all regions of the United States. The preceptorship is an intensive week-long experience followed by an open-book test designed primarily to emphasize the prevention or management of the most significant pitfalls in the perioperative management of the bariatric surgical patient.

The intensive week-long preceptorship requires the following requisites: involvement as a nonoperating participant at the operating table of at least three bariatric surgical procedures; participation in the preoperative selection and teaching process; participation in postoperative ward rounds; participation in follow-up care in the office or clinic setting; and participation in an organized support group. Ideally, any leisure time would be spent in an informal give-and-take concerning the challenges and rewards of bariatric surgery. Many, if not most, of these preceptor programs are pleased to include a new bariatric surgeon's primary staffer, physician's assistant, nurse practitioner, or nurse, who will be designated as the surgeon's principal training and follow-up person.

Whether a mentoring or a preceptor route is chosen, a new bariatric surgeon should attend the day-long Essentials of Bariatric Surgery course offered at the annual meetings of the ASBS and at other venues. This should be considered a global requirement. In subsequent ASBS meetings, a new bariatric surgeon can attend the yearly Masters Postgraduate Course, in which topics vary each year. In addition, the novice laparoscopic bariatric surgeon, who already has secure advanced laparoscopic skills, should attend a bariatric surgical training course of at least 2 days, which includes both didactic teaching and hands-on laboratory experience.

Many laparoscopic trainees leave these courses feeling that they are not yet ready to perform laparoscopic bariatric surgery. Increasingly, university teaching programs are offering minifellowships that are training programs in bariatric surgery and that last for more than 6 weeks and involve all aspects of bariatric education.[21] For the surgeon who may not have advanced laparoscopic surgery skills yet wants to perform laparoscopic bariatric surgery, a 1-year bariatric surgery fellowship may be the ideal training modality.

▶ SUMMARY

In summary, bariatric surgery is an exciting and dynamic field offering many opportunities for creativity, a surgical challenge, and the enormous reward that comes to the bariatric surgeon and his or her staff in following these patients for the next several years of their lives, observing not only the improvement or resolution of their comorbid conditions, but also the dramatic social and vocational changes that result. Dealing with bariatric patients day after day in the clinic offers to many of us a sense of accomplishment that no other area of surgery has been able to provide.

▶ REFERENCES

1. Lopez J, Sung J, Anderson M, et al: Is bariatric surgery safe in academic centers? Am Surg 2000;68:820-823.
2. Stunkard A, Wadden T: Psychological aspects of human obesity. In Bjorntorp P, Brodhoff B (eds): Obesity, pp. 352-360. Philadelphia, JP Lippincott, 1992.
3. Flanagan S: Obesity: the last bastion of prejudice. Obes Surg 1996;6:430-437.
4. American College of Surgeons: Recommendations for facilities performing bariatric surgery. Bull Am Coll Surg 2000;85:20-23.
5. Flanagan L: Fifteen-year experience with the gastric bypass procedure for the morbidly obese in community practice. Obes Surg 2000;10:128.

6. Wittgove A, Clark G, Schubert K: Laparoscopic gastric bypass, Roux-en-Y technique and results in 75 patients with 3-30 months follow-up. Obes Surg 1996;6:500-504.

7. Schauer P, Ikramuddin S, Hamad G, et al: The learning curve for laparoscopic Roux-en-Y gastric bypass is 100 cases. Surg Endosc 2003;17:212-215.

8. Higa KD, Boone KB, Ho T, et al: Laparoscopic Roux-en-Y gastric bypass for morbid obesity: technique and preliminary results of our first 400 cases. Arch Surg 2000;135:1029-1033.

9. DeMaria EJ, Sugerman HJ, Kellum JM, et al: Results of 281 consecutive total laparoscopic Roux-en-Y gastric bypasses to treat morbid obesity. Ann Surg 2002;235:640-645.

10. Provost D, Scott D, Jones DB: Laparoscopic Roux-en-Y gastric bypass procedure: defining the learning curve. Obese Surg 2001;11: 177(abstract).

11. Perugini R, Mason R, Czerniach D, et al: Predictors of complication and suboptimal weight loss after laparoscopic Roux-en-Y gastric bypass. Arch Surg 2003;138:541-545.

12. Kligman M, Thomas C, Saxe J: Effect of the learning curve on the early outcomes of laparoscopic Roux-en-Y gastric bypass. Am Surg 2003;69:304-309.

13. See C, Carter P, Elliott D, et al: An institutional experience with laparoscopic gastric bypass procedure complications seen in the first year compared with open gastric bypass complications during the same period. Am J Surg 2002;183:533-538.

14. Marshall JS, Srivastava A, Gupta SK, et al: Roux-en-Y gastric bypass leak complications. Arch Surg 2003;138:520-523.

15. Dresel A, Kuhn JA, Westmoreland MV, et al: Establishing a laparoscopic gastric bypass program. Am J Surg 2002;184:617-620.

16. Schwartz M, Drew R, Chazin-Caldie M: Laparoscopic Roux-en-Y gastric bypass: preoperative determinants of prolonged operative times, conversion to open gastric bypasses, and postoperative complications. Obes Surg 2003;13:734-738.

17. Reddy RM, Riker A, Marra D, et al: Open Roux-en-Y gastric bypass for the morbidly obese in the era of laparoscopy. Am J Surg 2002;184:611-615.

18. American Society for Bariatric Surgery, Society of American Gastrointestinal Endoscopic Surgeons: Guidelines for laparoscopic and open surgical treatment of morbid obesity. Obes Surg 2000;10: 378-379.

19. Buchwald H, Consensus Conference Panel: Bariatric surgery for morbid obesity: health implications for patients, health professionals, and third-party payers. J Am Coll Surg 2005;200:593-604.

20. Information concerning approved preceptorships for clinical bariatric surgical training. www.ASBS.org. Accessed May 20, 2004.

21. Society of American Gastrointestinal Endoscopic Surgeons. Available fellowships in surgical endoscopy and laparoscopy. http://www.SAGES.org/fellowships/index.php. Accessed May 20, 2004.

49

Nursing Care of the Bariatric Surgery Patient

Katherine Mary Fox, R.N., M.P.H.

Obesity is omnipresent in our society and its health risks are well known. Obese patients are becoming the norm; in fact, increasing numbers are being cared for in every service area. Morbid obesity is an incurable medical disease, and surgery is currently the only effective method for long-term control. Other patients with chronic, debilitating, life-threatening diseases are treated with compassion, unlike obese patients, who receive condemnation and rejection. Providing care for obese patients is physically and emotionally more difficult, stressful, and time consuming. These patients have needs and characteristics that are quite different from those of other patient populations. For the bariatric surgery staff, there is a triad of important challenges: (1) gaining expert knowledge related to the potential surgical complications; (2) providing a physically safe and comfortable environment; and (3) providing kind and supportive care. These challenges are the primary focus of this chapter.

Obese patients still encounter cultural prejudice and naïveté from the public and from medical professionals about the nature and causes of obesity. Many studies support the existence of this prejudice in physicians, medical students, and nurses. In a pertinent recent study, it was found that 24% of nurses said that they were "repulsed" by obese persons.[1] This, quite simply, must change. As we understand this disease, its impact on human lives, and the reasons behind our own negative responses, our capacity for compassion will increase. Knowledgeable bariatric surgery team members are given the opportunity to have a major and sometimes life-saving impact on the lives of these patients. This specialty can provide unparalleled meaningful and satisfying work.

OBJECTIVE

The objective of this chapter is to provide a guide to the care of clinically severe obese patients for the nursing community and other health care personnel who provide care before, during, and after bariatric surgery. The emphasis is largely on the information needed by nurses and other multidisciplinary team members within the hospital setting.

However, it is anticipated that this information will have value for administrators of bariatric programs and for those who encounter obese patients in other settings. For successful care of the bariatric surgery patient, it is necessary that providers possess special skills, understanding, and knowledge unique to this patient population.

FACILITIES AND EQUIPMENT

Specialized Environment

When a morbidly obese patient enters the hospital setting, it becomes the hospital's responsibility to ensure that safe care is provided. Safe care translates to well-qualified, experienced surgeons, educated and knowledgeable multidisciplinary staff, written procedures and protocols, facility modifications, equipment, and staffing levels specific to the needs of this patient population. Without these critical elements, safe care simply cannot be delivered, and the hospital assumes serious risk and liability. Table 49-1 lists recommended equipment and facility modifications to assist caregivers in providing optimally safe, efficient, and dignified care of the morbidly obese patient. Most minimally invasive surgical procedures (using laparoscopy) are performed in operating rooms originally designed for traditional open surgery. A group at Mount Sinai Medical Center, New York, has described a state-of-the-art suite for minimally invasive bariatric surgery, offered as a prototype for the next generation of operating facilities for laparoscopic procedures.[2]

Patient Clustering

Clustering bariatric surgery patients on the same unit and, if possible, dedicating a specific unit for bariatric surgery enables the safest care. Having a core of designated nurses who choose to specialize in the care of bariatric patients is optimal. The rationale and advantages are similar to those of other specialty areas: (1) staff understands the unique physical limitations and psychological needs of these patients, enabling better assistance and support; (2) staff is

Table 49-1	EQUIPMENT AND FACILITY REQUIREMENTS

Operating table(s) extra wide and capable of accommodating 800-1000 lb

Bariatric surgical instruments and retractors; laparoscopic instruments (43-46 cm long)

Footboards (for reverse Trendelenberg position) and knee rest (for laparoscopic procedures)

Long safety belt (for OR positioning)

Antiembolism socks and bariatric pneumatic sequential compression boots (extra-large)

Bariatric beds (accommodating weight of 800 lb or more) in sufficient numbers

Extra-wide, weight-bearing walkers, commodes, and wheelchairs (with facility accessibility)

Weight scales rated up to 850 lb or more

Overhead bar and trapeze

Extra-large patient gowns (with snap-open sleeves and wraparound backs)

Extra-large and large adult blood pressure cuffs

Assistive reaching and pulling devices (as used with CVA patients)

Size-accessible bathrooms and showers; floor-mounted toilets; handbars, and guardrails

Air-assisted transfer device such as the Hoverbed or lifting device (e.g., hoist)

Weight-bearing, wide, armless chairs; high, firm sofas or loveseats (in rooms and waiting areas)

Bariatric transport carts (stretchers) accommodating 800 lb

CT scanner capable of accommodating more than 500 lb

Examination tables (weight-rated and wide)

Extra-long phlebotomy needles and tourniquets

Long vaginal speculas

Note: Each area provides furniture, equipment, and space appropriate to the service rendered.

All weight-bearing equipment and furniture should be weight-rated to at least 500 lb.

CT, computed tomography; CVA, cardiovascular accident; OR, operating room.

better educated to recognize complications earlier, facilitating safer care; (3) nurses feel more competent, enhancing their job satisfaction; (4) administration is able to provide focused in-depth education and training to a specific group; (5) staff (based on the unique demands of this population) is more appropriate, providing greater satisfaction for patients and staff; (6) clustering the special equipment saves money by avoiding duplication and provides greater convenience of access; (7) staff is instructed in the proper body mechanics of turning, lifting, and transferring obese patients, decreasing potential for patient and personal job-related injuries; (8) staff participates in continuing education in the bariatric surgical field, enhancing their competency and their ability to teach other professionals or community members, providing service and hospital visibility; (9) litigation risk is decreased because of the safer care and environment; and (10) improved quality of care generates positive patient perceptions, subsequently impacting the hospital's community image and number of referrals.

▶ ORGANIZATION AND STAFF EDUCATION

Multidisciplinary Team

Candidates for surgery are selected carefully after evaluation by a multidisciplinary team with medical, surgical, psychiatric, and nutritional expertise. Ideally, this broad spectrum of expertise is available throughout all phases of patient care. In the context of the hospital setting, the multidisciplinary team that develops and monitors a critical pathway may consist of representatives from any department providing direct services to bariatric patients. Representatives from the support services departments, such as environmental services, purchasing, central supply, and engineering may be asked to participate in problem solving as part of the continuous quality-improvement process on an as-needed basis.

Staff Orientation, Inservice, and Continuing Education

Because obese patients seek hospital services other than bariatric surgery, it is essential that basic obesity and bariatric surgery education (including sensitivity and customer service) be provided to all existing hospital staff and be included in the initial orientation of all new personnel. Attendance at the surgeon's group discussion with prospective patients is an excellent adjunctive way to expose staff to basic information and to have the experience of being with morbidly obese individuals who are seeking to understand the surgical option. Davidson and Callery describe a method of converting the surgeon's patient-education and support-group sessions into continuing-education opportunities (with continuing education credit) for hospital staff.[3] To maintain state-of-the-art care in a cost-effective manner, ongoing bariatric continuing-education is targeted at the departments included in the multidisciplinary team, especially the nursing staff. As part of this education, these team members are made aware of the profound influence they have on the attitudes and behaviors of their coworkers and the importance of their positive role-modeling related to the bariatric patient.

▶ PHYSICAL AND EMOTIONAL SUPPORT

Physical Support

Physical considerations include being aware of and anticipating patients' reaching and bending limitations. Assistive reaching devices are purchased or constructed and kept on the unit to facilitate self-care, particularly perineal care. If assistance is necessary, it is provided compassionately, without reference to the disability. Assistance includes such things as placing the bedside stand, telephone, TV remote control, call light, and liquids within easy reach; helping the patient to remove or put on footwear; tying or snapping the back of the gown; pulling up the top sheet, blanket, and bedspread; positioning pillows; and picking up dropped items from the floor. Bariatric patients have special sensitivity to ambient air temperature. Obese patients tend to feel warmer and perspire more freely. They are much more comfortable in cooler rooms. Room fans are helpful, especially in warm weather. Patients who have experienced rapid weight loss following bariatric surgery tend to be cooler, and they prefer warmer rooms. If individual room temperature adjustment is not possible, provide extra blankets. Careful attention to simple comfort measures means a great deal to these patients. The following staff behaviors have been identified by preoperative patients (in focus groups conducted by the author) as their highest priorities: being treated with respect; informing support persons of the anticipated length of surgery and the location of the waiting room; and maintaining regular communication with support persons regarding patients' progress in the operating room, postanesthesia care unit (PACU), and nursing unit.

Emotional Support

PATIENT PERCEPTIONS

Although emotional support is important for any patient in a hospital setting, particular attention is given to this aspect of bariatric surgery because of the societal pressures obese patients routinely experience. Patients undergoing bariatric surgery continue to feel misunderstood and mistreated by medical and nonmedical personnel involved in the treatment of their obesity.[4] These reality-based perceptions stem from a combination of lack of knowledge, prejudice (which is learned at a very early age in our culture), the greater physical demands of providing care, and caregivers' personal fear of fatness projected onto the patient. Brilliant and comprehensive insight into these and other psychosocial issues is provided by Reto.[5] Patients feel nurtured when nurses appear to have time for them (even when, in reality, they do not) and when they listen attentively. Following through with promised medicine, water refills, and so forth can also have a great impact on patients' perceptions of acceptance. In fear of anticipated ridicule, nonsupport, and other negative responses, some patients may conceal their surgery from relatives, friends, and sometimes their spouses. Therefore, confidentiality in its broadest sense must be maintained.

STAFF BEHAVIORS

The most important provider behaviors include being respectful, nonjudgmental, and caring in all interactions. Patients are keenly sensitive to perceived ridicule, so whispering, giggling, and laughing is avoided in situations in which it might be misinterpreted (e.g., a patient walks past the nurses' station and two employees begin to whisper to each other while looking at the patient). Likewise, the word *fat* is not used because of its negative societal connotation. Many patients dislike like being referred to (in person) as *morbidly obese*, even if the term is applicable. Replacement terms such as *persons of weight*, *heavy (heavier)*, or *large (larger)* have a much kinder tone. Furthermore, it is wise for caregivers to avoid attempts to empathize with patients' overweight or to share personal dieting stories. There is risk that these well-intentioned remarks will be seen as patronizing and may enhance patients' feelings of inadequacy, isolation, and shame. Another very important component of emotional support involves neutralizing patient anxiety by making only positive, supportive comments about the surgery, the surgeon, and the patients' decisions. Unfortunately, in the past, it was common for patients to report that the opposite had occurred. Encouraging patients and showing enthusiasm for the positive changes they can expect in the future creates meaningful bonds.

Patients can be very sensitive to the staff's behavior because of their previous life experiences. Such things as unanswered call lights, overlooked care or comfort measures, and abrupt, impersonal comments or responses are often interpreted as personal rejection. Society has enculturated obese persons (consciously or unconsciously) to expect to be treated as disgusting, grotesque, slovenly, and emotionally and mentally deficient human beings. Patients may express this through anger, easily hurt feelings, demanding or controlling behaviors, apologetic requests, and defensive or other self-protective reactions. In addition, they often have a reverse bias against thin people, and feel that nonmorbidly obese caregivers cannot understand their plight.

These patient behaviors can be barriers to the staff's provision of compassionate care. However, responding to these patient behaviors with gentleness and kindness is often all that is needed. Appropriate touching is also therapeutic, reassuring, and comforting, and it implies acceptance. Patients have expressed a desire for these simple gestures, and they feel they are repulsive to the staff if touching is withheld.

Caregivers, once aware of the complex dynamics involved in caring for bariatric patients, can begin to acknowledge their own subtle or overt feelings, behaviors, and attitudes. This discovery can be an important turning point and can greatly influence providers' quality of care and positively impact other team members. Caregivers' responses also may be influenced by further understanding bariatric patients' socioeconomic, demographic, psychological, and lifestyle profiles.[6]

▶ PREOPERATIVE WORK-UP

Clinical Assessment

PHYSICAL EXAMINATION AND MEDICAL HISTORY

There are special considerations in assessing an obese patient. Blood pressure is best obtained using an appropriately-sized (large or extra-large) cuff that fits snugly. Using a cuff that is too small for the upper arm results in a falsely high reading and causes unnecessary patient embarrassment and discomfort. Although not ideal, a regular cuff can be used on the forearm or lower leg if a properly fitting cuff is not available. Listening for breath sounds can be difficult and may be best heard in the lower lung fields. If necessary, skin folds may be lifted or moved to gain better access to the chest. If the patient cannot sit up, heart sounds can usually be heard on the left lateral chest wall while the patient is turned toward the left side or at the second intercostal space next to the sternal border. Palpation of the abdomen is much more difficult in an obese patient; however, rebound tenderness can usually be detected. Bowel tones, if present, can usually be heard by applying more pressure with the stethoscope.

In taking a medical history, it is best to evaluate the common comorbidities associated with, or aggravated by, obesity. These include diabetes, hypertension, hypercholesterolemia, cardiopulmonary disease, asthma, sleep apnea, gastrointestinal disorders, gastroesophageal reflux disease, and arthritis. Urinary incontinence (due to pressure on the bladder from excessive weight) is also common. On admission, look for preexisting pressure ulcers, especially in the immobile superobese, and immediately report this finding to the surgeon, as surgery may be deferred until the ulcer is healed.

WEIGHT AND HEIGHT MEASUREMENTS

An accurate weight is taken on admission, using a scale designed to accommodate the morbidly obese individual. To avoid embarrassing the patient, obtain the weight discretely and privately and record it matter-of-factly, without comment, negative facial expressions, or other body language. Typically, hospital or clinic stand-up or sling scales provide accurate measurements only up to about 350 lb (159 kg).[7] Some bariatric beds incorporate scales. If the hospital does not have a scale that can accurately measure the weight of a superobese patient, the purchase of one should be a very high priority. To weigh a patient on the freight scale (as has been done in the past) is humiliating and insulting; the good will of the patient may be irretrievably lost. To ensure accuracy and consistency of results, all weight measurements are taken on the same specialized bariatric scale every time. Unless hospitalization is prolonged by a complication, the admission weight is sufficient.

Body mass index (BMI) is used today as the standard to determine a person's weight status. It is the most common method of expressing severity of obesity, even though it is not a true measure of body fat because it does not distinguish between muscle and fat. However, it correlates closely with the amount of obesity and is the most useful practical tool we have available. BMI values for individual patients are often obtained from height and weight tables such as those published by the National Heart, Lung, and Blood Institute (U.S. National Institutes of Health) or from a BMI calculator available from the same group. Some BMI calculators and formulas are quick to use but are not precise; the slight discrepancies can make a difference when rounding. Furthermore, there is no standard agreement among organizations regarding which formula is used. To manually calculate an *accurate* BMI, the formula in Figure 49-1 may be used. The patient's preoperative BMI is usually found in the physician's history and physical report.

BLOOD TESTS, CHEST RADIOGRAPHS, AND ECGS

Basic tests performed prior to surgery include a complete blood count, hemoglobin A_1c, a complete metabolic panel, thyroid testing (for hypothyroidism), urinalysis, and serum iron studies (serum ferritin, serum iron levels, and iron binding capacity). A serum intact parathormone test may be obtained to establish a baseline reading for evaluating long-term bone metabolism in gastric bypass patients. Most patients require a chest radiogram and an electrocardiogram.

CARDIOPULMONARY FUNCTION, SLEEP STUDIES, GASTROINTESTINAL TESTS

Other tests taken prior to bariatric surgery include standard pulmonary function tests and arterial blood gases, if indicated, and sleep studies if sleep apnea is suspected. Gastrointestinal tests may include an upper gastrointestinal radiographic series or an esophagogastroduodenoscopy, for hiatal hernia or reflux, and a gallbladder ultrasound. Preoperative testing serves to determine eligibility for surgery and the need for specialist consultations, as well as to document medical necessity for the insurance company. This testing also provides pretreatment reference points that enable postoperative evaluation of improvements in comorbidities.

PSYCHOLOGICAL EVALUATION

Psychological evaluation is done preoperatively to determine the patient's emotional status; psychiatric and family history; and capacity to understand the available surgical options, seriousness of the bariatric surgery, and ability to comply with the postoperative regimen. This evaluation usually includes written testing and an in-person interview by a licensed psychologist or psychiatrist, preferably one who understands obesity and is supportive of the surgery. Other testing may include a baseline quality-of-life questionnaire, and self-image and depression inventories.

Figure 49-1. Calculation formula for body mass index (BMI). For accuracy, keep two decimal places when calculating, and round the final number to one decimal place.

Formula for BMI = Weight (kg) ÷ Height (m²)

To convert pounds to kilograms, divide by 2.2

To convert inches to meters, divide by 39.37

To convert meters to meters square, multiply the number of meters by itself

To get the BMI, divide the weight in kilograms by the height in meters²

Example: The patient weighs 350 pounds and is 5'6" (66 inches) tall

1. Weight in pounds (350) divided by 2.2 = 159.09 kg

2. Height in inches (66) divided by 39.37 = 1.68 meters

3. Meters (1.68) multiplied by itself (1.68) = 2.82 meters squared

4. Weight in kg (159.09) divided by meters squared (2.82) = 56.41, or 56.4 BMI

Note: This formula equates to multiplying the weight in pounds by 702 and dividing that result by the height in inches; then dividing that result by the height in inches again.

Example: 350 x 702 = 245,700.00; 245,700/66 = 3722.73; 3722.73/66 = 56.41, or 56.4

Many testing options are available, and the choice of routine testing is commonly determined collaboratively by the surgeon and psychologist or psychiatrist.

Nutrition

Overweight patients are commonly undernourished, protein deficient, and lacking in the essential nutrients required for healing.[7] Changes in eyes, hair, lips, tongue, teeth, and gums may be indicators of poor nutritional status, and abnormalities are recorded in the preoperative assessment. Patients may be given preoperative nutritional supplementation by their surgeons prior to admission to enhance wound healing and nutritional status. Preoperatively, the dietitian discusses postoperative dietary and supplementation requirements and assesses patient understanding and potential compliance.

Informed Consent and Preoperative Teaching

Informed consent is usually obtained in the physician's office prior to surgery or immediately preceding surgery. Getting the patient's consent for the procedure involves more than a review of the risks-versus-benefits of the operation itself and of the short-term recovery period. It requires that the patient understand the necessity of *lifelong* compliance with: (1) dietary restrictions, (2) nutriment supplementation protocols, (3) laboratory work protocols, and (4) regular follow-up office visits. Adherence to appropriate protocols allows close monitoring of patient progress as well as the prevention or correction of abnormal findings. Staff is instrumental in reinforcing the need for this compliance and may also identify potentially noncompliant patients and those who need further teaching.

The surgeon thoroughly explains the risks of surgery; nurses provide in-depth explanations of what to expect prior to, during, and after surgery. The surgeon's office staff usually begins this process and the hospital staff continues it. The patient visits the preoperative clinic where thorough teaching related to the hospitalization and discharge occurs. Preoperative clinic nurses play a vital role in patient education, emotional support, and prevention of complications. They explain techniques, equipment, and routines and provide underlying rationale. Patients are taught to use flow-type incentive spirometry and the techniques of splinting with pillows, diaphragmatic breathing, coughing, leg and foot exercises, turning onto the side, and getting out of bed properly and safely. Emphasis is placed on the expectation of and need for early ambulation. Additionally, nurses explain the bed position, use of the patient-controlled analgesia (PCA) machine, the pain-assessment tool (pain scale), and pain management. The placements of the nasogastric tube, sequential compression hose, urinary catheter, drains, dressings, intravenous medications, and diet progression are also explained.

The potentials for such occurrences as infection, bowel problems, nausea, and blood clots are similarly reviewed. The possibilities of or plans for intensive care unit (ICU) admission immediately postoperatively, endotracheal intubation, continuous positive airway pressure or bilevel positive airway pressure are explained as are the move to the operating room, the time and place of arrival on the day of surgery, and the surgeon's preoperative preparation routine. Providing a tour of the pertinent hospital areas allows patients to become familiar with the surroundings and should decrease some of the stress and anxiety on admission. The preoperative clinic nurse also begins discharge teaching, an important contribution. Patients need repetition and reinforcement of discharge information and, after surgery, there is little time. Patients report that it is reassuring to be told that the hospital staff is familiar with bariatric surgery and that appropriate equipment and furniture are available.

Physical Preparation

Patients are expected to arrive the morning of surgery already showered and scrubbed. However, most patients perspire heavily and may have intertriginous dermatitis. Because these areas are difficult for patients to expose and reach, it is important to check and clean the axillary, neck, submammary, abdominal, inguinal, leg, and ankle folds as necessary. Patients should attempt to urinate and defecate prior to leaving the unit. Antiembolism stockings are applied and an appropriate doses of low-molecular-weight heparin are injected subcutaneously. The doses are repeated every 12 hours thereafter until patients are discharged.

Hydration

Preoperatively, patients are deprived of oral intake after midnight prior to surgery. Intravenous (IV) fluids are started on the nursing unit to hydrate patients. Because of the excess adipose tissue, IV access tends to be difficult to establish. It should be a written policy that *only a skilled IV nurse may start the IV*. IV antibiotics are usually administered in the operating room holding area.

Anesthesia

In morbidly obese patients, cardiac output, systemic and pulmonary artery pressures, and left and right ventricular pressure are all high.[8] General anesthesia with muscle paralysis causes a reduction in lung tidal volumes in all patients. In obese patients, these cardiorespiratory problems are exaggerated, and many morbidly obese patients cannot tolerate the supine position. The various positions routinely employed in surgery can further compromise cardiopulmonary function in these vulnerable patients. The reverse Trendelenburg position (RTP) is used during bariatric surgery. In a recent small study, this position was shown to have a marked effect on improving gas exchange and respiratory mechanics in 15 patients undergoing biliopancreatic diversion.[9]

▶ INTRAOPERATIVE CARE

Goals

The goals of intraoperative care as stated by McEwan are as follows: "Skilled perioperative nursing interventions afford patients safe and comfortable positioning during surgery, ensure optimal exposures of surgical sites, and prevent postoperative complications (e.g., pressure injuries, neuropathies, cardiovascular and respiratory compromises)."[10]

Procedures

In the operating room, the team helps to get the patient onto the table. A footboard prevents the patient from sliding down the table. The patient's arms are secured on padded armboards, palm upward, to protect the ulnar nerve. One or two long, padded safety belts are placed at least 2 inches above the knees to prevent the buckling of the knees while in reverse Trendelenburg position. A temperature-regulating blanket is placed over the patient's chest and arms to prevent the hypothermia that tends to develop with abdominal surgery. An electrosurgical unit dispersive pad is applied to the thigh to ground the electrocautery unit. Electrocardiogram electrodes, a pulse oximetry monitor, and an automatic blood pressure cuff (extra-large) are set up prior to anesthesia. The sequential compression device attached to the leg or foot compressors is turned on and checked. The roles of the scrub and circulating nurses (or operating room physician's assistant) are geared to the procedure to be performed and, of course, entail the use of the special equipment needed for bariatric surgery. After the operation, the patient is moved to a hospital bed and is taken to the PACU for recovery. Using the patient's bed eliminates transfer from operating room table to stretcher to hospital bed. The HoverMatt mattress is an effective and safe transfer device that is used in many hospitals. It suspends the patient's body by providing a frictionless pillow of air underneath the patient, which results in a very smooth and comfortable transfer. Fewer people are needed to make the transfer and, because lifting the patient is unnecessary during lateral transfers, it reduces the potential for injury.

▶ POSTOPERATIVE CARE

Postanesthesia Care

Waking up the bariatric surgery patient in the PACU has been described as a continual challenge.[11] Mechanical ventilation is sometimes required. However, newer anesthetic agents have facilitated quicker recovery and ambulation. Immediate care includes the use of an oxygen mask and subsequently a nasal oxygen cannula, coughing and deep breathing, provision of intravenous narcotics until the PCA pump is initiated, and monitoring vital signs, dressings, and urinary output. Giving encouragement and emotional support is also very important during this time. When the patient is stable, transfer to the nursing unit is accomplished.

Choi and colleagues evaluated the efficacy and safety of PCA in 25 morbidly obese patients following gastric bypass surgery.[12] They measured arterial blood gases, heart rate, mean arterial pressure, arterial oxygen saturation, respiratory rate, amount of opioid drug (morphine sulfate) used, patient satisfaction, visual analog scale for pain, and the incidence of nausea, vomiting, pruritus, and sedation. Visual analog scale pain scores were 5.4 ± 2.1 on the day of surgery but remained below 4 thereafter. Arterial oxygen saturation and vital signs were maintained, without significant changes, and side effects were minor and required no treatment.

Davidson and Callery reviewed nursing issues relating to the immediate postoperative care of obese patients referred to the ICU or the intermediate-level care (IMC) unit.[13] They include triage considerations, mobility, visiting, fluid resuscitation, management of sleep apnea, airway management, and transporting patients for procedures performed outside the ICU. Among the important points made in this article is that "all morbidly obese ICU patients are classified as higher acuity than routine ICU patients, because otherwise routine procedures take more time in the morbidly obese."[13] The rationale for higher-acuity classification is applicable to the care of the bariatric surgical patient, regardless of the nursing unit, and staffing should be adjusted accordingly.

Nursing Unit Care

ROUTINE

Routine care includes observation of vital signs, strict measurement and recording of fluid intake and output, control of pain and nausea, and monitoring of dressings for bleeding. With open procedures, the abdominal dressing is checked every 2 to 4 hours in the immediate postoperative period when hemorrhage is most likely to occur, and then every shift. Routine care also includes ensuring that "turn, cough, and deep-breathe" procedures (including frequent *observed* use of incentive spirometry), leg and foot exercises, and abdominal splinting (using pillows) are carried out properly by the patient.

BARIATRIC-SURGERY-SPECIFIC

When the patient arrives from PACU, the bed may again be put into the RTP, with the head of the bed elevated 14 inches (30cm) and a footboard in place. RTP is used to improve pulmonary function using gravity to pull the diaphragm down, thereby increasing tidal volume. The bed should not be flexed at the hips (although some bariatric beds cannot be completely straightened for RTP) because flexion impairs deep breathing and may promote pelvic venous pooling. Intravenous access is carefully maintained, including cautioning the patient to be careful not to dislodge the needle while ambulating, reaching, and turning. Often a peripherally inserted central catheter (PICC) line is used. The nasogastric tube (if present) is set to low suction power. If the tube comes out, absolutely no attempt at reinsertion on the nursing station is made. Reinsertion is performed under fluoroscopy only. It is critical that the nursing staff be made aware that suture lines and staple lines can be disrupted by "blind" reinsertion.

A bladder catheter placed at surgery is removed as soon as feasible, within 24 hours, if possible. Catheter retention is avoided whenever possible because catheters tend to discourage ambulation. To prevent urinary tract infection, diligent catheter care is necessary because personal hygiene is much more difficult for bariatric patients. Ambulation, as previously noted, is one of the most important aspects of care.

Table 49-2	COMPARISON OF ILEUS AND BOWEL OBSTRUCTION	
CATEGORY	ILEUS	BOWEL OBSTRUCTION
Abdomen	Distended and uncomfortable	Cramping abdominal pain (more severe than ileus)
Bowel sounds	Hypoactive or absent	Hyperactive
Flatus	Decreased or absent	Absent
Bowel movements	Absent	Absent
Appetite	Decreased or absent	Absent
Nausea and vomiting	Sometimes present	Always present
Temperature	Normal	Usually elevated
White blood count	Normal	Usually elevated
Diagnosis	Absence of bowel sounds with abdominal distention	Abdominal radiograph or CT scan: dilated loops of intestine

CT, computed tomography.

The following are nursing measures used to prevent postoperative ileus, constipation, obstipation, and bowel obstruction: decreasing pain medication (while maintaining good pain control), ambulating early, and encouraging adequate fluid intake (Table 49-2).

DIET

Depending on the surgeon's preference, ice chips and sips of water are started immediately and the diet is advanced to clear liquids given in frequent, small amounts (no more than an ounce) sipped slowly. Laparoscopic Roux-en-Y gastric bypass patients may have radiographic examination using water-soluble contrast media, to check for patency of the gastroenterostomy site and absence of leaks on the first postoperative day, prior to starting on clear liquids.[14] Once fluids are begun, several 1-ounce medicine cups are placed at the bedside so the patient can accurately measure amounts and manage intake without assistance from staff. The patient is cautioned to drink no more than 1 ounce every 5 minutes to prevent overfilling and creating pressure within the newly created small stomach (pouch). The dietitian plays a key role by ensuring that the dietary staff is familiar with the protocol and does not bring inappropriate food items to the patient. The patient, likewise, is told not to ingest inappropriate items if brought into the room by dietary staff (in error) or by visitors. The patient may remain on liquids following discharge at the preference of the surgeon or, alternatively, be advanced to purees prior to discharge. Patients are transitioned to full liquids, purees, semisolid, and then solid foods. Postoperatively, all bariatric patients require some degree of life-long, nutritional supplementation, which is begun during the first postoperative week. The more malabsorption created by surgery, the more supplementation is required.

MEDICATIONS

Typical medications used in patients undergoing bariatric surgery are antibiotics, anticoagulants, H_2 blockers, sedatives, and analgesics. Initially, IV pain medications are commonly delivered by PCA or, less commonly, by epidural catheter and incorporate the use of some form of pain-scale assessment. Patients transit from IV to oral analgesia prior to discharge. Other medications include those used to treat comorbidities, such as insulin or oral agents for diabetes, antihypertensives, and inhalation agents for asthma. Many patients on diabetic medication prior to surgery do not require it postoperatively. It is important to remember, in caring for morbidly obese patients, that many medications and most anesthetic agents are lipophilic, that is, they tend to accumulate in fatty tissue. Therefore, they are released irregularly into the circulatory system, depending on the kind of medication used and individual variances. Thus, resedation and oversedation can occur. Because these lipophilic drugs can have a cumulative effect, overdosage, which can cause respiratory depression and arrest, is the main concern. When giving intramuscular medications, a longer needle may be needed so as to avoid injecting into adipose tissue instead of muscle. Following operations wherein a small gastric pouch is created, large tablets can be crushed, chewed well, or taken in liquid form by the patient. Capsules can be broken apart and mixed with sugar-free Jell-O or a low-calorie liquid. The patient is told that nonsteroidal antiinflammatory drugs, some antibiotics, iron, and potassium are irritating to the stomach mucosa and are to be avoided. If there is no reasonable substitute route or drug available, the patient is instructed to use a liquid antacid prior to taking the medication.

ACTIVITY AND AMBULATION

Initially, attention is given to the appropriate bed position, the use of alternating pressure hose or foot compressors, and exercise of the lower extremities. Patients are provided with an overhead bar and trapeze to facilitate movement in bed. Abdominal binders are not routinely used because they constrict the lower costal margin and abdomen, which fosters splinting and atelectasis. The primary goal is early, independent, and frequent ambulation. The patient should be encouraged to get out of bed and move about to prevent respiratory complications and thrombophlebitis. Ambulation should occur within hours postoperatively and then every 2 to 4 hours while awake. Conscious patients admitted to the ICU/IMC have the same ambulation requirements as those on the surgical unit. ICU nurses may find the early and frequent ambulation order difficult to carry out because they are unaccustomed to caring for patients who are ambulatory. A further factor may be that "an estimated additional 1.5 hours of care are required per unconscious or full care morbidly obese patient."[15]

The first time the patient is out of bed, and as needed, the nurse should have an extra person in the room to assist in supporting the patient. The patient may feel weak or faint or have difficulty balancing and ambulating because of pain, medications, vertigo, or a fall in blood pressure caused by hypovolemia. Activities related to turning, positioning, and ambulating pose a genuine threat to nurse and patient safety. Anticipating and planning for the necessary equipment, sufficient number of staff, proper body mechanics, and moving techniques can help to prevent injury, fatigue, and accidents. Fortunately, many bariatric care products are available. The American Society for Bariatric Surgery, Gainesville, Florida (www.asbs.org), can provide help via a resource manual that identifies many vendors of care products.

RESPIRATORY CARE

Upper abdominal surgery predisposes a patient to the development of atelectasis. Incentive spirometry is used primarily to prevent or diminish atelectasis. The effectiveness of the effort is visible to the patient, thereby providing motivation to take deep inspirations. The measured volume is compared to the preoperative baseline, which is used as the goal. Staff must not assume that the patient is following the regimen properly. The patient is observed and coached throughout the postoperative stay to be sure incentive spirometry is being used frequently and with proper technique. If ordered, aerosol treatments are also observed by staff, and the patient is taught to understand the length of the treatment.

WOUND AND SKIN CARE

Generally, wound care in an uncomplicated patient is relatively simple and usually consists of observing the dressing for bleeding or hematoma; maintaining a dry, sterile dressing; observing the wound for healing or disruption and signs of infection; and assisting with staple removal. Closely related to wound care is the prevention of nausea and vomiting. "Abdominal wounds in obese patients have excess tension due to adipose and edema (sic). Vomiting can add intraabdominal pressure at the incisional area. Nasogastric tubes, antiemetics and keeping patient NPO are options."[16] Likewise, constipation should be avoided; subsequent straining increases intraabdominal pressure and can cause disruption of the wound.

Obese persons are more prone to infection than the nonobese. Adipose tissue is hypovascular, which impairs phagocytosis and decreases the body's ability to combat infection. In addition, diabetes is common in morbidly obese patients and may contribute to slow healing and infection.

Seriously infected wounds can occur in cases of intraabdominal leak and fistula formation and can be a nursing-care challenge. Consultation with nurses who specialize in wound care can be very helpful. Following discharge, seromas and minor wound dehiscences occur quite commonly and are usually easily treated. Pressure ulcers are uncommon in uncomplicated bariatric surgical patients. However, they can occur as a result of overhanging skin rubbing on wheelchair arms, bedside-rails, and other standard-sized equipment. If a patient with prolonged hospitalization is unable to ambulate, the nurse must be alert to the potential for pressure ulcers and should institute preventive measures such as frequent turning, positioning with pillows to provide support and prevent pressure, and special skin care. Specialized bariatric beds with variable air pressures may be used for selected patients. Urinary and fecal incontinence is also a potential cause of skin breakdown, as is chronic intertriginous dermatitis. Unexposed skin between skin folds is to be routinely cleaned and dried. Most often, this skin is excoriated, moist, warm, and odorous and is likely to be infected with *Candida albicans*.

Placing dry, absorbent gauze dressings or clean, dry washcloths or hand towels in the skin folds is an option. Absorbent powders, topical antifungal agents, and antibiotics are often ordered. When cleaning heavy skin folds, it may be necessary to obtain extra assistance. Similarly, wounds resulting from abdominal surgery heal more slowly in obese patients than in normal-weight individuals.

This puts patients at risk for complications such as incisional hernias, wound dehiscence, and evisceration. "Frequent dressing changes can place the bariatric patient at risk for epidermal stripping from frequent tape application and removal. Consider using an advanced wound caredressing (hydrocolloid, foam, or calcium alginate) that is changed less frequently than conventional dressings."[7] Dressings can be secured with Montgomery straps, tubular mesh, or mesh panties.

Sleep Patterns

Sleep apnea is very common in the obese. Snorers and patients with known sleep apnea are best located near the nurses' desk for closer observation because they are at higher risk for upper airway obstruction. There is also a risk for respiratory depression with administration of anesthesia or narcotics. Carbon dioxide narcosis can occur during the night and lead to respiratory arrest. For this reason, patients with sleep apnea and those weighing 300 lb or more are often best monitored in ICU/SCU overnight following surgery.

▶ COMPLICATIONS

Early Complications

Early complications are defined as those occurring during the surgical procedure or in the immediate postoperative period (usually prior to discharge). The nurse's assistive role in prompt recognition and reporting of the symptoms of complications (especially pulmonary embolism and anastomotic leak) is absolutely critical and can be life-saving for the patient. Hemorrhage manifests itself as excessive blood on the dressings or in the nasogastric tube, tachycardia, or a drop in blood pressure.[17] Respiratory insufficiency may be seen with pneumonia, atelectasis, pulmonary embolus, and even congestive cardiac failure.[18] Cyanosis, hemoptysis, hyperpnea, tachycardia, chest pain, blood pressure alterations, and diaphoresis may be indicative of either pulmonary embolism, adult respiratory distress syndrome, pneumonia, or pulmonary edema. Pulmonary embolism may be unavoidable despite prophylactic administration of heparin and early ambulation, but it is usually not fatal. Deep vein thrombosis may be indicated by swelling or pain in the legs, calf tenderness, and a positive Homan sign and is verified by Doppler studies. Wound infection (evidenced by redness, tenderness, pain, fever, and purulent drainage) and wound dehiscence (separation of wound edges) can be serious in the compromised obese patient.

In laparoscopic adjustable gastric banding, anastomotic or gastric perforation is not common and usually occurs during the surgeon's early learning curve. Indicative symptoms are persistent left shoulder pain, fever, tachycardia, tachypnea, and leukocytosis. In all bariatric procedures, the triad of fever, tachycardia (>120), and tachypnea should arouse suspicion of an anastomotic or staple-line leak. Other leak symptoms include shoulder pain, leukocytosis, blood pressure drop, oliguria, and signs of peritoneal irritation (generalized or localized abdominal pain, rigidity, distention, absence of bowel tones, and rebound tenderness).

Patients state that they "just don't feel right" or have a sense of impending doom. If a patient is found sitting cross-legged in bed ("the Buddha position") and having grunting respirations, leak is quite likely. Unfortunately, leaks can be difficult to diagnose, not always following a clear course or having positive diagnostic tests until sepsis is well established. A suspected leak, because of its potentially dire consequences, should prompt an order for immediate Gastrografin-swallow radiography and computed tomography (CT) scan with IV and oral contrast. If confirmed, reoperation or interventional radiologic drainage of the abscess (if localized) is necessary.

Late Complications

Late complications arise after the patient has left the hospital and has recuperated from the surgery. The major late complications in the various bariatric procedures are shown in Table 49-3. More specific potential complications related to malabsorption are anemia, bone demineralization, neurologic problems (e.g., peripheral neuropathy secondary to hypovitaminosis and Wernicke encephalitis), and protein malnutrition. These occur in proportion to (1) the amount of malabsorption created; (2) the quality of patient education; (3) the level of physician monitoring; and (4) the degree of patient compliance with follow-up office visits, laboratory testing, diet, and nutriment supplementation. Many late complications previously associated with the adjustable gastric band have been minimized. Reasons for this include individual and collective experience, improvements in the band and surgical technique, emphasis on follow-up care aspects, and improved adjustment technique.[19] When reviewing the complications in the various surgeries, it is important to remember that most patients do not experience major complications. The International Bariatric Surgery Registry indicates that 97.2% of patients have no major 30-day postoperative complications with a range of procedures, both complex such as

Roux-en-Y gastric bypass and simple such as vertical band gastroplasty and adjustable gastric banding.[20]

Patient Adjustments to Surgery

Patients inevitably must make physical, behavioral, and emotional adjustments to the surgery and thereby contribute to the avoidance of complications. These include such elements as the surgically-imposed new eating behaviors, compliance issues, and differences in lifestyle, body image, and social acceptance. To assist with these adjustments, support groups are provided by bariatric surgical practices as part of patients' comprehensive and life-long care commitment to the patient. Patients who regularly attend surgeon-sponsored support groups are likely to be more successful in losing and maintaining weight loss. Nurses can reinforce the importance of attending a group during discharge teaching. Some patients may desire or require additional support from a psychiatrist, psychologist, or other licensed mental health provider. An outstanding mental health workbook for postoperative gastric bypass patients has been written by Holtzclaw.[21]

▶ DISCHARGE TEACHING

Pain Management

The patient should be given a dose of pain medication just prior to discharge so that it will be effective during the journey home, and he or she should be instructed to take enough pain medication in the ensuing days to remain comfortable but active. It is helpful for the patient to know that the pain will decrease with each passing day and that the dose can be decreased accordingly. The patient should also be told the importance of maintaining a consistent level of pain relief rather than waiting until pain is severe before taking more medication. Most patients appreciate the

Table 49-3	**LATE COMPLICATIONS FOLLOWING BARIATRIC SURGERY**	
GB, DS, BPD	**VBG**	**AGB**
Staple-line breakdown (nontransected stomachs in GB)	Staple-line disruption	Band slippage (less common)
Peptic (marginal) ulceration	Reflux (esophagitis)	Reflux (esophagitis)
Adhesions	Adhesions	Adhesions (less)
Small bowel obstruction	Small bowel obstruction (rare)	Port complications
Stoma obstruction (stenosis)	Stoma obstruction (stenosis)	Stoma obstruction (stenosis)
Fatty-food and lactose intolerance	Some food intolerances	Some food intolerances
Dumping syndrome		
Nausea and vomiting	Nausea and vomiting	Nausea and vomiting
Abdominal pain	Bezoars (stomal)	Band erosion
Constipation or diarrhea		
Cholelithiasis	Cholelithiasis	Cholelithiasis
Incisional hernia (laparotomy)	Incisional hernia (laparotomy)	Incisional hernia (rare)
Pouch dilation	Pouch dilation	Pouch dilation
Volvulus		
Metabolic deficiencies (some severe or life-threatening)*	Some nutrient deficiencies	Some nutrient deficiencies
Depression	Depression	Depression

*Symptoms are directly related to the degree of malabsorption.
AGB, adjustable gastric banding; BPD, biliopancreatic diversion; DS, duodenal switch; GB, gastric bypass; VBG, vertical banded gastroplasty.
Note: Reoperation may be necessary in any bariatric procedure.

Table 49-4	BARIATRIC SURGERY DISCHARGE CRITERIA CHECKLIST

Hematocrit >25
Afebrile for previous 24 hours
No signs of wound inflammation or infection
Lungs clear; respirations normal
Nasogastric tube discontinued
Pain controlled; understands pain management
Nausea controlled
IV discontinued
Oral fluids tolerated
Ambulates frequently and independently
Prescriptions received
Medications from home returned to patient
Understands medications, dosages, and frequencies
Has surgeon's written phone numbers for problems, concerns, or questions
Verbalizes immediate postoperative dietary regime
Understands bathing, exercise, and lifting limitations
Understands potential bowel dysfunction and needed action
Able to name and describe the bariatric surgical procedure performed
Knows follow-up appointment date
Has transportation home provided by:
Signatures: (Nurse) (Patient)

reassurance that they will not become addicted to the medication during this short postoperative interval. The patient is told to contact the surgeon if the pain is not relieved adequately by the prescribed dosage (perhaps symptomatic of a complication) or if the supply of medication runs out prematurely.

Medications

New medications are reviewed with the patient prior to discharge, including any changes in medications previously taken for comorbidities. Remind the patient to inform the primary physician of the surgery and the likely improvements in comorbidities with weight loss. Medications may require dosage adjustments; they may be increased after malabsorptive operations (e.g., hormones), and they may be decreased or eliminated with loss of weight and improvement in comorbidities (e.g., insulin and antihypertensive agents).

Diet and Elimination

In general, most surgeons' office staff provide written and verbal pre- and postoperative dietary and elimination information. The hospital nurse is most effective in reinforcing these concepts. If the practice is hospital-based, the hospital nurses and dietitians assume greater roles in this teaching.

Wound Care

Usually, the abdominal dressing is removed prior to discharge. The patient is instructed to keep the wound clean and dry. Showering is permitted, using soap, gentle washing, and patting the wound dry. Baths, hot tubs, and swimming are not permitted until the wound is healed. The nurse instructs the patient regarding the signs and symptoms of inflammation, infection, seroma, dehiscence, and evisceration. The patient is also told to make an appointment to be seen in the office for a wound check in

about 10 days, at which time the remaining skin staples (if employed) will likely be removed.

Physical Activity and Limitations

Incisional hernias are relatively more common with open procedures. The patient is instructed to avoid lifting more than 10 lb. The patient is encouraged to climb steps and be actively moving and walking. Usually, the patient is allowed to drive unless taking medication that would interfere with mentation and reflexes. A patient from out of town who is flying home is taught exercises to use while on the plane and is told about the importance of getting out of the seat and moving around the plane every hour to decrease risk of deep vein thrombosis and pulmonary embolus. The patient is permitted to have sexual intercourse. The patient can return to work at the patient's discretion and level of stamina.

Late Complications

Signs and symptoms indicating wound infection, wound dehiscence or evisceration, seroma, thrombophlebitis, pulmonary embolus, pneumonia, ileus, marginal ulcer, bowel obstruction, myocardial infarction (uncommon), and leak or intraabdominal sepsis (also uncommon in the late postoperative period, but equally serious) are reviewed by the nurse to help the patient determine when to call the surgeon.

Follow-up Appointment with Surgeon

The discharge nurse establishes that the patient has a follow-up appointment with the surgeon. The patient and family are reminded of the importance of regular follow-up visits with the surgeon. The patient is strongly urged to attend the surgeon's support group. An out-of-town patient will return less frequently but will stay in contact with the surgeon via phone (according to the usual follow-up schedule) and via reports from the local primary care physician. Copies of all laboratory results are to be requested by the patient to be faxed directly from the patient's local laboratory to the surgeon's office. Out-of-town patients are encouraged to maintain (at a minimum) annual visits with the surgeon.

Bariatric Surgery Routine and Contact Information

Emergency and routine contact information is provided to the patient in writing. Depending on the hospital and surgeon relationship, the nurse provides the patient with nursing-unit phone numbers for nonemergent calls. A post-discharge follow-up phone call from a unit nurse to check on the patient's status can be beneficial in terms of rapport and early identification of problems.

▶ CONTINUOUS QUALITY IMPROVEMENT

Purpose

The basic principles of continuous quality improvement are to improve care, increase patient satisfaction, decrease costs, increase efficiency, and empower staff. The standard of care is determined by a composite of professional standards, patient expectations, surgical outcome criteria, safety and infection control outcomes, length-of-stay criteria, and (sometimes) accrediting or governmental criteria.

Process

The process is an evolution of problem-solving techniques and change theory. Empowering staff to resolve problems quickly at their levels in the organization and doing things right the first time are fundamental tenets of the process.

▶ CARE PLANS, CLINICAL PATHWAYS, PROTOCOLS, AND PRACTICE GUIDELINES

Overview

Individualized care plans are still being used in many facilities, although the trend is toward using clinical pathways. Care plans are based on the nursing process, critical-thinking skills, and the new North American Nursing Diagnosis Association taxonomy 11 (adopted in 2000) for nursing diagnoses. Standardized care plans save precious nursing time but still need to be individualized. "According to the guidelines from JCAHO, the client or family must be involved in the development of the care plan and it must be interdisciplinary. One reason the critical or clinical pathway is becoming more popular is the interdisciplinary approach involved in this system."[22] Both care plans and clinical pathways involve a problem-solving approach to care. Clinical pathways are most commonly developed for "high-risk or high-volume" patients (e.g., bariatric surgery) and work in concert with continuing quality of care. Variances can be documented on an individualized care plan until resolved. In today's managed-care environment, cost-effective services must be provided.

Rouse and colleagues described an optimal care path developed by their transdisciplinary team. By means of the optimal care path, both the length and the cost of stay decreased by about 17% while quality of care was unimpaired, as evidenced by a decreased percentage of wound infections and improved communication and collaboration among team members across the continuum of care.[23] Preserving quality while decreasing cost, length of stay, use of intensive care, and readmission were also cited in other studies.[24,25] Further, protocols and practice guidelines give specific sequential instructions for treating patients with particular problems and needs.[26] Protocols are especially helpful when there is extensive use of agency or float staff who are unfamiliar with the specialty.

Clinical Pathway Development

The multidisciplinary team develops the pathway using the hospital's pathway format and the physician's protocol or routine orders as a starting point. An additional category addressing the special emotional-support needs of the bariatric patient is essential. When developing the pathway, input related to the optimal plan of care and desired outcomes is sought from each department. A monitoring tool is used to track deviations in length of stay, expected outcomes, and resource utilization. The statistics used in the analysis of data obtained from the tool can range from simple to complex. Ultimately, the statistics will provide a means of identifying significant problems and, subsequently, prioritizing and planning improvements in care. The changes are implemented and evaluated. The cycle may be repeated until compliance with the standard is met.

▶ SUMMARY

Care of the bariatric surgery patient is infinitely rewarding when providers reflect on or witness the major lifestyle changes, improved quality of life, and joy that the compliant patient experiences. It is satisfying to know that the majority of patients have an uncomplicated clinical course and experience dramatic loss of excess weight, with marked improvement in health, appearance, self-esteem, employability, promotability, and physical, sexual, and social activity levels. Caregivers who provide safe, competent, supportive care make an immeasurably valuable and life-changing contribution to these patients. Administrators who support the bariatric surgery program make a significant impact on its quality, safety, and financial viability; their decisions also directly affect the overall satisfaction of the bariatric patients and caregivers.

▶ REFERENCES

1. Wellman NS, Friedberg B: Causes and consequences of adult obesity: health, social and economic impacts in the United States. Asia Pac J Clin Nutr 2002;11(suppl 8):S705-S709.
2. Herron DM, Gagner M, Kenyon TL, et al: The minimally invasive surgical suite enters the 21st century: a discussion of critical design elements. Surg Endosc 2001;15:415-422.
3. Davidson JE, Callery C: Making the most of your time: the benefits of converting patient education programs into continuing nursing education. Obes Surg 2000;10:482-483.
4. Kaminski J, Gadaleta D: A study of discrimination within the medical community as viewed by obese patients. Obes Surg 2002;12:14-18.
5. Reto CS: Psychological aspects of delivering nursing care to the bariatric patient. Crit Care Nurs Q 2003;26:139-149.
6. Fox KM, Taylor SL, Jones JE: Understanding the bariatric surgical patient: a demographic, lifestyle, and psychological profile. Obes Surg 2000;10:477-481.
7. Hahler B: Morbid obesity: a nursing care challenge. Medsurg Nurs 2002;11:85-90.
8. Brodsky JB: Positioning the morbidly obese patient for anesthesia. Obes Surg 2002;12:751-758.
9. Perilli V, Solazzi L, Bozza P, et al: The effects of the reverse Trendelenburg position on respiratory mechanics and blood gases in morbidly obese patients during bariatric surgery. Anesth Analg 2000; 91:1520-1525.
10. McEwen DR: Intraoperative positioning of surgical patients. AORN J 1996;63:1059-1063, 1066-1079.
11. Walter DA: Waking up the gastric bypass patient. Obes Surg 1997; 7:374-375.
12. Choi YK, Brolin RE, Wagner BK, et al: Efficacy and safety of patient-controlled anesthesia for morbidly obese patients following gastric bypass surgery. Obes Surg 2000;10:154-159.
13. Davidson JE, Callery C: Care of the obesity surgery patient requiring intermediate-level care or intensive care. Obes Surg 2001;11:93-97.
14. Wittgrove AC, Clark GW: Laparoscopic gastric bypass, Roux-en-Y: 500 patients: technique and results, with 3- 60-month follow-up. Obes Surg 2000;10:233-239.

15. Davidson JE, Kruse MW, Cox DH, et al: Critical care of the morbidly obese. Crit Care Nurs Q 2003;26:105-116.
16. Wilson JA, Clark JJ: Obesity: impediment to wound healing. Crit Care Nurs Q 2003;26:119-132.
17. Mason DS, Sapala A, Sapala JA: Roux-en-Y gastric bypass. AORN J 1993;58:1113-1140.
18. Shikora SA: Surgical treatment for severe obesity: the state of the art for the new millennium. Nutr Clin Prac 2000;15:13-22.
19. Fox SR, Fox KM, Srikanth MS, et al: The Lap-Band® System in a North American population. Obes Surg 2003;13:275-280.
20. Mason EE, Renquist KE, Jiang D: Perioperative risks and safety of surgery for severe obesity. Am J Cin Nutr 1992;55:573S-576S.
21. Holtzclaw TK: This is not brain surgery...but there *is* a magic pill! In Bellury P (ed): A Mental Health Companion for the Gastric Bypass Patient. Atlanta, The Storyline Group, 2003.
22. Client care plans and management. In Smith SF, Duell DJ, Martin BC (eds): Clinical Nursing Skills: Basic to Advanced Skills, ed 5, p. 30 . Upper Saddle River, Prentice Hall, 2000.
23. Rouse AD, Tripp BL, Shipley S, et al: Meeting the challenge of managed care through clinical pathways for bariatric surgery. Obes Surg 1998;8:530-534.
24. Huerta S, Heber D, Sawicki MP, et al: Reduced length of stay by implementation of a clinical pathway for bariatric surgery in an academic health care center. Am Surg 2001;67:1128-1135.
25. Roark MK: Critical pathways. J Health Care Res Manag 1997;15: 12-15.
26. Rich P, Brady C: Documentation. In Mayer B, Kowalak J (eds): Illustrated Manual of Nursing Practice, ed 3, p. 23. Springhouse, Penn., Lippincott Williams & Wilkins, 2002.

50

Patient Support Groups in Bariatric Surgery

Tracy Martinez, R.N., B.S.N.

At support group meetings, the ways patients introduce themselves vary. Patients are asked to tell the group about the comorbidities they no longer suffer from since their bariatric surgeries. Patients commonly disclose that they no longer need their blood pressure medications, that they can sleep without continuous positive airway pressure machines, and that they no longer require support to walk. They offer that they no longer suffer from diabetes, the terrible disease that literally whittles away the body. But most striking are the patients who state that they no longer suffer from "the worst comorbidity," that of loneliness. The psychological aspects of this disease are as important as the more publicized major medical comorbid conditions, especially when one considers the quality of life of the morbidly obese.[1]

All humans seek acceptance and love. Unfortunately, many of our patients who suffer from morbid obesity have endured a lifetime of loneliness and discrimination. Where does this bias and discrimination begin? Stunkard and Wadden conducted a study of children's attitudes toward obesity. They found that "children no more than 6 years of age describe silhouettes of an obese child as lazy, dirty, stupid, ugly, a cheater, and a liar.[1] Even more alarming, a survey of nursing attitudes toward the obese reported that nurses believed that the obese most likely have issues with anger and that they are lazy and overindulgent.[2]

Black-and-white line drawings of a normal-weight child, an obese child, and children with various handicaps, including missing hands and facial disfigurements, were shown to a variety of audiences. Both children and adults rated the obese child as least likable. It is unfortunate to observe that this prejudice extends across races and across rural and urban populations and, saddest of all, exists among the obese themselves.[3] Drawing an even grimmer picture of discrimination against this population, data suggest that these biases and discriminatory attitudes can be activated and subsequently conveyed without intention or conscious awareness.[4]

One of many misunderstandings about those who suffer from the disease of morbid obesity is that they have

an excessive prevalence of psychological illness. On the contrary, studies of severely overweight persons conducted before they underwent weight loss surgery have shown that there is no single personality type that characterizes the severely obese. This population does not report greater levels of psychopathology than the average weight-controlled population.[5] However, in our program's population, the prevalence of depression is quite high (80%), which is not surprising in a society that is overtly cruel to obese individuals.

Our society frequently demonstrates the ignorant belief that if patients ate less and exercised more, they could control their weight. In other words, patients "choose" to be obese. The fact is that morbid obesity is a disease of multi-factorial origin that is strongly associated with genetic predisposition. Studies of twins have shown that two thirds of the variations in body weight can be attributed to genetic factors.[6]

Morbid obesity is a chronic disease. Today there is no cure. Like any chronic disease, lifelong attention and ongoing effort are imperative to keep morbid obesity under control with weight loss and weight maintenance. Unfortunately, nonsurgical weight management does not demonstrate sustained weight loss in the long term in those suffering from morbid obesity.[7]

▸ PURPOSE OF A SUPPORT GROUP

There are numerous reasons for conducting support groups in bariatric programs. One is to educate prospective patients about the postoperative lifestyle they will encounter. Preoperative patients who attend support groups prior to surgery may have a significant advantage over those who do not; they experience less stress by becoming educated at a more leisurely pace than is possible for patients postoperatively. Seeing, interacting with, and listening to patients who have already undergone bariatric surgery may diminish anxiety for preoperative patients.

Having patients attend a support group preoperatively is one of the numerous ways in which a thoroughly informed consent is provided in addition to the traditional consultation and written informed consent. For this reason, some programs make attendance mandatory for preoperative patients. Further, many morbidly obese patients present to the program with a sense of isolation due to societal discrimination, as well as with a sense of shame and guilt resulting from years of failed dieting. Many individuals have damaged self-esteem and few friends. It is not uncommon for those who suffer from morbid obesity to put their needs on hold, often being supportive to others in order to gain acceptance and, thereby, neglecting their own needs.

A successful support group should provide an environment of self-identification and mutual understanding. Demonstrating empathy for patients as morbidly obese individuals in today's society and creating a sense of belonging reduces what is often a condition of chronic stress, and it enhances their self-image, a critical contribution of a support group.

A support group environment can facilitate learning if patients feel understood and comfortable. Education is an extremely important goal of a support group. Many practitioners in the field of bariatrics call bariatric surgery a tool, and they teach patients how to utilize this tool to maximize their postoperative success. The educational opportunities offered in support groups give patients the knowledge needed to take ownership of the decision to undergo surgery to treat their obesity and to enable them to accept the necessary lifestyle changes. Being involved with a group of peers who have common struggles with the chronic disease of morbid obesity creates an environment of knowledge, empowerment, and personal responsibility, all of which are necessary for the long-term success of a bariatric operation.

Educational needs change from the acute postoperative period (0 to 12 months) to the period that starts 12 months after surgery. During the acute phase, the needs commonly dealt with are diet advancement and food intolerances and stressing the importance of protein intake and vitamin supplementation. Other educational needs include mobility training; the role of exercise, particularly resistance training for the prevention of muscle-mass loss; body-image challenges; hair loss; and criticism from others for the decision to have surgery. Commonly, having failed at every other attempt at weight loss, patients express fears that surgery will not be successful.

Approximately 1 year after bariatric surgery, education and support needs change. New concerns emerge, including body-image changes and challenges, changes and stressors in family dynamics and friendships, the reactions of and attention from the opposite sex, coworkers' reactions, peer reactions, and concerns about excess skin. Spousal relationships may undergo major stress because patients' partners may feel threatened when patients achieve normal weight. As the patients' self-esteem increases, abusive relationships are often no longer tolerated, causing marital strife. Often, for the first time in a marital relationship, patients feel empowered and express their individuality and opinions without fear of repercussions.

Because of the distinct differences in the needs of patients during the acute period and the needs of patients after the first year, two separate support group meetings should be considered.

Another goal of a support group is to facilitate a social environment. As discussed earlier, many patients have isolated themselves from society, having few friends and date infrequently. There is research that documents employment discrimination as well as reduced acceptance by major colleges.[7] A successful support group can, for the first time in a patient's life, create a feeling of belonging and acceptance, as well as a sense of not being alone. The unfair burden of failure and shame is lightened; self-confidence and self-worth are potentiated.

Another purpose of a support group is to assist the long-term postoperative patient who is gaining weight to get back on track. As mentioned, there is no known cure for the chronic disease of morbid obesity. Sometimes, postoperative patients feel bulletproof and falsely assume, after experiencing successful weight loss at 1, 2, and even 3 years, that they need never concern themselves again with thoughts of weight maintenance. When patients return to the program with the chief complaint of weight gain, the postoperative guidelines of nutrition, vitamin supplementation, and the role of exercise and education must be reemphasized. All of these vital behaviors may be reaffirmed in the support group. The patient must accept the fact that maintaining weight loss is an ongoing, lifetime commitment and effort. Patients should not feel shame. On the contrary, patients should be congratulated for taking responsibility for reaching out for the necessary support.

▶ ORGANIZING SUPPORT GROUP MEETINGS

An ongoing connection between the bariatric patient and the bariatric program is essential. Programs should offer support group meetings at least once a month; to a postoperative patient seeking support, it can seem a long time between monthly meetings. One of the first steps in organizing a support group is to commit to a regular schedule so as to decrease the risk for confusion that causes patients to miss meetings. For example, meetings can be set up in a pattern such as the second Tuesday of each month, 7 to 9 pm. A predetermined schedule helps to increase attendance, and that contributes to patient compliance and the success of the group. We suggest that the program publish a calendar at, minimally, 6-month intervals. This calendar should include meeting time, date, location, facilitator, topic, and target audience, as well as any other special rules the program desires to invoke. Rules may exclude the presence of children, may allow the presence only of program patients, or may allow the presence only of patients for whom 1 year or more has passed since surgery, to name a few restrictions. Posting the support group calendars in convenient places in the clinic and making them accessible on the program's website is advisable (Table 50-1).

To create a safe environment in which patients can feel free to share their personal feelings and experiences is to address the subject of confidentiality. It is not uncommon for patients to discuss private and emotionally

Table 50-1	GENERAL SUPPORT GROUP SCHEDULE

July-December 2005
At (designated meeting place)
WHEN: The second Tuesday of each month from 7:00 pm to 8:30 pm
  (for example)
WHERE: Location, including address
WHO: Pre- and postoperative bariatric surgery patients of (program's
  or surgeon's name). Because this is an adult setting, we request that
  no children attend.

Confidentiality Statement:
Discussions held within the confines of this support group are to be
  honored, respected, and deemed confidential and are not to be
  shared in any manner outside of the group.

Format:
Introductions
Discussion (topic-driven/current events)
Open forum

Topics:

MONTH	DATE	TOPIC
July	07.12.2005	Keeping on Track While Traveling
August	08.09.2005	Exercise for Life
September	09.13.2005	Menu Sharing
October	10.11.2005	Patient Testimonies
November	11.08.2005	Surviving the Holidays
December	12.13.2005	Goal Setting

delicate feelings. Sometimes patients discuss sexual concerns, become tearful, or express certain vulnerabilities. A successful support group should convey and create a safe environment that facilitates such sharing and discussion. A code of ethics including confidentiality should be discussed and posted. Planning a meeting well in advance allows for the stability of a routine location and decreases the risk for having to change the meeting place in the middle of the year, which can cause confusion for patients.

When choosing the location for the support group meeting, there are several considerations. First, the location must be available on the dates desired. Second, the venue must offer comfort and be able to accommodate large patients; chairs must be armless and able to bear appropriate weight. There should be adequate handicapped parking nearby so patients do not have to walk too far from the parking lot to the meeting space. Handicapped-accessible bathrooms should be located within a reasonable distance to accommodate patients who are dependent on walkers, wheelchairs, or motorized scooters. Ideally, audiovisual equipment should be available for the use of speakers.

Meeting locations vary. Hospital conference rooms are ideal because they usually offer the special needs mentioned and are familiar to patients. If the hospital conference room is not an option, public libraries, churches, or community centers can provide adequate space, usually at a minimal charge or free. Another option is a local hotel meeting room. This, of course, would entail a monthly rental fee. The room's setup should be consistent. Chairs arranged in a circle convey a sense of inclusiveness and encourage involvement. Meeting-room doors should be kept closed to ensure privacy and confidentiality. A sign should be placed on the outside of the door simply stating "Private Meeting in Session." Although the focus of meetings is educational and support-oriented, some groups offer beverages and food as well.

A routine agenda helps to keep the group on schedule. An example of this might include introductions, followed by announcements, the guest speaker, questions and answers, and socialization.

▶ WHO SHOULD FACILITATE?

The facilitator plays a crucial role in the success of the support group. Thoughtful selection of the group facilitator is imperative. It is essential that the facilitator be a well-trained professional who represents the surgeon and the program in a unified mission; in other words, as an arm of the program. The leader should have training or experience in group facilitation and be capable of creating a consistent format for the meeting. The leader should set the tone, reinforcing the message of compassion and empathy.

The role of the group facilitator can be successfully fulfilled by a variety of professionals in the program's multidisciplinary team. The psychologist, registered nurse, registered dietician, and surgeon can be equally successful and effective. However, the designated individual should possess some basic characteristics of a qualified bariatric support group facilitator. The facilitator should:

- Demonstrate basic knowledge of the bariatric procedures performed in the program.
- Understand that he or she is a representative of the surgeon and the surgeon's program.
- Be able to distinguish normal as opposed to abnormal postoperative symptoms and be knowledgeable enough to defer questions and request immediate medical intervention if necessary and to know when to call upon the most qualified expert in the program.
- Be knowledgeable about group behavior and leadership and be capable of learning the personal views of the participants.
- Stay within the scope of his or her expertise and profession.
- Be respectful of the values of each member as a unique individual.
- Be able to initiate activities, interactions, and discussions.
- Be comfortable with expressions of emotion, conflict, and tension.
- Possess knowledge of and commitment to the self-help process.
- Be respectful of each member while being committed to the welfare of the group, focusing on building a sense of community, group cohesiveness, and consensus decision making when appropriate.
- Be punctual and dependable.

There are six basic and essential goals that the facilitator of a support group should promote and help participants to achieve:

1. Expression of emotions: empathy, understanding, acceptance, and a sense of self-worth and personal value.
2. Communication: good listening skills, emotionally supportive discussions, open and honest dialogue, self-disclosures.

3. Information: sharing of successful coping strategies, alternatives, options, and current scientific and medical facts.
4. Connection: conveying a sense of community; building supportive networks and a feeling of belonging and fellowship; building a sense of "you are not alone."
5. Opportunities: personal growth, with the encouragement of coping, adjusting, and overcoming.
6. Personal responsibility: reinforcing the importance of self-determination.

Postoperative bariatric patients are not ideal as group leaders for several reasons. First and most important, patients need to be patients. In other words, patients need their own recovery opportunities as well as long-term maintenance. Second, a professional working in the field of bariatrics has better knowledge to guide patients when real or perceived medical concerns inevitably arise. If a postoperative patient does assume the role of support group facilitator, he or she must be a successful patient and should be a role model who is at least 2 years postoperative.

▶ FOUR PATIENT PHASES

There are roughly four common phases that bariatric patients undergo. The support group facilitator should have some insight into these phases in order to best understand the group dynamics. These four phases are exhibited in various stages, from preoperative to a year or more after surgery.

The first phase is the *hope phase*. This phase consists of patients who have decided to have surgery and are preparing for it. They are extremely hopeful and are commonly full of questions for the group participants. They are, often for the first time in their lives, surrounded by a group of individuals who understand their plight, their sense of guilt, defeat, and hopelessness. The veterans in the group will eagerly share their experiences and give advice and encouragement. It is important, however, that the facilitator not allow a particular patient to monopolize the meeting, and that others are enabled to speak and voice their own questions and concerns. Sometimes the patient has a knowledge deficit, and it is appropriate to encourage such a patient to attend an informational lecture or consultation to gain basic knowledge about the surgery and its long-term ramifications.

The second phase is the *honeymoon phase*. This phase often occurs in the first through the ninth month following bariatric surgery. This is the time when patients, often for the first time ever, experience the sense of satiety. Commonly, depending on the procedure performed, patients may even experience anorexia. The scale continues to show lower numbers, often with little effort on the patient's part. You will hear words like *unbelievable* and *it's a miracle*. Reinforcement that this sensation is commonly experienced soon after surgery is important. In addition, this is the time to stress that compliance with the program guidelines, including nutrition, supplementation, and physical exercise, is imperative.

The third phase is commonly the *reality phase*. This occurs between the sixth and eighteenth months. One of the most common and fearful experiences shared by patients during this phase is that active hunger returns and dietary consumption increases. Patients often fear that their "tool" is not going to work for them. They can obsess about every food eaten; they often weigh themselves several times a day. Commonly, this group of patients wants reassurance that their experiences have been shared by others. It is appropriate to assure the patient that such feelings are common. Postoperative patients contribute their experiences of going through the same phase. Any symptoms of maladaptive behavior during this phase may require further investigation and treatment, even one-on-one treatment. Sometimes patients may do well to meet with the program nurse, the nutritionist, or even the psychologist if the individual is abnormally stressed or struggling.

The fourth and last phase occurs from the twelfth month on. This is called the *maintenance phase*. Although there is commonly a decline in support group attendance in this patient population, support group meetings are extremely beneficial for several reasons. Continual reinforcement of the idea that surgery is a tool, not a cure, and that constant, consistent lifestyle changes are needed for weight maintenance is essential. It is common for patients to want to be "normal" and to want to distance themselves from the memory of having had bariatric surgery at all. This attitude can be dangerous because weight gain as well as vitamin deficiencies can occur with noncompliance. For this reason, long-term follow-up and support group attendance should be taught and reinforced both pre- and postoperatively by the multidisciplinary team. This phase is when patients learn that they are not bulletproof and that surgery isn't the magic pill that it seemed to be in the first months after surgery.

Offering a multidisciplinary approach in the support group helps patients to maintain a healthy lifestyle emotionally as well as medically. The reinforcement they need to be able to assume personal responsibility is beneficial. Directing patients to the appropriate discipline within the program can be extremely helpful when a specific need is identified. This period can be extremely complex because patients have undergone a dramatic transformation medically, physically, and emotionally. Resolution of comorbidities are shared and celebrated. Relationships and body-image challenges are commonly presented to the group. For example, if a patient shares with the group that he or she has gotten off track with an exercise program, the support group can be a great help in several ways. Group members offer their ideas to the patient on how they maintain compliance with their exercise programs. This is a situation in which patients can be very effective teachers. The facilitator can reinforce the importance of exercise and should suggest that they meet with the program's exercise coordinator.

▶ SUPPORT GROUP TOPICS

A variety of topics can be enjoyable ways of providing a multidisciplinary approach to your support group. Preplanning and providing a schedule in advance allows patients to anticipate the topic. Patients in particular postoperative phases may choose to attend meetings that they find helpful in their own postoperative phases. Another benefit of preplanning is the confirmation of a speaker's attendance.

The topics and contents suggested here offer ideas for educating patients about psychological, medical, and emotional well-being through a variety of invited guest speakers and team members. They are intended to be engaging and to encourage interaction in the support group.

Exercise While Traveling

This meeting stresses the importance of exercising even while traveling. The exercise coordinator can demonstrate exercises that can be done in hotel rooms, including the use of resistance bands. He or she can also discuss planning vacations around activities such as hiking, canoeing, skiing, and so forth. Goal: To encourage patients to stay on track with exercise, even when out of their normal daily routines. Speaker: Exercise coordinator.

Weight Training for Weight Maintenance

This meeting educates participants about the importance of resistance training early postoperatively so as to minimize muscle loss during rapid weight loss, as well as the importance of muscle building for increased metabolic rate in the long term. This meeting can be conducted in the hospital physical therapy department or gymnasium for a thorough demonstration. Goal: To encourage muscle-mass building and increase basal metabolic rate. Speaker: Exercise coordinator.

Dining Out

This interactive topic can be presented in several ways. In planning this meeting, participants can be encouraged to bring menus from their favorite restaurants. The dietician can have an interactive question-and-answer session about which menu items are best for protein and which contain lower fat or hidden sugars. Goal: To educate patients that eating healthfully is possible in all settings, including restaurants, and how to find the best options. Speaker: Program dietitian.

Osteoporosis Prevention

Because several bariatric procedures can cause malabsorption of calcium, this topic is important. Asking a gynecologist to speak on this topic has several benefits: she or he has the requisite knowledge; patients may choose this individual for their care; and it educates the gynecologist about the success of bariatric surgery. Goal: The importance of vitamin supplementation after bariatric surgery. Speaker: Gynecologist or program nurse.

Patient Testimonials

This topic is always a favorite. At this meeting, selected patients are asked in advance to prepare 5- to 8-minute presentations that address what it was like living with the disease preoperatively, why they chose surgery, what their surgical experiences were like, and what life is like for them today. It is best to have as presenters patients who are at various postoperative stages. At the conclusion of the presentations, the participants are encouraged to ask questions and share comments. This stimulates interaction and can be very motivating for the group. Goal: To motivate patients by allowing them to hear successful patients' stories and to remind them that many others have similar experiences to share. Speakers: Patients scheduled ahead of time.

Panel of Experts

This meeting involves the attendance of all of the program's multidisciplinary team members, including surgeons, program nurses, registered dieticians, exercise physiologists, and program psychologists. Other panel experts may include a plastic surgeon, an internist, and a bariatrician. Patients are encouraged to ask questions that one or several experts answer. Goal: To make the entire team available to answer questions that patients haven't had the opportunity to ask or that have arisen postoperatively. Speakers: Program's multidisciplinary team.

Lean Protein Cooking

At this meeting, the registered dietician demonstrates low-fat, high-protein cooking ideas. She or he discusses innovative recipes that have reduced fat and high protein and are not too challenging to prepare. Ideally, a kitchen is available for demonstration. Along with a verbal presentation, samples can be offered. The question-and-answer session is usually very interactive after this meeting. Goal: To encourage patients to seek alternative cooking options instead of unhealthful preparations commonly learned in childhood. Speaker: Program dietitian.

Reconstructive Surgery After Weight Loss

The plastic surgeon chosen most likely has some kind of association with the program. It is important to choose one who has had experience operating on patients who have lost a significant amount of weight. Pre- and postprocedural photos are a common way to educate patients about the results of reconstructive surgery. The session may include questions submitted in advance. Goal: To educate patients about solutions for the excess skin that patients often have concerns about after weight loss. Speaker: Plastic surgeon.

When Friends Leave

It is common for the dynamics of relationships to change after patients lose significant amounts of weight. This can be hurtful and frightening for patients, and the changes and challenges can be stressful. Discussing this topic with a qualified professional is most beneficial. The psychologist shares his or her knowledge about the topic and the dynamics behind it, which opens up the group for sharing. Goal: To give patients education, tools, and support for this phenomenon that commonly occurs in patients' lives. Speaker: Program psychologist.

Body-Image Talk

We often notice that the patients' minds do not catch up with their bodies after weight loss. In other words, they still see themselves as 50, 75, or 100 pounds heavier. They share stories of going to the clothes rack and pulling out clothing four sizes larger then they currently wear. The program psychologist is well aware of this common behavior and can effectively educate patients on its dynamics. A presentation followed by group discussion can be very powerful. Sometimes patients may recognize that they need more one-on-one guidance and choose to see the psychologist individually for further guidance. Goal: To help patients recognize the challenges of altered body images and give them guidance to improve both body image and self image. Speaker: Program psychologist.

Self-Care

As discussed earlier in this chapter, patients commonly have suffered discrimination and self-blame for their disease. Many patients try hard to be accepted by doing things for others, often in excess. They forget or neglect their own needs. The goal of this meeting is to discuss self-care and self-love as well as to provide ways to experience them. There can be numerous presenters at these meetings. The psychologist discusses the psychological benefit of self-care. Others can share the benefits of self-care through massage therapy, facials, makeup consulting, and so forth. A yoga instructor can provide self-love through body care and the physical awareness that yoga encourages. Other speakers may include an exercise coordinator, a massage therapist, an aesthetician, a makeup artist, and a fashion consultant. Providing professionals who understand this population helps to break down barriers caused by altered self-image and fear. For example, it is much more likely that patients would get massages from a therapist who took the time to go and meet them at their support group. The common barrier patients share is a feeling of shame because of their size or loose skin. The massage therapist's attendance at the meeting has already, to some degree, broken down that barrier. Goal: To educate patients about the common issue of self-care and to provide examples of incorporating self-care into their lives. Speakers: Representatives of multiple disciplines.

These are just some of the unusual and innovative ways of educating patients in a support group. It is important to remember that many of the presentations should be reinforced by handouts. Encouraging patients to keep a binder or folder for support group educational materials allows them to refer to those materials when needed in the long term.

All guest speakers should be encouraged to discuss with the group facilitator the contents of their presentations and handouts well in advance of the meeting. It may be appropriate for the facilitator to give the proposed contents to the program nurse, surgeon, psychologist, or another multidisciplinary team member for review. All presentations should be accurate and within the program's guidelines. Ultimately, the surgeon holds this responsibility.

Table 50-2   SUPPORT GROUP RECORD

(Program's or Surgeon's Name)
Meeting Overview Record
Support Group:
- ☐ General
- ☐ Postop 1 Year or More
- ☐ Alternate Location 1
- ☐ Alternate Location 2
- ☐ Alternate Location 3
- ☐ Alternate Location 4

Date: _____
Facilitator: _____
Topic: _____
Overview of meeting: _____
_____
_____
_____

Attendance sign-in record completed: ☐ Yes
Handouts attached: ☐ Yes

DOCUMENTATION AND EVALUATION

It is important to organize and archive the information provided in support group meetings. This documentation should include an attendance record (Table 50-2). Validation of attendance may be a helpful tool in verifying one aspect of the informed-consent process. Another benefit is that it helps to build an e-mail list or correspondence list for support group announcements. It is also beneficial for recording the dates, topics, speakers, and handouts provided at each meeting. Documentation and record keeping are requirements of the Surgical Review Corporation for those seeking a Center of Excellence accreditation. Binders should be labeled by year, with documentation for archiving.

Because support group meetings are ultimately for the patients' benefit and satisfaction, yearly evaluations may be beneficial for ongoing improvement of the group meetings. Conducting an annual patient evaluation survey allows the facilitator to receive constructive information for planning future meetings. Helpful evaluation questions may include the comfort of the meeting space, the length and format of the meetings, and favorite and suggested topics for upcoming meetings. Patients are great teachers and everyone can learn a lot from them. The evaluations can be invaluable to facilitators while giving patients the opportunity to participate in the planning of the group meetings.

SUMMARY

In summary, bariatric patients go through dramatic transformations, both physically and emotionally. Often, the program's support groups are the only interactions available to individuals to discuss the disease and the lifestyle challenges they had experienced preoperatively, as well as the unique experiences they have had postoperatively. Support groups should be a priority for all bariatric programs, and surgery should not be performed without this support in place before patients undergo bariatric surgical procedures.

▶ REFERENCES

1. Stunkard AJ, Wadden TA: Psychological aspects of human obesity. Human Obes 1992;352-358.
2. Maroney D, Golub S: Nurses' attitudes toward obese persons and certain ethnic groups. Percept Mot Skills 1992;75:387-391.
3. Bessenoff GR, Sherman JW: Automatic and controlled components of prejudice toward fat people: evaluation versus stereotype activation. Soc Cogn 2002;18:329-353.
4. Stunkard AJ, Wadden TA: Psychological aspects of human obesity. Am J Clin Nutr 1992;55:5245-5325.
5. National Institutes of Health, Consensus Development Conference Panel: Gastrointestinal surgery for severe obesity. Ann Intern Med 1991;115:956-961.
6. Stunkard AJ, Froch TT, Hrubic Z: A twin study on human obesity JAMA 1986;256:51-54.
7. Canning H, Mayer J: Obesity: its possible effects on college acceptance. N Eng J Med 1966,275:1172-1174.

51

Multidisciplinary Team in a Bariatric Surgery Program

Michael L. Kendrick, M.D., Matthew M. Clark, Ph.D., Maria L. Collazo-Clavell, M.D., Jane L. Mai, R.N., Jeanne E. Grant, R.D., Michelle A. Neseth, and Michael G. Sarr, M.D.

Operative intervention is the most effective and durable treatment for medically complicated morbid obesity. Bariatric surgery represents a unique discipline for a number of reasons. First, the intent of a bariatric procedure is to alter *behavior* as well as physiology, as opposed to the typical extirpative or reconstructive surgical procedures. As such, a successful outcome is highly dependent on patient education and future adherence to healthful changes in behavior. Second, bariatric surgery includes elements not usually regarded as integral to a surgical procedure; the optimal outcome of a bariatric operation is dependent on continued changes in nutrition, exercise, and behavior and on receiving emotional and psychological support. Third, bariatric patients typically have multiple obesity-related comorbidities that affect operative risk and also require close medical surveillance postoperatively as many of these comorbidities improve, necessitating medication adjustment or discontinuation (the primary goal of the operation). For these reasons, bariatric patients represent a unique and complex group requiring a detailed, comprehensive, multidisciplinary preoperative evaluation, including education, and life-long postoperative follow-up to maximize the likelihood of safe and effective outcomes. A multidisciplinary team approach with sufficient expertise to manage the interplay of these behavioral, nutritional, psychological, medical, and surgical issues would therefore seem imperative.

The 1991 National Institutes of Health Consensus Conference brought to fruition established guidelines in the management of patients with severe obesity.[1] Among the recommendations concerning the management of patients being considered for bariatric operations was the firm consensus that a multidisciplinary team is an integral part of patient care. Most insurance providers have also embraced this concept, as have all recognized centers of excellence in bariatric surgery. This integrated, multidisciplinary approach appears intuitive in the setting of operations designed to result in significant improvement in medical comorbidities and quality of life issues through continual behavioral and nutritional surveillance. However, despite the apparent consensus, it is surprising to find that there is currently only a modicum of data effectively comparing the outcomes of multidisciplinary approaches over less comprehensive ones.[2] Most of the current literature concerning outcomes of bariatric surgery is generated by and published at centers utilizing multidisciplinary approaches to some extent.

We present the role of the multidisciplinary medical treatment team in bariatric surgery on the basis of the clinical practice at our institution. Our program has developed over the past 23 years, since the first concerted effort in this field was initiated at the Mayo Clinic in 1980. As have many other bariatric surgical groups, we have learned from our mistakes and those of others, and our group has evolved through experience and the implementation of new ideas.

▶ DEVELOPMENT OF THE TEAM

The history behind the development of the multidisciplinary team at the Mayo Clinic has been an interesting one and probably is reflected in changes in the models of health care delivery. I (MGS) have been involved for the past 18 years and have overseen the changes that have evolved. The prevailing impressions, beliefs, and interest of our medical community regarding bariatric surgery have changed markedly over the past 2 decades and exponentially in the past 5 years. Initially, the youngest and least experienced members of each division (endocrinology, psychiatry, surgery) were assigned the jobs of participating in the bariatric treatment team, even if they had no real interest in obesity as such. So it is not surprising that the results early on were not satisfactory[3]; but over the years, the players on this team have developed a true interest in obesity treatment or have been identified or recruited

Table 51-1	MULTIDISCIPLINARY MEDICAL TEAM MEMBERS AND TIMING OF INVOLVEMENT			
	PREOPERATIVE	IN-HOSPITAL	EARLY POSTOPERATIVE (FIRST 6 MONTHS)	LONG TERM
Surgeon	X	X	X	As needed
Internist/endocrinologist	X		X	X
NP/PA	X		X	X
Psychiatrist/psychologist	X		X	X
Dietitian	X	X	X	X
Bariatric coordinator	X	X	X	±

NP, nurse practitioner; PA, physician's assistant.

because of their specific interest in this area. In the past 5 years, the institution, from a financial standpoint, has also become very interested in the bariatric surgery program. In addition, society as a whole has been forced to embrace this concept because of the growing national epidemic of obesity and its social, financial, and medical implications. Thus, the development of a comprehensive, insightful, multidisciplinary team approach has evolved out of necessity and out of the genuine interest and dedication of most of the members of our current bariatric surgical team.

▶ THE TEAM

The goal of the multidisciplinary team approach is for each member to utilize his or her respective expertise and collectively orchestrate their efforts into optimal patient selection, education, and management. Table 51-1 lists various team members and the timing of their involvement in the evaluation of patients being considered for bariatric operations. Each phase of the process is discussed separately, highlighting the contributions of each discipline. We point out that our setting has an academic background, but the emphasis is first on patient care and only secondarily on academia. Because we are a large, tertiary care center (with a total of about 16,000 employees and 1500 inpatient beds), the expertise is quite concentrated, with many individuals impacting on the care of the bariatric patient. The preoperative care providers often differ from those within the hospital; thus, our organization may not be appropriate for smaller, more community-oriented programs. Nevertheless, with 16,000 employees and their families in a city of nearly 100,000, many of our patients hail from our local community and, thus, unlike much of our tertiary care surgical practice, a substantial percentage of the bariatric practice is community-based.

▶ PREOPERATIVE TEAM ASSESSMENT

Appropriate patient screening and preoperative education, preoperative evaluation and management of comorbidities and, finally, selection of the optimal procedure are paramount to the successful outcomes of bariatric operations.[4] With the increasing coverage of bariatric surgery by the lay press, many surgeons are confronted with self-referred patients who want to be considered for bariatric operations and often have unrealistic expectations. Ideally, however, a referral comes from an internist or primary care physician

familiar with the patient's weight and diet history as well as with the directly weight-related comorbidities of the patient. The referring physician also should have ensured that professionally supervised nonoperative methods of weight loss had been appropriately tried. Most important, the referral should reflect the importance of continued postoperative surveillance as medical comorbidities improve and medication changes become necessary, and it should provide an avenue for close surveillance to prevent nutritional deficiencies in the future.

Endocrinologist or Other Internist

In our practice, an endocrinologist or another interested internist (in conjunction with a dedicated nurse practitioner or physician's assistant) who has an interest in obesity treatment initially evaluates the prospective candidates referred for bariatric surgery. This evaluation may include a complete history and physical examination or a more focused evaluation of weight-related issues, depending on the referral source. Table 51-2 lists the major obesity-specific objectives of this initial evaluation. Detailed reviews of both supervised and unsupervised attempts at weight loss are imperative in assessing both patient motivation for and compliance with health behavior changes. Documentation of participation in recognized support groups, such as Weight Watchers, Jenny Craig, Overeaters Anonymous, or supervised therapeutic modalities such as Nutri-System, or even low-calorie liquid protein programs, show "buy-in" by the patient. A patient

Table 51-2	MAJOR OBJECTIVES OF INITIAL MEDICAL EVALUATION OF POTENTIAL CANDIDATES FOR BARIATRIC SURGERY

Obtain weight history, including:
    Maximum and minimum weights
    Previous experience with weight loss/regain
    Change in weight over time
    History of specific diets and outcomes (supervised, unsupervised)
    Identify use of pharmacologic weight-loss medications
    Assess daily activities and exercise (types, frequency, duration)

Identify and evaluate all medical comorbidities
    Screen for secondary causes of obesity if clinically indicated

Obtain complete social, behavioral, and psychiatric history

Determine patient objectives and motivation

who has not entered supervised programs or has a track record of poor short-term success or early drop-out rates should raise a definite red flag concerning behavioral and compliance issues that will require more intense behavior modification, education, and follow-up. During this initial evaluation, patients are also screened for medical causes of obesity such as disorders of metabolism, fully recognizing these to be unusual causes of severe obesity.

Detailed evaluation, recognition, and management of all medical comorbidities are an essential role of the internist. Adult-onset diabetes, hypertension, hyperlipidemia, degenerative joint disease, cardiopulmonary disease, and sleep apnea are common in the severely obese. All patients who are suspected, based on clinical history, of having obstructive sleep apnea undergo overnight oximetry and, when indicated, a sleep study. Utilization of continuous positive airway pressure (CPAP) in these patients in the perioperative period decreases perioperative pulmonary complications and prevents oxygen desaturation during the first several postoperative days when the patient is most susceptible to cardiac arrhythmias.[5] We mandate the institution of and the demonstration of adherence to some form of CPAP preoperatively in all patients with sleep apnea for at least 2 months in an attempt to recondition the untreated, "deconditioned" brainstem sleep center. Other specific cardiopulmonary evaluation is performed based on the clinical history (for instance, a screening set of pulmonary function tests is not a requisite part of the evaluation unless indicated by history and examination).

Dietitian

The main objectives of the dietitian in the preoperative setting are to obtain a detailed nutrition history, provide education, and establish realistic but objective nutrition goals. Eating patterns (binge eating, night eating, sweet eating) and energy and macronutrient intake are assessed and documented. Screening for evidence of eating disorders such as bulimia is performed as well but is further assessed during the psychological evaluation. The dietitian educates patients regarding caloric needs and record keeping and initiates a medical nutrition therapy program if one has not already been established. Patients are also educated regarding the specific nutritional implications of and expectations involved in bariatric operations. We have developed a nutrition education manual that details the nutritional guidelines that apply after bariatric surgery. This manual is given to patients preoperatively, enabling the patients and their families to plan for the necessary postoperative changes in eating and lifestyle habits. All patients participate in a multistage education and informational program and are initiated into medically supervised exercise and diet programs prior to surgery.

Psychiatrist or Psychologist

All patients considered for bariatric operations at the Mayo Clinic must have preoperative psychological evaluations that assess global psychosocial functioning and specific domains important in obesity treatment (Table 51-3). At present, our program relies heavily on the psychiatric

Table 51-3	**PSYCHIATRIC AND PSYCHOLOGICAL EVALUATION BEFORE BARIATRIC SURGERY**

Psychological Contraindications
  Axis I DSM-IV diagnosis: major depression, bipolar, schizoaffective disorder, bulimia nervosa, etc.: all must have been stable for 12 months
  No psychiatric hospitalization during the past 12 months
  Substance abuse: abstinent for the past 12 months

Other Psychological Factors
  Issues related to history of being the victim of sexual abuse or trauma: stable for 6 months
  Psychosocial stressors: judged to be manageable
  Positive aspects of being overweight: relationship or protective issues regarding weight
  Binge eating disorder and night eating syndrome: stable for 6 months

Positive Psychological Indications
  Participation in 3+ months of behavioral therapy (with no weight gain)
  Physically active lifestyle
  Social support: family, spouse, or friends

or psychological evaluation by dedicated psychologists and by selected individuals in psychiatry. Although our experience may be unique, the type of psychological evaluation initially conducted in our program was a general or standard psychological or psychiatric evaluation. Patients were screened for Axis I psychiatric disorders (depression, substance abuse, anxiety, bipolar disorder, etc.). Those with active disorders were first treated by a mental health professional and then reevaluated in 6 months. Unfortunately, having a lack of specific focus on obesity treatment caused us to overlook some important psychosocial domains. Indeed, the initial evaluations provided by our psychiatry department were unsatisfactory because the psychiatrists' interests were necessarily elsewhere. For example, several very difficult patients with borderline personality disorders slipped through the evaluation, causing considerable problems in the early postoperative period. Inherent in any procedure with a focus on behavioral modification is the requirement that the patient be capable of adherence to changes in health behaviors. For those with cognitive, language, or educational deficits, neurocognitive testing may be beneficial. Patients without the ability to understand the expectations or to comply with nutritional intake and necessary supplementation are not only likely to have a poor outcome but also are at increased risk for medical and nutritional complications.

The presence of suspected psychotic disorders (very unusual), unrecognized or untreated borderline personality disorders, uncontrolled behavioral disorders, uncontrolled depression, or active substance abuse is considered an absolute contraindication to bariatric surgery. Being a victim of sexual abuse is quite common in women with morbid obesity, especially in the absence of a family history of obesity, and should be probed for preoperatively. Weight loss can be problematic for trauma survivors. Binge eating disorder is related to depression and poor body image and may impact surgical outcome. These patients warrant careful psychiatric consultation based on the perceived inability of the patients to comply with the behavioral, physical, and nutritional expectations that are in place after a bariatric operation. If confirmed, the presence of a true untreated psychiatric disorder would, under most conditions, preclude further evaluation for bariatric surgery. Other disorders, such as marital or relationship issues, adjustment disorders, stress, or poor body image may require active psychiatric or psychological intervention as part of the preparation for surgery. Although major psychiatric disorders represent relative contraindications to bariatric surgery, the establishment of a working relationship with a mental health care provider and the documentation of both compliance and control allow many of these patients, on a selective basis, to become candidates for surgery. In fact, our clinical experience has been that actively engaging in appropriate mental health treatment can enhance the outcomes of treatments for obesity.[6]

The psychological evaluation has proven essential in identifying psychiatric and behavior disorders that would benefit from behavior modification. Patients must have appropriate motivation, be able to comply, understand the surgical risks, and have realistic expectations. The psychological evaluation also serves as an initial introduction to a licensed mental health professional. The multitude of psychosocial changes in the family, at the work place, and in social and sexual relations that occur as patients lose weight may mean that they will require professional help in the upcoming postoperative period.

Our health psychology group has also developed several group behavior programs to address aspects of behavior therapy and group support. This presurgical 16-week program involves review of a manual-based (partly self-learning) program titled LEARN (lifestyle, exercise, attitudes, relationships, nutrition).[7] We encourage local patients to attend this supervised group program at the Mayo Clinic or, if they live too far away, to review the manual with behavior psychologists in their own areas. There is also a 14-week binge eating disorder group for those who report experiencing more than 2 days per week of binge eating episodes. In terms of postsurgery programs, I (MGS) used to lead a bariatric support group one evening a month; however, this proved neither effective nor productive for several reasons. Quite possibly I, as a surgeon, was inadequately trained to moderate a truly functional support group. Help by the members of the support group in organizing and coordinating speakers and new patients was not forthcoming despite multiple offers and pleas, and the group degenerated into a social affair dominated by several patients.

At present, our psychologists lead a structured, twice per month, postsurgical support group. The group leaders review information from the LEARN manual, outline strategies for long-term behavior change, and foster discussion of the psychosocial changes experienced subsequent to surgery and weight loss. Many nonlocal patients utilize virtual support groups by participating in some of the many on-line Web sites and chat rooms. We have purposely avoided endorsing or even suggesting such on-line activity (because of our inability to monitor and validate on-line communications and information), but many prospective candidates and postoperative patients claim to have received considerable benefit from these functions.

Surgeon

Despite the excellent and thorough preoperative evaluation and education of a patient by the multidisciplinary presurgical team, the surgeon bears equal responsibility for ensuring appropriate patient selection, education, and preoperative preparation. As documented in the American College of Surgeons Statement on Principles Underlying Perioperative Responsibility, the surgeon is responsible for the preoperative preparation of the patient.[8] Minimizing the risks of operation while providing maximal opportunity for a satisfactory outcome requires a full appreciation by the surgeon of the patient's condition.

In our institution, the surgeon is initially consulted midway through the evaluation and only after the patient has been screened and identified as a potential candidate for a bariatric operation. This system of checks and balances protects the patient from the surgeon and vice versa. The surgeon's primary objective at the initial consultation is to ensure appropriate candidacy, educate the patient regarding surgical (and nonsurgical) options, describe the risks and potential short- and long-term complications, and reaffirm that the patient has realistic expectations. The possibility of future cosmetic surgery also merits discussion at this time.

Physician Extender

Each of our surgical teams includes a so-called physician extender (PE), a registered nurse with focused expertise and interest in bariatric surgery, who helps round out the preoperative, perioperative, and postoperative care by providing needed expertise in issues other than the operation, which is the primary specific concern of the surgeon. This nurse usually is more adept at recognizing family conflicts, educating the hospital nurses about the specifics of nursing care relevant to markedly obese patients, and serving as a necessary go-between for patients and their surgeons and internists.

Bariatric Coordinator

Equally important is the person who coordinates the timing of clinic visits, laboratory tests, specialty consultations, insurance approvals, operative dates, and a multitude of other scheduling details. Until now, this burdensome work has been handled in large part by the physician's secretary. However, as our bariatric practice has grown, we have noted increasing difficulties not only in arranging and scheduling the preoperative evaluations but, more important, also in ensuring that patients attend the long-term postoperative visits. Too many patients have fallen through the cracks and, on occasion, have developed potentially preventable postsurgical problems or complications. Therefore, we have recruited a dedicated bariatric coordinator whose job is to serve as the first contact for patients and referring physicians and to ensure organized and complete initial evaluations. In addition, the coordinator follows a defined protocol for pre- and postoperative medical tests and consultations to ensure regular follow-up visits and reminds those patients who have overlooked a surveillance test or follow-up visit of these responsibilities.

Table 51-4	PREOPERATIVE OBJECTIVES OF THE MULTIDISCIPLINARY TREATMENT TEAM

To assess comprehensively preoperative medical, psychological, behavioral, and nutritional status

To identify, evaluate, and optimize medical comorbidities

To ensure the absence of high-risk psychological, personality, or behavioral disorders

To ensure the patient's ability to understand and adhere to recommendations

To educate the patient about appropriate nutrition, realistic expectations, and the risks and benefits of the surgical intervention advised

To initiate appropriate medical, psychiatric, or behavioral treatment

To enroll the patient in diet, exercise, and behavioral programs

---

Use of a formal computerized database with a baseline preoperative structured evaluation and postoperative follow-up helps to ensure quality of care. Table 51-4 summarizes the preoperative objectives of the multidisciplinary medical team.

▶ IN-HOSPITAL TEAM APPROACH

Because of our local practice environment and institutional dynamics, the in-hospital team, although maintaining a multidisciplinary approach, is in large part composed of personnel different from the personnel of the preoperative outpatient team, except for the surgeon and nurse-PE who provides continuity throughout the operative phase. In some smaller bariatric programs, one can easily envision the same dietitian, psychologist, and internist following the patient through the hospitalization.

The in-hospital bariatric team is composed primarily of the surgeon, nurse-PE, relatively dedicated operating-room staff, dietitian, and nursing staff. In addition, of course, is an infrastructure that has the support personnel and facilities to meet the special needs of this weight-challenged patient population. Special chairs, wheelchairs, stretchers, patient beds and lifts, operating room tables, toilets, and related structural facilities are necessary for routine accommodation of people who weigh between 400 and 500 pounds. Most patients heavier than 500 pounds (230 kg) probably require care in specialized tertiary centers that have highly specialized facilities.[9] Several key members of the in-hospital bariatric team deserve special comment: operating room personnel, nursing services, and dietitians.

Operating Room Personnel

Although it is best that a broad spectrum of operating room nurses, technicians, and anesthesia staff have at least some experience with bariatric surgery, having a dedicated operating room staff promotes efficiency and avoids many foreseeable complications of inexperience. A dedicated staff is especially important for laparoscopic bariatric surgery, because many of the maneuvers during these operations are unique to the bariatric patient. Also especially important is an experienced anesthesia staff; again, the bariatric patient presents several anesthesia challenges, including pulmonary care, positioning unique to this population, dosing of anesthetics, cardiopulmonary monitoring, and so forth.

Nursing Services

Postoperative nursing care of the bariatric patient also provides several unique considerations. A dedicated patient floor or ward makes for efficiency in terms of use of the environment and facilities. The mobility of the postoperative bariatric patient requires both knowledge and appropriate facilities to avoid work-related injuries to the staff as well as to the patient. Similarly, working knowledge of sleep apnea and its treatment is important in the care of this population. However, the concept of a dedicated nursing unit, while theoretically ideal for best patient management, also provides a very real challenge for the hospital personnel department. Maintaining an adequate number of nurses can prove a significant challenge for several reasons. First, many younger nurses may not wish to deal exclusively with a bariatric surgery population; much of the general stigmata of obesity (albeit understandably) spills over onto the unenlightened nursing and paramedical support staff. Second, nurses have been injured (low back, shoulders, etc.) when working with the bariatric population in inadequate facilities, and they fear further injury. Third, the "glamour" of other services and the more attractive work schedules of outpatient units are understandable obstacles to staffing a dedicated bariatric unit. Many hospitals have developed unique approaches to this very real problem. We have addressed the problem by outfitting more than one patient care area to deal with this patient population, but continue to maintain these floors as general surgical areas.

Dietitians

Our program utilizes a different group of dietitians in the in-hospital setting. For our practice, this approach maximizes efficiency for the dietetics staff. Our hospital-based dietitians have developed extensive experience with the early postoperative refeeding period. Moreover, the reality of the postoperative setting and pending discharge is a prime time for the education of patients and their families concerning the step-by-step diet progression during the months after discharge. Indeed, we do not discharge our patients until our dietitian has reviewed with them the postoperative nutritional guidelines utilizing our nutrition education manual; we believe this session to be one of the most important parts of the early postoperative course.

▶ POSTOPERATIVE TEAM MANAGEMENT

Postoperatively, the multidisciplinary team approach is equally essential and is considered imperative for optimal short- and long-term outcomes. Significant areas of focus for the multidisciplinary team in the postoperative period are listed in Table 51-5.

In general, the postoperative team is the same as the preoperative team, at least in the overall specialties involved.

Table 51-5	POSTOPERATIVE OBJECTIVES OF THE MULTIDISCIPLINARY TREATMENT TEAM

To assess for evidence of subacute or chronic operative complications
To monitor preexisting medical conditions
To assess adherence to requirements for nutritional intake
To screen for nutritional deficiencies
To provide appropriate vitamin and mineral supplementation, as indicated
To continue behavioral therapy and support groups as necessary
To increase levels of physical activity and exercise
To monitor for psychosocial difficulties
To follow objective surveillance protocol

We do try to be flexible with postoperative follow-up and, as often as possible, we allow local physicians and psychologists to participate in postbariatric surgery care. We usually require a 6-week and 3-month visit to our clinic; however, we also very strongly encourage follow-up at our institution for, at the least, the first 6 months to 1 year. When patients are from greater distances (more than 200 miles), we are more flexible and coordinate with the home physicians to outline the primary medical and nutritional concerns specific to postbariatric surgical patients. Our follow-up questionnaires also help us to keep in touch with patients; these questionnaires are sent out at 3, 6, 12, 18, 24, 36, and 48 months postoperatively and detail symptoms, weight, medications, medical problems, and psychosocial concerns.

Endocrinologist or Other Internist

Bariatric procedures result in significant improvement in and often the resolution of many obesity-related medical comorbidities. Improvement in serum glucose control in diabetic patients is one of the earliest events, often occurring prior to significant weight loss. Monitoring for appropriate adjustments or often complete discontinuation of insulin or oral agents is imperative to avoid medication-induced morbidity. As weight loss continues, hypertension and hyperlipidemia improve in the majority of patients, allowing medication adjustment or allowing discontinuation (the ultimate goal). Sleep apnea resolves in many patients after significant weight loss, and the use of CPAP may become unnecessary. However, discontinuing the use of CPAP usually requires formal documentation of the reversal of sleep apnea and not just reliance on patients' symptoms.

The internist team and dietitian generally follow the patient closely for the first postoperative year. After that, annual assessment by the internist of nutritional status, weight trends, behavioral modification, and medical comorbidities typically suffice. Continued surveillance of nutritional indexes is important, with extent and frequency dependent on the specific procedure (restrictive as opposed to malabsorptive).[10] Assessment of adequate serum vitamin and mineral levels and appropriate supplementation may also be required. Our most common procedure is the vertical, disconnected, Roux-en-Y gastric bypass.[11] Patients undergoing Roux-en-Y gastric bypass routinely receive daily calcium and multivitamin-mineral supplements and

monthly vitamin B_{12} parenterally. Patients undergoing malabsorptive procedures require more detailed surveillance, concentrating on fat-soluble vitamins, and other supplements.[12]

Dietitian

The dietitian visits with the patient at 6 weeks to reconfirm understanding of nutritional goals (oral intake of fluids, calories, protein, advancement of food consistency, and so forth), provide additional education, and establish follow-up plans. Patients are then seen at varying intervals postoperatively for assessment of dietary and nutritional compliance.

Psychiatrist or Psychologist

Continued evaluation and follow-up with a psychologist are important. Ongoing behavioral therapy, assessment of compliance, and participation in support groups are beneficial for most patients. Recurrent or long-term behavioral therapy may be necessary in patients with poor compliance or other clinical indications, such as onset of relationship difficulties, changes in work status, and binge eating. Further evaluation or treatment of bariatric patients in the postoperative period by a psychiatrist is based on the preoperative assessment and is not considered routine.

Surgeon

The early postoperative care of the patient is the responsibility of the surgeon. Prompt recognition and treatment of postoperative complications are crucial. The importance of bariatric surgical follow-up is vital for several reasons. First, the direct bariatric surgical problems that may occur are not always evident to general surgeons who do not perform bariatric operations. Second, concerned follow-up shows the patient that the surgeon is also interested in how successful the patient is in weight loss and reversal of comorbidities. Patients are seen at 6 weeks postoperatively and again at 3 months. The surgeon monitors the postoperative recovery and identifies and manages the early postdischarge complications, should they occur.

The surgeon's role in the long term is variable; it is based on the institution, the surgeon's preference, and the effectiveness of the team approach. In our institution, the surgeon's role in long-term care is based on the presence of complications. Severe nutritional abnormalities, symptomatic cholelithiasis, incisional hernias, anastomotic strictures, and evaluation of failures for technical problems (pouch dilation, gastrogastric fistulas) all prompt surgical consultation.

▶ SUMMARY

Because bariatric surgery involves a unique patient population consisting of patients who have complex requirements that demand detailed preoperative and continual postoperative evaluation and management of medical, behavioral, and nutritional states, a multidisciplinary treatment team is essential to ensure appropriate patient and procedure selection, to reduce operative risk, and to ensure long-term success. Our program at the Mayo Clinic works, but it has an organizational structure unique to our institution. Other programs have different organizations, yet all should stress the need for multidisciplinary cooperation in virtually all aspects of the care of the bariatric patient.

▶ REFERENCES

1. National Institutes of Health Consensus Development Conference Panel: Gastrointestinal surgery for severe obesity. Ann Int Med 1991;115:956-961.
2. Cosmo LD, Vuolo G, Piccolomini A, et al: Bariatric surgery: early results with a multidisciplinary team. Obes Surg 2000; 10:272-273.
3. Hocking MP, Kelly KA, Callaway CW: Vertical gastroplasty for morbid obesity: clinical experience. Mayo Clin Proc 1986; 61:287-291.
4. Kral JG: Selection of patients for anti-obesity surgery. Int J Obes 2001;25(suppl 1):S107-S112.
5. Gupta RM, Parvizi J, Hanssen AD, et al: Postoperative complications in patients with obstructive sleep apnea syndrome undergoing hip or knee replacement: a case-control study. Mayo Clin Proc 2001;76: 897-905.
6. Clark MM, Balsiger BM, Sletten CD, et al: Psychosocial factors and 2-year outcome following bariatric surgery for weight loss. Obes Surg 2003;13:739-745.
7. Brownell KD: The LEARN® Program for Weight Management 2000. Dallas, American Health Publishing, 2000.
8. American College of Surgeons: ACS statement on principles underlying perioperative responsibility. Bull Am Coll Surg 1996; 81:39.
9. Sarr MG, Felty CL, Hilmer DM, et al: Technical and practical considerations involved in operations in patients weighing more than 270 kg. Arch Surg 1995;130:102-105.
10. Brolin RE, Leung M: Survey of vitamin and mineral supplementation after gastric bypass and biliopancreatic diversion for morbid obesity. Obesity Surg 1999;9:150-154.
11. Balsiger BM, Kennedy, FP, Abu-Lebdeh HS, et al: Prospective evaluation of Roux-en-Y gastric bypass as primary operation for morbid obesity. Mayo Clin Proc 2000;75:673-680.
12. Murr MM, Balsiger BM, Kennedy FP, et al: Malabsorptive procedures for severe obesity: comparison of pancreaticobiliary bypass and very very long limb Roux-en-Y gastric bypass. J Gastrointestinal Surg 1999;3:607-612.

52

Allied Science Team in Bariatric Surgery

Mary Lou Walen

Interest in the field of bariatric surgery has increased dramatically in recent years, along with the mounting incidence of morbid obesity in the United States[1-5] and globally,[6] as well as with the advent of laparoscopic procedures.[7,8] Bariatric surgery has achieved the status of being the "most effective"[9] treatment currently available for this tenacious life-long illness.[10-12] The need for allied health sciences to employ a multidisciplinary team approach resonates throughout written and spoken discussions regarding surgical treatment for the disease of morbid obesity. Dr. Henry Buchwald's statement that "the bariatric surgery patient is best evaluated and subsequently cared for by a multidisciplinary team"[9] is well founded in the data reporting long-term results of bariatric surgery.

This chapter outlines the various components of a bariatric multidisciplinary team and provides brief descriptions of their functions. It reviews the roles of the following team disciplines: internal medicine (encompassing the pulmonary, endocrine, musculoskeletal, hematologic, infections disease, gastroenterologic, and allergic/immunologic components); surgery; support groups; mental and behavioral health; exercise physiology; nutrition; and outcomes management.

The opportunity to offer interdisciplinary education and the experience of teamwork is intended to produce better patient outcomes that acknowledge the value of each team member's specialty-specific technical knowledge and skills.[13] As the number of operations and the variety of bariatric surgical techniques increase, the value to bariatric surgery of the multidisciplinary team approach becomes increasingly apparent. The model presented here constitutes the various disciplines required to enhance the long-term success of this unique surgical specialty. The allied health sciences or multidisciplinary team aspect of bariatric surgery (as contrasted with the operation itself) assumes an importance not ordinarily seen in the field of general surgery. This concept is becoming second nature to experienced bariatric surgeons yet may be a new concept for surgeons trained in the field of general surgery. Those who wish to become expert in bariatric surgery require education in the importance of surgical support services.[14]

▶ LONG-TERM, COLLABORATIVE MISSION OF THE ALLIED HEALTH TEAM

The allied health disciplines provide support for the framework of allied health.[13,14] An all-inclusive, programmatic approach is strongly recommended by the National Institutes of Health,[15-17] the American Society for Bariatric Surgery,[18] the American College of Surgeons,[19] and the Society of American Gastrointestinal and Endoscopic Surgeons.[20,21] These organizations provide guidelines and standards for the multidisciplinary approach to bariatric surgery that address the complexity of the disease and also take into account the exceptionally high surgical and anesthetic risk levels involved in bariatric surgery, as well as the level of patient compliance required for long-term success. Published standards underscore the need for a synergistic model of collaborative care[22] that will enable higher quality care and faster rates of recovery, the maximization of functional ability, timely return to normal activity, and a better quality of life.

The operation is preeminent in importance in the attainment of long-term results in many fields of surgery, but in bariatric surgery, it is quite different. In this case, the life-long achievement of improved health by the patient is defined by a team-based approach that yields effective results in a setting of mutual trust and credibility within the bariatric team. The core of every flourishing bariatric team resides in having a common purpose: the focus of every team member is continually on the long-term success of the patients.

Partnership With the Patient: Informed Consent

A common goal of the bariatric team is that a more thorough informed-consent process be required for bariatric surgery than is required for many other forms of surgery.[23] This is because of the elective nature of this surgery, its complexity, its long-term ramifications, and the necessity of patient compliance and cooperation with the team members to ensure safety and lifetime success. Informed consent for the bariatric patient is a process that provides the patient not only with sufficient information to allow for a reasonable decision about the surgery and its long-term ramifications, but also with an understanding of the importance of the involvement and education of family members.

Dr. Edward E. Mason recommended that each obesity surgeon periodically "review (a) what is known about the operation(s) recommended; (b) the materials available for education of patients; (c) the processes by which patients are informed and consent."[24] He has also stated, "The one person who is always present is the patient. There is information specific to each operation that can be life saving. The patient can, and should, learn about their new anatomy and the potential complications. A partnership between patient and surgeon is the best basis for lifetime care even though such a relationship is usually temporary."[24]

▶ MULTIDISCIPLINARY BARIATRIC TEAM

Interactive Specialized Care Providers

Under the direction of a skilled bariatric surgeon, the bariatric multidisciplinary team will include access to medical management of comorbidities, skilled nursing, people who have specialty-related dietary and nutritional skills, exercise training, experienced anesthesiologists, and psychosocial evaluation. The availability of interested and experienced pulmonologists and cardiologists, of rehabilitation facilities, and of home health care is essential. Guidelines for facilities[18] require sufficient institutional support and motivation within the hospital that involves cultural and physical enhancements so as to allow the operation to be performed safely and efficiently. Facilities, surgeons, and programs alike are expected to be knowledgeable and sophisticated in the collection and reporting of accurate outcomes data for accreditation requirements,[25,26] research purposes,[27] credentialing and privileging,[18,25,26] and sharing of outcomes data with patients.

Patient

As the most vital member of the team, the patient is encouraged to focus on education regarding not only the operation and the process, but also on knowledge of the lifestyle changes and commitment to lifetime exercise and proper nutrition. Because not all patients who suffer from morbid obesity are candidates for surgery, preoperative screening and education become a critical responsibility of the bariatric team. Proper bariatric care begins by acknowledging the individual needs of each patient who presents with an interest in the surgery. Combining commitment to surgical excellence with a caring, dignified, and focused approach by each team member is the foundation of any successful bariatric program.

Perhaps influenced by the widespread publicity stressing the obvious physical benefits of bariatric surgery, some patients may possess unrealistic expectations of success and limited understanding of the importance of their own personal contributions to that success. This situation must be addressed directly by bariatric surgeons and their allied health colleagues. Failure to do so may result in unacceptable complication rates, disgruntled patients and families, excessive costs, and treatment failures.

The allied health sciences approach provides for a clear delineation preoperatively of patients' responsibilities as well as the evaluation of patients' willingness to accept accountability for their participation in the process so it is as safe as possible medically for the operation and has the best opportunity to allow for achievement of long-term good health and longevity. The critical areas involved include: (1) lifestyle changes; (2) life-long exercise programs, preferably structured; (3) nutritional requirements, including knowledge about daily protein intake; (4) nutritional supplementation; (5) avoidance of aspirin and nonsteroidal antiinflammatory drugs; (6) avoidance of snacking between meals; and (7) willingness to do the necessary follow-up, including visits to the surgeon and participation in support group activities. The necessity of placing greater emphasis on the preconditioning phase of bariatric treatment is becoming increasingly important in engaging patients as team members.

Establishing and making available ongoing support groups provide strong bonds throughout the entire continuum of care. Exposure to the dynamic of support groups touches many phases of patients' recovery from morbid obesity and their concomitant physical, mental, and psychosocial limitations.

Operating Team

The team is most important to the bariatric patient during the operation itself. The surgeon, surgical assistant, scrub, and circulating personnel, along with the anesthesia providers, must offer the synchronized choreography necessary to care for this challenging patient at the most critical phase of his or her long journey toward lifelong weight management.

As discussed, the surgeon is the leader of this highly skilled team. The surgeon must be supported by the preoperative workup, the data collected, the patient's motivation, and the skill and dedication of the surgical team. It is imperative that the team work together from the beginning to bring their coordination, skills, and finesse to bear throughout this complicated procedure. It also requires specialized equipment and supplies.[18]

The capital outlay for this procedure is substantial but provision of these resources ensures a safe environment for the patient and a more efficient and effective surgical procedure. The operating table must be able to accommodate 850 to 1000 lb, with the patient supine and in reverse Trendelenburg position for much of the procedure. In addition to the operating table, instruments must be purchased that are of sufficient length for both the laparoscopic and the open approach. It is helpful to have a self-retaining retractor to provide optimal exposure of the operative field for the open procedure and for instances when laparoscopic procedures must be converted to open procedures. A good video tower for laparoscopic procedures provides adequate light, insufflation, video capability, and visualization of the field.

A dedicated surgical staff is preferable for a procedure of this magnitude. Providing consistent staffing enables a more efficient, smooth, and well-choreographed operation.

Staff members who are able to anticipate the needs of the surgeon and of their coworkers shorten operative time, decrease overall costs, and provide a greater degree of patient safety.

In addition to operating room staff, dedicated operating room block time is preferred for the bariatric service. Providing defined block time creates predictability for the patient, surgeon, and operative staff. In a successful and comprehensive bariatric program, the patient has worked diligently and cleared multiple hurdles in order to proceed with surgery. Delays on the day of surgery should be minimized so that the patient feels supported and comfortable.

Allowing the patient to feel comfortable begins with protecting the patient's dignity in all aspects of care. This is a patient population that has become accustomed to being treated as if they were second-class citizens. Society as a whole still does not view obesity as a disease. There are so many misconceptions about morbid obesity that it is understandable that this group of patients may need frequent communication, feedback, reassurance, and instruction. Simple things at the time of surgery, such as providing hospital gowns large enough to fit, chairs without armrests, scales that accommodate the morbidly obese patient, and wide-width wheelchairs are just a few of the ways in which a patient's dignity is maintained in a facility dedicated to the comprehensive care of the bariatric patient.

Bariatric Coordinator

A comprehensive program is one that incorporates all of the disciplines discussed. Providing a coordinator who monitors a patient's progress throughout the bariatric program not only ensures that the patient progresses appropriately but also ensures that the patient is optimally prepared for both the surgical procedure and the necessary lifestyle changes that follow it. The coordinator must work closely with the surgeon and the rest of the bariatric team. This individual is the touchstone for the bariatric patient and the liaison between the operative team and the patient. The coordinator should have clinical experience and a sincere desire to help this diverse patient population. The value of this role cannot be emphasized strongly enough.

Mental Health Providers

The mental health and behavioral medicine components of the bariatric team are vital elements if the surgical intervention is to produce the desired effects. For the patient undergoing bariatric surgery, where success is measured by short- and long-term results, mental health and behavioral health approaches to the psychological condition of the patient are essential. They rely on a relational approach and effective communication, not only among the professionals of the treatment team, but also with the patient and his or her support system.

Nutritionists

Both the original 1991 National Institutes of Health Consensus Statement on Gastrointestinal Surgery for Severe Obesity[28] and the 2004 American Society for Bariatric Surgery Consensus Conference Statement on Bariatric Surgery for Morbid Obesity,[29] stress the need for a multidisciplinary team approach to determining candidacy for undergoing weight loss surgery. A valuable member of this team is a nutritionist or registered dietitian who specializes in weight-loss surgery. A preoperative nutritional assessment is a way to determine whether the patient will be able to comply with the postoperative diet and the precise vitamin and mineral supplementation needed.

The function of the nutritionist goes far beyond preoperative approval. The responsibility extends into long-term care of the patient. This includes educating, counseling, encouraging, and supporting the patient throughout the surgical weight-loss experience. Helping patients to understand why surgery requires a change in their eating behaviors and motivating them to make these changes is vital to their success with the surgery. Careful explanation needs to be addressed to the concept that weight loss surgery is only a tool that will aid them in losing weight. The nutritionist's role is to explain that they will have to follow specific nutritional guidelines, exercise, and take the vitamin and minerals that are recommended if they are to lose weight and remain healthy.

Exercise Physiology

A main focus of the multidisciplinary bariatric team is to give physical and emotional support to all patients, as well as making them aware of the important changes that will affect their lives after surgery. Physical activity provides many benefits for bariatric patients, including improvement in their cardiorespiratory systems, strength levels, muscular endurance, and flexibility.

Physical activity is essential to obese individuals, and it must be done under supervision. These individuals commonly lead sedentary lifestyles; they are not used to and, in some instances, not capable of the least strenuous physical activity. Starting a fitness program without any orientation is likely to cause physical injuries and result in more harm than benefit. It is essential to provide some physical activities that patients are capable of performing, after proper evaluation that takes into account the physical and anthropometric characteristics of the specific patients. Ideally, exercise is started preoperatively, is maintained perioperatively, and becomes an essential element of postoperative management.

Support Groups

Support groups offer circumstances wherein patients may share ideas and tips about healthful eating choices and exercise while experiencing the comfort of being able to express their hopes and fears and interact socially without feeling judged because of their obesity. There is a common bond and understanding that intertwines people who have faced years of prejudice by society. Emotionally and physically, many severely obese people have isolated themselves in attempts to avoid being hurt and humiliated.

Many patients who have had surgery to achieve weight loss find themselves conflicted about their new body image and life changes. Following surgery, excessive eating is no longer an option as a means of achieving emotional comfort. It is during this time that support groups are particularly beneficial to patients. These groups allow patients to interact with other patients who have shared similar life experiences and can provide peer-based, nonclinical encouragement and motivation. Patients describe support groups as situations in which they feel accepted and as though they belong. Studies show that patients who attended support group meetings regularly tended to lose more weight than those who did not. In group meetings patients can communicate with and gather knowledge from patients in all postoperative stages. It is an opportunity for the program to reinforce principles, lifestyle changes, and commitment to a new way of life.

▶ TEAMWORK IN BARIATRIC OUTCOMES MANAGEMENT

With the dramatic increase in the frequency with which bariatric surgery has been performed in recent years there has been a subsequent demand for a greater amount of timely, high-quality data concerning the clinical outcomes of these procedures. Regulatory, contractual, and financial influences as well as public demand can influence the amount of data that must be collected by a bariatric program. Information systems have been impacted by expectations that data from bariatric programs are unique and can provide information that has been unknown until now. These data must be collected from disparate information systems, and that requires teamwork and coordination among the multiple entities that possess the data.

The high surgical and anesthetic risk levels involved in bariatric surgery have an impact on the amount and unique quality of the data that must be collected to answer the complex questions surrounding the clinical outcomes of bariatric patients. Furthermore, the number of operations and the variety of surgical techniques have increased at a pace that challenges the ability of any information system to capture correct data.

Teamwork is strongly involved at the information systems level because there is demand for various skills that one person alone may not possess. For example, a technical information systems person may be able to build the system for data capture but may not have enough clinical knowledge to understand which data are needed to answer clinical-outcomes questions. Technical and clinical personnel have to work as a team to determine the best and most efficient ways of capturing the data needed to support a successful, highly visible, and heavily data-rich bariatric program.

There must be sufficient institutional support and motivation within the hospital setting to make data capture, collection, and analysis a priority. It is especially important to provide clear definitions of priorities to all personnel involved in producing data when contractual relationships with outside hospitals or health management organization are involved. Some bariatric data are not easily captured by existing systems, such as when a procedure is converted from a laparoscopic to an open-access technique or when a patient is returned to the operating room for management of a complication. These data may not be available until the existing information systems are altered and the human processes are redesigned to best capture that information.

▶ SUMMARY

The multidisciplinary bariatric team is characterized by the long-term synergistic efforts of specialized allied health providers. Their mission is to prepare comprehensively the morbidly obese patient for life-long lifestyle changes that begin well before the day of surgery; to optimize short- and long-term postoperative success; to realize the greatest safety for patients; and to meticulously record outcomes data to pave the way for ongoing improvements in bariatric surgery.

▶ REFERENCES

1. Peskin GW: Obesity in America. Arch Surg 2003;138:354-355.
2. Klein S, Wadden T, Sugerman H: American Gastroenterological Association (AGA) technical review on obesity. AGA J 2002;123:883-932.
3. Flegal KM, Carroll MD, Ogden CL, et al: Prevalence and trends in obesity among US adults, 1999-2000. JAMA 2002;288:1723-1727.
4. Damcott CM, Sack P, Shuldiner AR: The genetics of obesity. Endocrinol Metab Clin North Am 2003;32:761-786.
5. Zimmerman RL: The obesity epidemic in America. Clin Fam Pract 2005;4:229-247.
6. World Health Organization: Obesity: preventing and managing the global epidemic. WHO Technical Report Series 2000. 894. Geneva. http://whqlibdoc.who.int/trs/WHO_TRS_894.pdf. Accessed June 1, 2006.
7. Clark GW, Wittgrove AC: Laparoscopic Roux-en-Y gastric bypass. Surg Laparosc Endosc 1998;8:406-407.
8. Steinbrook R: Perspective: surgery for severe obesity. N Engl J Med 2004;350:1075-1079.
9. Buchwald H: Bariatric surgery for morbid obesity: health implications for patients, health professionals, and third-party payers. J Am Coll Surg 2005;200:593-604.
10. Schauer PR, Ikramuddin S, Ramanathan R: Outcomes after laparoscopic Roux-en-Y gastric bypass for morbid obesity. Ann Surg 2000;232:515-529.
11. Buchwald H, Avidor Y, Pories W, et al: Bariatric surgery: a systematic review and meta-analysis. JAMA 2004;292:1724-1737.
12. Christou N, Sampalis JS, Liberman M, et al: Surgery decreases long-term mortality, morbidity, and health care use in morbidly obese patients. Ann Surg 2004;240:416-424.
13. Finch J: Interprofessional education and teamworking: a view from the education providers. BMJ 2000;321:1138-1140.
14. Saltzman E, Anderson W, Apovian C, et al: Criteria for patient selection and multidisciplinary evaluation and treatment of the weight loss surgery patient. Obes Res 2005;13:234-243.
15. National Institutes of Health: Consensus Development Conference on Surgical Treatment of Morbid Obesity. Dec 4-5, 1978: Bethesda, Md.
16. National Institutes of Health: Health implications of obesity. NIH Consensus Development Conference Statement 1985;5.
17. National Institutes of Health: Gastrointestinal surgery for severe obesity. NIH Consensus Development Conference. March 25-27, 1991; Bethesda.
18. American Society for Bariatric Surgery: Guidelines for Surgery. www.asbs.org. Accessed June 2, 2005.
19. American College of Surgeons: Recommendations for facilities performing bariatric surgery: Bull Am Coll Surg 2000;85.
20. American Society for Bariatric Surgery/Society of American Gastrointestinal and Endoscopic Surgeons: Guidelines 2000. www.asbs.org/html/lab_guidelines.htm. Accessed June 1, 2006.
21. The Society of American Gastrointestinal and Endoscopic Surgeons: www.sages.org/sagespublication.php?doc=30. Accessed, 2005.

22. Henneman EA, Lee JL, Cohen JL: Collaboration: a concept analysis. J Adv Nurs 1995;21;103-109.
23. Chaney JM: Implementing team approaches in primary and tertiary care settings: applications from the rehabilitation context. Fam Syst Health 1999;17:413-426.
24. Mason EE, Hesson W: Informed consent for obesity surgery. Obes Surg 1998;8:419-428.
25. Surgical Review Committee: www.src.org. Accessed, May 25, 2006.
26. American College of Surgeons: Bariatric Surgery Center Network Accreditation Program. www.facs.org. Accessed May 20, 2005.
27. National Institute of Diabetes and Digestive and Kidney Diseases (NIDDK) Bariatric Surgery Clinical Research Consortium: Request for Applications. www.grants.nih.gov/grants/guide/rfa-files/RFA-DK-03-006.hrml. Accessed November 1, 2002.
28. National Institutes of Health: Gastrointestinal Surgery for Severe Obesity, NIH Consensus Statement. NIH 1991;9:1-20.
29. Buchwald H, Consensus Conference Statement: Bariatric surgery for morbid obesity: health implications for patients, health professionals, and third-party payers. J Am Coll Surg 2005;200:593-604.

53

Requisite Facilities
for Bariatric Surgical Practice

John J. Gleysteen, M.D.

The initial coinage of the term *morbid obesity* in the mid-1960s was prompted by the need for a unique description of persons suitable for the "new" weight-reducing jejunoileal bypass surgery, an operation first performed in the early 1950s. Originally the term referred to persons who were more than 100 lb over their calculated insurance-table "ideal weight,"[1] or twice the normal weight predicted for the individual age, sex, body build, and height.[2] Even later, to distinguish the extremely obese from those who were marginally qualified for inclusion, the terms *super-obesity* and *super superobesity* were coined. The yardstick of measurement changed to body mass index in kg per m[2]. The population numbers have grown since surgical attention was directed toward obesity, and in the United States the prevalence of class 3 obesity (a body mass index above 40) has increased from 1% in the 1960s to over 3% currently.[3] Some U.S. population groups have percentages as high as 6%.

Today, bariatric surgery is the treatment of choice for morbid obesity. The successful conduct of this specialized surgery is dependent on surgeons well trained in this field, a multidisciplinary team approach, a dedicated in-hospital and outpatient environment, and the facilities appropriate to a bariatric practice. In this chapter, we review the specifics of these requisite facilities.[4]

▶ OFFICE FACILITIES

Introduction of the patient to the surgical team must occur in the office or clinic setting, whether the practice is a private-independent or an academic university-affiliated group. In addition to having the necessary technical expertise in gastrointestinal and biliary surgery, bariatric surgeons need to look upon morbid obesity as a disease, and they must also have an intimate knowledge of the numerous conditions and illnesses induced or aggravated by morbid obesity. The American Society for Bariatric Surgery Executive Committee has developed guidelines for credentialing surgeons in the field.[5] The office practice

is dependent on the dedicated bariatric surgery team, which includes the receptionist, the administrator, the nursing personnel, the dietitian, and others, each of whom must have a certain fund of knowledge about obesity and bariatric surgery.[6]

The physical aspects of the office or clinic require special consideration to make them suitable for large patients. Obese people are sensitive to their accommodations and will criticize or avoid situations in which they feel uncomfortable or derided by others. Some chairs should have no arms, and all chairs and sofas should be firm and high enough to ensure that heavy patients can arise from them easily. There should be at least 6 to 8 inches between each chair or sofa.[7] A few extrawide wheelchairs should be available for patients with limited mobility. Thus, the waiting area must be large enough to accommodate this furniture without crowding and yet with allowance for a sufficient number of people to attend at any one time. Clinic doors and hallways may have to be wider than usual (about 40 inches) to accommodate wheelchairs and scooters.[7]

The examination rooms must be spacious and must have tables that are wide enough for the patients and are bolted to the floor or wall so that they do not tip forward when patients sit on the edges of the tables. Other accessories in the room should include sturdy step stools, wide blood pressure cuffs, and superlarge examining gowns.

Obviously, weight and height measurements must be made, but there is no need to place a scale in each examination room. The scale does need to be conveniently and privately positioned, away from the presence of other patients and staff; and weight should be silently recorded, free of any commentary.[7] The scale should be counter-balanced, digital (ideally), and have a capacity as high as 1000 lb.

Visual aids should be available for patient education. They can include a television monitor with sound and a VCR and DVD player. Appropriate tapes or CDs made commercially or recorded by office staff expedite the education of patients and make the time spent during preoperative visits useful. The visual aids may focus on dietary instructions or show reports of patients' experiences during postoperative visits.

HOSPITAL FACILITIES

The team concept is just as important in the hospital setting as it is in the private office. The participants on the hospital team are more numerous and include the surgeons and their assistants; nursing staff, in and outside of the operating room; dietitians; clerical personnel; specialty consultants; and the anesthesia staff. To perform anesthesia adequately and safely in the morbidly obese, not only are special skills required, but special equipment may be necessary too.[8] For patients who are preoperatively disabled or encounter postoperative difficulties, medical specialists in nutrition and endocrine management, rehabilitation, and physical therapy may be asked to play a brief but intensive role.

Operating Room

The operating room and its equipment must be prepared for bariatric surgery. Both patient size and the required equipment demand a large room, although size requirements are not specific. The operating table (various brands are available) must accommodate weights above 800 lb and must have extendable side pieces for use in occasional cases of girth peculiarities.[9] Generally, the standard-sized table (75 × 20 in) with heavier weight capacity is suitable and is preferred by the surgeons and assistants who stand around it. The extraheavy (>500 lb) patients may be able to help themselves to transfer from gurney to operating room table before the operation, but they can be of no assistance afterwards. The task of moving patients off the table in those cases cannot be left to aides with strong arms and backs. An air mattress-type of transfer system (e.g., Hovermatt, HoverTech International, Bethlehem, Pa.) can be helpful in facilitating the transfer of patients from operating room table to gurney or, preferably, directly onto a patient bed.[9]

Surgical equipment in the bariatric operating room may not be different from that in other rooms in which gastrointestinal and laparoscopic general surgery is conducted. However, instrument packs, for both open and laparoscopic procedures, must include several items on the side that are extralong, so they can be available when needed for use in some patients. In particular, laparoscopic trocars must to be long enough so that an approximately equal length can be inside and outside of the abdominal wall; this allows the instruments traversing it to be maneuverable with technical precision. Failure to have long enough trocars on hand is one well-recognized cause for conversion from laparoscopic to open gastric bypass.[10]

Morbidly obese patients who are sent from recovery areas to patient rooms should arrive on or be transferred onto beds that maximize their comfort and accommodate their weight. Bari-beds are available as heavy-duty, extrawide (for 350 to 600 lb), and extraheavy-duty (for >600 lb). These beds are generally wider and have better mattresses

and stronger spring assemblies that increase their weight tolerance. A 500-lb patient who spends 4 days in a regular hospital bed after surgery may break the bed. The wider bariatric bed has to be able to roll along hallways and through doors that are sufficiently wide and also must fit into elevators that are wide enough. The big-enough hospital room should, preferably, be a single room for accommodation reasons. Attention must be given to the toilet facilities, which commonly are suspended from the bathroom wall. Massive weight may detach the toilet suddenly; a portable commode with a 750-lb capacity provides a safe alternative.

The same requirements apply as in the office setting: on-floor scales and gurneys with nearly 1000-lb capacities, extrawide wheelchairs, and wide blood pressure cuffs must be readily available. For deep vein thrombosis prophylaxis during and after operation, pneumatic compression devices must make allowance for extrathick legs; some companies such as Venodyne (Microtek Medical Holdings, Alpharetta, Ga.) have extralarge or bariatric sleeves to fit large legs. These are items that should be purchased, not rented.

Support Facilities

Other items of special equipment for the management of obese patients merit comment. Especially with any volume of bariatric patients in the hospital, the radiology department should have at least one general table that can hold and position patients up to 750 lb, especially for gastrointestinal contrast studies.[9] Most computed tomography scanners have upper limits of about 350 lb, but extralarge-capacity scanners are available; a hospital with an active bariatric program should invest in one or have access to one.

Intensive care units often are compartmentalized into small patient rooms with a central nursing access point; one room should be prepared or enlarged to accommodate the occasional critically ill postoperative obese patient in a large bariatric bed, along with requisite patient care equipment.

The dietary department should review the facilities, especially with respect to menu selections appropriate for postoperative patients. It should be able to provide liquid diets free of sugar and diets of exceedingly soft substances. Registered dietician consultants must be available to the patient before discharge.

CENTERS OF EXCELLENCE

It may seem to be a short leap from having an active hospital bariatric surgical program to being a center of excellence, but it is an important step and is certainly the path advocated by the American Society for Bariatric Surgery.[11] The establishment of a center of excellence involves expansion of the support facilities in the hospital and in the clinic or office. Expansions may occur in the management of nutrition and dietary requirements, in the handling of diabetes and metabolic diseases, in the arena of physical medicine and rehabilitation, and also in hospital public relations and the development of informatics.

Hospitals with high volume and active bariatric surgical programs, whether academic or private, begin to attract patients who are at higher risk and so are more costly. All hospitals confront varied demands by managed care programs and must pay close attention to costs, even while sponsoring lucrative clinical practices. Designed to avoid cost variations and reduce unnecessary costs in hospitals, by surgeons, and in surgical training programs in many surgical arenas, the use of *clinical pathways* has emerged as a way of organizing care pragmatically.[12] The pathways are written so that what is necessary is defined, and extravagances and variations that are not cost-effective are avoided. They standardize patient care, which improves quality while reducing cost. They may well be considered a requisite element in the improvement of bariatric surgical care.

A clinical pathway was proposed in 1999 at the University of California, Los Angeles, to manage bariatric surgery.[12] It involved a format for preoperative preparation, perioperative care, and a 3-day postoperative stay. A committee of attending surgeons, nurses, intensive care physicians, nutritionists, quality-assurance specialists, and administrators wrote it. Compared to the data for patients managed the year before its implementation, it reduced the average length of stay by a day, the length of stay in the intensive care unit by 0.3 day, and average hospital costs per admission by 40%; it even reduced the readmission rate from 4.2% to 3.2%.[12] Operative morbidity rates were unaffected. The mundane task of writing postoperative orders was facilitated by standardized forms, and the forms were believed to reduce the risk for errors in patient management. The expenses avoided by using such a pathway intensify the appeal for any hospital management administration of incorporating a support-encompassing specialized program and of maintaining a center of excellence in bariatric surgery.

The additional personnel found in a center-of-excellence hospital would include a medical director who represents bariatric surgery and who has a vote in the relevant administrative decisions concerning the institution.[11] Consultative personnel, who may have a small presence in a hospital affiliated with a bariatric program, may become more important and integral to maintaining the levels required of a center of excellence. This expansion might be found in the pulmonary and critical care areas, in the nutrition and metabolic disorders sections, and in rehabilitation; all of these areas focus on the complete care of patients during the pre- and postoperative periods and on the detection of difficulties and their correction in order to enhance the quality of life of the patients.

The establishment of patient support groups sponsored by the hospital is another characteristic of the concept of centers of excellence. This support should be integrated with the support efforts of an aligned surgical practice. The hospital usually supplies the meeting area and is also the resource for the nonsurgical personnel who participate in support group meetings: nutritionists, exercise physiatrists and therapists, and psychologists. Through its medical illustration and media services, the hospital may be the resource for informational brochures, interview-film creation, operation-film editing, and other educational videos useful for patient support.

Through the hospital's public relations and informatics departments, the creation and programming of a bariatric Web site may be combined with patient support efforts. It can be closely aligned with the hospital support group and can be a resource for referring physicians that can educate them regarding patient and surgical criteria and chronic postoperative care issues and to acquaint them with available bariatric surgeons.

A popular component of a patient-support Web site is a chat room. This takes additional Web organization, but it can allow local patients to get to know each other and can indirectly popularize the support group by publicizing the meeting schedules and enhancing attendance at the meetings. The ready availability of information can reduce the time support staff spends answering repetitive questions, thus improving staff efficiency.[6] There are national examples of such Web sites that have features that can be copied locally, but a local site does more than a national program to enhance and popularize the center-of-excellence hospital and its physicians. Patients tend to be supportive of each other and to share information regarding types of foods that can be tolerated and where to get clothes as they lose weight. Communication among pre- and postoperative patients can enable those who will soon undergo surgery to be comforted and to better understand what their experiences will be like.[9]

▶ CONCLUSION

The requisite facilities and equipment of a bariatric surgery program or center of excellence are those that make the surgical program competent, efficient, and competitive. In turn, these are the attributes that translate into the provision of competent and compassionate care for the bariatric patient. Perhaps the inscription on the lamp outside Albert Schweitzer's jungle hospital at Lambarene might be a fitting final annotation for the bariatric surgery facility: "Here, at whatever hour you come, you will find light and help and human kindness."[13]

▶ REFERENCES

1. Payne JH, DeWind LT: Surgical treatment of obesity. Am J Surg 1969;118:141-145.
2. Scott HW, Sandstead HA, Brill AB, et al: Experience with a new technique of intestinal bypass in the treatment of morbid obesity. Am J Surg 1971;174:560-565.
3. Freedman DS, Khan LK, Serdula MK, et al: Trends and correlates of class 3 obesity in the United States from 1990 to 2000. JAMA 2002; 288:1758-1761.
4. Recommendations for facilities performing bariatric surgery. Bull Am Coll Surgs 2000;85:20-23.
5. American Society for Bariatric Surgery: Guidelines for granting privileges in bariatric surgery. Obes Surg 2003;13:238-239.
6. Schirmer B: Operative principles: setting up a bariatric program. SAGES Postgraduate Course Syllabus 2001;13-17.
7. National Association to Advance Fat Acceptance: Guidelines for healthcare providers in dealing with fat clients. www.naafa.org/ documents/brochures/healthguides. Accessed November, 2003.

8. Boyce JR, Ness T, Castroman P, et al: Preliminary study of the optimal anesthesia positioning for the morbidly obese patient. Obes Surg 2003;13:4-9.

9. Livingston E: So you think you want to add bariatric surgery to your practice: what do you need? American College of Surgeons Postgraduate Course Syllabus 2002; October, 2002.

10. Wittgrove AC, Clark GW: Laparoscopic gastric bypass, Roux-en-Y: 500 patients: technique and results, with a 3-60 month follow-up. Obes Surg 2000;10:233-239.

11. American Society for Bariatric Surgery: Bariatric centers of excellence. Obes Surg 2003;13:240.

12. Huerta S, Heber D, Sawicki MP, et al: Reduced length of stay by implementation of a clinical pathway for bariatric surgery in an academic health care center. Am Surg 2001;67:1128-1135.

13. Brailler JM (ed): Medical Wit and Wisdom, p. 222. Philadelphia, Running Press, 1993.

54

Laparoscopic Suites and Robotics in Bariatric Surgery

Matthew E. Newlin, M.D. and W. Scott Melvin, M.D.

As surgery finally enters the computer age, the 20th century concept of the operating room is being replaced by a setting that provides better instrumentation, communication, ergonomics, efficiency, and information management. For more than 100 years, the operating theater consisted of a single room equipped with a table that had limited mobility, a strong overhead light, and mechanical tools manipulated by the surgeon's hands under direct vision. This arrangement has served the surgical community very well for almost every type of open surgery. With the advent of better lenses, better light delivery, and fiberoptic technology, minimally invasive surgery flourished. At the end of the 20th century, these changes joined with the emergence of computers to transform the operating room's capabilities. As the 21st century begins, advanced digital, optical, and computer technologies have created and will continue to create operating rooms and surgical devices that can better serve the surgeon, the hospital, and the patient.

▶ ESSENTIALS OF THE LAPAROSCOPIC SUITE

The laparoscopic suite must combine various factors to provide an environment in which the surgeon can interact with the surgical instruments, the nurses, and the technology to provide safe, efficient, and comfortable care for the morbidly obese patient. The ideal laparoscopic suite and its advantages are described herein.

General Configuration

The operating room designed for laparoscopic surgery, and specifically bariatric surgery, should be large enough to accommodate the necessary equipment as well as the operating room personnel and a large and heavy patient. Minimum clear working space in the room should be at least 20 × 20 ft. Ideally, the room should measure closer to 25 × 25 ft so as to accommodate all of the equipment and to allow for adequate working space. The doorways to the operating room must be extra wide to allow for passage of

extra large hospital beds. The operating table must be large and capable of supporting patients in excess of 500 lb. The table should be highly adjustable (in order to allow changes in position) as well as radiolucent (to allow for intraoperative radiographs). Ceiling-based arms or columns should be strategically placed to support cameras, monitors, insufflation lines, and other equipment.

Two camera systems should be available. The second camera or video input serves as a backup system and may also be used if two intraoperative images are needed. For example, if an intraoperative endoscopy is performed during a laparoscopic procedure, it can be displayed on some of the operating room monitors. With digital capabilities, the modern operating room can accommodate rapid transmission of live images as well as the display of the patient's medical records, radiographic images, or other previously performed procedures such as endoscopy. This allows the surgeon to utilize this information quickly, in a real-time fashion, so as to better tailor the surgical procedure.

Ultrasound and fluoroscopy inputs can be built in to the room's systems. The monitors should be flat and digital and should articulate freely to provide the viewing of a sharp image in an ergonomically advantageous position. Insufflation gas is hard-wired from the hospital gas lines through the suspended arms to provide a continuously available flow of gas. Equipment, such as at least one insufflator, light source, electrosurgical unit, and harmonic scalpel power module, rests on one of the suspended arms and can be moved freely into various positions. This general operating room configuration allows for a highly adaptable environment where laparoscopic surgery and bariatric procedures can be performed efficiently (Fig. 54-1).

Instrumentation

Bariatric surgery patients require modified laparoscopic instrumentation. Because of their large size, these patients may require extra long graspers, staplers, and laparoscopes. The supply rooms that house these instruments as well as

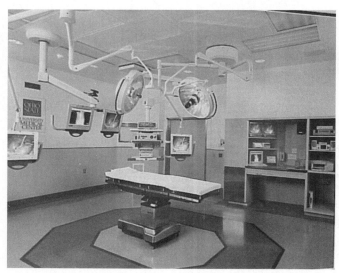

Figure 54-1. The modern laparoscopic suite features suspended equipment, voice-activated functions, and digital communication systems.

the stapler cartridges and other essential equipment should be located very close to the operating room.

Communication

One of the greatest advantages of the modern laparoscopic suite lies in its ability to enhance communication. Voice-activated wireless computer control allows the surgeon to adjust, set up, and perform many tasks common to laparoscopic surgery. For example, the surgeon, using a headset that is linked to a voice-activated computer, can tilt or rotate the operating table, adjust the lights, white-balance the camera, or place a telephone call. Luketich and others showed that such a system eliminated an average of 15 physician-directed nursing commands per case and significantly improved the satisfaction of the operating room personnel.[1]

Because of the number and quality of the monitors in the operating room, all operating room staff can more easily observe what is transpiring within the abdomen. This may allow those in a supportive role better to anticipate what the surgeon may require next and improve response times to the surgeon's needs.

Teaching

Closely related to communication, the teaching capabilities of the surgeon improve in a laparoscopic suite. Not only can the student, resident, or visiting surgeon more easily observe a surgical case, but also the digital nature of the image can be transmitted to remote locations. Images, live or delayed, can be transmitted to a conference room via a closed circuit or across the world with the use of high-capacity Internet or satellite links.

This ability to provide instantaneous communication presents the opportunity for what has become known as telementoring. In telementoring, the surgeon can demonstrate a particular procedure to a number of other surgeons who are trying to learn new skills. Alternatively, the

mentoring surgeon can observe another surgeon who may be performing a procedure for which he or she needs guidance or verbal advice. The ethical and medicolegal ramifications of telementoring have not been completely determined. Is the mentor liable for the opinions expressed? Should the mentor be participating in the care of a patient he or she has never met or examined? Are those who are being taught adequately educated by observing from a remote site? These questions remain unanswered.

Ergonomics and Efficiency

The traditional operating room, when poorly adapted to minimally invasive surgery, creates many ergonomic problems. Cables, pedals, and tubing rest on the floor where they can interfere with walking and the movement of carts. Cables can become frayed by the passage of wheeled carts. Large and heavy carts occupy valuable floor space and may compromise access to the patient, especially in the case of an emergency. Breaks in sterility can occur when controls for some of this equipment rest too close to the surgical field and require manipulation by nursing staff.

The surgeon's ability to concentrate on the task at hand improves with better ergonomics. Surgeon fatigue has been shown to increase when monitors do not rest in the direct sight line of the surgeon or operating personnel.[2] Suspended, mobile, small-profile monitors allow well-placed, unobstructed views of the operative field.

The modern laparoscopic suite should strive to improve the ergonomics and maximize the efficiency of the operating team and the facility. The use of a voice-activated computerized operating room can result in a shorter average length of time for each procedure.[3] Hard-wired gas insufflation lines rather than portable gas tanks that require moving and frequent replacement help to avoid operating room delays and interruptions in surgical procedures. By avoiding bulky and heavy carts laden with video and insufflation equipment, and instead utilizing suspended equipment, the facility's room turnover becomes easier and faster. Video setup times and put-away times can be reduced significantly with the use of a laparoscopic suite, and this may translate into an associated cost savings.[4]

Information Management

In an era of digital images, electronic collection of data, and broadband transmission of this information, the modern operating room lends itself well to producing educational videos and photos, easily accumulating data during surgical procedures, and providing live demonstrations that can be used in telementoring. However, privacy becomes a major concern. The Health Insurance Portability and Accountability Act of 1996 establishes national standards for electronic health care transactions and also addresses the security and privacy of health data.[5] Steps must be taken by the facility and the surgeons to protect patients' privacy while taking advantage of the modern operating room's ability to record and share data.

The digital nature of information input also allows prompt and efficient documentation of surgical procedures. Information can be captured via voice-directed programs that create sound or video clips. More commonly, the information management system uses a software application with standard menu items, including photo documentation, to allow for quick and easy integration of details of the procedure to form standard reports of routine procedures. These systems are also sophisticated enough to allow real-time production of billing data and notification to referring doctors. Most of these systems can be located directly in or adjacent to the operating or procedure room.

As these management systems become further developed and mature, they can be integrated into the operating room supply system, documenting the equipment used and monitoring the inventory in ordering systems. The goal of seamless and integrated multidisciplinary information flow is elusive and ever changing, but great strides are being made.

Summary

Minimally invasive surgery, whether utilized for gastrointestinal surgery or elsewhere in the abdomen or body in general, introduces a new set of requirements and issues when compared with traditional open surgery. If surgeons, hospitals, and surgical centers are to adapt to these issues, they must embrace the new technologies of infrastructure. In some manner, the modern laparoscopic operating room must incorporate the elements discussed in order to achieve an efficient and ergonomic environment that is both safe and cost-effective, thereby optimizing the care of the bariatric surgery patient.

▶ ROBOTICS

Robots have progressed from the pages of science fiction books to become an integral part of many manufacturing industries. As computers have become more powerful and smaller, robots are being used to improve safety, precision, and the results of many tasks, especially those that involve a high degree of repetitiveness. The concept of a robot in the surgical suite may frighten many people. Robots engender an image of an autonomous machine performing preprogrammed tasks without direct human control. The dictionary broadly defines a robot as a device that automatically performs complicated and often repetitive tasks, or as a mechanism guided by automatic controls.[6] In this regard, the devices used in the operating room are not robots because they still remain under the direct control of the surgeon and they do not perform preprogrammed maneuvers automatically. For this reason, the field may be better served if the term *robot* were replaced by the more precise term *computer-enhanced telemanipulator device*. However, the term *robot* will most likely remain the more widely accepted term, and for the purposes of this chapter, the term *robot* will be used.

Surgery using robots is, in reality, telerobotic surgery. This implies that a surgeon can perform surgery in a patient from a remote location. This location may be the other side of the operating room or, with the use of high-speed data transmission, the other side of the world.[7,8] The possibility of remote-site surgery has spawned two more terms: *telementoring* (previously discussed) and *telepresence*.

Telepresence utilizes the telerobot from an off-site location to perform surgery without the surgeon's being present with the patient. Although still a medicolegal and ethical question, telepresence surgery may become feasible in battlefield surgery where a surgeon behind the front lines can perform surgery in a wounded soldier on the battlefield.

The Food and Drug Administration has approved several robotic systems for use in the United States in intraabdominal surgery. These systems, regardless of their manufacturers, share several features: (1) a remote surgeon's console where a three-dimensional image is viewed, and the surgeon manipulates levers, pedals, or instruments to control the robot's arms (Fig. 54-2); (2) a surgical cart where the arms of the robot interface with the patient in a sterile manner; and (3) a control tower housing light sources as well as computer equipment that combines the stereoscopic video image into a three-dimensional image that is seen by the surgeon at the console. These traits combine to form a central control platform that allows the surgeon to maintain control of the operating instruments while utilizing the advantages provided by the system (Fig. 54-3).

It is important to note that the surgeon and robot work in a master-slave relationship. The surgeon's commands are translated into movements of the robot's working instruments. The surgeon sits at the console, physically separated from the patient. The surgeon may require an assistant, in sterile surgical garb, to pass equipment such as suture or a Penrose drain into the abdominal cavity through an accessory port (Fig. 54-4).

Telerobotic surgery changes the direct doctor-patient contact and allows computer enhancement of the surgeon's activities. This enhancement includes elimination of any tremor, wrist movement of the robotic arms with six degrees of freedom plus grasp, motion scaling, and imaging using a stereoscopic view. The surgeon, using the

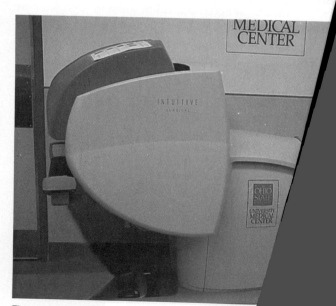

Figure 54-2. The robotic console is a movable unit [...] sits to control the robotic arms.

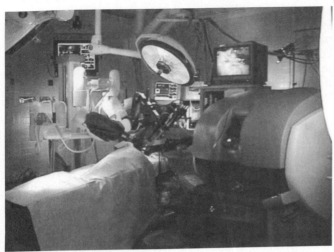

Figure 54-3. The robotic system is positioned over the operating room table.

robot, can perform complex surgical maneuvers that may be more difficult using standard laparoscopic techniques, which limit range of motion of the surgical instrument to four degrees of freedom plus grasp. The robot provides more degrees of freedom because of its ability to articulate the instruments in a wrist-like manner that is unavailable with standard laparoscopic instruments.

raabdominal Applications

ot-assisted surgery devices have received approval
e Food and Drug Administration and have been used
numerous intraabdominal procedures. Robot assis-
cholecystectomy, esophagectomy, fundoplication,
yotomy, pyloroplasty, splenectomy, pancreatec-
colectomy have all been described.[9,10] Cadiere
es reported a series of 146 cases from a single
Marescaux and colleagues[7] described a series
s undergoing robot-assisted laparoscopic
y and found that results and operative

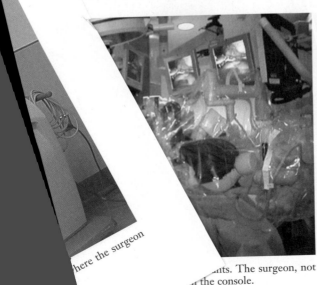

here the surgeon

nts. The surgeon, not
the console.

times were similar to laparoscopic cases. Robot-assisted laparoscopic Nissen fundoplication was also studied and found to result in similar perioperative courses and outcomes, albeit with a longer operating time than that required by the laparoscopic technique.[13] Robotic assistance, especially when used in a small operative field and in areas where movement and vision would otherwise be limited, seems to add value when magnification of the field and precision movements are essential. For example, during a Heller myotomy or antireflux surgery, the esophageal hiatus and fibers of the esophagus can be viewed clearly so esophageal injury can be avoided and, if committed, can be recognized and repaired more easily than when standard laparoscopic techniques are used.[11,14]

It has been suggested that robot-assisted laparoscopic surgery works best in small, confined spaces.[11] Thus, the limited dissection around the gastroesophageal junction necessary for the performance of a laparoscopic adjustable gastric band placement lends itself well to the use of the robot. Indeed, robot-assisted laparoscopic gastric banding has been described.[15] However, changing the field of view during a procedure from the gastroesophageal junction to the ligament of Treitz, as may be required during a Roux-en-Y gastric bypass, would require the removal of the robotic arms from the patient, movement of the robotic cart, and reinsertion of the arms in a more appropriate location or orientation. This introduces a time delay, as well as safety issues.

Despite these drawbacks, the performance of Roux-en-Y gastric bypass using telerobotic devices has been reported. Various techniques have been described for these procedures. Horgan's group described completion of the gastrojejunostomy utilizing a sutured anastomosis under computer-assisted control.[16] The initial steps of the operation were undertaken using standard laparoscopic instrumentation, and the robot was applied for the gastro-jejunostomy anastomosis. This portion of the operation requires precise suturing in a very confined environment.

An alternative approach has been described in which both the gastrojejunostomy and the enteroenterostomy are completed using robotic assistance. After completion of a sutured jejunojejunostomy, the operating room table and patient are repositioned in relation to the robot. Sudan describes the technique of duodenal switch in which the proximal anastomosis is performed with the aid of the robot (personal communication; Sudan R, Creighton University, July 2003).

Despite having been applied safely to bariatric surgery, robotic-assisted bariatric surgery has not been compared to standard laparoscopic or open bariatric surgery in a prospective, randomized manner. The excellent results and efficient operating room times reported by many open and laparoscopic centers set high standards for quality that current robotic devices may not be able to improve upon significantly.

Future Directions

The use of robotics in bariatric surgery will continue to mature. Robotic devices will include a broad spectrum of devices and procedures that will increase the safety and efficacy of current procedures. With proper sensing and programming, it is conceivable that independent preprogrammable devices could be assembled after insertion through natural orifices to complete the predefined surgical intervention. Although these kinds of procedures and structures are not soon to be realized, progress will continue toward integrating advanced technology into bariatric surgery.

▶ REFERENCES

1. Luketich JD, Fernando HC, Buenaventura PO, et al: Results of a randomized trial of HERMESTM-assisted versus non-HERMESTM-assisted for laparoscopic anti-reflux surgery. Surg Endosc 2002;16: 1264-1266.
2. Berguer R, Rab GT, Abu-Ghaida H, et al: A comparison of surgeon's postures during laparoscopic and open surgical procedures. Surg Endosc 1997;11:139-142.
3. Kaeding C: Study shows efficiency of computerized operating rooms. Ohio State University Release, Aug 12, 2002.
4. Kenyon TAG, Urbach DR, Speer B, et al: Dedicated minimally invasive surgery suites increase operating room efficiency. Surg Endosc 2001;15:1140-1143.
5. Health Insurance Portability and Accountability Act: www.cms.hhs.gov/hipaa. Accessed July 19, 2003.
6. Merriam-Webster: www.m-w.com. Accessed July 20, 2003.
7. Marescaux J, Leroy J, Rubino F, et al: Transatlantic robot-assisted telesurgery: feasibility and potential applications. Ann Surg 2002; 235:487-492.
8. Larkin M: Transatlantic, robot-assisted telesurgery deemed a success. Lancet 2001;358:1074.
9. Melvin WS, Needleman BJ, Krause KR, et al: Computer-enhanced "robotic" telesurgery: initial experience in foregut surgery. Surg Endosc 2002;16:1790-1792.
10. Talamini M, Campbell K, Stanfield C: Robotic Gastrointestinal surgery: early experience and system description. J Laparoendosc Adv Surg Tech 2002;12:225-232.
11. Cadiere GB, Himpens J, Germay O, et al: Feasibility of robotic laparoscopic surgery: 146 cases. World J Surg 2001;25:1467-1477.
12. Melvin WS, Krause KR, Needleman BJ, et al: Computer enhanced versus standard laparoscopic anti-reflux surgery. J Gastrointest Surg 2002;6:32-35.
13. Gould JC, Melvin WS: Computer-assisted robotic antireflux surgery. Surg Laparosc Endosc Percutan Tech 2002;12:26-29.
14. Melvin WS, Needleman BJ, Krause KR, et al: Computer-assisted robotic Heller myotomy: initial case report. J Laparoendosc Adv Surg Tech A 2001;11:251-253.
15. Cadiere GB, Himpens, J, Vertruyen M, et al: The world's first obesity surgery performed by a surgeon at a distance. Obes Surg 1999;9: 206-209.
16. Horgan S, Vanuno D: Robots in laparoscopic surgery. J Laparoendosc Adv Surg Tech A 2001;11:415-419.

55

Liability Issues in Bariatric Surgery

Otto L. Willbanks, M.D., F.A.C.S.

The mere thought of a personal injury liability lawsuit causes apprehension and anxiety in the minds of most bariatric surgeons. Generally prevailing thought still questions the legitimacy of the field of bariatric surgery, in spite of overwhelming evidence to the contrary. Because of this, many bariatric surgeons are defensive in matters relating to their patients and to patient care. Reinforcing this defensive mode is the unquestionably litigious quality of present-day society, the ready availability of experienced personal injury attorneys, and a certain group of physicians who are only too willing to offer themselves as expert witnesses in cases against surgeons.

The obvious first line of defense for the surgeon is to provide no basis for a lawsuit—that is, to avoid committing malpractice. Theoretically, three essentials are required for a valid cause of action against a physician, and all three must be present for an incident to be judged to be malpractice. First, there must be negligence on the part of the physician. Willful intent is not required and, in fact, if the harming activity is willful, the matter may become a criminal act (assault). Second, there must be damage, and that damage must be quantifiable or measurable. Third, it must be shown that the negligence actually caused the damage. All three elements must be demonstrated.

It should be understood that incidents containing all three of these characteristics rarely go to trial; they are usually settled by negotiation between the parties and their attorneys. The concept of the three essential characteristics is accurate, but a casual glance tends to lure the physician into a state of oversimplification. Actually, other factors come into play when considering what constitutes negligence. For example, not obtaining informed consent is a form of negligence, as is the use of an unproven or a previously disproven technique. These and other matters must, then, be considered.

On a more positive note, the most important way to minimize risk is to know the standard of care, stay up-to-date on this standard and on the medical literature, and then always live up to the principles of the standard of care. High-quality care is most likely to generate positive outcomes and minimize the risk for injury, poor results, and dissatisfaction, each of which leads to lawsuits. The best way to keep up with the field is to develop an intimate

knowledge of and familiarity with the literature and to attend meetings at which recent advances are presented and evaluated.

A lawsuit, even one that is won by the doctor, can be very expensive. Adequate insurance to cover a major adverse judgment is essential, regardless of what is required by the hospital. Further, the surgeon must be sure to know what is covered and what is not and be certain that adequate coverage has been purchased.

▶ INFORMED CONSENT

Virtually all medical malpractice suits allege lack of informed consent. Therefore, the bariatric surgeon should anticipate that allegation. It has long been known that patients' recall of the informing process is faulty, even when a large monetary award is not a factor. Robinson and Merav, in 1976, published a study in which potential cardiac surgery patients' informing sessions were recorded, and then recall was evaluated at 4 and 6 months after operation.[1] Six different categories were evaluated, with an average recall of only 29%. The worst category, recall of potential complications, was only 10%. Of the patients, 65% alleged fabrication or falsehood on the part of the informing doctor, and 85% recalled less than half of what they had been told. The range of recall was 3% to 57%. Knowing that recall is so unreliable, even when secondary gain (as in a lawsuit) is not involved, suggests that accurate documentation of the complete disclosure of the pros and cons and complications of a bariatric procedure is essential.

A simple progress note stating, "Full disclosure of the advantages and disadvantages of surgery, all possible results, complications, and alternative methods of treatment were disclosed, and the patient accepts these and requests surgery" does not hurt, but is not adequate documentation. More specific documentation is needed so that the specific problems disclosed are in the record.

Recording the interview is one option, but it must be kept in mind that any omissions will also be documented. A taped interview that is inadequate could then become evidence that could be used against the surgeon.

Many surgeons use information booklets. These booklets were, for a long time, written and printed up by the surgeons who use them, and they remain a viable method of informing patients. More recently, the American Society for Bariatric Surgeons published such a booklet, one that had been reviewed and approved by recognized bariatric surgeons. This booklet is probably about as accurate a representation of the accepted standard of care as is currently available. Copies of this booklet are available for purchase from the American Society for Bariatric Surgeons (www.asbs.org). However, giving the booklet to the patient is not enough. A surgeon should conduct a personal interview session during which questions are asked and answered. The potential patient's individual concerns should be specifically discussed, frankly and forthrightly. All of this must then be meticulously documented in the permanent record. Only then can it be established that informed consent was achieved.

One surgeon has printed an initial interview sheet, to be filled in at the time of the interview, listing those present, the patient's history and the results of the physical examination, previous weight-loss attempts, and obesity-aggravated medical problems. It also lists across the bottom of the page single-word reminders of each point to be disclosed and discussed, and they are to be checked off as discussed. This is made part of the permanent record and is evidence that full disclosure was made. Other surgeons give a multiple-choice, true-or-false, or other written test that is kept in the record to show that the patient had a realistic working knowledge of what to expect. Whatever the mechanism, it is important to document the informing process. Items not documented are considered by the courts not to have happened.

CHOICE OF PATIENTS

There are several types of patients that should arouse a sense of caution in the surgeon. A few of these are noted here. Beware the patient who presents complaining that his or her previous surgeon or physician was negligent, had poor bedside manner or was rude, or that his or her office staff was rude or insulting. In general, one who is "bad-mouthing" his previous surgeon or other professionals. In such cases, the earlier physician should be contacted. There are several reasons for this action. If a change of physicians is going to occur, the new doctor must know the details of the patient's previous care and how the patient responded to that treatment. Further, the prior doctor can supply information such as drug-seeking, belligerent, or complaining behavior, as well as the patient's bill-paying habits, all characteristics that will have to be considered prior to accepting the patient.

Beware the poly-substance abuser and the alcoholic. These people are prone to be demanding and are likely to be bariatric surgery failures. Alcohol, for example, is a three-way loss. It has a lot of calories (gram for gram, the same as sugar); it stimulates appetite; and it takes the edge off inhibitions. It can make a substantial difference when small bites, well chewed, swallowed slowly, and consumed in tiny amounts, are the necessary goals of full patient compliance with food.

Whether or not the potential patient has been the plaintiff in a lawsuit, especially a medical malpractice lawsuit, may be important information. This subject should be diplomatically and carefully explored in the initial interview session.

MARKETING

The surgeon should be extra cautious in the use of marketing techniques. The legal right to advertise is well established and no organization or person can prohibit marketing, provided it is true and not misleading. On the other hand, a certain amount of restraint and good judgment is called for.

The American College of Surgeons guidelines condemns the use of testimonials, considering them misleading and, frequently, self-aggrandizing. In general, hucksterism in any form has no place in a surgeon's ethical practice. Be careful that huckster-like comments do not appear in advertising or marketing formats. It is very important to avoid any statement that could be interpreted as a guarantee or an implied guarantee or promise of a specific outcome. A plaintiff's attorney, when considering a case, would make note of this sort of comment and it does not bode well for the surgeon when it is presented to a jury.

Quite a number of bariatric surgeons do not market the procedure, believing that to be a red flag they do not want to wave. In any case, there seems to be quite an abundance of morbidly obese patients available, and many surgeons consider advertising to be unnecessary.

INNOVATIVE TECHNIQUES

Bariatric surgeons are, by nature, innovative and imaginative. These characteristics raise problems in the minds of plaintiffs' attorneys, who are constantly probing for practices that fall "outside the accepted standard of care."

The prudent surgeon, conceiving a new technique or a modification of a previously established technique, uses caution in its application. Prior evaluation in the animal laboratory is good science and indicates a basic concern for the safety and effectiveness of a new technique. After establishing favorable results in animals, the proposed modification should be evaluated by the Institutional Review Board (IRB) of the hospital and receive approval prior to use in an actual patient. The patient should have the evaluative nature of the operation explained in detail, and written consent that includes a description of the evaluative nature of the operation should be obtained prior to its use.

The plaintiff's attorney may try to establish that the surgeon is experimenting on the patient, and this possibility must be confronted by the surgeon in advance. Consultation with other surgeons and the support of other doctors will blunt such an attack, but in this regard the surgeon should have his defense planned out and supported by other colleagues.

Use of well-established techniques for which reliable statistics are available in the literature is the safest and most prudent course to take. Of course, surgical progress demands that modifications and evaluations be carried out. The use of such modifications should be cautious, well-founded in concept, supported by research, approved by the relevant IRBs and should be used in concert with adequate informed consent and ample consultations. Otherwise, the surgeon risks appearing capricious and arrogant or simply irresponsible, qualities that will not favorably impress a jury. Simply holding an academic appointment or a professorship does not render a surgeon immune to this type of attack. Caution and care should always be used when instituting improvements, modifications, and new techniques.

ATTITUDES

In general, it is the unhappy patient with a poor result who brings suit. There is an occasional "dedicated plaintiff" that is determined to find a reason to sue, but usually it is an unhappy patient and usually one with a poor result. The most common reason for filing a lawsuit is perceived physician indifference. Most patients will not sue a surgeon they like personally. This is not a hard rule but, for the most part, it applies.

Patients should be made to feel welcome, their comments and complaints answered fully in an environment that is not hurried or rushed. They should be made to feel they are in a friendly environment and are appreciated. The three most important words in patient relations are rapport, rapport, and rapport. This must be genuine, though. Patients are good at sensing when a friendly attitude is false or manufactured. Even the attitude of office personnel can be a major source of hostility and of a subsequent lawsuit. Office staff must understand this clearly and be dedicated to treating patients with respect and courtesy.

Leaving the impression of being too busy to answer a patient's questions must be avoided at all costs. The perception that a doctor is too rushed to respond to a patient's concerns or that a doctor or the staff is arrogant represents one of the leading causes of malpractice suits.[2]

A considerable amount of restraint should be used in marketing activities. Legally, marketing and advertising cannot be prohibited by any organization or person. This is deemed restraint of trade, and it violates the first amendment. However, as stated, overzealous marketing can mislead patients and result in unpleasant public relations and even criminal charges under some circumstances.

The American College of Surgeons (www.facs.org) and the American Medical Association (www.ama-assn.org) have ethical guidelines that are detailed and specific about marketing, stating that self-aggrandizing and misleading statements are off limits. The use of testimonials is considered misleading and is to be avoided. Advertising or marketing can and will be used by a plaintiff's attorney to indicate a self-enriching attitude on the surgeon's part and will be brought up in any court proceeding. The time to consider these factors is before launching a Web site, television or newspaper marketing program, or seminar. After the statements are out there, it is too late to cover these contingencies.

It may seem a little like walking on eggs, and to some extent it is. The individual surgeon needs to understand the full implications of each activity. Many patients have been helped by bariatric surgery, and there are many more who could be helped. Common sense coupled with in-depth thought can keep this surgery available and avoid a lot of unpleasantness.

AFTER BEING SUED

Once a suit is filed or even looks like it might be filed, it is critical that the record not be altered in even the most insignificant way. Any attempt to do so will immediately be seized by the plaintiff's attorney and used to make the defendant appear deceptive and at fault.

The best advice that can be offered to a doctor against whom a suit has been brought is to "get over it." Rarely is a lawsuit a personal matter, and it should not be considered a valid attack on a doctor's character or capabilities. The problem should be approached rationally, after thought and not in haste or when emotionally upset over the matter. The liability carrier should be notified as soon as it is apparent that a problem exists, even if a suit has not been filed. A meeting will be scheduled with an experienced liability defense attorney and the defendant must be brutally frank with that attorney. It must be remembered that the defense attorney cannot be of help if all aspects of the case are not known.

An evaluation of the case will be scheduled with a recognized expert, usually one who is not personally known by the defendant. After that, a decision will be made as to whether to look for a settlement or to fight the action. The defendant ordinarily participates in this decision. The carrier may or may not encourage a settlement, and the defendant will have to consider all of the advice offered. The carrier will weigh the cost of settlement against the cost of a court fight and will consider the possibility of losing entirely.

Actions settled out of court are reported to the National Practitioners Data Bank as are adverse court judgments. The surgeon must decide which course to follow. Most liability carriers do not cover exemplary or punitive damages, so a surgeon will have to decide whether it is advisable to hire a personal attorney for advice along the way. A defendant in a malpractice action should look to the legal professionals who are trying to be of assistance, just as a surgeon expects patients to rely on his or her medical or surgical skills and judgment.

No one likes to consider being a defendant in a malpractice or liability matter, but in today's litigious environment, the chances of escaping that experience are not good. One must be prepared and must think ahead, with this possibility in mind. If a lawsuit does occur, that is what one's professional liability insurance is there for.

REFERENCES

1. Robinson G, Merav A: Informed consent: recall by patients tested postoperatively. Ann Thor Surg 1976;22:209-212. Reprinted in Bull Am Coll Surg 1977;62:7-9, 30.
2. Hickson G, Federspiel J, Richert J, et al: Patient complaints and malpractice risk. JAMA 2002;287:2951-2957.

56

Requirements for Medical Writing: Reporting Bariatric Surgical Outcomes

Mervyn Deitel, M.D., F.I.C.S., C.R.C.S.C., F.A.C.N., D.A.B.S.

Scientific communication is a responsibility and obligation of the surgeon in his or her effort to enrich and advance knowledge. Reporting in journals (print and on-line) is the primary means of achieving this interaction, which is particularly important in the developing field of bariatric surgery.

▶ UNIVERSAL REQUIREMENTS FOR MEDICAL JOURNALS

The editors of the major medical journals, who make up the *International Committee of Medical Journal Editors*, met in Vancouver, Canada, in 1978, where they drew up uniform requirements for manuscripts submitted to biomedical journals. These requirements have been updated at four additional meetings of that group; the most recent update was completed in October 2004.[1]

Most peer-reviewed medical journals follow these requirements, although individual journals may make changes to suit their particular readerships. Usually, a clear, author-friendly format is selected as the style for a surgical journal.

The ritual for the reference section is particularly important. Some journals require listing the first seven authors, followed by *et al*; if there are more than seven authors, those journals usually drop back to three authors, followed by *et al*, whereas other journals give the first three authors only, followed by *et al*. References must be accurate and complete, according to the journal's requirements. Authors should always consult the Instructions to Authors page of the journal to which they are submitting a manuscript. The precise format followed by a journal should be observed: a cover letter should include a declaration of originality; it should be followed by a title page, an abstract, and a body-text structure that has clear and consistent headings and organization. The manuscript may be submitted by mail, on disk or CD or, in many instances, electronically via email attachment. When writing about studies, it is important to present the statistical methods employed. For studies involving humans or animals, institutional review board approval of the ethics involved must be obtained initially and stated in the manuscript. In reporting studies involving questionnaires, the response rate must be given.

Randomized, Controlled Trials

A report of a clinical trial requires adequate descriptions of the design and analysis in order to determine the strength of the findings. Eligibility criteria, prospectivity, the specific method of randomization, treatment arms, statistical power, and masking (i.e., whether the person assessing outcomes was blind to the treatments) must be described.[2] The statistical software package or statistical tests employed must be identified. The authors should provide sufficient information so that the reader, if given the data, could replicate the results.[3] The clinical trial should be large enough to detect important differences.

Author Requirements and Common Errors

Conflicts of interest, financial relationships, and sponsoring agencies must be disclosed.[4,5] Publishers require that a form be signed by the corresponding author or, in many journals, by all of the authors, attesting to the originality of the work and transferring copyright to the publisher. The principal or corresponding author is responsible for ensuring that the manuscript has been reviewed and approved by all the other authors. Some publishers request that the cover letter and the copyright assignment be signed by all of the authors.

Published letters to the editor likewise require a signed copyright transfer form. For acknowledgements or personal communications, it is now usually necessary to provide written permission from all individuals named. For case reports, written informed consent for publication is now commonly required from the patient being reported, if there is identifying information, or from the parent, guardian, or legal power of attorney. If the patient is identifiable because of the uniqueness of the case, permission requires that the patient be shown the manuscript that is to be published.

Reproduction of figures and tables from other sources, even if modified, requires that the author provide written permission from the copyright holder (usually a publisher); credit is acknowledged in the figure legend or table footnote. As a courtesy, permission may also be obtained from the original authors.

Some commonly misspelled words in submitted papers concerning obesity surgery are *anastomosis, laparoscopic,* and *absorption.* Current medical literary dogma prefers *before* instead of *prior to, because of* or *on the basis of* instead of *due to, compared with* rather than *compared to,* and so forth. However, most good journals endeavor to get the message across clearly through the application of contemporary and grammatical English. Some journals prefer to maintain the author's personality in the reporting, yet most journals prefer bland uniformity in style.

An appropriate table or illustration is preferred to text because it usually provides a more succinct overview of the data at a glance, and it adds variety to the article's layout. Specific data in tables and figures should not be duplicated in the text, and vice versa.

Some Points on Content

Articles should be presented with brevity. The title should be precise, yet informative, and should contain no abbreviations. Research articles generally are preceded by a structured *abstract* of fewer than 250 words. The abstract must correspond precisely with the text: nothing should be included in the abstract that is not in the article. Empty narration in the abstract should be avoided. Do not write, "*x* is described, *y* is discussed," but instead give specific hard data.[6]

Case reports of novel observations are accepted by most journals if they make a point for use in clinical practice. They are usually preceded by a short unstructured abstract of one paragraph (fewer than 150 words). For *editorials, commentaries,* and *correspondence,* abstracts are not required.

The *methods* section must not be flawed. The *results* section must make sense, and the data must add up. In scientific writing, Systéme Internationale (SI) metric units are used. Also, generic names of drugs (e.g., warfarin) and sutures (e.g., polypropylene) are used; the product name may follow in parentheses. In a study that has follow-up, the proportion of patients who completed the study must be indicated.

In the *discussion* section, the introduction should not be repeated. The discussion should consider the results of the study in the context of other reported studies. The conclusions should be substantiated by the data. The authors should avoid using an excess number of *references* and should not overload the references with citations of their own publications unless they are integrally relevant to the immediate manuscript. As noted previously, the reference style of the journal must be followed consistently.[7] All references should be checked for accuracy and put in the order cited in the text (or, if required by the target journal, in alphabetical order according to authors' surnames). Authors should not cite references that they themselves have not read. References to papers not yet accepted for publication (*unpublished data*) and to *personal communications* are not acceptable in the references; they should be included in parentheses in the text. Citations in the references of presentations at meetings are to be avoided unless the paper emanating from this presentation has been published and can be cited.

Letters to the editor regarding articles published should be written in a polite fashion, even if indicating disagreements or legitimate questions. They can provide lively and useful interchanges. However, the letter writer should be aware that the author of the article has the right to reply in the same issue and receives the last word. Also, letters to the editor that do not pertain to a previous article can express an opinion or provide a brief communication. However, caution and sober reflection should be used before writing a letter to the editor: assume that every piece of writing will be read by an adversary in the context of litigation, that is, by an unfriendly lawyer.

The author line under the title of an article should contain only authors who have directly contributed to the work or to the development of the manuscript and those who are in agreement with its publication. In editorials, letters, and commentaries, the authors' names may appear at the end, rather than at the beginning of the text, depending on the style of the specific journal. Headings that do not follow the organization of research articles may be inserted, if they are helpful, within editorials, reviews, and correspondence.

Language and Formatting

Manuscripts must be double-spaced throughout, including the references, tables, and figure legends, to enable editing. Right margins should be unjustified (ragged). Sentences that are too long are to be avoided. Upon receipt, each manuscript is assigned its own manuscript code number, which is transmitted to the authors; for prompt retrieval, this number should be cited in all communications, including on the final disk. It is very helpful for authors whose first language is not English to have their papers undergo manuscript review by an expert in the English language, preferably an editor, before submission. With the globalization of surgical communication, English has emerged as the dominant language in scientific communication.[8] When an accepted manuscript is being formatted, it is beneficial if the journal's expert copy editor is also an experienced surgeon, so that meanings will not be changed if words must be reordered.

Manuscript Selection Process

The editor in chief of the journal usually distributes each paper to two members of the editorial board for objective peer review, to be returned in a timely fashion. When there is discord regarding a manuscript's merit for acceptance, a third reviewer is consulted. Most editors also invite outside expert referees into the review process. The reviewers grade the papers with respect to originality, importance, scientific accuracy, and style and format, and they provide an opinion regarding priority for publication, a confidential report to the editor, and recommendations to the authors. If the paper is accepted, a minor revision may be needed or the paper may have to be restructured. Major revision may require more studies or longer study follow-up that may facilitate attainment of statistical significance by the time of the manuscript's resubmission.

Some articles require a second review by the editorial board to make sure that the concerns have been addressed. A further revision may still be necessary by the authors before final acceptance. An *invited commentary* may be necessary to balance the discussion of a paper. The authors should regard the members of the editorial board as helpful colleagues, not adversaries.

◗ COPYRIGHT AND DOCUMENTATION

Copyright law provides for the protection of the rights of parties involved in the creation and dissemination of intellectual property. The authors transfer or assign the copyright of the paper, including the figures and tables, to the publisher. Copyright legally protects authorship and publication. Duplicate publication of articles is not permitted and would constitute a violation or infringement of the copyright law.[5] Dual publication and multiple publications using parts of one study ("salami slicing") are forms of academic dishonesty and fraud.[9]

The publisher maintains the copyright and has control over reprints. However, a specific copyright is generally not necessary for guidelines intended for multiple publications, but their sources should be acknowledged. Works created by the U.S. government are in the public domain and can generally be reproduced for fair use.

If a paper has previously appeared on an Internet site, submission for print publication is considered duplication. Some journals expedite papers accepted for print publication by placing them immediately on their own Web sites. If Internet publication elsewhere is to follow journal publication of an article, journal consent should be obtained first, and the publication should be clearly referenced. However, after a paper is published, its abstract is part of the public domain.

As noted, all authors listed under the title of an article should have made contributions to the article. Each author's specific contribution may be requested or required by the editor or publisher before publication.

◗ PUBLISHING IN THE MODERN ERA

Because of the rapid advances in electronic media over the past 10 to 15 years, every paper should be mailed to the editorial office with its disk (or CD), or it may be sent by e-mail attachment as a Word document. The papers may then be submitted to the reviewers as e-mail attachments, with review forms to be filled in electronically and returned by email.[10]

Submission of Figures

High-quality, relevant, helpful figures may be included. Figures must be provided for publication in tagged image file format (TIFF) or encapsulated PostScript (EPS) files, or as clear hardcopy pictures for scanning. JPEG and PowerPoint files are not, at this time, used in medical publication. Colored pages in the text section require special production, which entails significant extra cost by the printer, and this cost usually must be passed on to the authors. Therefore, if colored illustrations are accepted, most journals require that the extra cost for them be prepaid by the authors. However, most colored figures reproduce well in black-and-white format, thus averting costs by the authors.

Portable Document Format

Page proofs must be reviewed by the authors. In the past, proofs were sent by fax or costly express courier. The proofs could not be sent by e-mail unless the recipient owned the publisher's formatting program (e.g., QuarkXpress) and could open the files.

Now, using the (Adobe) portable document format (PDF) program, proofs can be sent as an e-mail attachment and can be downloaded using the Adobe Acrobat Reader software (downloaded free of charge from the Internet site: *www.adobe.com*). The publisher distills the QuarkXpress files into PDF files, and the proofs are expedited to the corresponding author by e-mail attachment, accompanied by the copyright transfer and reprint order forms.

The proofs in PDF format retain the designer's layout, graphics, colors, and fonts. The corresponding author can view the formatted paper (including any color figures) on a computer screen and can print it out for hardcopy review. The authors check the edited, formatted paper for any errors in meaning and for typographic errors.[10] The PDF file cannot be modified by the author, and no new material or corrections can be added at the proof stage. Manual corrections on hardcopy proofs should be sent promptly to the publisher by fax, avoiding making notations too close to the pages' margins where they may be cut off in transmission.

Consolidation Among Publishers and Rising Journal Prices

Changes in medical journal publishers over the years have been frequent. As an example, *Obesity Surgery* was first published by Rapid Communications of Oxford, England, in 1991; the firm subsequently moved to London as International Thomson Publications. As many of the large, older publishing houses in the United States fell because of rising costs, the merged company of Lippincott Williams & Wilkins acquired a part of International Thomson Publications. This conglomerate then came under the ownership of Wolters Kluwer of Amsterdam.

In the midst of an ongoing strike at Pergamon Press in Oxford in the early 1990s, Elsevier of Amsterdam obtained Pergamon and later Reed, to become Reed Elsevier, which subsequently acquired Harcourt Press and produces 1700 scientific journals—about one third of the established medical journals. A number of their nonprofit journals were dropped. In 1998, Elsevier called off a planned acquisition of Wolters Kluwer after European regulators raised concerns. Elsevier has acquired Churchill Livingstone, Butterworth, Mosby, and W.B. Saunders. The remaining major scientific journal publishers are John Wiley & Sons, based in New York, Springer Verlag, with a head office in Germany, and the British publisher Blackwell. With all the mergers and expansions, the prices of these journals might be anticipated to fall; however, the prices of the acquired medical journals have risen precipitously. Annual subscription prices include about $2500 for the neuroscience favorite *Synapse*, about $4000 for *Anatomical Record*, and about $20,000 for Elsevier's combined neurology journal *Brain Research*.[11]

Although medical libraries' budgets are growing, the libraries are slashing subscriptions and book buying to meet the rising costs of scholarly journals. Publishers claim that owning hundreds of journals enables them to serve scholars better because they have the financial resources to invest in digital technology; yet experience has shown that when publishers own large numbers of journals, prices rise.

Since 1986, as the number of publishers has dwindled, the average journal price has more than tripled, rising far more steeply than the rate of inflation. Meanwhile, libraries increased their journal spending by 130% but cut the number of subscriptions by 6% and the number of books they buy annually by 26%.[11] Journals are the lifeblood of scholarship. However, rising journal prices contribute to the escalating costs of higher education.

Internet Publication

In the mid 1990s, a move began to publish journals on the Internet, but peer review and good quality were lacking. Furthermore, on-line publication does not overcome the high costs of a trained staff, editing, formatting, and equipment. The four major medical print journals placed their publications on the Internet free of charge, with major financial loss, and they were subsequently forced to charge substantial fees for entry into their Web sites. Now, most major print journals are also available on-line in standard generalized markup language (SGML) and PDF formats, but with a subscription cost. A password and username must be used for entry. The articles on the Internet may be downloaded free of charge by subscribers or on a pay-per-view basis by nonsubscribers. The Internet provides an extremely compact means of on-line access to full articles, and it has the advantage of linking its references to the cited papers elsewhere (e.g., clicking on the references to access a paper cited from another journal).

Regarding the World Wide Web, it has been said that we are entering an era of paperless media. However, more trees are being chopped down today for the print media than ever before.

▶ RECOMMENDATIONS FOR REPORTING WEIGHT LOSS IN BARIATRIC SURGERY

Reports providing the absolute weight loss (or the percent of initial weight lost) as the sole descriptive index (i.e., operative weight minus the weight at a point in time) are not acceptable as the sole measure of weight loss. The initial weights differ in various studies. Furthermore, after a bariatric operation in the superobese, the number of kilograms lost tends to be greater, but the percent of excess weight loss tends to be less than in the morbidly obese. For comparative bases, weight loss is preferred as percent of *excess* weight lost (%EWL) or change in body mass index (BMI). Metric units (i.e., kilograms, meters, etc.) are necessary in all scientific publication.

Ideal Body Weight and Excess Weight

Ideal weight is derived from the 1983 Metropolitan Height and Weight Tables,[12-17] and is the weight for each height at which mortality is lowest and longevity is highest. The ideal weight is less than the average weight for a specific height in the population. The tables are based on the 1979 Build Study,[18] which was the result of an 18-year mortality study derived from the pooled data of 4.2 million individuals from 25 life insurance companies in the United States and Canada. The tables provide the weight that was found to be associated with maximum life expectancy. These weights are given in a range for body frame (small, medium, and large), based on elbow width, measured with calipers.[12,13,19] The middle 50% of the elbow breadths (25th to 75th percentiles) was designated as the medium frame, with 25% falling within the categories of small and large frames. Generally, the midpoint of the range of weights for a medium frame is chosen as the ideal weight.

Ideal weight may be calculated by using the formula shown in Table 56-1, which gives values corresponding to the midpoint of the range for the medium frame on the Metropolitan tables, with a margin of error that is less than 1%.[20] There were a number of criticisms of the Metropolitan tables[13]: (1) minorities were underrepresented in the insurance-purchasing population; (2) 10% of the weights were self-reported; (3) the insured population was part of a higher economic group than the general population; (4) weights were taken while participants were wearing indoor clothing (allowing 5 lb for males and 3 lb for females, with 1-inch heels for both sexes); (5) applicants with major disease (e.g., heart disease, cancer, or diabetes) at the time of insurance policy issuance were excluded so as to provide an indication of the effect of weight alone on mortality; (6) applicants were 25 to 59 years of age, although the ideal weight for survival increased up to age 50. However, there is no other study on weight survival based on so vast a sample.

Excess weight is defined as the actual weight minus the ideal weight (Table 56-2). In turn, the excess weight forms the basis for calculating the %EWL (see Table 56-2).

Table 56-1	FORMULA FOR CALCULATION OF IDEAL WEIGHT

Adult female: 5 ft tall = 119 lb. For each additional inch, add 3 lb.
Adult male: 5 ft 3 inches tall = 135 lb. For each additional inch, add 3 lb.
1 foot = 30.4 cm; 1 inch = 2.54 cm.
Divide lb by 2.2 to change to kg.

The formula corresponds to the midpoint of a medium frame in the Metropolitan Tables, with accuracy within 1%. To convert to ideal weight for a small or large frame, decrease or increase the result by 10%. Patients are to be without shoes.

Table 56-2

Excess weight = Actual weight − Ideal weight

Percent excess weight loss =

$$\left[\frac{(\text{Operative weight} - \text{Follow-up weight})}{\text{Operative excess weight}} \right] \times 100.$$

Body Mass Index

BMI is regarded as the most accurate method of comparing obesity. It gives a number that indicates the degree of weight for all heights. It is calculated from the formula weight/height^2 for men and weight/height$^{1.5}$ for women, where the body weight is in kilograms (kg) and the height is in meters squared (m^2).[21] However, the formula for women is somewhat difficult to use, so the formula for men (weight/height^2) is used for all patients. BMI has a very high correlation with body density and skinfold thickness measurements and is the best indicator for "fatness."[22,23]

Disease and mortality studies that have used the BMI have generally been based on population studies of fewer than 50,000 individuals. Thus, BMI may actually provide less accuracy in providing an ideal measure for survival than does the Metropolitan study, which included 4.2 million people and on which the lowest-mortality BMI was originally based.

A BMI of 20 to 25 kg per m^2 is associated with lowest mortality rates, and mortality rates rise as the BMI rises or falls beyond the range of these numbers.[24] A BMI of 20 to 25 indicates normal weight; a BMI between 25 and 29.9 indicates overweight; a BMI of 30 indicates obesity, 40 indicates morbid obesity, and 50 has been designated as superobesity. A BMI below 17.5 is among the criteria for anorexia nervosa and is commonly seen in such states of malnutrition as cancer cachexia.

Percent Excess BMI Loss

The percent of BMI loss has been used in bariatric surgery publications as well (Table 56-3). Since the National Institutes of Health/National Institute of Diabetes and Digestive and Kidney Diseases defined excess weight as starting at a BMI above 25,[25] BMI units higher than 25 have been defined as percent excess BMI loss (%EBMIL)[26] by the following formula:

$$\%\text{EBMIL} = 100 - \left[\left(\frac{\text{Follow-up BMI} - 25}{\text{Beginning BMI} - 25} \right) \times 100 \right].$$

For example, if an individual has an initial BMI of 45, then the 20 BMI units above the upper limit of the normal

Table 56-3

$$\text{Percent BMI loss} = \left[\frac{\text{Operative BMI} - \text{Follow-up BMI}}{\text{Operative BMI}} \right] \times 100.$$

BMI of 25 BMI units represents a %EBMIL of 100; a loss of 10 BMI units (to a BMI of 35) would be a %EBMIL of 50. It is possible that %EBMIL may become the standard for presenting weight loss data in clinical studies of the overweight and obese.

Patient Follow-up

Changes in %EWL, BMI, or %EBMIL are frequently shown in graphic form as a curve, with bars on one side of each time point indicating the standard deviation; the number of patients followed and the number eligible for follow-up at each time point should be shown. However, a curve generally denotes longitudinal analysis which, according to purist statisticians, requires 100% follow-up at each time point.[27]

Cross-sectional analysis is appropriate for studies of incomplete follow-up, using a table or bar graph. The bar or histogram y axis indicates the weight-loss parameter chosen, with the time points reported on the x axis. Again, the number of patients followed and the number eligible for follow-up at each time point should be indicated. Standard deviation may be indicated on top of each bar.[28]

▶ REFERENCES

1. International Committee of Medical Journal Editors: Uniform requirements for manuscripts submitted to biomedical journals. Ann Intern Med 1997;126:36-47. www.icmje.org
2. Schumm LP, Fisher JS, Thisted RA, et al: Clinical trials in general surgical journals: are methods better reported? Surgery 1999;125:41-45.
3. Rennie D: How to report randomized controlled trials. The CONSORT statement. JAMA 1996;276:649.
4. International Committee of Medical Journal Editors: Conflicts of interest. Ann Intern Med 1993;118: 646-647.
5. Juerson C, Flanagin A, Fontanarosa PB, et al: American Medical Association Manual of Style: a Guide for Authors and Editors, ed 9. Philadelphia, Lippincott Williams & Wilkins, 1998.
6. Deitel M: The requirements for medical writing. Obes Surg 2002; 12:151-153(editorial).
7. Patreas K: Recommended Formats for Bibliographic Citation. Bethesda, Md., National Library of Medicine, Reference Service, 1991.
8. Tompkins RK, Ko CY, Donovan AJ: Internationalization of general surgical journals. Arch Surg 2001;136:1345-1352.
9. Schein M, Paladuga R: Redundant surgical publications: tip of the iceberg? Surgery 2001;129:662-663.
10. Deitel M, Ahmed MS, Bandong R: Publishing in the modern era. Obes Surg 2001;11:1(editorial).
11. As publishers perish, libraries feel the pain. New York Times, November 3, 2000:C1, C5.
12. Metropolitan Life Foundation: Metropolitan height and weight tables. Stat Bull Metrop Insur Co 1983;64:2-9.
13. Deitel M: Indications for surgery for morbid obesity. In Deitel M (ed): Surgery for the Morbidly Obese Patient, pp. 69-79. Toronto, FD-Communications, 1989.
14. Standards Committee, American Society for Bariatric Surgery. Guidelines for reporting results in bariatric surgery. Obes Surg 1997;7:521-522.
15. ASBS Standards Committee: Surgery for Morbid Obesity: What Patients Should Know, ed 3, pp. 27-28. Toronto, FD-Communications, 2001. www.asbs.org
16. National Bariatric Surgery Registry: NBSR Database Instructional Manual, Version 2.3, p. 173. Iowa City, Iowa, Department of Surgery, University of Iowa Hospital & Clinics, 1987.
17. International Bariatric Surgery Registry. University of Iowa Hospitals, Iowa City, Iowa. www.surgery.uiowa.edu/ibsr
18. Society of Actuaries and Association of Life Insurance Medical Directors of America: Build Study, 1979. Chicago, Society of Actuaries, 1980.

19. Frisancho AR, Flegel PN: Elbow breadth as a measure of frame size for US males and females. Am J Clin Nutr 1983;37:311-314.

20. Miller MA: A calculated method for determination of ideal body weight. Nutr Supp Serv 1985;5:31-33.

21. White F, Pereira L: In search of the ideal body weight. Ann R Coll Phys Surg Can 1987;20:129-132.

22. Keys A, Fidanza F, Karvonen MJ, et al: Indices of relative weight and obesity. J Chron Dis 1972;25:329-343.

23. Womersley J, Durnin JVGA: A comparison of the skinfold method with the extent of "overweight" and various weight-height relationships in the assessment of obesity. Br J Nutr 1977;38:271-284.

24. MacLean LD: Surgery for obesity: where do we go from here? Am Coll Surg Bull 1989;74:20-23.

25. Kuczmarski RJ, Flegal KM: Criteria for definition in overweight in transition: background and recommendations for the United States. Am J Clin Nutr 2000;72:1074-1081.

26. Greenstein RJ, Belachew M: Implantable gastric stimulation (IGS™) as a therapy for human morbid obesity: report from the 2001 IFSO Symposium in Crete. Obes Surg 2002;12(supp 1):S3-S5.

27. Jeng G, Renquist K, Doherty C, et al: A study on predicting weight loss following surgical treatment for obesity. Obes Surg 1994;4:29-36.

28. Deitel M, Greenstein RJ: Recommendations for reporting weight loss. Obes Surg 2003;13:159-1560(editorial).

Index

Page numbers followed by f refer to figures and by t refer to tables.

H

I